Advances in Inflammatory
Bowel Diseases

Advances in Inflammatory Bowel Diseases

Edited by

P. Rutgeerts

Department of Gastroenterology
University Hospital
B-3000 Leuven
Belgium

J.-F. Colombel

Department of
Hepatogastroenterology
Hôpital Huriez
CHRU Lille
F-59037 Lille
France

S.B. Hanauer

University of Chicago
Department of Medicine,
Gastroenterology Section
Chicago
IL 60637, USA

J. Schölmerich

Klinik und Poliklinik für Innere
Medizin
Klinikum der Universität
Regensburg
D-93042 Regensburg
Germany

G.N.J. Tytgat

Department of Gastroenterology
Academic Medical Center
NL-1105 AZ Amsterdam-
Zuidoost
The Netherlands

A. van Gossum

Gastroenterologie
Hôpital Erasme
B-1070 Brussels
Belgium

Proceedings of the Falk Symposium 106 held in Brussels, Belgium, June 18–20, 1998

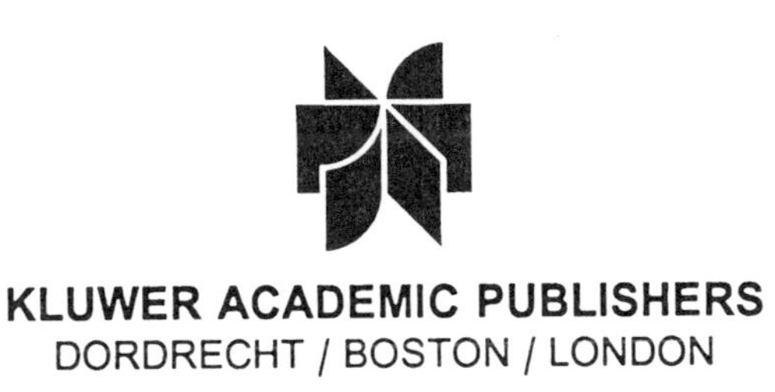

KLUWER ACADEMIC PUBLISHERS
DORDRECHT / BOSTON / LONDON

Library of Congress Cataloging in-Publication Data is available.

ISBN 0–7923–8750–3

Published by Kluwer Academic Publishers,
P. O. Box 17, 3300 AA Dordrecht, The Netherlands

Sold and distributed in North, Central and South America
by Kluwer Academic Publishers
101 Philip Drive, Norwell, MA 02061, U.S.A.

In all other countries, sold and distributed
by Kluwer Academic Publishers,
P. O. Box 322, 3300 AH Dordrecht, The Netherlands

Printed on acid-free paper

Printed and bound in Great Britain by MPG Books, Bodmin, Cornwall.

Contents

List of Principal Authors   viii

Preface   xi

SECTION I: AETIOLOGICAL FACTORS IN IBD

1.   Susceptibility genes in inflammatory bowel diseases   3
JP Hugot, JF Colombel, G Thomas

2.   Genetic heterogeneity within inflammatory bowel disease   17
J Satsangi, D Jewell

3.   Inflammatory bowel disease and genetics: What to tell our patients?   24
M Peeters, S Vermeire, S Joossens, P Rutgeerts

4.   The importance of environment in inflammatory bowel disease: New data   34
J Cosnes

5.   Nicotine in the treatment of ulcerative colitis   43
WJ Sandborn

SECTION II: PATHOGENESIS OF IBD

6.   Inflammatory lesions of the myenteric plexus in Crohn's disease   55
K Geboes, P Rutgeerts

7.   The infectious track in inflammatory bowel diseases   68
J-F Colombel, P Bulois, E Lederman, P Desreumaux, A Darfeuille-Michaud, HJ Van Kruiningen, A Cortot

CONTENTS

8.   The role of nutrition in the pathogenesis of inflammatory bowel disease   **80**
MA Gassull, E Cabré

9.   Role of nutritional therapy in IBD   **89**
DBA Silk

SECTION III: IMMUNOLOGICAL BASIS OF IBD

10.   Animal models of IBD: Impact on understanding immunologically mediated intestinal inflammation   **105**
RB Sartor

11.   The role of IFN-γ in inflammation and immunopathology   **112**
A Billiau, P Matthys, K Vermeire, H Heremans

12.   The role of interleukin-12 in inflammatory bowel disease   **130**
F Pallone, G Monteleone, R Marasco, L Biancone, T Parrello

13.   Cytokines and inflammatory bowel disease   **135**
PCF Stokkers, SJH van Deventer

14.   Immunomodulation therapy in inflammatory bowel diseases: Cytokines and anti-cytokines   **145**
LC Karp, SR Targan

SECTION IV: CANCER IN IBD

15.   Risk factors for development of colorectal cancer in inflammatory bowel disease   **159**
TA Brentnall

16.   Early detection of cancer in inflammatory bowel disease: What should be done?   **168**
A Forbes, D Rowlands

17.   Utility of IBD classification: Is it helpful from a therapeutic standpoint?   **185**
DB Sachar

18.   Aetiopathogenesis of IBD: Where do we stand?   **188**
C Fiocchi

SECTION V: STANDARD THERAPIES IN IBD

19.   Aminosalicylates in the treatment of ulcerative colitis and Crohn's disease   **201**
LR Sutherland

CONTENTS

20. How to use steroids in inflammatory bowel disease   210
R Löfberg

21. Immunosuppression therapy in ulcerative colitis and Crohn's disease   218
DH Present

22. Sequential therapy for inflammatory bowel disease   227
SB Hanauer

SECTION VI: SURGERY FOR IBD

23. Surgery for Crohn's disease: When to operate, how to operate   233
VW Fazio

24. Natural history of Crohn's recurrence at the ileocolonic anastomosis   244
G D'Haens

25. Relapse prevention strategies in Crohn's disease   251
H. Lochs

26. Changes in prognosis for patients with inflammatory bowel disease   257
RG Farmer

SECTION VII: IBD: A SYSTEMIC DISEASE

27. Trefoil peptides and inflammatory bowel disease   269
DK Podolsky

28. Functional neuroimmune interactions in IBD and their therapeutic implications   275
SM Collins, B Qiu, F Galeazzi

29. Inflammatory arthropathy and inflammatory bowel disease   280
M De Vos, H Mielants, F De Keyser, C Cuvelier, EM Veys

30. Refractory anaemia and iron deficiency in IBD   288
C Gasche

31. Manipulation of intestinal microflora   297
M Campieri, P Gionchetti

32. Pathogenesis and treatment of pouchitis   301
DP Jewell

Index   311

List of Principal Authors

A. Billiau
Laboratory of Immunobiology
Rega Institute
University of Leuven
Minderbroedersstraat 10
B-3000 Leuven
Belgium

T. A. Brentnall
Division of Gastroenterology
Department of Medicine
University of Washington
Medical Center
Box 356424
Seattle
WA 98195
USA

M. Campieri
Istituto di Clinica Medica I
Policlinico S Orsola
Via Massarenti 9
I-40138 Bologna
Italy

S. M. Collins
Division of Gastroenterology – 4W8
Digestive Diseases Research
  Program
Department of Medicine
Faculty of Health Sciences
McMaster University
1200 Main Street West
Hamilton
ONT L8N 3Z5
Canada

J-F. Colombel
Clinique des Maladies de l'Appareil
  Digestif
Hôpital Claude Huriez

Centre Hospitalier Universitaire
  (CHetU)
F-59037 Lille
France

J. Cosnes
Service de Gastroentérologie et
  Nutrition
Hôpital Rothschild
33 boulevard de Picpus
F-75571 PARIS Cedex 12
France

G. D'Haens
Department of Internal Medicine
University Hospital Gasthuisberg
Herestraat 49
B-3000 Leuven
Belgium

M. De Vos
University Hospital
Department of Gastroenterology
De Pintelaan 185
B-9000 Gent
Belgium

R. G. Farmer
Georgetown University Medical Center
3800 Reservoir Road NW
Washington DC 2307-2197
USA

V. W. Fazio
Department of Colorectal Surgery
The Cleveland Clinic Foundation
9500 Euclid Avenue
Cleveland
OH 44195
USA

LIST OF PRINCIPAL AUTHORS

C. Fiocchi
Case Western Reserve University
School of Medicine (BRB)
Gastroenterology Division
10900 Euclid Avenue
Cleveland
OH 44106-4952
USA

A. Forbes
St Mark's Hospital and Academic
  Institute
Northwick Park
Watford Road
Harrow
Middlesex HA1 3UJ
UK

C. Gasche
Klinik für Innere Medizin IV
Abteilung Gastroenterologie und
  Hepatologie
Währinger Gürtel 18-20
A-1090 Wien
Austria

M. A. Gassull
Department of Gastroenterology
Hospital Universitari Germans Trias i
  Pujol
Carretera del Canyet s/n
E-08916 Badalona
Spain

K. Geboes
Gastrointestinal Pathology Unit
University Hospital St Rafael
K.U. Leuven
Minderbroedersstraat 12
B-3000 Leuven
Belgium

S. B. Hanauer
University of Chicago
Department of Medicine
Gastroenterology Section
5758 South Maryland Avenue
MC9028, Room DCAM 6601
Chicago
IL 60637
USA

D. P. Jewell
Gastroenterology Unit
The Radcliffe Infirmary
Woodstock Road
Oxford
OX2 6HE
UK

H. Lochs
IV. Medizinische Klinik
Schwerpunkt Gastroenterologie
Medizinische Fakultät (Charité)
Humboldt Universität zu Berlin
Schumannstr. 20–21
D-10117 Berlin
Germany

R. Löfberg
Department of Gastroenterology
Karolinska Institute at
Huddinge University Hospital
S-14186 Stockholm
Sweden

F. Pallone
Unitá di Gastroenterologia
Dip. Medicine Sperimentale
Policlinico Univ. 'Mater Domini'
Via T. Campanella
I-88100 Catanzaro
Italy

M. Peeters
Department of Internal Medicine
Division of Gastroenterology
University Hospital Gasthuisberg
Herestraat 49
B-3000 Leuven
Belgium

D. K. Podolsky
Gastrointestinal Unit (GRJ-719)
Massachusetts General Hospital
32 Fruit Street
Boston
MA 02114-2620
USA

D. H. Present
Mount Sinai Medical Center
12 East 86th Street
New York
NY 10028
USA

D. B. Sachar
Division of Gastroenterology
The Mount Sinai Medical Center
Box 1069
One Gustave L Levy Place
New York
NY 10029-6574
USA

W. J. Sandborn
Mayo Clinic
200 First Street SW
Rochester
MN 55905
USA

R. B. Sartor
University of North Carolina at Chapel
  Hill
Division of Digestive Diseases
CB #7038 – Glaxo Building
Chapel Hill
NC 72599-7038
USA

J. Satsangi
Gastroenterology Unit
The Radcliffe Infirmary
Woodstock Road
Oxford
OX2 6HE
UK

D. B. A. Silk
Department of Gastroenterology and
  Nutrition
Central Middlesex Hospital NHS Trust
Acton Lane
London
NW10 7NS
UK

L. R. Sutherland
Department of Community Health
  Sciences
The University of Calgary
3330 Hospital Drive N.W.
Calgary
ALB T2N 4N1
Canada

S. R. Targan
Cedars–Sinai Division of
  Gastroenterology and IBD Center
8700 Beverly Boulevard Suite D4063
Los Angeles
CA 90048
USA

G. Thomas
Fondation Jean Dausset
INSERM U. 434
27 rue Juliette Dodu
F-75010 Paris
France

S. J. H. van Deventer
Department of Experimental Internal
  Medicine
Academic Medical Centre
University of Amsterdam
Meibergdreef 9
NL-1105 AZ Amsterdam Zuidoost
The Netherlands

Preface

The Falk Symposia dedicated to Inflammatory Bowel Disease have brought the leading researchers and clinicians in the field together for many years in order to summarize the current state of our understanding of aetiopathogenesis and therapeutic options. In this manner they contribute greatly to the prompt dissemination of advances amongst all those involved in IBD research and patient care.

In this book are published the proceedings of the Falk Symposium No. 106 held in Brussels, Belgium, June 18–20, 1998.

It is striking that complete darkness persists concerning the cause of both Crohn's disease and ulcerative colitis, whereas insights into the pathogenesis of the inflammatory changes progress almost daily. The focus of today's research is mainly on genetic susceptibility for IBD, on mucosal immunopathological mechanisms and on the development of immunomodulation strategies for treatment.

We still do not understand the basic difference between ulcerative colitis and Crohn's disease. During the symposium a working party pursued its attempts to develop a reliable classification for comprehending the heterogeneity of Crohn's disease. The final report was presented at the World Congress of Gastroenterology in Vienna, September 6–11, 1998. It now seems established that two susceptibility loci for IBD are present on the genome, one on chromosome 16 (*IBD1* gene) and one on chromosome 12 (*IBD2* gene). They would, however, account for only a small fraction of the increased risk of developing the disease for siblings of IBD patients in Crohn's families. Moreover several groups do not confirm the linkage and it is not at all clear whether the same genes would be involved in the pathogenesis of sporadic IBD.

CD4+ T-cells play a crucial role in the pathogenesis of IBD. The hypothesis of the dichotomy of ulcerative colitis being a 'T-helper-2' type of disease and Crohn's disease a 'T-helper-1' type of disease remains as yet unconfirmed. In early Crohn's lesions cytokine patterns associated with preponderance of Th2 effects have been detected. Moreover the concept of a clear-cut difference between Th1 and Th2 response as found in mice does not stand uniformly in man. The findings in the many experimental models of IBD therefore cannot simply be applied to the human situation. However, the monoclonal antibody against tumor necrosis factor, a pivotal Th1 cytokine, turns out to be a major breakthrough in the treatment of refractory Crohn's disease and allows temporary closure of longstanding perianal and abdominal wall fistulae. Other immunomodulation therapies including rhIL10, rhIL11, antisense oligonucleotide to ICAM-1 and many others are under study. For long-term control of IBD, immunosuppression with azathioprine or 6-mercaptopurine is now generally acknowledged to be standard therapy.

The prevalence of IBD is increasing rapidly in our western societies and the diseases represent a challenging medical problem. The seriously jeopardized quality of life in these patients and the risk for the development of cancer are only a few of the reasons to make research in the field a priority and to allocate to it more means.

The Editors

Section I
Aetiological factors in IBD

1
Susceptibility genes in inflammatory bowel diseases

J. P. HUGOT, J. F. COLOMBEL and G. THOMAS

INTRODUCTION

Chronic inflammatory bowel diseases (IBDs) are lifelong diseases which evolve either intermittently or with a more chronic mode of evolution. They include two main entities: Crohn's disease (CD) and ulcerative colitis (UC). Most of the time, differential diagnosis between CD and UC is easy. However, a precise classification for about 10% of inflammatory colitis remains difficult in practice. There have been time and geographic variations of the incidence of these diseases, indicating a role of environmental factors which may be associated with the western life style. Among them, tobacco has been well documented. Infectious agents, in particular mycobacteria and measles virus, although suspected, have not yet been fully demonstrated. Other physiopathological mechanisms that have been proposed include mucus abnormalities, increased intestinal permeability, vascular abnormalities, abnormal local immune response, autoantibodies, etc. However, the actual involvement of any of these different factors in the aetiology has not yet been definitely proven. A genetic predisposition to IBDs has been long suspected, given the existence of ethnic and familial aggregations of these diseases. This genetic predisposition appears to be at least in part common to both types of diseases. Identification of the relevant susceptibility genes would be a critical step in the understanding of the pathogenesis of these diseases and for the development of new targeted therapies. With this aim, the two most frequently used strategies are: association studies and linkage studies. It is likely that a combination of both strategies will be successful in the future.

GENETIC EPIDEMIOLOGY OF IBD

Epidemiology

The maximal incidence of CD is observed in young adults between 20 and 30 years old. For UC, the incidence is highest and remains approximately constant between 20 and 50 years of age. A second peak of incidence is often observed between 60 and 70 years. The average age at onset of the disease is 8 years younger for CD (26 years) than for UC (34 years). IBD may be observed in children most frequently after 10 years of age. Females are slightly more frequently affected by CD (sex ratio female/male: 1.2). In contrast, UC has a reverse sex ratio (sex ratio male/female: 1.2).

IBDs are observed throughout the world but do not have homogeneous distribution. In most studies, the frequency of UC is higher than that of CD. Thus, for UC, published prevalence rates are between 80 and 157 per 100 000 inhabitants and the incidence rates are between 1.5 and 25 per 100 000 inhabitants. For CD, the prevalence varies between 27 and 106 per 100 000 inhabitants and the incidence between 0.8 and 9.8 per 100 000 inhabitants. The large differences observed between studies may in part be explained by geographic, ethnic or time-dependent variations of incidence. In Europe, the average incidence rate at present is 5.6 per 100 000 for CD and 10.4 per 100 000 for UC[1]. In the north of France, where a large registry has collected data from most IBD cases, the incidence is 4.9 per 100 000 and 3.2 per 100 000 for CD and UC, respectively[2]. A north-to-south gradient for IBD incidence has been observed in Europe and in North America. A recent European study, however, demonstrated that the variation remains small: 1.5 fold higher in the north than in the south[1]. Finally, there are some regional concentrations of cases which are not well understood at present.

Differences in incidence for ethnic groups living in the same geographical region are in support of a major impact of ethnic factors predisposing to IBDs[3]. The white population of European origin appears to be at the highest risk. Striking differences in incidence are observed between the white and black populations living in the United States or in South Africa, and between the Caucasian and Maori populations in New Zealand. Throughout the world, within those of Caucasian origin, the highest incidence of IBD is observed in the Jewish population where it is 2–5 times higher. This difference is highest for the Ashkenazi population from central Europe (rather than eastern Europe).

Most epidemiological studies have reported an increasing incidence of IBD with time. More specifically, it appears that the incidence of CD has at least doubled since the mid-twentieth century in most European countries. Currently, it remains uncertain whether this increase has stopped or whether it is still rising. It is likely that this variation of incidence occurred earlier in the northern part of Europe and could thus contribute to the north-to-south gradient. IBD has been described as more frequent in urban regions compared with rural ones. However, this higher incidence in urban environments was mainly mentioned in studies performed before 1960. Similarly, the lower frequency of IBD in unfavourable socioeconomic environments has also been discussed. It is tempting to relate these different epidemiological data to the modification in urban life style of western societies since the 1950s/1960s. The improvement in socioeconomic level and the diffusion of this modern life style coincide with the time and geographic variations of incidence.

Although epidemiological observations strongly suggest a role for environmental factors in the initiation of IBD, these studies have seldom provided precise hypotheses on the factors and mechanisms that may be at work. Oral contraceptives have been implicated but this is not fully confirmed. Food regimen has been suspected but no specific nutrient may be retained as a risk factor today. Among the environmental risk factors that have been proposed for IBD, the most clearly established is tobacco[4]. Smokers are at a higher risk of developing CD than non-smokers. Persistent tobacco smoking appears to be a risk factor for relapse and increases the therapeutic score in a dose-dependent manner, suggesting an aetiological role[5]. The deleterious effect of tobacco in CD could be due to the modification of the microcirculation of the intestine, a hypothesis which would be in line with the vascular theory of the disease based on the discovery of vascular lesions within the affected regions. In contrast, in UC, tobacco appears to be beneficial[6]. Nicotine patches have been proposed as an adjuvant to the classical treatment of UC[7]. The beneficial role of tobacco has been related to the stimulation of mucus secretion in the colon.

Given the similarities between CD and intestinal tuberculosis and Johns' disease observed in bovines, an aetiological role of mycobacteria has been investigated on several occasions. Mycobacteria have been observed in affected tissues but in an erratic manner which does not provide a definitive demonstration of their aetiological involvement[8]. More recently, several observations have suggested a role for measles virus. In the UK, there appears to be an increased prevalence of IBD in subjects who were vaccinated with an attenuated strain of measles virus[9]. In Sweden, it was possible to identify individuals who were born, 40 years earlier, after their mothers had developed clinical symptoms of measles during the third trimester of pregnancy[10]. In this group, 75% of individuals were affected by CD. In addition, an electron microscopic analysis of tissues from CD patients showed evidence of viral particles which resemble those of measles[11]. It should be noted, however, that most of these observations have not yet been replicated by independent groups of investigators[12].

Family studies

At present, the most important known risk factor for IBD is a familial history of the disease[13–17]. For CD, 8–10% of affected individuals have one or more relatives with the disease. For UC, familial aggregations appear slightly less frequently and, in most studies, on average 6% of individuals with UC have at least one affected relative. Familial aggregations are more frequent when the disease was diagnosed before 15 years in the proband. Although, in most families, concordance for the same disease is observed, mixed families with both UC and CD are not uncommon. For many authors, the frequency of mixed families is higher when the proband has developed CD, rather than UC.

The demonstration of ethnic or familial aggregations of IBD suggests the existence of genetic factors that predispose to the disease. However, these aggregations may, at least in part, be due to environmental factors that are shared by members of the same community. The relative contribution of genetic and environmental factors may be evaluated using sophisticated methods developed by genetic epidemiology. The most important observation in favour of the existence of a genetic predisposition to IBD is found in twin studies: twins who have grown up together usually share the same environment but may be either genetically identical (monozygotic twins) or semi-identical (dizygotic twins).

Comparison of the concordance rates for the disease between the two categories of twins reveals differences between the two categories that are significant for CD and suggestive for UC[18–20]. It is noteworthy that the concordance rate for IBD is comparable to that observed for diseases such diabetes and asthma, for which genetic susceptibility has been well documented.

The risk of developing IBD for first-degree relatives of an IBD patient is 1.2% for CD and 1.0% for UC. The relative risk of IBD for patients' relatives can be computed as the prevalence of IBD in relatives divided by the prevalence of the disease in the population. The risk of CD in first-degree relatives of a CD patient is 10–14 times higher than in the general population[14,15]. The relative risk of UC for a first-degree relative of a UC patient is about 8[14]. The relative risk of developing UC for a first-degree relative of a CD patient is close to 4. Interestingly, the risk of developing CD for a first-degree relative of UC patient is very little higher than that of the general population[14]. For both diseases, the risk of family members developing the disease increases with the number of cases within the family.

Affected first-degree relatives of CD patients are more frequently siblings and the prevalence of CD is twice as high in siblings as it is in parents of the proband. For UC, the risks in siblings and parents are approximately the same. The risk of transmission of the disease to children is more difficult to evaluate because the follow up is often too short and the children are usually younger than the average age at onset. For CD, even after correction for age, published results are extremely variable[15,16]. The previously mentioned secular variation in incidence rates may, at least in part, explain these observations. The risk of a child of an affected individual developing the disease is probably in the range of 1 to 3%. A younger age at onset in familial cases and an onset which progresses to the younger ages from generation to generation is often reported.

The relative risk decreases sharply with the distance from affected relatives on the pedigree. The relative risk for second-degree relatives of affected individuals is 5–10 times less than that of the first-degree relatives. Interestingly, children of couples with two affected parents are at a high risk for the same disease. This correlation is strongest for CD[17]. Interestingly, however, an increased incidence of CD in children of parents who are both affected by UC has been observed.

ASSOCIATION STUDIES

One strategy to identify genes that contribute to genetic susceptibility is based on the known or hypothesized physiopathological mechanisms that are responsible for the disease. This consists of searching for genetic polymorphisms that may be present in the genes putatively involved and measuring, in groups of affected and control individuals, the frequency of each allele. Such genes are called 'candidate genes'. Given the prominent chronic inflammation of these diseases, the first candidate genes studied were those involved in immune regulation. The HLA system has been most studied but the data remain uncertain.

HLA genes

The contribution of major histocompatibility complex genes has received considerable attention in IBD. In Japanese and Jewish patients, HLA DRB1*1502 is associated with susceptibility to UC[21,22]. Studies in other ethnic groups have revealed conflicting results[23,24]. The explanation for these discrepancies can be provided by documented ethnic variability in HLA Class II frequencies: in Japanese and Jewish populations, DRB1*1502 is the most common allele, but this allele is rare in non-Jewish Caucasians and appears to play little part in IBD pathogenesis in this group[25]. More consistent results suggest that HLA plays an important role in determining UC phenotype. Data from Oxford showed that HLADRB1*0103 was strongly predictive of need for surgery[24]. This association was greatest in patients with extensive disease, extraintestinal manifestations (EIMs), particularly aphthous stomatitis, arthritis and uveitis. In contrast, the frequency of DRB1*04 allele was reduced in patients with distal colitis and EIMs[26]. The DRB1*0301 DQB*201 haplotype was predictive of extensive colitis, particularly in female patients[24]. HLA associations in CD are even more conflicting than in UC. A highly significant association with the allele DRB3*03 was observed in a small group of patients and controls[27]. A significant association with the DRB1*01 allele was found in two studies from the United States and France[22,28]. In the former, the association was strongest with the HLADRB1*01-DQB1*0501 haplotype. Two studies in large populations from northern Europe have shown a positive association with HLADRB1*07[28,29]. Interestingly, the DRB1*07 allele was also associated with psoriasis[30] and the concurrence of psoriasis and CD in both subjects and families has been described[31]. The most impressive result observed in the French study was an important decrease in HLADRB1*03 in CD[28]. The estimated strength of the negative association between carrying these alleles and CD was odds ratio (OR) 0.46. This variation has also been described in Germany[29] and the Netherlands[32], although, in the latter study, the result was only significant in a subgroup of patients with peri-anal disease. It might even be a general characteristic of IBD since it was also observed in UC[33]. This suggests that HLADRB1*03 alleles mediate resistance to IBD. The mechanisms underlying this protective effect are still speculative and require functional studies. It may be a consequence of a high affinity of the putative antigenic peptide of IBD for the DRB1*03 molecule. This affinity may competitively inhibit the effective presentation by another adequate molecule to immunocompetent cells. The association may also result from a linkage disequilibrium between DRB1*03 and a functional gene located in its vicinity.

Other genes from the HLA region

Alteration in the production of the tumour necrosis factor alpha (TNFα), encoded by a gene which lies between C2 of Class III and HLA-B of Class I, is well described in IBD and, recently, treatments with two anti-TNFα monoclonal antibodies have proved to be effective, in comparison with placebo, in chronic active CD[34,35]. Two different approaches have been used to study the association between TNF locus and IBD. The group from Los Angeles, using five microsatellite sequences within the TNF locus, determined TNF microsatellite allele frequencies at 5 loci. There were no differences in individual TNF microsatellites allele frequencies between IBD patients and controls. However, there was a CD-associated allelic combination TNF a2b1c2d4e1[36]. This haplotype was associated with the previously described HLA-DR1/DQ5 combination. Several groups studied the polymorphism at position −308 in the promoter region of the TNFα gene. The results were discordant: the frequency of the TNF2 allele (associated with a higher level of TNFα transcription) was found to be decreased in patients with UC in the Netherlands[37] and decreased in CD and females with distal colitis in England[38]. No significant results were observed in other studies[26,39]. It is so far difficult to reconcile these results and it appears unlikely that these loci are important overall determinants of disease susceptibility. However, two promising aspects should be further tested: (1) the group from Amsterdam recently described specific combinations of 4 alleles in the TNFα and LTα genes which may be markers for altered TNFα production in IBD subgroups[40]; and (2) there is recent evidence that TNF microsatellites can identify CD patients with poor response to anti-TNF (cA2) therapy[41].

Two genes encoding the transporter associated with antigen processing (TAP) proteins, TAP 1 and TAP 2, are located between HLA-DP and HLA-DQ. These molecules are involved in endogenous antigen processing. In CD, no association was found with overall disease, but a significant decrease of TAP2AA genotype was found in patients who did not respond to steroid therapy[42].

Interleukins

Clinical studies and animal models provided evidence that the balance between proinflammatory cytokines, IL-1a and IL-1b, and their endogenous inhibitor IL-1ra is an important factor in the regulation of intestinal inflammation[43]. A decrease in IL-1ra/IL-1a+b ratio has been found in inflamed colonic mucosae from patients with IBD but also from inflammatory controls[44–46]. The genes for IL-1a and IL-1b are located on the long arm of chromosome 2, in close linkage with the gene encoding IL-1ra. Mansfield *et al.* reported that, in a UK population, IL-1ra allele 2 was more frequent in UC patients than in controls (35% vs. 24%)[47]. They found an OR of 2.0 for UC in carriers for at least one copy of this allele when compared with healthy controls. This finding suggests that the allele 2 of IL-1ra is a genetic marker for UC susceptibility. A moderate increase in the prevalence of IL-1ra genotype 2 in affected patients was confirmed in some, but not all, subsequent studies[39,46,48–51]. The explanation for these differences between studies is not clear. It may be due to the small numbers of patients. Bioque *et al.* were able to show a significant difference in the frequency of allele 2 carriers between CD, UC and controls only by combining their data from a Dutch population with data from Mansfield's study[50]. Disease heterogeneity may be extremely relevant to these discrepancies. Allele 2 of the IL-1ra may be associated exclusively with a particular subgroup of UC patients with extensive colitis and need for surgery[47]. However, this classification remains controversial since disease extent in UC may vary considerably over time. A Taq1 RFLP has been described in exon 5 of IL-1b. The IL-1b allele frequencies of IBD patients may not differ from controls[50,51]. However, IL-1b allele 2 was significantly increased in non-carriers of IL-ra allele 2[50,51] and IL-1ra allele 2–IL-1b (Taq1) allele 2 association was significantly decreased in CD and UC patients compared with controls[50]. The mucosal imbalance of the IL-1 system in IBD may be thus genetically determined: allele 2 of the IL-1ra has been associated with an impaired increase in IL-1ra in colonic mucosae[46] and IL-1b allele 2 represents an IL-1b high secretor phenotype[52]. In conclusion, there is mounting evidence that genes of the IL-1 system are important in overall susceptibility to IBD. Functional studies of cytokine production in different subgroups of patients, defined by the IL-1ra/IL-1b genotypes, are now needed to further clarify disease heterogeneity[50,51].

Studies involving T-cell receptor, IL-10, IL-2 and mucin genes have given inconsistent results or are still preliminary.

Intercellular adhesion molecule-1 (ICAM-1)

ICAM-1 is a receptor for the major group of human rhinoviruses and a ligand for lymphocyte-function-associated (LFA) antigens. It serves multiple functions in the propagation of inflammatory processes, the best characterized being facilitation of leukocyte migration from the intervascular space in response to inflammatory stimuli. Preliminary studies suggest that ICAM-1 monoclonal antibodies may be useful in CD[53]. ICAM-1 gene polymorphisms at codon 241 and at codon 469 (chromosome 19) have been studied by Yang *et al.*[54]. These two polymorphisms were not associated with CD or UC, but, after stratification for pANCA status, some weak associations were found which might suggest that this polymorphism is associated with some subsets of IBD.

DNA mismatch repair

A provocative association has been recently put forward between IBD and the DNA mismatch repair gene MLH1 on 3p which is associated with hereditary non-polyposis rectal cancer (HNPCC)[55]. Polymerase chain reaction products were analysed by single-strand conformation polymorphisms (MLH1 exons 9, 11, 14, 15 and 16) and polyacrylamide gel electrophoresis (markers D3S1611 and D3S1768). CD, UC and familial IBD were significantly associated with different MLH1 exon 15/D3S1611 haplotypes. D3S1611/D3S1678 haplotype was associated with CD whereas MLH1 exon 15/D3S1611 haplotype AA was protective. This study raises the question of whether family members of HNPCC kindreds are at risk for IBD. Interestingly, some pathological patterns (reduction in the colonic crypt in the presence of an excess of macrophages) observed in the colonic biopsies of HNPCC family members are reminiscent of IBD[56] and a member of one family, considered not at risk for HNPCC by genetic analysis, developed UC[57]. However, the number of patients in Pokorny *et al.*'s study[55] was small and their findings need to be reproduced by other centres. Meanwhile, clinicians should continue to explore the possibility of familial associations between IBD and HNPCC[58].

Future developments in association studies

Although much effort has been devoted to searching for associations, at present the results are still meagre. In the future investigations may be improved along two different lines: better categorization of patients, and more rigorous selection of controls through a modified design of the analysis.

Emerging evidence points to distinct clinical patterns and heterogeneity within CD and UC[59]. Power to detect susceptibility genes might be magnified considerably by studying disease subgroups: different susceptibility genes may underlie specific phenotypic traits in IBD. Thus, identification of a particular phenotype should help the search for a corresponding gene. However, clinical classification of IBD is not yet standardized. There is great interest in the hypothesis that monitoring the presence of pANCA and ASCA (anti-*Saccharomyces cerevisiae* mannan antibodies) may help to stratify patients and to define homogeneous subgroups. Vasiliauskas *et al.* have suggested that, in patients with CD, serum pANCA expression characterizes a UC-like clinical phenotype[60]. This important finding was not reproduced in the French population[61], but the technique used to identify pANCA was different. An increased prevalence of pANCA was noted in unaffected UC family members in some[62] but not all studies[63] and, consistent with genetic heterogeneity, a relationship between ANCA status and genotype has been recently confirmed: 92% of patients with the DR3 DQ2 TNF2 were pANCA positive vs. 73.9% of the DR3 DQ2 TNF2 negative patients[64]. Data concerning ASCA are still preliminary[65]. Their presence in 20% of healthy relatives of patients with CD suggests that ASCA may also represent a serological marker of genetic heterogeneity[66]. ASCA has been associated with a younger age at onset of CD and small bowel location and the TNF a2b1c2d4e1a haplotype has been associated with the presence of ASCA[67].

Spurious associations between candidate genes and disease can result from ethnic differences between cases and non-related controls. This can occur when there exist both ethnic differences in candidate gene allele frequencies and ethnic differences in disease incidence. This type of ethnic variation, often referred to as population stratification, can result from the preferential breeding of individuals with similar ethnic background. To overcome this potential limitation of association studies, it has been proposed to use parental genotypes of the affected cases instead of those provided by unrelated controls. In this approach, the frequency of the presence of a particular allele among the cases versus among the controls is still compared. However, now the controls are no longer the unrelated individuals but are the two parental alleles that are not transmitted to the affected child. Among this group of methods, the most popular is called the transmission disequilibrium test (TDT). Several groups are currently collecting affected sibs and their parents to perform such tests in order to evaluate the previously proposed associations.

WHOLE GENOME SEARCH

Due to the development of a precise genetic map of the human genome, it is now possible to perform a systematic screening of the entire human genome in search of a region that would demonstrate a genetic linkage with a disease. Due to the complex mode of inheritance which characterizes the genetic contribution to IBD aetiology, model-free analysis of the segregation data has to be utilized. The prototypic method of such an approach is the measurement of the proportion of alleles shared identically by descent among affected sib pairs. Due to the small number of meioses that relates two sibs (2 meioses), the typing of no more than 400 highly polymorphic loci is required to explore the entire genome. Because this number of loci is small, it is no longer necessary to target the genetic studies to candidate genes. Thus, this approach does not require a prior assumption about the nature of susceptibility genes. Identification of specific regions which are more often shared by affected individuals than expected from Mendel's laws provides the location of the susceptibility locus. This approach has, however, two drawbacks. First, it provides only a rough estimation of the location (at least 20 cM in the present reports), making the subsequent steps of positional cloning difficult. Second, it may be somewhat less powerful than those methods based on the candidate gene approach so that large numbers of families and sibships should be investigated. Recent studies have emphasized the importance of access to large numbers of multiply-affected families and rigorous statistical design and analysis.

So far, two such original studies have allowed the localization of yet-unidentified susceptibility genes to IBD on chromosomes 12 and 16[68,69], thus demonstrating that alterations in at least two different genes are involved in genetic susceptibility to IBD. It is of interest to note that, within these regions, several genes appear to be good candidate genes. Such genes can now be investigated in search of genetic polymorphism or mutations that may be associated with IBD.

Chromosome 16 locus

A European collaborative study (using the identity by descent method) enabled the assignment of linkage to the pericentromeric region of chromosome 16 of a first CD-susceptibility locus named IBD1[68]. This finding has been replicated in independent data sets by four groups – the most important test of validity for linkage analysis in complex traits[70–73]. The linkage does not appear to apply to Jewish patients which further indicates heterogeneity within CD patients[70]. Fine mapping has recently narrowed the linkage to a 10-cM segment with a maximum lod score at D16S416 and D16S3117[74]. IBD1 contributes a relative risk to siblings of 1.3 and therefore probably accounts for only a fraction of inherited susceptibility to CD. Whether this region also contributes to UC susceptibility is still being debated[70,71,75]. Evidence of linkage was detected in the families affected only with UC but not in mixed (CD–UC) families. This suggests that the disease locus may be involved in both diseases but that the alleles predisposing to UC and CD are different.

Chromosome 12 locus

A second susceptibility locus to both UC and CD was mapped on the long arm of chromosome 12 in a 41-cM region around D12S83 with a locus-specific relative risk to siblings of 2.0[69]. Promising positional candidate genes in the vicinity of tested markers include the genes encoding interferon-γ, vitamin D receptor and integrin $\beta7$. This localization was further confirmed by two independent groups in Caucasian populations[76,77]. Whether the susceptibility genes on chromosomes 16 and 12 act independently or synergistically is not known.

Other loci

In a UK data set of non-Jewish European Caucasians with UC, the sharing of alleles among affected sibling pairs provided evidence of linkage with the DRB1 locus contrasting with the weakness of the overall associations previously noted[7,24]. Negative results were subsequently reported[78,79]. In the study by Hugot *et al.*[68], the initial screen identified a possible CD locus close to D1S236 on chromosome 1 but the linkage result for this marker was not significant in a second family panel. In the study from Oxford, two additional regions on chromosomes 3 and 7 were identified; they provide a locus-specific relative risk of 1.8 and 1.9, respectively[69]. Furthermore, a region on chromosome 2 and a marker within the HLA region on chromosome 6 showed positive linkage to UC[69]. These observations have not been replicated. It is likely that other genes that have not been identified or even localized may contribute to the genetic susceptibility to IBD.

It has been shown that IBD is diagnosed earlier in life among offspring than among affected parents, an observation that has been interpreted as evidence of genetic anticipation[80]. A recent study in a US population suggests that anticipation may be restricted to CD Jews families[81]. The list of genetic conditions exhibiting anticipation is growing rapidly and is associated with triplet nucleotide repeat expansion. Recently, CAG repeat expansions have been observed in a subset of families with CD[82]. However, these findings have not yet been reproduced. Epidemiological data for genetic anticipation are subject to many biases. Changes in the environment that have occurred during the last 50 years have been proposed to account at least in part for the age difference at diagnosis between parents and children[83,84].

In recent years, the large number of observations that has built up has led to improved understanding of the mechanisms implicated in the development of IBD. The existence of genetic factors is now clearly established, and the implication of environmental factors is highly likely.

Interestingly, new candidate genes are being identified through animal studies. Several genetic manipulations in the mouse have resulted in inflammatory damage to the digestive tract which share at least some of the manifestations of CD or UC[85]. In most cases, the discovery of an IBD-like disease in these manipulated animals had not been anticipated. Manipulations of genes involved either in immunity or in epithelial integrity and functions may cause IBD in the animals. These observations reflect the complexity of the mechanisms that maintain the homeostatic equilibrium of the immune system on the epithelium of the digestive tract. For several models, the IBD-like manifestations are only expressed in the presence of bacteria in the intestinal lumen, thus underscoring the importance of environmental factors.

Due to methodological problems inherent in the search for association using unrelated case–control individuals in heterogeneous populations, the currently proposed candidate genes have to be confirmed. Theoretical considerations and recent experimental studies suggest that the power of association studies increases when disease heterogeneity is taken into account. Definition of homogeneous subgroups may rely upon precise phenotypic characterization and the use of serological markers[59].

The candidate gene approach and genome-wide scanning are two methods that have, until recently, been used independently in search of genes involved in the development of IBD. Their combined use on large data sets should lead to definitive results in the near future. Such progress in identifying IBD-susceptibility genes relies on the registration of a large number of families and patients and is thus critically dependent on collaboration between groups that include both trained clinicians and experienced geneticists.

Acknowledgements

The work of the authors is supported in part by the Association F. Aupetit, the European Community (Contract BMH4-CT97-2098) the Ministère de l'Enseignement Supérieur et de la Recherche, the Ministère de la Santé et de l'Action Humanitaire (Direction Générale de la Santé), INSERM, Fondation Jean Dausset, CH et U de Lille, and the Ferring and Astra companies.

References

1. Shivananda S, Lennard-Jones J, Logan R et al. Incidence of inflammatory bowel disease across Europe: is there a difference between north and south? Results of the European collaborative study on inflammatory bowel disease (EC–IBD). Gut. 1996;39:690–7.
2. Gower-Rousseau C, Salomez JL, Dupas JL et al. Incidence of inflammatory bowel disease in Northern France (1988–1990). Gut. 1994;35:1433–8.
3. Sonnerberg A, Wasserman IH. Epidemiology of inflammatory bowel disease among U.S. military veterans. Gastroenterology. 1991;101:122–30.
4. Tobin MV, Logan RFA, Langman MJS, McConnell RB, Gilmore IT. Cigarette smoking and inflammatory bowel disease. Gastroenterology. 1987;93:316–21.
5. Cosnes J, Carbonnel F, Beaugerie L, Le Quintrec Y, Gendre JP. Effects of cigarette smoking on the long-term course of Crohn's disease. Gastroenterology. 1996;110:424–31.
6. Merrett MN, Mortensen N, Kettlewell M, Jewell DO. Smoking may prevent pouchitis in patients with restorative protocolectomy of ulcerative colitis. Gut. 1996;38:362–4.
7. Pullan RD, Rhodes J, Ganesh S et al. Transdermal nicotine for active ulcerative colitis. N Engl J Med. 1994;330:811–15.
8. Sanderson JD, Moss MT, Tizard MLV, Hermon-Taylor J. Mycobacterium paratuberculosis DNA in Crohn's disease tissue. Gut. 1992;33:890–6.
9. Thompson NP, Montgomery SM, Pounder RE, Wakefield AJ. Is measles vaccination a risk factor for inflammatory bowel disease? Lancet. 1995;345:1071–4.
10. Ekbom A, Daszak P, Kraaz W, Wakefield AJ. Crohn's disease after in-utero measles virus exposure. Lancet. 1996;348:515–17.
11. Levin J, Dhillon AP, Sim R, Mazure G, Pounder RE, Wakefield AJ. Persistent measles virus infection of the intestine: confirmation by immunogold electron microscopy. Gut. 1995;36:564–9.
12. Haga Y, Funakoshi O, Kuroe K et al. Absence of measles viral genomic sequence in intestinal tissues from Crohn's disease by nested polymerase chain reaction. Gut. 1996;38:211–15.
13. Gilat T, Hacohen D, Lilos P, Langman JS, and the International IBD Study Group. Childhood factors in ulcerative colitis and Crohn's disease. Scand J Gastroenterol. 1987;22:1009–24.
14. Orholm M, Munkholm P, Langholz E, Nielsen OH, Sorensen TIA, Binder V. Familial occurrence of inflammatory bowel disease. N Engl J Med. 1991;324:84–8.
15. Peeters M, Nevens H, Baert F et al. Familial aggregation in Crohn's disease: Increased age-adjusted risk and concordance in clinical characteristics. Gastroenterology. 1996;111:597–603.
16. Roth MP, Petersen GM, McElree C, Vadheim CM, Panish JF, Rotter JI. Familial empiric risk estimates of inflammatory bowel disease in Ashkenazi Jews. Gastroenterology. 1989;96:1016–20.
17. Bennett RA, Rubin PH, Present DH. Frequency of inflammatory bowel disease in offspring of couples both presenting with inflammatory bowel disease. Gastroenterology. 1991;100:1638–43.

18. Tysk C, Lindberg E, Järnerot G, Flodérus-Myrhed B. Ulcerative colitis and Crohn's disease in an unselected population of monozygotic and dizygotic twins. A study of heritability and the influence of smoking. Gut. 1988;29:990–6.
19. Thompson NP, Driscoll R, Pounder RE, Wakefield AJ. Genetics versus environment in inflammatory bowel disease: results of a British twin study. BMJ. 1996;312:95–6.
20. Orholm M, Binder V, Sorensen TIA, Kyvik KO. Inflammatory bowel disease in a Danish twin register. Gut. 1996;39(suppl 3):A187.
21. Futami S, Aoyama N, Honsako Y et al. HLA-DRB1*1502 allele, subtype of DR15, is associated with susceptibility to ulcerative colitis and its progression. Dig Dis Sci. 1995;40:814–18.
22. Toyoda H, Wang SJ, Yang HY et al. Distinct associations of HLA class II genes with inflammatory bowel disease. Gastroenterology. 1993;104:741–8.
23. Duerr RH, Neigut DA. Molecularly defined HLA-DR2 alleles in ulcerative colitis and an anti-neutrophil cytoplasmic antibody-positive subgroup. Gastroenterology. 1995;108:423–7.
24. Satsangi J, Welsh KI, Bunce M et al. Contribution of genes of the major histocompatibility complex to susceptibility and disease phenotype in inflammatory bowel disease. Lancet. 1996;347:1212–17.
25. Parkes M, Satsangi J, Jewell DP. Mapping susceptibility loci in inflammatory bowel disease: why and how? Mol Med Today. 1997;3:546–53.
26. Roussosmoustakaki M, Satsangi J, Welsh K et al. Genetic markers may predict disease behavior in patients with ulcerative colitis. Gastroenterology. 1997;112:1845–53.
27. Forcione DG, Sands B, Isselbacher KJ, Rutsgi A, Podolsky D, Pillai S. An increased risk of Crohn's disease in individuals who inherit the HLA class II DRB3*0301 allele. Proc Natl Acad Sci USA. 1996;93:5094–8.
28. Danzé PM, Colombel JF, Jacquot S et al. Association of HLA class II genes with susceptibility to Crohn's disease. Gut. 1996;38:69–72.
29. Reinshagen M, Loeliger C, Kuehnl P et al. HLA class II gene frequencies in Crohn's disease: a population based analysis in Germany. Gut. 1996;38:538–42.
30. Schmitt-Egelnolf M, Boehncke WH, Ständer M, Eiermann TH, Sterry W. Oligonucleotide typing reveals association of type I psoriasis with the HLA-DRB1*0701/2, -DQA1*0201, -DQB1*0303 extended haplotype. J Invest Dermatol. 1993;100:749–52.
31. Hughes S, Williams SE, Turnberg LA. Crohn's disease and psoriasis. N Engl J Med. 1983;308:101.
32. Bouma G, Poen AC, Garcia-Gonzalez MA et al. HLA-DRB1*03, but not the TNFα-308 promoter gene polymorphism confers protection against fistulising Crohn's disease. Immunogenetics. 1998;47:451–5.
33. Heresbach D, Colombel JF, Danzé PM, Semana G. The HLADRB1*03016DQB1*0201 haplotype confers protection against inflammatory bowel disease. Am J Gastroenterol. 1996;5:1060.
34. Stack WA, Mann SD, Roy AJ et al. Randomised controlled trial of CDP 571 antibody to tumour necrosis factor-a in Crohn's disease. Lancet. 1997;349:521–4.
35. Targan SR, Hanauer SB, Van Deventer SJH et al. A short term study of chimeric monoclonal antibody cA2 to tumor necrosis factor-a for Crohn's disease. N Engl J Med. 1997;337:1029–35.
36. Plevy SE, Targan SR, Yang H, Fernandez D, Rotter JI, Toyoda H. Tumor necrosis factor microsatellites define a Crohn's disease-associated haplotype on chromosome 6. Gastroenterology. 1996;110:1053–60.
37. Bouma G, Xia B, Crusius JBA et al. Distribution of four polymorphisms in the tumour necrosis factor (TNF) genes in patients with inflammatory bowel disease (IBD). Clin Exp Immunol. 1996;103:391–6.
38. Louis E, Satsangi J, Rousosmoustakaki M et al. Cytokine gene polymorphisms in inflammatory bowel disease. Gut. 1996;39:705–10.
39. Heresbach D, Ababou A, Bourienne A et al. Etude du polymorphisme des microsatellites et des gènes du tumor necrosis factor (TNF) au cours des maladies inflammatoires chroniques de l'intestin. Gastroenterol Clin Biol. 1997;21:555–61.
40. Bouma G, Crusius JBA, Odkerk Pool M et al. Secretion of tumor necrosis factor a and lymphotoxin a in relation to polymorphism in the TNF genes and HLA-DR alleles. Relevance for inflammatory bowel disease. Scand J Immunol. 1996;43:456–63.
41. Plevy SE, Taylor K, DeWoody KL, Schaible TF, Shealy D, Targan SR. Tumor necrosis factor (TNF) microsatellite haplotypes and perinuclear anti-neutrophil cytoplasmic antibody (pANCA) identify Crohn's disease (CD) patients with poor clinical response to anti-TNF monoclonal antibody. Gastroenterology. 1997;112:1062A.

42. Heresbach D, Alizadeh M, Bretagne JF *et al.* TAP gene transporter polymorphism in inflammatory bowel disease. Scand J Gastroenterol. 1997;32:1022–7.
43. Cominelli F, Pizarro TT. Interleukin-1 and interleukin-1 receptor antagonist in inflammatory bowel disease. Aliment Pharmacol Ther. 1996;10(Suppl 2):49–53.
44. Nishiyama T, Misuyama K, Toyonaga A, Sasaki E, Tanikawa K. Colonic mucosal interleukin 1 receptor antagonist in inflammatory bowel disease. Digestion. 1994;55:368–73.
45. Casini-Raggi V, Kam L, Chong YJ, Fiocchi C, Pizarro TT, Cominelli F. Mucosal imbalance of IL-1 and IL-1 receptor antagonist in inflammatory bowel disease. J Immunol. 1995;154:2434–40.
46. Andus T, Daig R, Vogl D *et al.* Imbalance of the interleukin 1 system in colonic mucosa – association with intestinal inflammation and interleukin 1 receptor agonist genotype 2. Gut. 1997;41:651–7.
47. Mansfield JC, Holden H, Tarlow JK *et al.* Novel genetic association between ulcerative colitis and the anti-inflammatory cytokine interleukin-1 receptor antagonist. Gastroenterology. 1994;106:637–42.
48. Duerr RH, Tran T. Association between ulcerative colitis and a polymorphism intron 2 of the interleukin-1 receptor antagonist. Gastroenterology. 1995;108:A812.
49. Tountas NA, Yang H, Coulter DI, Rotter JI. Increased carriage of allele 2 of IL-1 receptor antagonist (IL-1ra) in Jewish populations: the strongest known genetic association in ulcerative colitis. Gastroenterology. 1996;110:A1029.
50. Bioque G, Crusius JBA, Koutroubakis I *et al.* Allelic polymorphism in IL-1b and IL-1 receptor antagonist (IL-1Ra) genes in inflammatory bowel disease. Clin Exp Immunol. 1995;102:379–83.
51. Heresbach D, Alizadeh M, Dabadie A *et al.* Significance of interleukin-1b and interleukin-1 receptor antagonist genetic polymorphism in inflammatory bowel diseases. Am J Gastroenterol. 1997;92:1164–9.
52. Pociot F, Molvig J, Wogensen L. A. Taq 1 polymorphism in the human inteleukin-1b (IL-1b) gene correlated with IL-1b secretion *in vitro*. Eur J Clin Invest. 1992;22:396–402.
53. Yacyshyn B, Woloschuk B, Yacyshyn MB *et al.* Efficacy and safety of ISIS 2302 (ICAM-1 antisense oligonucleotide) treatment of steroid-dependent Crohn's disease. Gastroenterology. 1997;112:1123A.
54. Yang H, Vora DK, Targan SR, Toyoda H, Beaudet AL, Rotter JI. Intercellular adhesion molecule 1 gene associations with immunologic subsets of inflammatory bowel disease. Gastroenterology. 1995;109:440–8.
55. Pokorny RM, Hofmeister A, Galandiuk S, Dietz AB, Cohen ND, Neibergs HL. Crohn's disease and ulcerative colitis are associated with the DNA repair gene *MLH1*. Ann Surg. 1997;6:718–25.
56. Cristofaro G, Lynch HT, Caruso ML *et al.* New phenotypic aspects in a family with Lynch syndrome II. Cancer. 1987;60:51–8.
57. Caruso ML, Cristofaro G, Lynch HT. HNPCC-Lynch syndrome and idiopathic inflammatory disease. A hypothesis on sharing of genes. Anticancer Res. 1997;17:2647–50.
58. Sandborn WJ. Inflammatory bowel disease and hereditary nonpolyposis colorectal cancer: is there a genetic link? Gastroenterology. 1998;114:608–9.
59. Coche JC, Colombel JF. Heterogeneity of inflammatory bowel disease: clinical subgroups of patients. Research and Clinical Forums. IBD and Salicylates-3. 1997;20:P136–45.
60. Visiliauskas EA, Plevy SE, Landers CJ *et al.* Perinuclear antineutrophil cytoplasmic antibodies in patients with Crohn's disease define a clinical subgroup. Gastroenterology. 1996;110:1810–19.
61. Jamar-Leclerc N, Reumaux D, Duthilleul P, Colombel JF. Do pANCA define a clinical subgroup in patients with Crohn's disease? Gastroenterology. 1997;112:316.
62. Shanahan F, Duerr RH, Rotter JL *et al.* Neutrophil autoantibodies in ulcerative colitis: familial aggregation and genetic heterogeneity. Gastroenterology. 1992;103:456–61.
63. Reumaux D, Delecourt L, Colombel JF, Noel LH, Duthilleul P, Cortot A. Antineutrophil cytosplasmic autoantibodies in relatives of patients with ulcerative colitis (letter). Gastroenterology. 1992;103:1706.
64. Satsangi J, Landers CJ, Welsh KI, Koss K, Targan SR, Jewell DP. The presence of anti-neutrophil antibodies reflects clinical and genetic heterogeneity within inflammatory bowel disease. Inflamm Bowel Dis. 1998;4:18–26.
65. Quinton JF, Sendid B, Reumaux D *et al.* Anti-*Saccharomyces cerevisiae* mannan combined with antineutrophil antibodies in inflammatory bowel disease: prevalence and diagnostic role. Gut. 1998;42:788–91.

66. Sendid B, Quinton JF, Charrier G *et al.* Anti-*Saccharomyces cerevisiae* mannan antibodies (ASCA) in familial Crohn's disease. Am J Gastroenterol. 1998;93:1306–10.
67. Vasiliauskas EA, Plevy SE, Targan SR. Stratification of Crohn's disease by antineutrophil cytoplasmic antibodies (ANCA) and anti-*Saccharomyces cerevisiae* antibody (ASCA) distinguishes phenotypic subgroups. Gastroenterology. 1997;112:1112A.
68. Hugot JP, Laurent-Puig P, Gower-Rousseau C *et al.* Mapping of a susceptibility locus for Crohn's disease on chromosome 16. Nature. 1996;379:821–3.
69. Satsangi J, Parkes M, Louis E *et al.* Two stage genome wide search in inflammatory bowel disease provides evidence for susceptibility loci on chromosome 3, 7 and 12. Nature Genet. 1996;14:199–202.
70. Ohmen JD, Yang HY, Yamamoto KK *et al.* Susceptibility locus for inflammatory bowel disease on chromosome 16 has a role in Crohn's disease, but not in ulcerative colitis. Hum Mol Genet. 1996;5:1679–83.
71. Parkes M, Satsangi J, Lathrop GM, Bell JI, Jewell DP. Susceptibility loci in inflammatory bowel disease. Lancet. 1996;348:1588.
72. Cho JH, Fu Y, Kirshner BS, Hanauer SB. Confirmation of a susceptibility locus, for Crohn's disease on chromosome 16. Inflamm Bowel Dis. 1997;3:186–90.
73. Cavanaugh J, Wilson S, Srami M *et al.* Affected sib-pair analysis of pericentromeric chromosome 16 markers in inflammatory bowel disease families. Gastroenterology. 1997;112:A946.
74. Hugot JP, Zouali H, Colombel JF *et al.* Fine mapping of the inflammatory bowel disease susceptibility locus 1 (IBD) in the pericentromeric region of chromosome 16 [abstract]. Gastroenterology. 1998; (in press).
75. Mirza MM, Lee J, Teare D *et al.* Evidence of linkage of the inflammatory bowel disease susceptibility locus on chromosome 16 (IBD1) to ulcerative colitis. J Med Genet. 1998;35:218–21.
76. Hampe J, Stokkers P, Nürnberg P *et al.* Linkage to a susceptibility region on chromosome 12 but not 16 in the north central European family sample by multipoint non-parametric linkage analysis. Gastroenterology. 1997;112:A990.
77. Duerr RH, Zhang L, Preston RA *et al.* Further evidence for an inflammatory bowel disease susceptibility locus on chromosome 12. Gastroenterology. 1997;112:A963.
78. Naom I, Lee J, Ford D *et al.* Analysis of the contribution of HLA genes to genetic predisposition in inflammatory bowel disease. Am J Hum Genet. 1996;59:226–33.
79. Mathew C, Easton D, Lennard-Jones J. HLA and inflammatory bowel disease. Lancet. 1996;348:68.
80. Polito II JM, Rees RC, Childs B, Mendeloff AI, Harris ML, Bayless TM. Preliminary evidence for genetic anticipation in Crohn's disease. Lancet. 1996;347:798–800.
81. Akolkar D, Heresbach D, Lesser M *et al.* Anticipation in Crohn's disease may be influenced by ethnicity of the transmitting parent. Gastroenterology. 1998; (in press).
82. Cho JH, Fu Y, Pickles M, Kirschner B, Hanauer SB. CAG repeat expansion in subsets of families with Crohn's disease. Gastroenterology. 1997;112:948A.
83. Grandbastien B, Peeters M, Franchimont D *et al.* Anticipation in familial Crohn's disease. Gut. 1998;42:170–4.
84. Hugot JP, Colombel JF, Bélaïche J *et al.* Date of birth in familial Crohn's disease suggests environmental factors [abstract]. Gastroenterology. 1998; (in press).
85. Elson CO, Sartor RB. Tennyson GS, Riddell RH. Experimental models of inflammatory bowel disease. Gastroenterology. 1995;109:1344–67.

2
Genetic heterogeneity within inflammatory bowel disease

J. SATSANGI and D. JEWELL

INTRODUCTION

In recent years, the importance of genetic susceptibility in the pathogenesis of Crohn's disease and ulcerative colitis has been re-assessed. Both genetic epidemiological and molecular data suggest that the use of the single unifying term 'inflammatory bowel disease', although convenient, has limited scientific basis: the model of inheritance which appears to best explain the data is that Crohn's disease and ulcerative colitis are in fact a group of polygenic diseases sharing some, but not all, susceptibility genes. This model appears to explain the clinical variability of disease presentation – a specific disease phenotype may result from the interaction between environmental stimulus with the products of specific allelic mutations in a number of susceptibility loci. Considerable progress is being made in identifying the number and identity of susceptibility genes and the mutations involved. In the present review, the data supporting the model of genetic heterogeneity are reviewed, and the results of recent molecular studies are discussed.

THE GENETIC MODEL

Recent epidemiological studies, notably the systematic review of the Swedish twin registry performed by Tysk and colleagues[1], have provided considerable insight into the genetic model most pertinent to Crohn's disease and ulcerative colitis. In the Swedish study, 80 twin pairs were identified in whom at least one twin had a definite diagnosis of inflammatory bowel disease. The health of the other member of the twin pair was then ascertained. Monozygotic twins were concordant for Crohn's disease in 8 of 18 twin pairs but concordance was only found in 1 of 26 dizygotic pairs. In twins with one proband having ulcerative colitis, 1 of 16 monozygotic pairs was concordant for disease but all 20 dizygotic pairs were discordant. The authors derived a coefficient of heritability in Crohn's disease, higher than that previously demonstrated in schizophrenia or asthma, and equivalent to that in insulin-dependent diabetes mellitus and multiple sclerosis. The coefficient of heritability in ulcerative colitis was less than that in Crohn's disease, arguing for a stronger environmental component in susceptibility. Thus, these data demonstrated heterogeneity between Crohn's disease and ulcerative colitis, and also the combined effect of environmental and genetic factors. Subsequent studies from Denmark and the United Kingdom have reflected the results described in the Swedish data set.

The twin studies have been supplemented by many studies of the prevalence of familial inflammatory bowel disease in relatives of patients with Crohn's disease and ulcerative colitis. Large data sets have been studied in Scandinavia[2], United Kingdom[3] and in the United States of America[4]. In Oxford[3], 433 patients with Crohn's disease were studied. In 78 families (18%), at least one first- or second-degree relative also had inflammatory bowel disease. Both Crohn's disease and ulcerative colitis occurred in the multiply affected pedigrees. First-degree relatives were most commonly affected (11.5%). Siblings were most at risk (33 siblings in 29 families). Crohn's disease was more common than ulcerative colitis in affected siblings.

Assuming population prevalences of 70/100 000 for Crohn's disease, and 100/100 000 for ulcerative colitis, the authors calculated the relative risk in siblings of patients with Crohn's disease to be 36.5 for Crohn's disease, 16.6 for ulcerative colitis, and 24.7 for inflammatory bowel disease.

These data reflect the results from studies in Europe and the United States of America. The prevalence rates of familial inflammatory bowel disease derived from these studies are not consistent with the models of Crohn's disease and ulcerative colitis as simple Mendelian disorders. Although complex segregation analyses have suggested simple models may be pertinent to a small proportion of patients with Crohn's disease and ulcerative colitis, a more complex model is necessary to explain the concurrence of both diseases in multiply affected families, and the heterogeneity of clinical presentation.

In subsequent studies[5], the investigators in Oxford compared the clinical characteristics of disease (disease type, extent, age of onset, need for surgery and presence of extraintestinal manifestation) in affected individuals in multiply affected families. High degrees of concordance were noted for disease type, extent, extraintestinal manifestations, and smoking history in affected sibling pairs and in parent–child pairs. Again, these data reflect those from other Western populations.

The model of disease inheritance most consistent with these epidemiological data is that Crohn's disease and ulcerative colitis each consist of a number of related polygenic disorders. Interaction between susceptibility genes and environmental stimuli would give rise to disease phenotype. The full disease phenotype would be determined, according to this model, not only by the number and identity of genes involved, and the number and identity of environmental agents, but also by specific mutations of disease genes involved.

Although the model of disease inheritance is complex, this model has allowed detailed molecular genetic studies to investigate the contribution of specific candidate genes to disease susceptibility and behaviour. Moreover, recent studies have identified novel susceptibility loci in inflammatory bowel disease using genome-wide scanning techniques. The results of the molecular studies have largely been consistent with heterogeneity, not only between Crohn's disease and ulcerative colitis, but also within these conditions.

Moreover, both candidate-gene-directed studies and genome-wide scanning have pointed to important differences between ethnic groups in genetic susceptibility. Thus, the difference in prevalence rates of inflammatory bowel disease and familial inflammatory bowel disease between Jews and non-Jews has already been supplemented by data which have demonstrated differing contributions of both HLA and non-HLA related genes in these ethnic groups.

CANDIDATE GENE STUDIES PROVIDE EVIDENCE FOR HETEROGENEITY BETWEEN AND WITHIN CROHN'S DISEASE AND ULCERATIVE COLITIS

Genes involved in the regulation of the specific immune response and in the maintenance of epithelial integrity are currently under investigation as susceptibility genes in inflammatory bowel disease. The genes of the major histocompatibility complex (in man the human leukocyte antigen (HLA) region on chromosome 6) have received most attention. Early studies involving serological typing, small numbers of patients, and poorly matched controls, led to inconclusive results. However, recent data involving molecular genotyping of large numbers of patients and matched controls point towards considerable heterogeneity in the contribution of the HLA system in Crohn's disease and ulcerative colitis. To date, it appears that the relative contribution of the HLA region to genetic susceptibility is stronger in ulcerative colitis than in Crohn's disease. Linkage analyses in European non-Jewish populations suggest that the HLA region encodes important determinants of susceptibility and behaviour in ulcerative colitis. Moreover, allelic association studies have demonstrated that specific alleles encode susceptibility to ulcerative colitis, and may predict disease severity. Consistent with the concept of heterogeneity between ethnic groups, allelic associations differ between Japanese[6], Jewish[7] and non-Jewish[8] patients. In Japanese and Jewish patients, DRB1*1502 is an important susceptibility allele in ulcerative colitis[7,9]. However, this allele is uncommon in non-Jewish European populations in whom DRB1*103 and DRB1*12 encode susceptibility alleles[8]. Furthermore, in the non-Jewish European population, HLA DRB1*0103 and HLA DRB1*0301 may predict the severity and extent of disease, respectively. It is particularly noteworthy that allelic associations, initially demonstrated in the Oxford population, have been replicated in other European and North American populations with ulcerative colitis.

In Crohn's disease, the contribution of the HLA system to disease susceptibility and severity remains controversial. Although investigators in Northern Europe[10] have been unable to demonstrate linkage between susceptibility to Crohn's disease and the HLA system, investigators in North America, who have studied mixed Jewish/non-Jewish populations, have reported a significant contribution of the HLA system to disease susceptibility in Crohn's disease[11].

Two recent studies underline the importance of genetic heterogeneity and provided further evidence for a relationship between specific allelic variations of the HLADRB1 locus and disease phenotype. Roussomoustakaki and co-workers in Oxford[12] studied 107 patients requiring colectomy for ulcerative colitis. In these patients, the HLA DRB1*0103 allelic frequency was significantly increased (14.1% vs. 3.2%, $p < 10^{-5}$), particularly in the presence of extraintestinal manifestations (22.8% vs. 3.2%, odds ratio = 8.95).

Orchard and colleagues[13] have undertaken detailed studies of the clinical and immunogenetic characteristics of patients cared for in Oxford, with particular respect to the presence of extraintestinal manifestations. On the basis of these studies[13], the association of arthropathy with Crohn's disease has been classified as either a pauci-articular asymmetrical arthropathy (type 1) associated with active intestinal inflammation, or a symmetrical polyarthropathy (type 2), associated with either active or inactive disease. This clinical characterization of the arthropathy has been reinforced by the demonstration that the pauci-articular arthropathy has distinct immunogenetic characteristics compared with both a control group and the patients with polyarthropathy[14]. Thus, the acute pauci-arthropathy (type 1) was associated with DRB1*0103 (40% vs. 3%, relative risk 12.1), B35 (relative risk 2.2), and B27 (relative risk 4.0). the polyarthropathy (type 2) was associated with HLA B44 (relative risk 2.1).

Studies of other candidate genes reinforce the importance of heterogeneity within inflammatory bowel disease, and between different ethnic groups. Genes encoding cytokines have been subject to study in European and North American populations. It seems likely that ethnic differences underlie the discrepant results in these populations. Whereas data from Europe do not point towards the gene encoding the interleukin-1 receptor antagonist as an important determinant of behaviour or susceptibility in ulcerative colitis[15], data from California provide strong evidence for the importance of allelic variation in this gene[16]. There is considerable interest in the contribution of the genes encoding tumour necrosis factor-α, interleukin-2 and interleukin-10[17], in view of the animal models of inflammatory bowel disease produced by manipulation of these loci.

Allelic variations of genes encoding proteins involved in mucosal integrity have received less attention than immunoregulatory genes. However, the genes encoding the intestinal mucins (MUC2 and MUC3) have been implicated in disease susceptibility in preliminary linkage and association studies[18,19]. The attractive hypothesis that the length of variable number of tandem repeat sequences encoded within these genes may alter protein function (and thus intestinal permeability) remains to be proven.

GENOME-WIDE SCANNING: RECENT PROGRESS

Screening of the entire human genome for novel susceptibility loci in complex disorders such as Crohn's disease and ulcerative colitis has been practicable only in recent years. The development of linkage maps of the human genome, based on the wide-spread presence of anonymous microsatellite markers on each chromosome, has allowed a systemic analysis of the contribution of the entire human genome to susceptibility. Studies in other complex disorders, notably insulin-dependent diabetes, multiple sclerosis and schizophrenia, have emphasized, not only the potential benefits of this methodology, but also the difficulties. Access to large numbers of multiply affected families is necessary to overcome the formidable statistical challenges associated with this technique. In turn, considerable financial resources are required, not only for identification of such families and for collection of genetic material, but also for the laboratory tests, statistical analysis and replication studies.

Nevertheless, progress in inflammatory bowel disease has been notable. Hugot and colleagues[20] reported the first genome-wide scanning in inflammatory bowel disease, involving a total of 78 multiply affected families with Crohn's disease. These investigators identified a putative susceptibility locus in the pericentromeric region of chromosome 16 which they designated IBD1. The sibling relative risk (λs) attributed to this locus by the authors was only 1.3. The authors themselves estimated that this region would account for only a relatively small proportion of genetic contribution to susceptibility to Crohn's disease. In spite of this reservation, it is remarkable that the linkage has been replicated widely in Europe[21], North America[22] and Australia[23]. Studies are underway to identify the susceptibility gene or genes within this region.

Subsequently, investigators in Oxford[19] reported the results of a two-stage genome-wide search involving 186 affected sibling pairs with inflammatory bowel disease. In 81 sibling pairs, both had Crohn's disease; in 64, both had ulcerative colitis; and in the remaining 41, one sibling had Crohn's disease and the other ulcerative colitis. The data provided strong evidence for the model of genetic heterogeneity. Evidence for linkage with regions on chromosomes 12, 7 and 3 was noted in both Crohn's disease and ulcerative colitis. In addition, individual markers on chromosomes 2 and 6 (D6S273 in the HLA region) were linked with susceptibility to ulcerative colitis, whereas a microsatellite marker close to the IBD1 locus designated by Hugot and colleagues was linked to susceptibility to Crohn's disease. Again, it is noteworthy that linkage with the potential susceptibility locus on chromosome 12 has been readily replicated in studies involving European[21] and American[22] populations.

The investigators in Oxford have further investigated the contribution of the region on chromosome 12[23]. Linkage disequilibrium tests involving microsatellite markers within this region have allowed fine mapping of the putative susceptibility locus on chromosome 12. Recent data suggest that this locus may now be mapped to within 1 centiMorgan of a microsatellite marker, a distance suitable for the construction of physical maps.

As the results of genome-wide scanning are being reported from other centres, novel susceptibility loci are being reported. Lessons from studies in other complex disorders suggest that inconsistency between studies may result, not only from statistical methodological differences, but also from real heterogeneity of the populations and disease phenotypes studied. Recent data from Vermeire and colleagues[24] underline this point – DNA from affected Belgian sibling pairs was genotyped in Oxford using the microsatellite markers which had been used to identify susceptibility loci on chromosomes 3, 7, 12 and 16. In these Belgian sibling pairs with Crohn's disease, no convincing evidence for linkage with these regions was evident, and genome-wide scanning is being completed in these families.

The clinical, epidemiological and molecular genetic data now available suggest strongly that Crohn's disease and ulcerative colitis are related polygenic disorders. There is increasing confidence that identification of susceptibility genes is likely to be possible in the near future. Perhaps of greatest benefit will be an increase in basic understanding of the pathophysiology of these diseases. Many fundamental questions remain to be answered, including the simple question of how many diseases are truly represented by the term 'inflammatory bowel disease'.

References

1. Tysk C, Lindberg E, Järnerot G, Flodérus-Myrhed B. Ulcerative colitis and Crohn's disease in an unselected population of monozygotic and dizygotic twins. A study of heritability and the influence of smoking. Gut. 1988;29:990–6.
2. Orholm M, Munkolm P, Langholz E, Nielsen OH, Sorensen TI, Binder V. Familial occurrence of inflammatory bowel disease. N Engl J Med. 1991;324:84–8.
3. Satsangi J, Rosenberg WMC, Jewell JP. The prevalence of inflammatory bowel disease in relatives of patients with Crohn's disease. Eur J Gastroenterol Hepatol. 1994;6:413–16.
4. Roth M-P, Petersen GM, McElree C, Vadheim CM, Panish JF, Rotter JI. Familial empiric risk estimates of inflammatory bowel disease in Ashkenazi Jews. Gastroenterology. 1989;96:1016–20.
5. Satsangi J, Grootscholten C, Holt H, Jewell DP. Clinical patterns of familial inflammatory bowel disease. Gut. 1996;38:738–41.
6. Asakura H, Tsuchiya M, Aiso S et al. Association of the human leukocyte DR2 antigen with Japanese ulcerative colitis. Gastroenterology. 1982;82:413–18.
7. Toyoda H, Wang S-J, Yang H et al. Distinct association of HLA Class II genes with inflammatory bowel disease. Gastroenterology. 1993;104:741–8.
8. Satsangi J, Welsh KI, Bunce M et al. Contribution of genes of the major histocompatibility complex to susceptibility and disease phenotype in inflammatory bowel disease. Lancet. 1996;347:1212–17.
9. Asakura H, Sugimura K. HLA, antineutrophil cytoplasmic autoantibody and heterogeneity in ulcerative colitis. Gastroenterology. 1995;108(2):597–9.
10. Hugot JP, Laurent-Puig P, Gower-Rousseau C et al. Linkage analyses of chromosome 6 loci, including HLA, in familial aggregations of Crohn's disease. Am J Med Genet. 1994;52:207–13.
11. Plevy SE, Targan SR, Yang H, Fernandez D, Rotter JI, Toyoda H. Tumor necrosis factor microsatellites define a Crohn's disease-associated haplotype on chromosome 6. Gastroenterology. 1996;110:1053–60.
12. Roussomoustakaki M, Satsangi J, Welsh KI et al. Genetic markers may predict disease behaviour in patients with ulcerative colitis. Gastroenterology. 1997;112(6):1845–53.
13. Orchard TR, Wordsworth BP, Jewell DP. Peripheral arthropathies in inflammatory bowel disease (IBD): their natural history and articular distribution. Gut. 1998;42:387–91.
14. Orchard TR, Thiyagaraja S, Welsh KI, Wordsworth BP, Jewell DP. HLA genes are important phenotype determining genes in the peripheral arthropathies of inflammatory bowel disease (IBD). Gastroenterology. 1998;114:A1056.
15. Louis E, Satsangi J, Roussoumoustakaki M et al. Cytokine gene polymorphisms in inflammatory bowel disease. Gut. 1996;39(5):705–10.
16. Tountas NA, Yang H, Coulter DL, Rotter JI, Cominelli F. Increased carriage of allele 2 of IL-1 receptor antagonist in Jewish populations: the strongest known genetic association in ulcerative colitis. Gastroenterology. 1996;110(4):A1029.
17. Parkes M, Satsangi J, Jewell DP. Contribution of the IL-2 and IL-10 genes to inflammatory bowel disease (IBD) susceptibility. Clin Exp Immunol. 1998;113:28–32.
18. Parkes M, Satsangi J, Simmons J, Bell JI, Lanthrop GM, Jewell DP. Preliminary evidence links the MUC2 gene to inflammatory bowel disease susceptibility. Gastroenterology. 1997;112(4):A1059.
19. Satsangi J, Parkes M, Louis E et al. Two-stage genome-wide search in inflammatory bowel disease: evidence for susceptibility loci on chromosomes 3, 7 and 12. Nature Genet. 1996;14(2):199–202.
20. Hugot JP, Laurent-Puig P, Gower-Rousseau C et al. Mapping of a susceptibility locus for Crohn's disease on chromosome 16. Nature. 1996;379:821–3.

21. Curran ME, Lau KF, Cardon L *et al.* Genetic analysis of inflammatory bowel disease in a large European patient population supports linkage to human chromosomes 12 and 16. Gastroenterology. 1998;115:1066–71.
22. Duerr RH, Zhang L, Preston RA *et al.* Further evidence for an inflammatory bowel disease susceptibility locus on chromosome 12. Gastroenterology. 1997;112(4):A2050.
23. Parkes M, Satsangi J, Merriman A, Jewell DP. Precision mapping of chromosome 12 linkage in IBD: evidence for a haplotype association. Gastroenterology. 1998;114:A902.
24. Vermeire S, Peeters M, Vlietinck R *et al.* No evidence for linkage on chromosomes 16-12-7 and 3 in the Belgian population may reflect genetic heterogeneity of inflammatory bowel disease. Gastroenterology. 1998;114:A784.

3
Inflammatory bowel disease and genetics: what to tell our patients?

M. PEETERS, S. VERMEIRE, S. JOOSSENS and P. RUTGEERTS

INTRODUCTION

Over the last few years, patients have become more interested in the familial and genetic aspects of their disease. They confront their physicians, general practitioners and specialists, with up-to-date information which they obtain on internet, in the newspapers, in the increasing number of available patients' guides and sometimes in the specialized medical press. Faced with this increased knowledge, physicians must be prepared to answer key questions about the aetiology, diagnostic procedures, therapeutic options and prognosis of their patient's disease. In the USA, this way for a patient to deal with his disease is already common. Europe is more conservative and it is uncommon to see a patient entering the consultation room with a New England article under his arm. Although these geographical differences still exist, physicians the whole world over will soon be treating well-informed and critical patients.

In addition to this changing attitude among patients, the medical world has experienced in the last decade a real genetic revolution. In 1992, Weisenbach et al.[1] were able to report the development of the first linkage map of the human genome. Semiautomatic techniques for genotyping the markers, adequate statistical interpretation and sufficient numbers of affected relatives have allowed genome-wide searches in different polygenic disorders. A rapidly increasing number of (susceptibility) genes have been identified. For example, the genetic mutations in several rare dominant and recessive inherited syndromes, such as familial adenomatous polyposis (FAP)[2], multiple endocrine neoplasia type (MEN1,2), Fanconi's anaemia, have been recently described. Moreover, susceptibility genes in more common diseases such as breast (BRCA1,2)[3,4] and colon cancer (MSH2, MLH1, PMS1,2)[5,6] were identified. This increasing knowledge of the human genome creates the option to develop diagnostic tests to identify individuals at highest risk and it certainly may speed up the development of more specific prevention strategies in certain diseases. The ability to identify those of high risk for a certain disease might also result in therapeutic diversification. Knowledge about the functions of newly identified genes might result in the development of new therapies directed towards specific molecular targets.

Most of the recent advances were made by studying familial forms of disease. They represent only a small fraction (5–10%) of common diseases such as colon cancer. In sporadic cases, the gene–environment interaction probably plays a more important role in pathogenesis. Moreover, genetic polymorphism or low penetrance in genes may influence the individual reaction to environmental factors. Also in the field of inflammatory bowel disease (IBD), clinicians and researchers witness these 'revolutions'. Case reports on IBD families, i.e. families with more than one member affected by ulcerative colitis (UC) or Crohn's disease (CD), were already published soon after the description of both diseases. More recently, large-cohort studies and epidemiology data have become available providing objective figures on family history. Risk estimates in high- (Ashkenazi Jews) and low-risk populations have been published over the last two years, loci of susceptibility genes for IBD were discovered and research in this field is continuing its explosive pace. Moreover, markers such as antineutrophil cytoplasmic antibodies (ANCA), anti-*Saccharomyces cerevisiae* antibodies (ASCA), increased small bowel permeability etc. might also play an important role in the identification of healthy family members at risk and/or patient subgroups. Therefore, this is an update of the available data and a summary of the information which, at present, it is relevant to discuss with our patients.

IBD AND GENETICS: A LOT OF QUESTIONS – WHAT ABOUT THE ANSWERS?

Patients with IBD must cope with a chronic illness as, today, no therapeutic intervention can cure them. Therefore, they question their physicians about recent therapeutic advances and new basic findings in the field, hoping that one day, their disease may be cured and that it will be prevented in their family members.

Is my disease really hereditary?

Most IBD patients, when they are first diagnosed, are questioned about other family members affected by the disease. Moreover, a lot of patients' guides include a section on genetics and IBD. Patients are also concerned about their offspring and about planning new pregnancies. These are reasons enough for patients to have open discussions about this topic with their physicians.

What are the facts to support the involvement of genetics in IBD? Already in 1934 Crohn reported a 14-year-old boy with ileitis whose sister developed the same condition soon afterwards[7]. Over the years, several studies have been published on the increased prevalence of IBD among relatives of patients with Crohn's disease and ulcerative colitis. Although the early studies were mostly anecdotal, over the last decade, several hospital and population-based studies in different ethnic groups have confirmed the high frequency of a strong family history in these diseases. The reported prevalence varies between 4.5 and 18.8% in CD and between 1.1 and 14.6% in UC. Some families with remarkable histories have been reported[8], especially in CD.

Other data, mostly epidemiological, support the importance of genetic predisposition in susceptibility to IBD. First, there is a considerable difference in prevalence between racial and ethnic groups. CD and UC are most common in white people, especially the Ashkenazi Jews of western Europe, United States, and Cape Town[9]. Moreover, this increased prevalence persists after migration to another continent. Second, probably the most convincing data come from studies of twins. Tysk *et al.*[10] reported a systematic analysis of the Swedish twin registry. Eighty pairs with at least one twin affected by IBD were identified. All pairs were brought up in the same environment. Concordance for the disease was higher (44%) in monozygotic CD twins than dizygotic (4%) and UC twins. The calculated coefficient of heritability corrected for familial environment was, respectively, 1.0 (95% CI 0.34–1.0) and 0.53 (95% CI 0.24–1.0) for CD and UC. Third, there is the impression that the frequency of occurrence of IBD in couples is low. Finally, there is an increased occurrence of IBD in genetic syndromes such as Turner's and Hermansky-Pudlak syndrome. It's also well known that the frequency of HLA-associated diseases, such as ankylosing spondylitis (HLA-B27) and primary sclerosing cholangitis (HLA-B8DR3), is higher in IBD than predicted. Recently, all these indirect data pointing to a role of genetics in the pathogenesis of IBD were supported by the discovery of the IBD1 gene on chromosome 16[11]. Today, there is enough indirect and direct evidence that genes play a part in the pathogenesis of IBD. But, how do we explain heredity to our patients?

'Hereditary' in IBD. Is it like haemophilia? Since my father has it, do I have a 50% chance of getting it too?

The answer is no. Crohn's disease and UC do not have a simple Medelian mode of inheritance. The recent advances in our knowledge of pathophysiological mechanisms and the clinical impression of different behaviour of certain subtypes of IBD, makes the traditional classification into Crohn's disease and ulcerative colitis insufficient. It is important to introduce the concept of heterogeneity. Inflammatory bowel disease is no longer one disease entity but a group of multifactorial diseases. The phenotypic presentation is the expression of an interaction between environmental and genetic factors. A specific set of susceptibility genes influences the individual response to environmental factors.

Patients have to know that 'hereditary' in IBD does not mean that a defective gene, one for UC and one for CD, is being passed from one generation to another. 'Hereditary' is more a predisposition which is determined by an individual set of genes. The different combinations of genes and the possible interactions with environmental factors result in diseases with specific characteristics. Formerly, these were grouped in CD and UC. An exact identification and stratification of the patient populations becomes extremely important with regard to clinical course, therapeutic adjustments and underlying pathophysiological mechanisms.

If my disease runs in families, what is the risk that a first-degree relative will become affected?

Early studies showed an 8–15-fold increase in risk for first-degree relatives. More recently, risk estimates based on a positive family history were calculated for high- (Ashkenazi Jews[12,13]), intermediate- (North America[13], Europe[14,15]) and low-risk (South Asians[15]) IBD populations. Three studies[12-14] used the same method to calculate the age-corrected empirical risks. The risks for IBD were high for relatives of Jewish patients, 7.8% and 4.5% for CD and UC, respectively. Relatives of non-Jewish probands have risks of 5.2% and 1.6%, respectively. These latter are in agreement with those found in a European non-Jewish population. In Europeans, the overall IBD risk for first-degree relatives of CD probands was 4.8%. The risks were 10.4%, 6.1% and 2.0% for offspring, siblings and parents respectively. Daughters of CD probands had a risk which was almost twice that of sons. Probert *et al.* compared the family risk in Europeans and South Asians in a well-defined area in England[15]. In Caucasians, the risk of first-degree relatives of UC patients developing UC is increased 15-fold. No increased risk for developing CD was detected among relatives of UC patients. Relatives of CD probands are at a 27-fold risk of CD and a slightly increased risk of UC. In contrast, there is a lack of risk in relatives of South Asian patients with CD, both for CD and for UC. Only a small increase in risk in relatives of patients with UC was detected. Two Scandinavian studies[16,17] reported a 10–15-fold increased risk of developing UC among patients' relatives. Similarly, the risk of developing CD in first-degree relatives of CD patients was increased.

We can conclude that the risk in relatives, especially in fist-degree relatives, is increased. The highest risk is found in offspring and mostly the same type of disease will develop. Ethnic differences exist, with the highest risk in Ashkenazi Jews. But, due to heterogeneity, these estimates might only reflect the risk in a subset of patients and it cannot be extrapolated to the global IBD population.

Is there a test available to identify those relatives at increased risk?

Although the answer is no today, some progress has been made. Before 1996, research was especially focused on the HLA complex located on chromosome 6. Methodological differences and heterogeneity in study populations led initially to controversial conclusions. Recent well-designed studies suggest that HLA genes are important determinants of disease susceptibility in UC, but less so in CD[18,19]. Heterogeneity between ethnic groups seems to exist. For example, in Japanese[20] and Jewish patients[18], HLA DRB1*1502 (DR2) is implicated in susceptibility to UC. World wide, different groups, using new genetic technology, are now working on the identification of susceptibility genes. Hugot *et al.*[11] were the first to report the results of a genome-wide search, using a non-parametric two-point sibling-pair linkage method. They localized a susceptibility locus for CD within the pericentromeric region of chromosome 16, named IBD1. Recently, the same authors were able to better define the localization of this locus[21]. A two-stage genome-wide search performed by Satsangi *et al.*[22] on 186 affected sibling pairs, provided evidence for linkage between IBD and regions on chromosomes 12, 7 and 3. Furthermore, individual markers on chromosomes 2 and 6 were linked with UC but not CD. A region on chromosome 16 was linked with susceptibility to CD. In our own IBD population[23], we found no evidence for linkage with loci described on chromosomes 3, 7, 12 and 16. A possible explanation for the discrepancies is the heterogeneity within CD and UC, which may lead to different datasets containing different proportions of disease subgroups or phenotypes. Moreover, to replicate the results of previous linkage studies, a large number of siblings is needed. Studies to detect ANCA in healthy first-degree relatives of patients with UC compared with healthy controls have shown conflicting results. Studies have reported positivity in first-degree relatives of between 15 and 30%[24]. In contrast, Lee *et al.*[25] found no increased frequency compared with controls. Moreover, the frequency of pANCA was not significantly increased in healthy monozygotic twins with UC compared with healthy controls[26]. This study did not support the hypothesis that pANCA is a subclinical marker of genetic susceptibility to UC. Intestinal permeability is increased in patients with Crohn's disease and a proportion of their healthy relatives. Already by 1986, Hollander *et al.*[27] reported an increased permeability in 78% of healthy relatives of patients with CD. Results of additional studies were controversial, mainly due to the lack of standardization in methodology. Recent studies detected an increased permeability index in 10–25% of healthy relatives[28, 29]. Reports on an increased sensitivity of healthy first-degree relatives to NSAID challenge were interesting. A significantly higher proportion of relatives showed an increased permeability compared with controls[30]. One can speculate that there may be a genetically determined hypersensitivity of the bowel mucosa to environmental factors. This hypothesis, however, conflicts with the finding that permeability is also increased in 30% of spouses of CD patients[29].

Today, none of the available markers is useful for screening unaffected relatives. Patients and their relatives must understand that blood samples are only serving research purposes and that they cannot identify individuals at risk. Hopefully, this will change in the near future. Due to disease heterogeneity, it might be necessary to use a set of markers to detect relatives at risk or a marker may be specific for a subtype of disease. There is also the question of whether it makes sense to identify relatives at risk for a disease which we cannot prevent or cure. We must consider the psychological impact for the patient and the identified relative.

My daughter or my brother recently developed an IBD. How will the disease evolve?

With large numbers of families becoming available, several groups have focused on clinical patterns in these families. Relatives of patients with CD and UC are at increased risk of the concordant disease type. Reported rates range between 77%[31] and 89%[14]. Until two years ago, only anecdotal and conflicting reports on similarities of clinical characteristics within multiply-affected families were available. In a study of 10 families in which 32 cases of IBD occurred, it was noted that 3 of 4 affected siblings had similar disease patterns[32]. The three concordant siblings had identical HLA haplotypes. In contrast, Weterman and Pena, analysing the clinical patterns and the histopathological features of siblings both suffering from CD, found no difference in clinical pattern compared with unrelated CD patients[33]. Over the last two years, several studies in the USA and

Europe have provided important data on clinical characteristics of familial IBD, such as disease extent, age at onset (diagnosis), presence of extraintestinal manifestations, need for surgery and exposure to environmental factors. Concordance for clinical type and site of disease was reported for CD. A French study[34], reported concordance for disease location of 56% and for disease type of 49%. Concordance became more striking in families with more than two members affected, with almost 80% concordance for location and type. These findings are in contrast to the study of Lee *et al.*[35]. In their study of 67 IBD families with three or more affected first-degree relatives, the authors could not identify any significant differences between familial and sporadic cases. An interesting observation was that significantly more non-smokers had UC than CD. Our own study of 68 families[14], confirmed the French data with a high level of agreement, especially in siblings. Greater-than-expected concordance for site and clinical type of CD was also reported by Bayless *et al.*[36]. By using a conditional logistic model, they could predict site and clinical aggressiveness in another relative with Crohn's disease. For a specific site, the odds ratio for another family member with CD ranged 3.5 to 37.6. For example, the probability of ileal disease in a second patient from a family with CD and ileal disease based on the conditional logistic model would result in an odds ratio of 37.6 because of concordance. The data on concordance in clinical characteristics in UC are scarce. Although high concordance for the presence of extraintestinal manifestations (74 and 89%) was observed in these patients, concordance for colonic involvement was only 53% in parent–child pairs and 68% in affected siblings[37].

Most of the data available today are highly suggestive for similarities within families. In general, disease type is the same in IBD families. Data on the other characteristics such as disease location and aggressiveness are more controversial, although we have the impression that they are specific for a given family. New studies using strict definitions of clinical characteristics might further support the previous data.

My son developed CD at an early age and the course of the disease is more aggressive than mine. What is the reason?

In disorders with a genetic component, such as hereditary non-polyposis colorectal carcinoma, cases tend to present at an earlier age. The association between familial CD and early age at onset or diagnosis has been extensively studied. A familial aggregation study performed in Italy found an almost identical mean age at onset in patients with and without a positive family history[38]. Also, Lee *et al.*[35] did not find any differences between the median age at diagnosis of familial cases of CD (25 years) and UC (27 years) compared with 27 and 33 years, respectively, in a large epidemiological study. In contrast, the French study[34] observed a significantly younger age at onset in their familial CD patients (22 years) than in sporadic cases (26.5 years). Polito *et al.* published a provocative paper in 1996[39]. They studied 27 pairs of two-generation first-degree relatives. In 85% of the pairs, the member of the later generation was younger at diagnosis than the member of the preceding generation. Moreover, disease was more extensive in 56% of the children, with male parents accounting for almost all of the generation differences. These findings led to the hypothesis of genetic anticipation in Crohn's disease. Genetic anticipation is a term that denotes increase in severity or decrease in the age at onset as a disease is passed through generations. It has been described in monogenic neurological diseases, such as Huntington's disease[40] and myotonic dystrophy[41]. The molecular basis for this phenomenon involves the progressive amplification of unstable triplet repeats of DNA. These contribute to DNA instability. A recent study[42] looked for anticipation in 57 parent–first affected child pairs. Age at diagnosis of the offspring was younger in 84% of pairs, with a median difference of 16 years. Satsangi *et al.*[37] found that the parent at onset was more than five years older than the child in 78.8% of pairs. Discordance in the calendar years of onset for parent and offspring was observed in both studies. In contrast to the study of Polito[39], these two studies found a high degree of concordance in disease extent and severity between generations. Moreover, Grandbastien *et al.*[42] observed no influence of parental sex, as evidence of imprinting, on clinical characteristics in their children. In conclusion, most of the studies reported anticipation for age at diagnosis, but it is not clear whether this can be explained by genetic alterations or by the influence of environmental factors as suggested in a recent abstract by Hugot *et al.*[43].

If IBD is not one disease, can patients be stratified into different prognostic and therapeutic groups?

Although we must answer that it is premature for most of the data to be used in the clinic, some stratification markers can serve in the decision tree. We have already mentioned the location of determinants of disease susceptibility within the HLA complex for UC. In northern Europeans, HLA DR3 and HLA DR103 are, respectively, associated with extensive and more severe colitis requiring surgery[44]. Subclinical markers may help to stratify the population of patients. Two autoantibodies have been associated with CD and UC. The first is antineutrophil cytoplasmic antibody with perinuclear staining (pANCA). This IgG_1 antibody is present in sera of 50–80% of patients with UC and 10–30% of patients with CD. Recently, Targan[45] proposed a stratification of CD and UC by a number of clinical, subclinical and genetic parameters in different subgroups. First, the pANCA-producing UC population has an even greater MHC Class II allele association than the UC population as a whole[46]. Secondly, clinical evidence suggests that the presence of pANCA may be related to expression of a different form of inflammation that may not be as responsive to the standard therapies. In CD, pANCA-producing patients with an 'UC-like' phenotype appear to represent a CD/UC overlap syndrome[47].

The first report on the presence of systemic antibodies against the yeast *Saccharomyces cerevisiae* (ASCA) in patients with CD was published in 1988[48]. Recently, Colombel and co-workers[49] found ASCA positivity in 66% of patients with CD and in 12% of patients with UC. A high positive predictive value was observed by combining ASCA and pANCA. Our own study showed, respectively, 48 and 8% ASCA positivity in patients with CD and UC[50].

An interesting field of research is the role of mucin glycoproteins in the normal intestine and in IBD. These glycoproteins can be classified in 6 different species (I to VI)[51]. A deficiency in mucin subclass IV was reported in patients with UC. Moreover, in monozygotic twin pairs with one sibling having UC, both siblings had reduced mucin subclass IV[52]. This finding supports the idea of a primary mechanism increasing host susceptibility. Normal patterns were found in CD. Of all the markers tested, pANCA and ASCA are the most likely to be used routinely in the stratification of our IBD population. It will be interesting to determine other serum and genetic markers allowing the identification of patients who will respond to a certain treatment or may be associated with a poor prognosis. With disease heterogeneity, a set of markers will be probably necessary for adequate stratification.

CONCLUSION

Nowadays, patients are well informed about the characteristics of their disease. Patients are reading about the progress in the field of IBD genetics, including the identification of susceptibility genes. Confronted with that knowledge, they are concerned about their family and have several practical questions about this topic for their physicians.

Although our understanding of the role of genetics in IBD has progressed, individual screening is not possible today. The main difficulty is the heterogeneity of the disease. Nevertheless, recent data on the risks of the disease, clinical characteristics and markers make family counselling possible, important and useful. It is of extreme interest to identify multi-affected families and to collect DNA for future testing. Inflammatory bowel disease in families has undergone an evolution from pure description to real counselling. Hopefully, we will be able, in the near future, to screen relatives and to stratify our patients.

References

1. Weissenbach J, Gyapay G, Dib C *et al.* A second generation linkage map of the human genome. Nature. 1992;359:794–801.
2. Bodmer WF, Bailey CJ, Bodmer J *et al.* Localization of the gene for familial adenomatous polyposis on chromosome 5. Nature. 1987;328:614–16.
3. Miki Y, Swensen J, Schattuck-Eidens D *et al.* A strong candidate for the breast and ovarian cancer susceptibility gene BRCA1. Science. 1994;266:66–71.
4. Wooster R, Neuhausen SL, Mangion J *et al.* Localization of a breast cancer susceptibility gene, BRCA2, to chromosome 13q12-13. Science. 1994;265:2088–90.
5. Peltomaki P, Aaltonen LA, Sistonen P *et al.* Genetic mapping of a locus predisposing to human colorectal cancer. Science. 1993;290:610–12.
6. Lindbolm A, Tannergard P, Werelius B, Nordenskjold M. Genetic mapping of a second locus predisposing to hereditary non-polyposis colon cancer. Nature Genet. 1993;5:279–82.
7. Crohn BB. The broadening conception of regional ileitis. Am J Dig Dis. 1934;1:97–9.
8. Van Kruiningen HJ, Colombel JF, Cartun RW *et al.* An in-depth study of Crohn's disease in two French families. Gastroenterology. 1993;104:351–60.
9. Gilat T, Grossman A, Fireman Z, Rosen P. Inflammatory bowel disease in Jews. In: McConnel R, Rozen P, Langman M, Gilat T, editors. The Genetics and Epidemiology of Inflammatory Bowel Disease. Basel, New York: Karger; 1986:135–40.
10. Tysk C, Lindberg E, Jarnerot G, Floderus-Myrhed B. Ulcerative colitis and Crohn's disease in an unselected population of monozygotic and dizygotic twins. A study of heritability and the influence of smoking. Gut. 1988;29:990–6.
11. Hugot JP, Laurent-Puig P, Gower-Rousseau C *et al.* and The Groupe d'Etude Thérapeutique des Affections Inflammatoircs Digestives. Mapping of a susceptibility locus for Crohn's disease on chromosome 16. Nature. 1996;379:821–3.

12. Roth MP, Petersen GM, McEltree C, Vadheim CM, Panish JF, Rotter JI. Familial empiric risk estimates of inflammatory bowel disease in Ashkenazi Jews. Gastroenterology. 1989;96:1016–20.
13. Yang H, McElree C, Roth M-P, Shanahan F, Targan SR, Rotter JI. Familial empirical risks for inflammatory bowel disease: differences between Jews and non-Jews. Gut. 1993;34:517–24.
14. Peeters M, Nevens H, Baert F et al. Familial aggregation in Crohn's disease: increased age adjusted risk and concordance in clinical characteristics. Gastroenterology. 1996;111:579–603.
15. Probert CSJ, Jayanthi V, Hughes AO, Thompson JR, Wicks ACB, Mayberry JF. Prevalence and family risk of ulcerative colitis and Crohn's disease: an epidemiological study among Europeans and South Asians in Leicestershire. Gut. 1993;34:1547–51.
16. Orholm M, Munkholm P, Langholz E, Nielsen OH, Sorensen TIA, Binder V. Familial occurrence of inflammatory bowel disease. N Engl J Med. 1991;324:84–8.
17. Monsen U, Berglund M, Brostom O. Prevalence of inflammatory bowel disease amongst relatives of patients with ulcerative colitis. Scand J Gastroenterol. 1987;22:214–18.
18. Toyoda H, Wang SJ, Yang H, Redford A, Magalong D, Tyan D. Distinct association of HLA Class II genes with inflammatory bowel disease. Gastroenterology. 1993;104:741–8.
19. Satsangi J, Welsh KI, Bunce M et al. Contribution of genes of the major histocompatibility complex to susceptibility and disease phenotype in inflammatory bowel disease. Lancet. 1996;347:1212–17.
20. Futami S, Aoyama N, Honsako Y et al. HLA-DRB1.1502 allele, subtype of DR15, is associated with susceptibility to ulcerative colitis and its progression. Dig Dis Sci. 1995;40:814–18.
21. Hugot JP, Zouali H, Colombel JF et al. and GETAID, EPIMAD and the European Concerted Action on the Genetics of IBD. Fine mapping of the inflammatory bowel disease susceptibility locus 1 in the pericentromeric region of chromosome 16. Gastroenterology. 1998;114:A4093.
22. Satsangi J, Parkes M, Louis E et al. Two stage genome-wide search in inflammatory bowel disease provides evidence for susceptibility loci on chromosomes 3, 7 and 12. Nat Genet. 1996;14:199–202.
23. Vemeire S, Peeters M, Vlietinck R et al. No evidence for linkage of IBD to chromosome 16, 12, 7 and 3 in the Belgian population. Gastroenterology. 1998;114:A4539.
24. Shanahan F, Duerr RH, Rotter JI et al. Neutrophil autoantibodies in ulcerative colitis: familial aggregation and genetic heterogeneity. Gastroenterology. 1992;103:456–61.
25. Lee JCW, Lennard-Jones JE, Cambridge G. Antineutrophil antibodies in familial inflammatory bowel disease. Gastroenterology. 1995;108:423–7.
26. Yang P, Järnerot G, Danielson D, Tysk C, Lindberg E. pANCA in monozygotic twins with inflammatory bowel disease. Gut. 1995;36:887–90.
27. Hollander D, Vadheim CM, Brettholz E, Petersen GM, Delahunty T, Rotter JI. Increased intestinal permeability in patients with Crohn's disease and their relatives – a possible aetiological factor. Ann Intern Med. 1986;105:883–5.
28. May GR, Sutherland LR, Meddings JB. Is small intestinal permeability really increased in relatives of patients with Crohn's disease? Gastroenterology. 1993;104:1627–32.
29. Peeters M, Geypens B, Claus D et al. Clustering of increased small intestinal permeability in families with Crohn's disease. Gastroenterology. 1997;113:802–7.
30. Hilsden RJ, Meddings JB, Sutherland LR. Intestinal permeability changes in response to acetylsalicylic acid in relatives of patients with Crohn's disease. Gastroenterology. 1996;110:1395–403.
31. Satsangi J, Grootscholten C, Holt H, Jewell DP. Clinical patterns of familial inflammatory bowel disease. Gut. 1996;38:738–41.
32. Kemler BJ, Glass D, Alpert E. HLA studies with multiple cases of inflammatory bowel disease. Gastroenterology. 1980;78:A1194.
33. Weterman IT, Pena AS. Prevalence of Crohn's disease in first-degree relatives of patients with Crohn's disease. In: McConnel R, Rozen P, Langman M, Gilat T, editors. The Genetics and Epidemiology of Inflammatory Bowel Disease. Basel, Switzerland: Karger; 1986:27–34.
34. Colombel JF, Grandbastien B, Gower-Rousseau C et al. Clinical characteristics of Crohn's disease in 72 families. Gastroenterology. 1996;111:604–7.
35. Lee JCW, Lennard-Jones JE. Inflammatory bowel disease in 67 families each with three or more affected first-degree relatives. Gastroenterology. 1996;111:587–96.
36. Bayless TM, Tokayer AZ, Polito II JM, Quaskey SA, Mellits ED, Harris ML. Crohn's disease: concordance for site and clinical type in affected family members – Potential hereditary influences. Gastroenterology. 1996;111:573–9.

37. Satsangi J, Grootscholten C, Holt H, Jewell DP. Clinical patterns of familial inflammatory bowel disease. Gut. 1996;38:738–41.
38. Meucci G, Vecchi M, Torgano G *et al.* and the IBD Study Group. Familial aggregation of inflammatory bowel disease in Northern Italy: a multicenter study. Gastroenterology. 1992;103:514–19.
39. Polito II JM, Rees RC, Childs B, Mendeloff AI, Harris ML, Bayless TM. Preliminary evidence for genetic anticipation in Crohn's disease. Lancet. 1996;347:789–800.
40. Adams P, Falek A, Arnold J. Huntington disease in Georgia: age at onset. Am J Hum Genet. 1988;43:695–704.
41. Harper PS, Harley HG, Reardon W, Shaw DJ. Anticipation in myotonic dystrophy: a new light on an old problem. Am J Hum Genet. 1992;51:10–16.
42. Grandbastien B, Peeters M, Franchimont D *et al.* Anticipation in familial Crohn's disease. Gut. 1998;42:170–4.
43. Hugot JP, Colombel JF, Belaiche J *et al.* and EPIMAD, GETAID and the European Concerted Action on Genetics of IBD. Date of birth analysis suggests environmental factors in familial Crohn's disease. Gastroenterology. 1998;114:A4092.
44. Roussomoustakaki M, Satsangi J, Louis E *et al.* Genetics of ulcerative colitis: HLA DRB1*103 (DR103) is associated with extra-intestinal manifestations and need for surgery. Gastroenterology. 1997:112;1845–53.
45. Targan SR. Ulcerative colitide(s) and Crohn's diseases: stratification of classically diagnosed diseases. In: Caprilli R, editor. Inflammatory Bowel Disease – Trigger Factors and Trends in Therapy. Stuttgart: Schattauer; 1997:49–55.
46. Yang H, Rotter JI, Toyoda H *et al.* Ulcerative colitis. A genetically heterogeneous disorder defined by genetic (HLA Class II) and subclinical (ANCAs) markers. J Clin Invest. 1993;92:1080–4.
47. Vasiliauskas E, Plevy SE, Landers CJ *et al.* Perinuclear cytoplasmic antibodies (pANCA) in patients with Crohn's disease define a clinical subgroup. Gastroenterology. 1996;110:1810–19.
48. Main J, McKenzie H, Yeaman GR *et al.* Antibody to Saccharomyces cerevisiae (baker's yeast) in Crohn's disease. Br Med J. 1988;297:1105–6.
49. Quinton JF, Sendid B, Reumaux D *et al.* Anti-Saccharomyces cerevisiae mannan combined with antineutrophil cytoplasmic autoantibodies in inflammatory bowel disease: prevalence and diagnostic role. Gut. 1998;42:788–91.
50. Peeters M, Vermeire S, Dantonio R *et al.* Anti-Saccharomyces cerevisiae antibodies and ANCA status in a large Flemish IBD population. Gastroenterology. 1998;114:A4337.
51. Podolsky DK, Isselbacher KJ. Glycoprotein composition of the colonic mucosa. Specific alterations in ulcerative colitis. Gastroenterology. 1984;87:991–8.
52. Tysk C, Riedesel H, Lindberg E, Panzini B, Podolsky K, Järnerot G. Colonic glycoproteins in monozygotic twins with inflammatory bowel disease. Gastroenterology. 1991;10:419–23.

4
The importance of environment in inflammatory bowel disease: new data

J. COSNES

The aetiopathogenesis of inflammatory bowel disease (IBD) remains unknown. Among the factors which predispose to the development of IBD, only two have been clearly identified: family history and smoking status. These factors act in different ways. Whereas having a relative with IBD increases the risk of Crohn's disease and ulcerative colitis[1], current smoking increases by two-fold the risk for Crohn's disease but actually decreases the risk for ulcerative colitis[2]. Regarding the clinical spectrum of the disease, patients with a family history of IBD may have a younger age at onset[3] but do not have a more severe course than patients with sporadic disease (Carbonnel *et al.*, submitted for publication). Smoking has different effects. Studies of sib pairs with IBD and discordant for smoking status have shown that smoking influences the phenotype of IBD. Smokers develop Crohn's disease and non-smokers develop ulcerative colitis[4]. In ulcerative colitis, current smoking and nicotine use may be beneficial[5,6] but, in Crohn's disease, smoking is associated with a more marked clinical activity[7], a lower quality of life[8], more frequent complications[9], an increased need for immunosuppressive drugs[10], and faster recurrence after surgery[11,12]. Thus, smoking appears as a major factor which may influence the severity of the disease. Many questions remain, however. In ulcerative colitis, is the apparently beneficial effect of smoking prolonged, and should we advise a smoker to quit? In Crohn's disease, a common finding was that women of child-bearing age were especially vulnerable to the harmful effect of smoking[10-12], which raised the question of whether the use of oral contraceptives is a confounding variable. Finally, as colonic Crohn's disease has many features in common with ulcerative colitis, and in certain cases the two diseases may be associated[13] or consecutive[14], it is not clear whether smoking is harmful to Crohn's patients who have colonic lesions only.

SMOKING AND LONG-TERM COURSE OF ULCERATIVE COLITIS

Some anecdotal observations have suggested that smoking may decrease symptoms and improve colonic lesions of some patients with ulcerative colitis[15,16], and nicotine patches have some efficacy in mild forms of the disease[6]. However, the effect of smoking upon the long-term course of ulcerative colitis is not well known. The best criterion to assess retrospectively the severity of ulcerative colitis is the need for colectomy. Using that end point, ulcerative colitis in smokers does not appear to be less severe than that in non-smokers in most[17–21], but not all[22], retrospective studies. In fact, the small proportion of smokers (usually about 10%) compromises the validity of the comparison between smokers and non-smokers, and the absence of a difference between the groups may be linked to a lack of statistical power, with a large beta error. Therefore, we studied retrospectively a large series of patients with ulcerative colitis, including 85 smokers[23].

Patients and methods

Among 644 patients with ulcerative colitis seen consecutively in our unit between January 1974 and February 1997, criteria for definite diagnosis of ulcerative colitis were lacking in 30 and smoking habits were unknown in 58. Five hundred and fifty-six patients were thus studied. Patients were classified as smokers ($n = 85$) if they had smoked more than 7 cigarettes per week for at least the six months following diagnosis of ulcerative colitis. This definition therefore included patients who smoked throughout the duration of the disease ($n = 52$), patients who started smoking after diagnosis ($n = 2$), and patients who stopped during the disease ($n = 31$). Non-smokers ($n = 471$) were those who never smoked ($n = 335$), smoked a little or occasionally ($n = 6$) or had stopped smoking before ulcerative colitis was diagnosed ($n = 130$).

Overall severity of the disease was assessed retrospectively, using three criteria: (a) onset of complications (toxic megacolon, fulminant colitis, etc.), (b) importance of medical therapy, i.e. the need for topical or systemic glucocorticoid and immunosuppressive drugs, and (c) incidence of colectomy.

Data for smokers and non-smokers were compared using Students t-test or χ^2 test as appropriate. For actuarial analysis, the Kaplan–Meier model was used, with the date of diagnosis as the starting point. The curves were compared by the log rank test.

Results

Smokers and non-smokers did not differ significantly according to age (mean 31 vs. 34 years), sex ratio (1.42 vs. 0.95) or family history (6 vs. 7%) but mean duration of disease was longer in smokers (mean 116 vs. 87 months, $p = 0.01$). Fulminant colitis and/or toxic megacolon were observed in 8 smokers (9%) and 63 non-smokers (13%, difference not significant). Colonic dysplasia and/or cancer were observed in one smoker and 10 non-smokers (NS). Sclerosing cholangitis and pouchitis were observed in non-smokers only (in 7 and 6 patients, respectively).

Need for systemic medical therapy is indicated in Table 1. Fewer smokers than non-smokers required systemic glucocorticoids. Cortico-dependency was observed in two smokers out of the 44 who received systemic corticosteroids (5%), vs. 29 non-smokers out of 297 (10%, NS). Twenty-four smokers (29%) had to be colectomized vs. 156 non-smokers (33%, NS). Figure 1 gives the

Table 1 Cumulative systemic medical therapy in a retrospective series of patients with ulcerative colitis according to smoking status

	Smokers (n = 85)	*Non-smokers (n = 471)*	*p*
Salicylates	83 (98%)	461 (98%)	NS
Steroids *per os*	44 (52%)	297 (63%)	0.05
Intravenous steroids	17 (20%)	114 (24%)	NS
Immunosuppressive drugs	3 (4%)	36 (8%)	NS

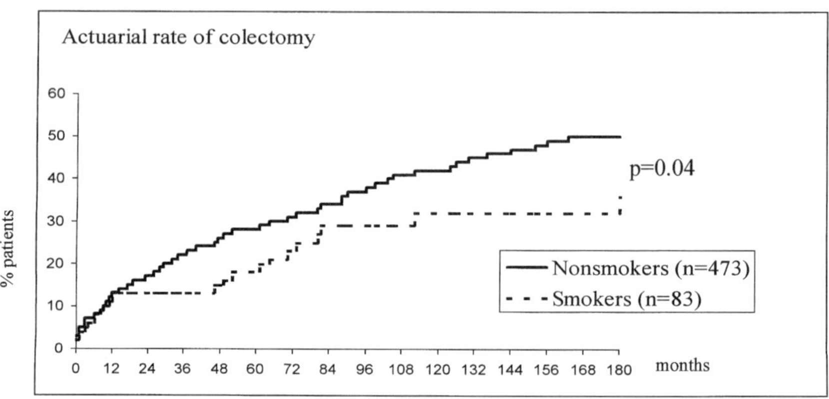

Figure 1 Cumulative actuarial rate of colectomy in smokers and non-smokers. The two curves were compared using log rank test. Adapted from Mokbel *et al.*[23] with permission

actuarial rate of colectomy in the two groups. At 10 years, the proportions of smokers and non-smokers who had been colectomized were 32 ± 12% and 42 ± 6%, respectively. The two curves were significantly different according to log rank test ($p = 0.04$).

Comment

The lower need for oral glucocorticoid and the lower actuarial rate of colectomy in smokers suggest that ulcerative colitis in smokers is characterized by a less severe clinical presentation and a better long-term prognosis than in non-smokers. These results confirm and extend previous findings that smoking has beneficial effects on the course of ulcerative colitis. It should be noted, however, that the frequencies of severe forms (requiring intensive intravenous treatment, fulminant colitis, or toxic megacolon) were not significantly different in smokers and non-smokers. For one individual, the advantage of a reduction of 10% of the risk for colectomy may be debated when compared with the numerous and serious consequences of continuing smoking[24]. It is not clear whether or not smoking cessation may worsen the course of ulcerative colitis and further studies are needed to assess this point. In our opinion, the adverse effects of smoking far outweigh the potential, but unproved, ability of continued smoking to decrease the colectomy rate. Therefore, patients with ulcerative colitis should be encouraged to stop smoking: attempts should be performed under strict supervision of both a gastroenterologist and a trained physician specialized in smoking cessation, and should probably use the transdermal nicotine patch.

SMOKING, ORAL CONTRACEPTIVE USE AND CROHN'S DISEASE

In studies assessing the effect of smoking in Crohn's disease, young women appear to be especially vulnerable[7-12]. This vulnerability may be linked to an effect of oral contraceptive use, either additive or confounding. To assess the respective effects of current smoking and oral contraceptive use on the clinical course of Crohn's disease, we performed a prospective one-year cohort study in a large series of young women with Crohn's disease[25].

Patients and methods

Three hundred and eighteen women of child-bearing age with Crohn's disease and CDAI < 200, who attended our unit consecutively during the year 1995, were included prospectively. Patients were classified as current smokers if they smoked > 7 cigarettes per week and as oral contraceptive users if, at inclusion, they were using and thereafter continued oral contraceptives for a period longer than 6 months. The end-point was whether or not the patient developed active Crohn's disease (flare-up episode, chronic active evolution, or disabling anoperineal disease) during the year of follow-up.

Results were analysed using logistic regression. The variables recorded at inclusion were sex, age, CDAI value, disease activity the previous year, anoperineal disease, small bowel lesions, colonic lesions, immunosuppressive therapy, smoking and oral contraceptive use.

Results

Twenty-seven patients were excluded from analysis because they became pregnant ($n = 23$) or were lost to follow-up ($n = 4$). Among the 291 others, 165 were smokers and 126 used oral contraceptives. Among the latter, 14 used a

Table 2 Cohort study of young women with Crohn's disease. Comparison of characteristics at inclusion according to the activity of the disease during the year of follow-up

	Active disease *(n = 133)*	*Inactive disease* *(n = 158)*	*p*
Age (years)	31 ± 8	32 ± 7	NS
Duration of disease (years)	6.5 ± 5.5	7.3 ± 6	NS
CDAI at inclusion 150–200	26 (20%)	15 (10%)	0.02
Active disease the previous year	103 (77%)	62 (39%)	0.0001
Small bowel lesions	77 (58%)	91 (58%)	NS
Colonic lesions	83 (62%)	63 (40%)	0.0001
Anoperineal lesions	41 (31%)	21 (13%)	0.0005
Immunosuppressive therapy	37 (28%)	36 (23%)	NS
Cigarette smoking	87 (65%)	79 (50%)	0.008
Oral contraceptive use	61 (46%)	65 (41%)	NS

progestational agent without oestrogen, 107 a low-oestrogen formulation, and five a 50-μg oestrogen formulation. At baseline, the proportion of oral contraceptive users was not significantly different between patients whose disease was in sustained remission and those whose disease was not, or between smokers and non-smokers. During the year, 133 patients (46%) developed active disease. The percentage of active disease was higher in smokers (52%) than in non-smokers (37%, $p = 0.008$) but not different in oral contraceptive users (48%) vs. non-users (44%, NS). In smokers, the percentage of active Crohn's disease was identical in oral contraceptive users (52%) and non-users (53%, NS). Table 2 gives the comparison of baseline characteristics of patients according to the activity of the disease during the year of follow-up. Logistic regression selected three covariates associated with active disease: active disease during the previous year (odds ratio 4.73 [2.78–8.06]), presence of anoperineal lesions at entry (odds ratio 2.13 [1.3–4.03]), and current smoking (odds ratio 1.77 [1.05–2.99]). The same covariates were selected when the analysis was restricted to the 219 women who were not receiving immunosuppressive therapy. Thus it can be concluded that the use of oral contraceptives had no significant effect on the activity of the disease and did not enhance the effect of smoking (Figure 2).

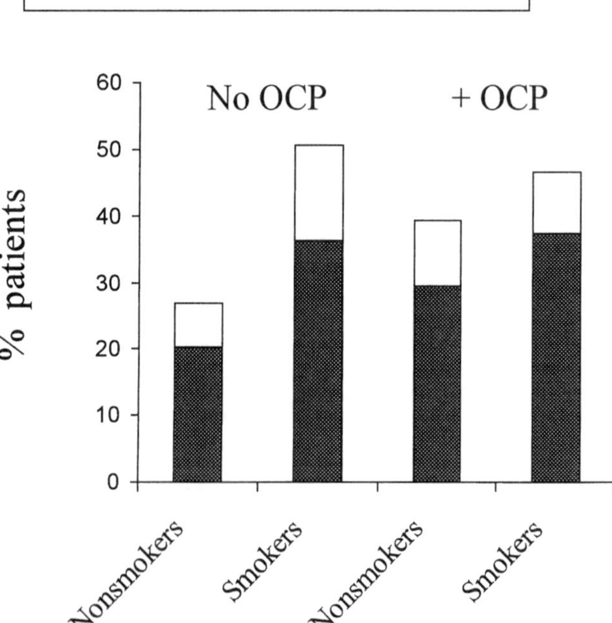

Figure 2 Percentages of patients who developed a flare-up episode or chronic active disease during the year of follow-up according to smoking status and oral contraceptive (OCP) use at inclusion. In patients not taking oral contraceptives, more smokers than non-smokers had active disease ($p < 0.01$). This difference was not significant in patients taking oral contraceptives

Comment

This prospective study demonstrates that smoking is an independent risk factor for active Crohn's disease in young women. By contrast, oral contraceptive use was not associated with a more severe evolution of Crohn's disease. When considering this result, different biases may be of concern[26,27]. First, patients receiving immunosuppressive therapy were advised to use effective contraception. Second, patients with recently active disease may be more likely to take oral contraceptives than those with quiescent disease in order to prevent a pregnancy that might affect their clinical status. Third, it has been suggested that smokers are more likely to take oral contraceptives than non-smokers[26] and that oral contraceptive users are more likely to smoke[28]. In fact, in the present study, the proportions of oral contraceptive users did not differ significantly depending on whether or not Crohn's disease had been active during the year preceding inclusion, and were similar among smokers and non-smokers. The pill was still innocuous when analysis was restricted to patients who were not receiving immunosuppressive drugs. Finally, there was no significant interaction between oral contraceptive use and smoking. In view of the striking synergy between oral contraceptives, including low-oestrogen formulations, and smoking as regards the risk of haemorrhagic stroke[29] and myocardial infarction[30], this negative result argues against the importance of thromboembolic events in the pathogenesis of Crohn's disease and its complications. Besides, a retrospective study[31] showed that oral contraceptive use was not associated with an increased risk of recurrence after surgery for Crohn's disease. Therefore, from a practical point of view, there is no reason connected with Crohn's disease to advise a woman to consider other methods of contraception than low-oestrogen oral contraceptives, even if she cannot stop smoking.

SMOKING AND CROHN'S COLITIS

The effect of smoking is of special interest in patients with Crohn's colitis because current smoking has a protective effect on the development of ulcerative colitis[32] and may improve colitis-related symptoms in some patients[33]. Moreover, it has been suggested that smoking may affect disease location by protecting against colonic inflammation[34]. Thus, a beneficial effect of smoking in Crohn's colitis is conceivable. Actually, a retrospective analysis of the long-term course of the disease in our series of patients with Crohn's colitis did not show that smokers were doing better than non-smokers. The need for immunosuppressive drugs and the colectomy rate were not different between the two groups, and more smokers required steroids (Table 3). To assess more precisely the effect of smoking in patients with Crohn's colitis only, we performed a one-year prospective study according to the same design as the study of the respective effects of smoking and oral contraceptive use.

Patients and methods

One hundred and fifty-eight patients who had Crohn's colitis, with or without anal involvement, and who attended our unit consecutively during the year 1995 were

Table 3 Comparison of the therapeutic needs in a retrospective series of patients with Crohn's colitis according to smoking status. Mean duration of the disease was 90 ± 75 months and 87 ± 91 months in smokers and non-smokers, respectively (NS)

	Smokers (n = 235)	*Non-smokers (n = 188)*	*p*
Steroids	211 (90%)	148 (79%)	0.002
Immunosuppressive drugs	85 (36%)	52 (28%)	0.06
Nutritional support	65 (28%)	41 (22%)	NS
Colectomy	61 (26%)	58 (31%)	NS
Iterative excisional surgery	17 (7%)	14 (7%)	NS

Table 4 Main events during the year of follow-up in a prospective cohort of 158 patients with Crohn's colitis, according to status at baseline

	Smokers (n = 85)	*Non-smokers (n = 73)*	*p*
Flare-up episode	27 (32%)	17 (23%)	NS
Chronic active disease	14 (16%)	3 (4%)	0.01
Disabling anoperineal disease	4 (5%)	7 (10%)	NS
Quiescent disease	40 (47%)	46 (63%)	0.04
Intensification of medical therapy[*]	36 (42%)	25 (34%)	NS
Excisional surgery	3 (4%)	4 (5%)	NS
Hospitalization	27 (32%)	22 (30%)	NS
Work cessation >3 days	29 (43%)	17 (36%)	NS

[*] Re-initiation of steroids or immunosuppressive therapy

included prospectively. Criteria for exclusion were previous or active small bowel lesions, and CDAI >200. Patients were classified as current smokers if they smoked >7 cigarettes per week. The end-point was again whether or not the patient developed active Crohn's disease (flare-up episode or chronic active evolution) during the year of follow-up. Results were analysed using logistic regression.

Results

More smokers than non-smokers developed active disease ($p = 0.04$, Table 4). However, the need for intensification of medical therapy, the hospitalization rate, and the proportion of patients who had to stop working for more than 3 days, were not significantly different between the two groups. Finally, the effect of smoking was not significant according to logistic regression (odds ratio 1.58 [95% confidence interval, 0.77–3.24]).

Comment

This prospective study showed that, compared with non-smokers, more smokers with Crohn's colitis developed active disease during the year. However, other indicators of disease severity did not show differences between the groups, and, after adjustment for important variables such as the activity of the disease during the year before inclusion, sex and presence or absence of anoperineal disease, smoking was no longer associated with active disease. This negative result may have been due to a lack of statistical power or because too large a proportion of these patients were in an active phase of their disease at baseline. Alternatively, a minority of patients with Crohn's colitis may have ulcerative colitis-like lesions which might benefit from nicotine impregnation. Further studies are needed to test these hypotheses. In any case, as a whole, the response of Crohn's colitis to smoking differs from that of ulcerative colitis, and the same advice to stop smoking should be given to Crohn's patients, whether or not they have colonic involvement.

CONCLUSIONS

Among the various environmental factors which have been proposed to play a role in IBD, smoking is at present the best recognized and the most determinant. Our studies confirm that smoking influences disease severity both in the short term and long term. In Crohn's disease, smoking cessation has probably to be recognized as a major therapeutic goal. Although the benefit on the clinical course of the disease may be delayed, digestive symptoms improve usually in a few months, and, in some patients, surgery may be avoided[10]. Crohn's disease is a lifelong disease and patients who stop smoking will benefit one day.

Acknowledgements

The author thanks all the physicians working in Hôpital Rothschild, and particularly Pr J. P. Gendre and Drs F. Carbonnel and L. Beaugerie who participated in the management of these patients and the preparation of the studies mentioned in this paper.

References

1. Peeters M, Nevens H, Baert F *et al.* Familial aggregation in Crohn's disease: increased age-adjusted risk and concordance in clinical characteristics. Gastroenterology. 1996;111:597–603.
2. Calkins BM. A meta-analysis of the role of smoking in inflammatory bowel disease. Dig Dis Sci. 1989;34:1841–54.
3. Colombel JF, Grandbastien B, Gower-Rousseau C *et al.* Clinical characteristics of Crohn's disease in 72 families. Gastroenterology. 1996;111:604–7.
4. Bridger S, McGregor C, Forgacs IC, Bjarnasson I, MacPherson AJS. The effects of smoking on the development of inflammatory bowel disease. Gastroenterology. 1998;114:A943.
5. Tobin NV, Logan RFA, Langman MJS, McConnell RB, Gilmore IT. Cigarette smoking and inflammatory bowel disease. Gastroenterology. 1987;93:316–21.
6. Sandborn WJ, Tremaine WJ, Offord KP *et al.* Transdermal nicotine for mildly to moderately active ulcerative colitis. A randomized, double-blind placebo-controlled trial. Ann Intern Med. 1997;126:364–715.
7. Duffy LC, Zielezny MA, Marshall JR *et al.* Cigarette smoking and risk of clinical relapse in patients with Crohn's disease. Am J Prev Med. 1990;6:161–6.
8. Russel MG, Nieman FH, Bergers JM, Stockbrugger RW and the South Limburg IBD Study Group. Cigarette smoking and quality of life in patients with inflammatory bowel disease. Eur J Gastroenterol. 1996;8:1075–81.
9. Lindberg E, Jarnerot G, Huifeldt B. Smoking in Crohn's disease: effect on localization and clinical course. Gut. 1992;33:779–82.
10. Cosnes J, Carbonnel F, Beaugerie L, Le Quintrec Y, Gendre JP. Effects of smoking on the long term course of Crohn's disease. Gastroenterology. 1996;110:424–31.
11. Sutherland LR, Ramcharan S, Bryant H, Fick G. Effect of cigarette smoking on recurrence of Crohn's disease. Gastroenterology. 1990;98:1123–8.

12. Cottone M, Rosselli M, Orlando A *et al.* Smoking habits and recurrence in Crohn's disease. Gastroenterology. 1994;106:643–8.
13. Vasiliauskas EA, Plevy SE, Landers CJ *et al.* Perinuclear antineutrophil cytoplasmic antibodies in patients with Crohn's disease define a clinical subgroup. Gastroenterology. 1996;110:1810–19.
14. Langevin S, Menard DB, Haddad H, Beaudry R, Poisson J, Devroede G. Idiopathic ulcerative proctitis may be the initial manifestation of Crohn's disease. J Clin Gastroenterol. 1992;15:199–204.
15. Jick H, Walker AM. Cigarette smoking and ulcerative colitis. N Engl J Med. 1983;308:261–3.
16. De Castella H. Non-smoking: a feature of ulcerative colitis. Br Med J. 1982;284:1706.
17. Rudra T, Motley RJ, Rhodes J. Does smoking improve colitis? Scand J Gastroenterol. 1989;170(suppl):61–3.
18. Boyko EJ, Perera DR, Koepsell TD, Keane EM, Inui TS. Effects of cigarette smoking on the clinical course of ulcerative colitis. Scand J Gastroenterol. 1988;23:1147–52.
19. Benoni C, Nilsson A. Smoking habits in patients with inflammatory bowel disease. Scand J Gastroenterol. 1984;19:824–30.
20. Holdstock G, Savage D, Harman M, Wright R. Should patients with inflammatory bowel disease smoke? Br Med J. 1984;288:362.
21. Srivasta ED, Newcombe RG, Rhodes J, Avramidis P, Mayberry JF. Smoking and ulcerative colitis: a community study. Int J Colorectal Dis. 1993;8:71–4.
22. Fraga XF, Vergara M, Medina C, Casellas F, Bermejo B, Malagelada JR. Effects of smoking on the presentation and clinical course of inflammatory bowel disease. Eur J Gastroenterol Hepatol. 1997;9:683–7.
23. Mokbel M, Carbonnel F, Beaugerie L, Gendre JP, Cosnes J. Effet du tabac sur l'évolution à long terme de la rectocolite hémorragique. Gastroentérol Clin Biol. 1998;(in press).
24. Bartecchi CE, McKenzie TD, Schrier RW. The human costs of tobacco use (first of two parts). N Engl J Med. 1994;330:907–12.
25. Cosnes J, Carbonnel F, Carrat F, Beaugerie L, Gendre JP. Effects of smoking and oral contraceptive use on the clinical course of Crohn's disease. Gastroenterology. 1998;114:A956.
26. Katschinski B, Fingerle D, Scherbaum B, Goebell H. Oral contraceptive use and cigarette smoking in Crohn's disease. Dig Dis Sci. 1993;38:1596–600.
27. Lashner BA, Kane SV, Hanauer SB. Lack of association between oral contraceptive use and Crohn's disease: a community-based matched case-control study. Gastroenterology. 1989;97:1442–7.
28. Sandler RS, Wurzelmann JL, Lyles CM. Oral contraceptive use and the risk of inflammatory bowel disease. Epidemiology. 1992;3:374–8.
29. Petitti DB, Sidney S, Bernstein A, Wolf S, Quesenberry C, Ziel HK. Stroke in users of low-dose oral contraceptives. N Engl J Med. 1996;335:8–15.
30. Hennekens CH, MacMahon B. Oral contraceptives and myocardial infarction. N Engl J Med. 1977;296:1166–7.
31. Sutherland LR, Ramcharan S, Bryant H, Fick G. Effect of oral contraceptive use on reoperation following surgery for Crohn's disease. Dig Dis Sci. 1992;37:1377–82.
32. Motley RJ, Rhodes J, Kay S, Morris TJ. Late presentation of ulcerative colitis in ex-smokers. Int J Colorect Dis. 1988;3:171–5.
33. Roberts CJ, Diggle R. Non-smoking: a feature of ulcerative colitis. Br Med J. 1982;285:440.
34. Russel MG, Volovics A, Schoon EJ, Shivananda S, Stockbrugger RW. Clinical characteristics at diagnosis in 724 smokers and 638 nonsmokers with inflammatory bowel disease: results of the European collaborative study on IBD. Gastroenterology. 1997;112:A1078(abstract).

5
Nicotine in the treatment of ulcerative colitis

W. J. SANDBORN

INTRODUCTION

New first-line therapies which provide alternatives to the mesalamine class of drugs in patients with ulcerative colitis (UC) and which can be used in treatment-refractory patients are needed. Nicotine is a candidate drug for this role. Epidemiology studies have shown that smoking protects against developing UC and placebo-controlled trials have demonstrated that transdermal nicotine is effective for active UC. This article reviews the rationale, mechanisms, pharmacology and clinical results of nicotine treatment for UC.

RATIONALE

In the early 1980s, it was reported that the prevalence of UC in non-smokers was greater than in current smokers, and that former smokers were at even greater risk than life-time non-smokers[1–9]. A meta-analysis of these studies gave the following odds ratios (95% CI) for UC risk: current smokers vs. life-time non-smokers 0.42 (0.34–0.48); and former smokers vs. life-time non-smokers 1.73 (1.36–1.98)[10] (Figure 1). Clinical patterns relating smoking and UC disease activity include: UC onset after stopping smoking and UC remission with resuming smoking; remission of active UC after starting smoking in never-smokers followed by a flare of UC with stopping smoking; and a flare of UC in remission after stopping smoking[11–13]. These observations led to the treatment of UC with nicotine[13].

MECHANISMS

There are many possible mechanisms for a therapeutic effect of nicotine in UC[14] (Figure 2). One study reported no effect of smoking on humoral immune function in smokers with UC compared with non-smoking healthy controls[15]. Other

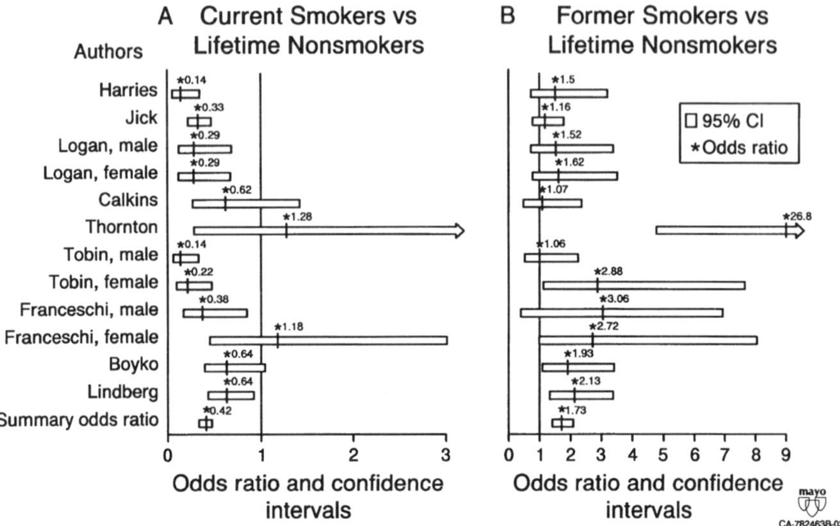

Figure 1 Individual and summary odds ratios and 95% confidence intervals for ulcerative colitis studies included in meta-analysis. **A.** Current smokers compared with life-time non-smokers; **B.** Former smokers compared with life-time non-smokers. Modified and reproduced with permission from Reference 10: Calkins BM. A meta-analysis of the role of smoking in inflammatory bowel disease. Dig Dis Sci. 1989;34:1841–5

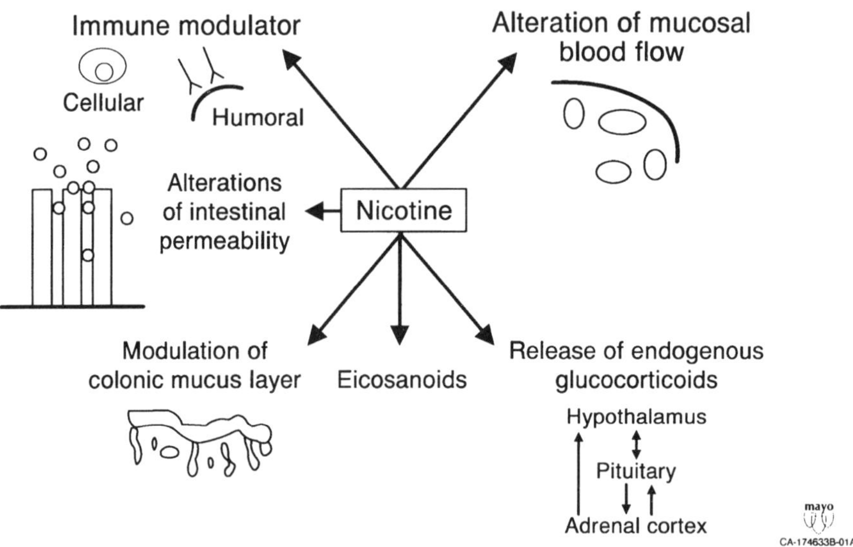

Figure 2 Proposed mechanisms of the 'protective effect' of nicotine in ulcerative colitis. Reproduced with permission from Reference 14: Cohen RD, Hanauer SB. Nicotine in ulcerative colitis. How does it work and how can we use it? Clin Immunother. 1996;3:169–74

studies have reported that nicotine, tobacco, and smoking alter cellular immune function by inhibiting production of various cytokines including IL-1B, IL- 2, IL-8, IL-10, and TNFα in controls and patients with UC[16–18]. Nicotine and smoking decrease colonic mucosa production of eicosanoids including prostaglandin E, 6-keto-PGF$_{1a}$, leukotriene B$_4$, leukotriene C$_4$/D$_4$/E$_4$, prostaglandin F$_{1\alpha}$, prostaglandin F$_{2\alpha}$, and 15-hydroxy-eicosatetraenoic acid in human and animal controls[19–20]. The effect of nicotine on eicosanoid production in UC is unknown. Colonic mucus is decreased in patients with UC and smokers with UC have increased mucus production[21–22]. However, nicotine has minimal or no effect on mucus production in human controls or patients with UC[18,23,24]. Smoking and nicotine both increase circulating ACTH and plasma cortisol concentrations[25,26]. Increases in endogenous corticosteroids could potentially benefit UC. Finally, patients with UC have increased intestinal permeability to chromium-51-labelled ethylenediaminetetra-acetic acid ([^{51}Cr]EDTA) and smoking decreases intestinal permeability to ^{51}Cr-EDTA in healthy controls[27,28]. However, smoking does not decrease [^{51}Cr]EDTA in patients with UC[29].

NICOTINE GUM AND TRANSDERMAL PATCHES

Clinical pharmacology

Polacrilex gum containing 4 mg of nicotine results in peak blood nicotine concentrations which are approximately two thirds of those observed with cigarettes and smokeless tobacco[30]. However, nicotine administered in gum results in variable absorption[31]. To avoid this variability, a nicotine patch has been developed for transdermal administration. Transdermal nicotine administration provides steady plasma nicotine concentrations that are also two thirds of those observed during smoking[32]. Nicotine is primarily metabolized in the liver[33]. The major nicotine metabolites are cotinine and nicotine-*N*-oxide, neither of which is pharmacologically active[33]. Orally administered nicotine has low bioavailability due to first-pass hepatic metabolism[34,35].

Results

Uncontrolled studies reported that nicotine gum 4 mg 5–7 sticks per day or transdermal nicotine 15 mg/24 h and 22 mg/24 h was beneficial in patients with active UC[13,36–40]. Never-smokers were said to tolerate nicotine poorly[36,38]. Controlled trials were subsequently performed to determine the safety and efficacy of nicotine therapy for UC.

Six controlled trials of nicotine gum or patch therapy for UC have been performed (Table 1). An 'N of 1' study in seven patients with active UC demonstrated that nicotine gum 2 mg administered 5–7 times per day was effective compared with placebo in 3 of 7 patients with active UC[41]. Two randomized double-blind placebo-controlled trials of transdermal nicotine for active UC reported that the highest tolerated dose of nicotine (up to 25 mg/24 h and 22 mg/24 h) was effective compared with placebo[42,43]. Both studies increased the nicotine dose from 11 mg or 15 mg up to 22 mg or 25 mg over 1–2 weeks in order to allow the subjects to develop tolerance to nicotine side-effects. A fourth

Table 1 Patient response in six controlled trials of nicotine administered as gum or as a transdermal patch for ulcerative colitis

Reference	Total no. of patients	Response (%)				Indication for treatment	Treatment (%)		
		Nicotine	Placebo	Steroids*	p		Type of administration	Dose	Duration
Lashner et al.[41]	7	43%	0%			Active	Gum	2 mg, 5–7/day	2 weeks
Pullan et al. [42]	72	49%	24%		0.03	Active	Patch	25 mg/24 h	6 weeks
Sandborn et al.[43]	64	39%	9%		0.01	Active	Patch	22 mg/24 h	4 weeks
Thomas et al.[44]	61	20%		45%	0.08	Active	Patch	25 mg/16 h	6 weeks
Guslandi and Tittobello[45]	38	71%		88%	>0.05	Active	Patch	15 mg/24 h	5 weeks
Thomas et al.[46]	80	45%	50%		0.28	Remission	Patch	15 mg/16 h	26 weeks

* Steroids: in the Thomas et al. study[44], prednisolone 15 mg/day was administered for 6 weeks; in the Guslandi and Tittobello study[45], prednisone was administered at a dose of 30 mg/day and tapered over 5 weeks

randomized controlled trial which compared transdermal nicotine at the highest tolerated dose (up to 25 mg/16 h) with prednisolone 15 mg/day in active UC demonstrated equivalence of the two therapies, although there was a trend towards the prednisolone being more efficacious[44]. A fifth randomized controlled trial which compared transdermal nicotine 15 mg/24 h for 5 weeks with prednisone 30 mg/day tapered over 5 weeks also showed equivalence, although again there was a trend towards prednisone being more efficacious[45]. The sixth randomized double-blind placebo-controlled trial showed that a lower dose of transdermal nicotine (15 mg/16 h) was not effective for maintaining remission in patients with UC[46].

There may be a dose–response relationship between the transdermal nicotine dose (dose + duration) and both plasma concentrations of nicotine and clinical response. In the two placebo-controlled trials where transdermal nicotine demonstrated efficacy in active UC, the 22 mg/24 h dose resulted in a mean trough serum nicotine concentration of 11.3 ± 8.4 ng/ml[43] and the 25 mg/24 h dose resulted in a mean trough plasma nicotine concentration of 8.2 ± 7.1 ng/ml[42]. In contrast, in the placebo-controlled trial where transdermal nicotine did not demonstrate efficacy for maintaining remission in UC, the 15 mg/16 h dose resulted in a mean trough plasma nicotine concentration of 5.3 ng/ml[46].

Adverse events

Nicotine binds to nicotinic acetylcholine receptors resulting in a variety of neurological actions and physiological changes, including tachycardia, increased blood pressure and increased alertness[47]. The adverse events reported in clinical trials of transdermal nicotine for UC include contact dermatitis, light-headedness or dizziness, nausea and vomiting, headaches, sleep disturbance or violent/sexual dreams, central nervous system stimulation, diaphoresis or sweating, shakiness or tremor, and tachycardia[42,43]. Tolerance to nicotine develops rapidly[48].

Of greater concern are the serious diseases associated with smoking, including addiction, cardiovascular disease and cancer. Nicotine addiction occurs when nicotine is inhaled in cigarette smoke, resulting in a rapid rise in plasma nicotine concentrations[47,49]. Transdermal nicotine results in a gradual rise in plasma nicotine, and peak concentrations are lower than those occurring during smoking[31,32]. While transdermal nicotine can relieve the withdrawal symptoms of nicotine addiction, it is not addictive itself[47,49,50]. Nicotine addiction did not occur following 6 months of transdermal nicotine (15 mg/16 h) administered to maintain remission in patients with UC[46]. Animal studies and mechanistic studies suggest that nicotine could accelerate atherosclerosis but human evidence is inconclusive[51]. Nicotine does not promote thrombosis in humans[51]. When compared with placebo, transdermal nicotine 15 mg/16 h lowered plasma fibrinogen concentrations and did not affect markers of platelet activation, endothelial damage, or serum lipids when administered to maintain remission in patients with UC[52]. The association between cigarette smoke and cancer has been attributed to the *N*-nitrosamines, such as 4-(methylnitrosoamino)-1-(3-pyridyl)-1-butanone (NNK), and to benzopyrene and other polycyclic aromatic hydrocarbons[53]. Nicotine itself is not a carcinogen but is a precursor of

N-nitrosamines[53]. Whether there is endogenous formation of these *N*-nitrosamines in humans with exposure to non-tobacco sources of nicotine is unknown[54].

TOPICAL ADMINISTRATION OF NICOTINE TO THE COLON

Topical administration of nicotine directly to the colon as an enema or delayed-release oral capsule could decrease systemic absorption and side-effects, and be clinically beneficial.

Clinical pharmacology

Pharmacokinetic studies in healthy volunteers and patients with UC have demonstrated that liquid enemas containing nicotine tartrate at a dose of 45 μg nicotine base/kg (approximately 3 mg nicotine base) or 6 mg nicotine base complexed to carbomer (an acrylic acid polymer) have low systemic absorption and are well tolerated after a single dose[35,55]. Similarly, a dose-ranging pharmacokinetic study in healthy volunteers demonstrated that delayed-release oral nicotine tartrate capsules containing 3 mg or 6 mg nicotine base have low systemic absorption and are well tolerated[56]. Extensive first-pass hepatic metabolism of both nicotine enemas and delayed-release oral nicotine has also been reported[55,56].

Results

Two pilot clinical studies of 6 mg nicotine tartrate or 6 mg nicotine carbomer liquid enemas in patients with active distal UC demonstrated that colonic administration of nicotine may be efficacious[57,58]. Peak and trough concentrations of nicotine as determined at 4 weeks were low or undetectable[57]. These data suggest that nicotine administered directly to the colon can result in a local treatment effect in the absence of therapeutic serum nicotine concentrations. A randomized double-blind placebo-controlled dose-ranging trial of nicotine administered directly to the colon is warranted.

Adverse events

Nicotine enemas and delayed-release oral nicotine were well tolerated, both in three single-dose pharmacokinetic studies[35,55,56] and two 28-day pilot clinical trials[57,58]. The most frequent adverse events were light-headedness and nausea. These adverse reactions were of short duration (<30 min in the single-dose studies and <1–2 h during the first 1–2 days in the 28-day studies) and of minor severity. Patients did not discontinue the studies prematurely because of these adverse events. Given the very low or undetectable peak serum nicotine concentrations in one of the 28-day studies[57], it seems unlikely that the observed minor adverse events were caused by nicotine. These findings are in contrast to a previous study of transdermal nicotine in which adverse reactions to nicotine occurred frequently (77% of nicotine-treated patients) and were severe enough to result in discontinuation of the nicotine in 13% of the nicotine-treated patients[43].

CONCLUSIONS

Ulcerative colitis is primarily a disease of non-smokers. Randomized placebo-controlled trials of transdermal nicotine for active UC have demonstrated efficacy with the highest tolerated dose of nicotine (up to 22–25 mg/24 h). A placebo-controlled trial using a lower dose of transdermal nicotine (15 mg/16 h) to maintain remission in patients with UC did not demonstrate efficacy. Side-effects from transdermal nicotine were frequent, including contact dermatitis, nausea and light-headedness. In order to reduce systemic absorption and side-effects, nicotine has been administered directly to the colon. Pharmacokinetic studies demonstrated that nicotine enemas and delayed-release oral nicotine have low systemic absorption (due to first-pass hepatic metabolism) and are well tolerated. Two uncontrolled pilot studies reported that nicotine enemas may be of clinical benefit in patients with active left-sided UC. Placebo-controlled trials are warranted to confirm these uncontrolled observations.

References

1. Harries AD, Baird A, Rhodes J. Non-smoking: a feature of ulcerative colitis. Br Med J. 1982;284:706.
2. Jick H, Walker AM. Cigarette smoking and ulcerative colitis. N Engl J Med. 1983;308:261–3.
3. Logan RFA, Edmond M, Somerville KW, Langman MJS. Smoking and ulcerative colitis. Br Med J. 1984;288:751–3.
4. Calkins B, Lilienfeld A, Mendeloff A, Garland C, Monk M, Garland F. Smoking factors in ulcerative colitis and Crohn's disease in Baltimore. Am J Epidemiol. 1984;120:498.
5. Thornton JR, Emmett PM, Heaton KW. Smoking, sugar, and inflammatory bowel disease. Br Med J. 1985;290:1786–7.
6. Tobin MV, Logan RFA, Langman MJS, McConnell RB, Gilmore IT. Cigarette smoking and inflammatory bowel disease. Gastroenterology. 1987;93:316–21.
7. Franceschi S, Panz E, La Vecchia C, Parazzini F, Decarli A, Porro GB. Non-specific inflammatory bowel disease and smoking. Am J Epidemiol. 1987;125:445–52.
8. Boyko EJ, Koepsell TD, Perera DR, Inui TS. Risk of ulcerative colitis among former and current cigarette smokers. N Engl J Med. 1987;316:707–10.
9. Lindberg E, Tysk C, Andersson K, Jarnerot G. Smoking and inflammatory bowel disease. A case control study. Gut. 1988;29:352–7.
10. Calkins BM. A meta-analysis of the role of smoking in inflammatory bowel disease. Dig Dis Sci. 1989;34:1841–5.
11. De Castella H. Non-smoking: a feature of ulcerative colitis. Br Med J. 1982;284:1706.
12. Jick H, Walker AM. Cigarette smoking and ulcerative colitis. N Engl J. Med. 1983;308:1477–8.
13. Roberts CJ, Diggle R. Non-smoking: a feature of ulcerative colitis. Br Med. J 1982;285:440.
14. Cohen RD, Hanauer SB. Nicotine in ulcerative colitis. How does it work and how can we use it? Clin Immunother. 1996;3:169–74.
15. Srivastava ED, Barton JR, O'Mahony S *et al.* Smoking, humoral immunity, and ulcerative colitis. Gut. 1991;32:1016–19.
16. Madretsma S, Wolters LMM, Van Dijk JPM *et al.* In-vivo effect of nicotine on cytokine production by human non-adherent mononuclear cells. Eur J Gastroenterol Hepatol. 1996;8:1017–20.
17. Madretsma GS, Donze GJ, Van Dijk APM, Tak CJAM, Wilson JHP, Zijlstra FJ. Nicotine inhibits the in vitro production of interleukin 2 and tumor necrosis factor-α by human mononuclear cells. Immunopharmacology. 1996;35:47–51.
18. Louvet B, Buisine MP, Desreumaux P *et al.* Transdermal nicotine decreases mucosal IL-8 expression but has no effect on mucin gene expression in ulcerative colitis (UC). Gastroenterology. 1998;114:A1028(G4209).
19. Motley RJ, Rhodes J, Williams G, Tavares IA, Bennett A. Smoking, eicosanoids and ulcerative colitis. J Pharm Pharmacol. 1990;42:288–9.

20. Zijlstra FJ, Srivastava ED, Rhodes M *et al*. Effect of nicotine on rectal mucus and mucosal eicosanoids. Gut. 1994;35:247–51.
21. Podolsky D, Isselbacher KJ. Glycoprotein composition of colonic mucus. Gastroenterology. 1984;87:991–8.
22. Cope GF, Heatley RV, Kelleher J. Smoking and colonic mucus in ulcerative colitis. Br Med J. 1986;293:481.
23. Ryder SD, Raouf AH, Parker N, Walker RJ, Rhodes JM. Abnormal mucosal glycoprotein synthesis in inflammatory bowel diseases is not related to cigarette smoking. Digestion. 1995;56:370–6.
24. Finnie IA, Campbell BJ, Taylor BA *et al*. Stimulation of colonic mucin production by corticosteroids and nicotine. Clin Sci. 1996;91:359–64.
25. Kershbaum A, Pappajohn DJ, Bellet S, Hirabayashi M, Shafiiha H. Effect of smoking and nicotine on adrenocortical secretion. JAMA. 1968;203:275–8.
26. Wilkins JN, Carlson HE, Van Vunakis H, Hill MA, Gritz E, Jarvik ME. Nicotine from cigarette smoking increases circulating levels of cortisol, growth hormone, and prolactin in male chronic smokers. Psychopharmacology. 1992;78:305–8.
27. Jenkins RT, Jones DB, Goodacre RL *et al*. Reversibility of increased intestinal permeability to ^{51}Cr-EDTA in patients with gastrointestinal inflammatory diseases. Am J Gastroenterol. 1987;82:1159–64.
28. Prytz H, Benoni C, Tagesson C. Does smoking tighten the gut? Scand J Gastroenterol. 1989;24:1084–8.
29. Benoni C, Pyrtz H. Effects of smoking on the urine excretion of oral ^{51}Cr EDTA in ulcerative colitis. Gut. 1998;42:656–8.
30. Benowitz NL, Porchet H, Sheiner L, Jacob P. Nicotine absorption and cardiovascular effects with smokeless tobacco use: comparison with cigarettes and nicotine gum. Clin Pharmacol Ther. 1988;44:23–8.
31. Benowitz NL, Peyton J, Savanapridi C. Determinants of nicotine intake while chewing polacrilex gum. Clin Pharmacol Ther. 1987;41:467–73.
32. Bannon YB, Corish J, Corrigan OI, Devane JG, Kavanagh M, Mulligen S. Transdermal delivery of nicotine in normal human volunteers: a single and multiple dose study. Eur J Clin Pharmacol. 1989;37:285–90.
33. Benowitz NL, Kuyt F, Jacob P, Jones RT, Osman AL. Cotinine disposition and effects. Clin Pharmacol Ther. 1983;34:604–11.
34. Benowitz NL, Jacob P, Denaro C, Jenkins R. Stable isotope studies of nicotine kinetics and bioavailability. Clin Pharmacol Ther. 1991;49:270–7.
35. Zins BJ, Sandborn WJ, Mays DC *et al*. Pharmacokinetics of nicotine tartrate after single-dose liquid enema, oral, and intravenous administration. J Clin Pharmacol. 1997;37:426–36.
36. Perera DR, Janeway CM, Feld A, Ylvisaker JT, Belic L. Smoking and ulcerative colitis. Br Med J. 1984;288:1533.
37. Watson JP, Lewis RA. Ulcerative colitis responsive to smoking and to nicotine chewing gum in a patient with α1 anti-trypsin deficiency. Resp Med. 1995;89:635–6.
38. Srivastava ED, Russel MAH, Feyerabend C, Williams GT, Masterson JG, Rhodes J. Transdermal nicotine in active ulcerative colitis. Eur J Gastroenterol Hepatol. 1991;3:815–18.
39. Guslandi M, Tittobello A. Steroid-sparing effect of transdermal nicotine in ulcerative colitis. J Clin Gastroenterol. 1994;18:347–50.
40. Guslandi M, Tittobello A. Pilot trial of nicotine patches as an alternative to corticosteroids in ulcerative colitis. J Gastroenterol. 1996;31:627–9.
41. Lashner BA, Hanauer SB, Silverstein MD. Testing nicotine gum for ulcerative colitis patients. Experience with single-patient trials. Dig Dis Sci. 1990;35:827–32.
42. Pullan RD, Rhodes J, Ganesh S *et al*. Transdermal nicotine for active ulcerative colitis. N Engl J Med. 1994;330:811–15.
43. Sandborn WJ, Tremaine WJ, Offord KP *et al*. Transdermal nicotine for mildly to moderately active ulcerative colitis. A randomized, double-blind, placebo-controlled trial. Ann Intern Med. 1997;126:364–71.
44. Thomas GAO, Rhodes J, Ragunath K *et al*. Transdermal nicotine compared with oral prednisolone therapy for active ulcerative colitis. Eur J Gastroenterol Hepatol. 1996;8:769–76.
45. Guslandi M, Tittobello A. Outcome of ulcerative colitis after treatment with transdermal nicotine. Eur J Gastroenterol Hepatol. 1998;10:513–15.

46. Thomas GAO, Rhodes J, Mani V *et al*. Transdermal nicotine as maintenance therapy for ulcerative colitis. N Engl J Med. 1995;332:988–92.
47. Benowitz NL. Pharmacologic aspects of cigarette smoking and nicotine addiction. N Engl J Med. 1988;319:1318–30.
48. Porchet HC, Benowitz NL, Scheiner LB. Pharmacodynamic model for tolerance: application to nicotine. J Pharmacol Exp Ther. 1988;244:231–6.
49. Henningfield JE, Keenan R. Nicotine delivery kinetics and abuse liability. J Consult Clin Psychiatry. 1993;61:743–50.
50. Pickworth WB, Bunker EB, Henningfield JE. Transdermal nicotine: reduction of smoking with minimal abuse liability. Psychopharmacology. 1994;115:9–14.
51. Benowitz NL, Gourlay SG. Cardiovascular toxicity of nicotine: implications for nicotine replacement therapy. J Am Coll Cardiol. 1997;29:1422–31.
52. Thomas GAO, Davies SV, Rhodes J, Russell MA, Feyerabend C, Sawe U. Is transdermal nicotine associated with cardiovascular risk? J R Coll Phys Lond. 1995;29:392–6.
53. Hecht SS, Hofmann D. The relevance of tobacco-specific nitrosamines to human cancer. Cancer Surveys. 1989;8:273–94.
54. Carmella SG, Borukhova A, Desai D, Hecht SS. Evidence for endogenous formation of tobacco-specific nitrosamines in rats treated with tobacco alkaloids and sodium nitrite. Carcinogenesis. 1997;18:587–92.
55. Green JT, Thomas GAO, Rhodes J *et al*. Pharmacokinetics of nicotine carbomer enemas: a new treatment for ulcerative colitis. Clin Pharmacol Ther. 1997;61:340–8.
56. Compton RF, Sandborn WJ, Laswon GM *et al*. A dose-ranging pharmacokinetic study of nicotine tartrate following single-dose delayed-release oral and intravenous administration. Aliment Pharmacol Ther. 1997;11:865–74.
57. Sandborn WJ, Tremaine WJ, Leighton JA *et al*. Nicotine tartrate liquid enemas for mildly to moderately active left-sided ulcerative colitis unresponsive to first-line therapy: a pilot study. Aliment Pharmacol Ther. 1997;11:663–71.
58. Green JT, Thomas GAO, Rhodes J *et al*. Nicotine enemas for active ulcerative colitis – a pilot study. Aliment Pharmacol Ther. 1997;11:859–63.

Section II
Pathogenesis of IBD

6
Inflammatory lesions of the myenteric plexus in Crohn's disease

K. GEBOES and P. RUTGEERTS

INTRODUCTION

The wall of the gastrointestinal system is composed of four layers: the mucosa, the submucosa, the muscularis propria and the serosa with subserosal connective tissue or adventitia. The enteric nervous system (ENS) is embedded within these four layers. It differs functionally and structurally from any other region of the peripheral nervous system. The ENS is composed of ganglionated plexuses in the submucosa (Meissner and Henle's plexus) and in the fibrous septum between the two layers of the muscularis propria (myenteric plexus) and aganglionated plexuses in the mucosa and muscularis propria. Collagen is excluded from the enteric plexuses and support for neuronal elements is provided by enteric glial cells. Enteric glia differ from Schwann cells in that they do not form basal laminae and they ensheath axons, not individually, but in groups[1]. Yet, like Schwann cells, they can synthesize and express MHC molecules[2,3]. The presence of MHC Class II molecules suggests that they may act as antigen-presenting cells (APC). It has been suggested that Schwann cells can present *Mycobacterium leprae* antigens to T cells and hence play an active role in the inflammatory responses of nerves seen in tuberculoid leprosy[4]. Extrinsic autonomic nerves are present in the bowel wall, mainly in the subserosal connective tissue.

Structural alterations of the different layers of the bowel wall are common in chronic idiopathic inflammatory intestinal disorders. They can be recognized sometimes on gross inspection but in general, microscopy allows better detection and, for some alterations, more sophisticated techniques, such as immunohistochemistry, are needed. The latter, furthermore, allow study of correlations with functional alterations and the inflammatory reaction. Microscopic alterations, such as an irregular pseudovillous mucosal surface, the occurrence of irregular, shortened and bifid crypts with loss of parallelism and variability of the intercryptal distance, are common in ulcerative colitis (UC) and Crohn's disease (CD). Distortion of the mucosal architecture is therefore one of the major diagnostic microscopic features[5]. Alterations of the smooth muscle tissue in the muscularis mucosae and muscularis propria are commonly observed in diseases such as necrotizing enterocolitis in infants, ischaemic bowel disease, systemic sclerosis and following therapeutic interventions, such as surgery and chemo- or radiotherapy[6]. Fibromuscular obliteration of the lamina propria is observed in the solitary rectal ulcer syndrome and in chronic gastritis. In UC and CD, the smooth muscle cell alterations appear as irregular thickening of the muscle tissue due to oedema or actual increase in smooth muscle cell mass; as irregular connections between the muscularis propria and muscularis mucosae; as fragmentation of smooth muscle bundles, as an additional muscle coat and as an interruption of the smooth muscle tissue with loss of smooth muscle cells and fibrosis. Ultrastructural studies show smooth muscle cell hypertrophy, myofibroblast transformation, necrosis and increased collagen content in the immediate vicinity. An increased collagen content and alterations of the types of collagen are a feature of many inflammatory and fibroproliferative diseases including CD[7]. Immunohistochemical studies have demonstrated an increased type V collagen content in CD[8]. Extrinsic nerves are also affected by chronic inflammatory processes, since a relative increase in sympathetic nerve fibres has been reported in the diseased gut. Alterations of the ENS can also be observed. In some conditions, such as paraneoplastic pseudo-obstruction associated with small cell carcinoma of the lung, systemic sclerosis, inflammatory axonopathy, Chagas's disease and some viral diseases (CMV, EBV), they are definitely related to perineural inflammation[9]. In other conditions, such as achalasia of the oesophagus, they are probably related to inflammation.

Structural alterations of the bowel wall are a major feature of Crohn's disease, a condition characterized by transmural inflammation. They include alterations of the ENS in addition to mucosal, muscular and connective tissue changes. The frequency and possible functional consequences of the structural ENS abnormalities occurring in CD, as well as their relation to inflammation, have not received wide attention and therefore have not been established clearly. The aim of the present paper is to review the neural changes occurring in CD and discuss their relationship with inflammation and possible functional consequences.

STRUCTURAL ABNORMALITIES OF THE ENTERIC NERVOUS SYSTEM IN HUMAN CD

Routine microscopical observations

The occurrence of structural abnormalities of the enteric nervous system (ENS) in CD was recognized already in the early descriptions of the disease[10]. It was noted that 'neural changes, characterized by increased prominence of nerve fibers and ganglia, that were not discernible in the early phase, were detectable in the intermediate phase of the disease' and that 'in the chronic phase, the submucous and myenteric nerve plexuses appear prominent'[11]. This observation suggests a relationship of the nervous changes to inflammation and the duration and evolution of the disease.

The structural abnormalities of the ENS occurring in the CD include architectural alterations of the plexuses, alterations of the neural cell bodies (damage, hypertrophy and hyperplasia), nerve fibre hypertrophy (increase in size) and hyperplasia (increase in number) and alterations of the enteroglial cells[12]. An increase in the number of ganglion cells is found in the myenteric plexus in inflamed areas and in adjacent overtly non-inflamed areas of the intestine[13].

In order to examine the frequency of the lesions we have studied the surgical specimens of 40 CD patients, 10 patients operated for UC and 10 patients operated for adenocarcinoma of the caecum. The mean age ± SD of the patients with CD (21 women, 19 men) was 34.7 ± 12.5. Their Crohn's disease had been diagnosed at the age of 26.6 ± 10.4. For 24 patients, the surgical specimen came from the first operation. Twenty-one patients were operated on for obstructive disease, 17 for perforating complications. Abnormalities of the ENS were detected with routine microscopy in 37/40 patients with CD (93%), in 2/10 cases with UC and in none of the samples from patients operated for carcinoma. In a study comparing the diagnostic value of a large series of microscopic parameters, nervous changes were found in 10/19 (52%) patients with CD and 2/23 (8%) with UC. It was concluded that these changes were highly suggestive for CD with a significant difference between UC and CD. Furthermore, they were shown to to be well reproducible (88% agreement)[14]. The occurrence of nerve fibre hypertrophy and hyperplasia in CD has been confirmed by objective measurements using point-count morphometry[15]. Similar lesions do occur in UC and, although they are certainly far more common in CD, they are therefore not entirely specific.

While nerve fibre hypertrophy in the submucosa can be reliably assessed on routinely stained histological slides, mucosal nerve fibre hypertrophy can only be demonstrated using immunohistochemistry with antibodies directed against nerve fibre components, such as synaptophysin and nerve growth factor receptor. In CD, mucosal nerve fibre hypertrophy is common but appears only in areas overlying submucosal fibre hypertrophy. In UC, an increase of mucosal nerve fibres can be demonstrated using antibodies directed against synaptophysin but staining for NGF receptor was negative. In contrast, in samples from normal mucosa and from cases with non-specific colitis, mucosal fibres were rare and usually small[16]. The observed nerve cell and fibre hyperplasia may thus reflect a nerve growth factor-stimulated proliferative process as the receptor for this peptide is significantly increased in CD. The upregulation of the NGF receptor in CD has been confirmed and its neuronal and enteroglial expression was found to be associated with enhanced expression of CD27, another member of the NGF receptor family, occurring in many neurons and glial cells but mainly on T cells and mucosal plasma cells, supporting a relationship with the inflammatory reaction[17]. CD27 is present on the cell surface as a homodimer and binds to CD70, which is present on activated lymphocytes.

Ultrastructural studies

Electron microscopic studies of CD, UC and control samples have demonstrated the presence of swollen, structureless, empty nerve fibres or axons. The axons appear as large lucent structures, sometimes with large membrane-bound vacuoles, swollen mitochondria and concentrated neurofibrils. The changes can be focal or diffuse. They are widespread and extensive and can occur in macroscopically affected or non-affected areas and in samples from section margins. The axonal changes are not limited to areas with concurrent inflammation. Their specificity for CD has, however, not been confirmed. A mean of 77.8% abnormal axons (range 52–98%) was found in a study of eight cases with CD[18]. Yet, in another study, a mean of 29.9% (range 12.2–60%) abnormal axons was found in samples from patients with CD while, in samples from UC cases, a mean of 21–25% abnormal axons was counted. In the same study, a mean of 12–63% of abnormal axons was also found in controls, including one case of diverticulitis[19]. The axonal changes are considered a sign of axonal damage and necrosis. Plasma cells, macrophages, mast cells and eosinophils are associated with the abnormal nervous structures. It has therefore been suggested that the destruction of nervous system axons could be the result of immunological effector cells and their products. The presence of similar findings in areas remote from gross damage suggests the possibility that the damage may be produced by an agent(s) capable of travelling along axons. The hypothesis that CD may be an autonomic neuropathy was proposed[20].

In addition to axonal necrosis, we observed increased collagen deposition in the immediate vicinity of axon fibres (Figure 1).

Immunohistochemical data

An increased and aberrant expression of MHC Class II antigens on enteric glial cells and glial cell sheaths of nerve fibres has been detected in samples from

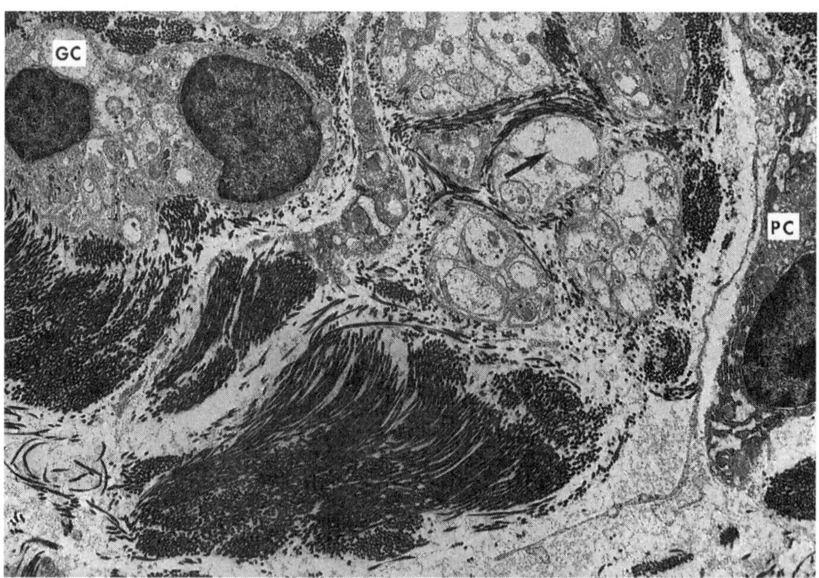

Figure 1 Transmission electron microscopy: Crohn's disease – ileum – myenteric plexus – section margin – pretreatment with tannic acid for identification of collagen; the photograph shows a myenteric ganglion with glial cells (GC) and axon bundles. The axon bundles are partially composed of normal axons and partially of swollen empty axons (arrow). In between the axon bundles, a dense irregular deposition of collagen is present. Immediately adjacent to the ganglion lies a plasma cell (PC). ×2500

patients with CD. Increased membranous expression of HLA-DR is present in macroscopically involved and uninvolved areas, in the colon and ileum, and correlates with aberrant or increased epithelial expression. A relationship exists also with the presence of inflammatory cells, especially CD8+ T lymphocytes[21]. The induction of HLA-DP and DQ antigens is restricted to areas of moderate and high inflammatory activity[22].

Peptidergic nerves are probably more predominant in the enteric nervous system than in any other neural tissue and neuropeptides are known to be important in normal intestinal motility. Substance P and vasoactive intestinal peptide (VIP) have been studied extensively in human inflammatory bowel disease, because of their established role in inflammation at other sites of the body[23]. Abnormalities of the VIP innervation pattern have repeatedly been reported in CD[24]. Substance P levels are increased in both CD and UC. The significance of these findings remains unclear but they provide evidence for alterations in the peptidergic innervation. They could be related to gastrointestinal motility disorders occurring in patients with active and inactive CD[25]. In this context mention should also be made of changes in the nitrergic innervation, which has emerged in the past years as an important inhibitory pathway. There is evidence that the inducible form of the enzyme involved in the synthesis of nitric oxide is affected by inflammation. In the guinea-pig, TNBS-induced ileitis is accompanied by the induction of inducible NO synthase in a subset of myenteric neurons. In resection specimens of patients with toxic megacolon, a notorious complication of colitis, inducible NO synthase is markedly elevated[26].

In order to examine the possible relationship between motility disturbances and lesions of the ENS we have studied the distribution of NO synthesizing neurons in surgical specimens from human normal ($n = 12$) and CD small intestine ($n = 12$) utilizing a histochemical method for the detection of NO-synthase-dependent NADPH diaphorase activity and immunohistochemistry for NO synthase. Patients with CD included in the study were operated for stricturing disease. The control patients were operated for abdominal trauma ($n = 7$), colonic adenocarcinoma ($n = 3$) and an appendiceal tumour ($n = 2$). After opening the specimen, samples were obtained from normal and from inflamed areas, snap frozen in liquid nitrogen precooled isopentane and stored until use at $-70°C$. Perpendicular cryostat sections of these biopsies were used for enzyme- and immunohistochemistry. The presence of the constitutive form of NO synthase was revealed by the reduction of tetrazolium dye in the presence of reduced nicotinamide adenine dinucleotide phosphate (NADPH).

Immunohistochemistry, following a three-step indirect immunoperoxidase technique, was used for the detection of NO synthase and for neurofilaments with antibodies directed against the 68- and 200-kDa neurofilaments (Sanbio, Uden, The Netherlands). The primary and secondary antisera were prescreened to eliminate crossreactivity. Endogenous peroxidase was blocked by incubating the sections for 30 min in 0.3% H_2O_2 in methanol. The biopsies were analysed in a blinded manner for: the pattern of distribution of neurons and extensions in the submucosa, muscularis propria and myenteric plexus; the types of neurons present, NO-positive vs. NO-negative; the average number of cell bodies for the ganglia of the submucous and myenteric plexuses and the ratio of NO^+ neurons over the total number of neurons (NO^+/NO^+ and NO^-) for the ganglia of the submucous and myenteric plexuses. Cells were quantified by counting the number of neuronal cell bodies per ganglion using 100× or 40× objectives, in sections stained with antibodies directed against neurofilaments, and the proportion of NADPH diaphorase-positive cell bodies was determined in double-stained preparations.

In samples from controls, occasional NADPH diaphorase-positive neuronal cell bodies were found. Overall an average of 2.2 cell bodies per ganglion was

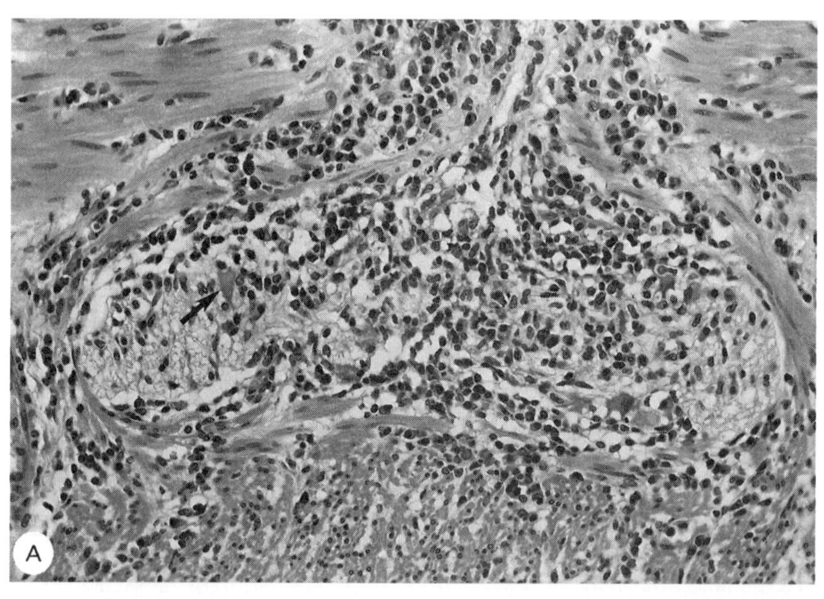

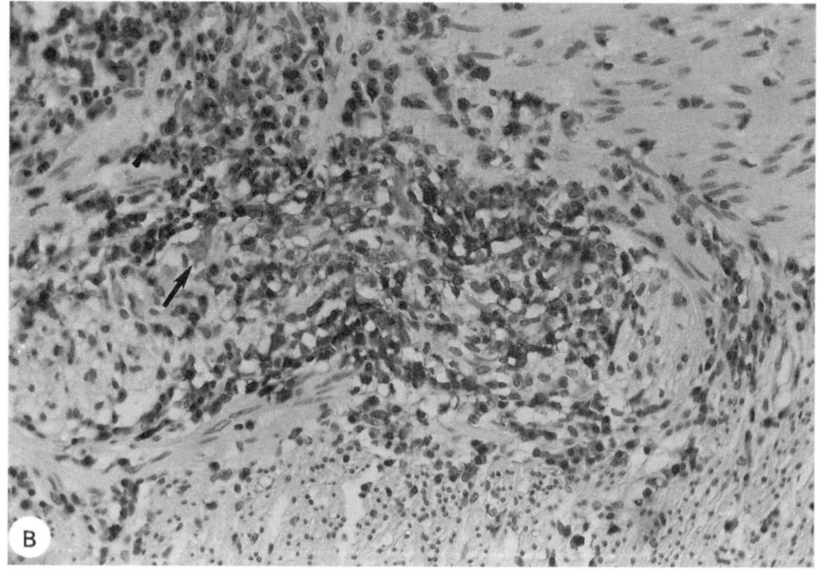

counted in the submucosal plexuses (total number of ganglia counted = 200) and 39% of the cell bodies showed a positive staining with NADPH. In the myenteric plexus all ganglia contained positively labelled cells. An average of 3.29 cell bodies was counted (total number of ganglia counted = 78); 47% of the cell bodies showed a positive NADPH diaphorase staining. Using combined staining with antibodies against neurofilaments, it was possible to distinguish between two types of NO-positive neuronal cell bodies and NO-negative cells. NO-positive cells were either negative or positive for antibodies against the neurofilaments. Enzyme activity was also present in abundant fibres in the longitudinal and circular muscle layers.

In Crohn's disease specimens, NO-positive neuronal cell bodies show a distribution similar to that seen in control specimens. The average number of cell bodies in the ganglia of the submucous plexus was 5 (160 ganglia counted) with 58.7% positive for NADPH. In the myenteric plexus an average of 7.6 cell bodies per ganglion was found (120 ganglia) with 62.8% of the cell bodies staining positive for NADPH diaphorase[27]. This phenomenon was later more extensively studied and confirmed[28]. This means that, in CD, there is a relative increase of NO-positive cells in the myenteric plexus in inflamed and non-inflamed areas, when compared with normal controls. So, while NO derived from inflammatory cells in CD may be involved in hyperaemia and tissue injury and mediate some of the alterations in intestinal motility associated with IBD,

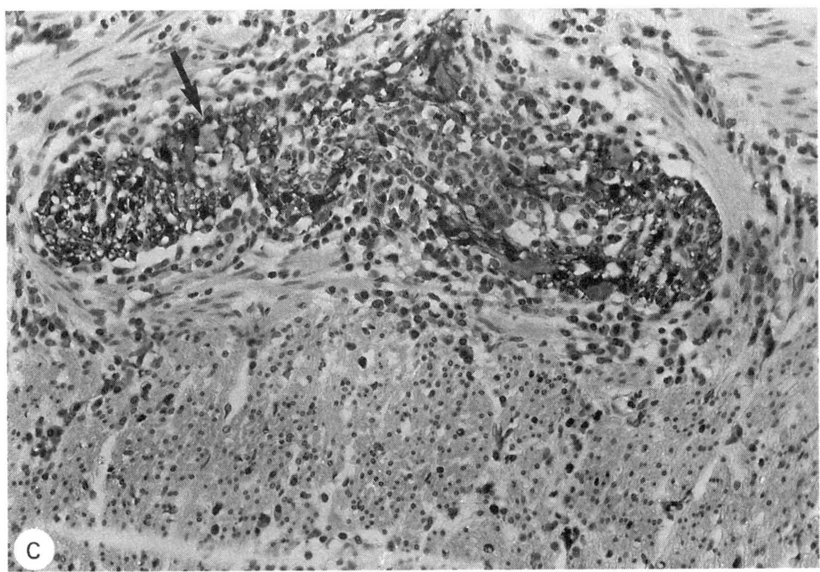

Figure 2 Ganglion in the myenteric plexus – sample obtained in macroscopically involved area from a specimen with Crohn's disease. Arrows indicate the presence of neurons. The microphotograph shows a ganglion with neuronal cell bodies and axon bundles infiltrated by lymphocytes and plasma cells. **A**: routine haematoxylin & eosin staining; **B**: immunohistochemistry using an antibody directed against LC (common leucocyte antigen – CD45); **C**: immunostaining using antibodies against S100 indicating enteroglia. ×220

the motility disturbances might also be the result of the production of NO by neuronal cells in the ENS and especially of the relative increase of NO-positive neuronal cells[29].

NERVOUS CHANGES AND INFLAMMATION

Nerve fibre hypertrophy and axonal damage in CD are associated with the presence of a cellular inflammatory infiltrate composed of plasma cells, lymphocytes, eosinophils and mast cells which may be closely apposed to nerves[30,31] (Figure 2). A dense infiltrate of inflammatory cells can be present around small ganglia of the submucosal plexuses. Granulomas in close contact with and causing distortion of the myenteric plexus, can be observed in the septum between the inner and outer layer of the muscularis propria (Figure 3). In an immunohistochemical study of surgical ileal biopsies from 10 patients with CD and 6 controls (normal = 4, UC = 2), we demonstrated the presence of T lymphocytes and CD45RO-positive monocytes in the vicinity of nerve fibres and ganglia[32]. The highly prominent nervous changes observed in the submucosa and called 'neuromatous lesions' are mainly seen in areas with more deeply situated inflammatory lesions[33]. Yet, axonal damage and necrosis is also seen in uninvolved section margins[20]. So, it is at present still unknown whether the nervous changes are simply secondary to inflammation or not. The occurrence of lesions in macroscopically uninvolved areas may indeed indicate a more primary event, preceding mucosal inflammation, as suggested by Dvorak[20]. An alternative might be that the neuronal network may provide a pathway for transmural

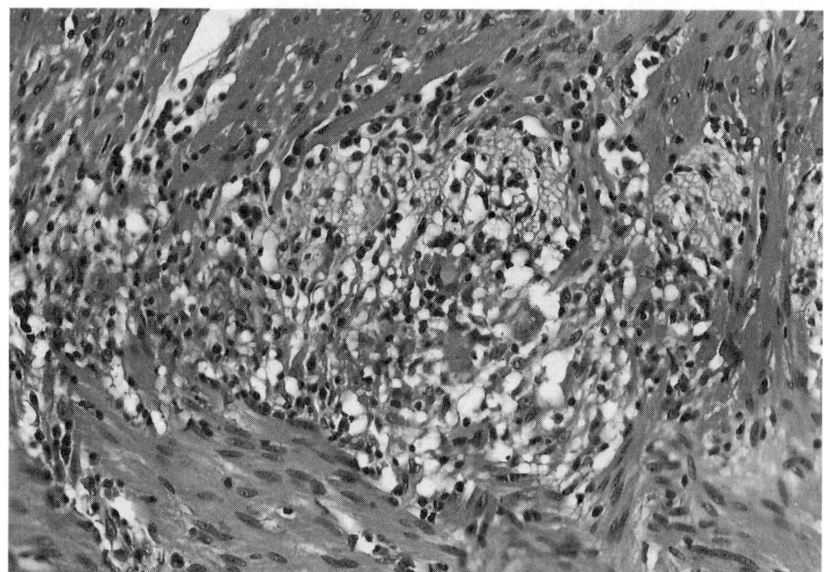

Figure 3   Granulomatous inflammation of the myenteric plexus (H&E ×220)

and lateral spreading of the disease. In order to examine this hypothesis, we have studied the section margins of 40 right ileocolectomy surgical specimens obtained from CD patients operated for perforating complications ($n = 17$), stricturing disease ($n = 21$) and medically intractable inflammation ($n = 2$). Neural lesions were found in the ileal section margins in 22/40 cases. In these cases, small numbers of inflammatory cells or solitary cells were found in close contact with individual nerve fibres in the muscularis propria or nerve fibre bundles in the myenteric plexus. Occasionally, inflammatory cells were also found within a ganglion or nerve fibre bundle. The inflammatory infiltrate consisted of eosinophils or mast cells in 50%, of lymphocytes in 27% and was mixed in 23% of cases. The close proximity between eosinophils and mast cells and fascicles of axons has also been reported with electron microscopy. In addition, electron microscopic findings suggestive of release of eosinophil granule products have been noted. Release of potent cytotoxic and neurotoxic materials from the eosinophil granules might contribute to the axonal damage[20]. It seems thus more likely that the nervous changes occurring in CD are related to inflammation and result from inflammation. The morphologically observed neural changes can therefore best be understood as degenerative (axonal damage) and secondarily regenerative (nerve cell and fibre hypertrophy and hyperplasia). Whether they are a primary event, or in other words, whether nervous structures are a primary target for the inflammatory reaction, or just a secondary target, being affected as a bystander, in the whole process is not clear.

NERVOUS CHANGES, INFLAMMATION AND RECURRENCE

Early endoscopic recurrence and a high rate of endoscopic recurrence following ileocolectomy are characteristic for CD. Recurrent lesions are mostly confined to the neoterminal ileum[34]. The early recurrent lesions occurring in the neoterminal ileum apparently do not originate from identifiable pre-existing mucosal inflammation. In an immunohistochemical study of biopsies obtained in 14 patients (7 with CD; 7 non-CD controls) in the neoterminal ileum during surgery and 4–6 months after surgery, we did not observe microscopic lesions in the peroperative biopsies[35]. Endoscopic lesions, left in place after 'curative surgery' have no influence on early endoscopic anastomotic recurrence in CD[36]. Macroscopic or microscopic evaluation of the section margins has poor predictive value for the recurrence rate and, although postoperative recurrence may be higher in patients with microscopic involvement, negative section margins do not predict absence of recurrence[37,38]. Yet, in most cases, evaluation of the section margins has focussed on the presence or absence of mucosal inflammation. Very few studies have examined the possible relationship between neural inflammation and the pathway of recurrence. In a preliminary study, we examined neural MHC Class II expression and lymphocytic neuropathy in section margins from 12 patients with CD and 4 controls. The sections were stained with a panel of antibodies including LC (leukocytes), MB1 and MB2 for the identification of B cells, MT1, OKT4 and OKT8 for the identification of T lymphocytes and subsets, S100 for the identification of enteroglial cells, neurofilaments for the identification of nerves and HLA-DR and TAL1B5 for the

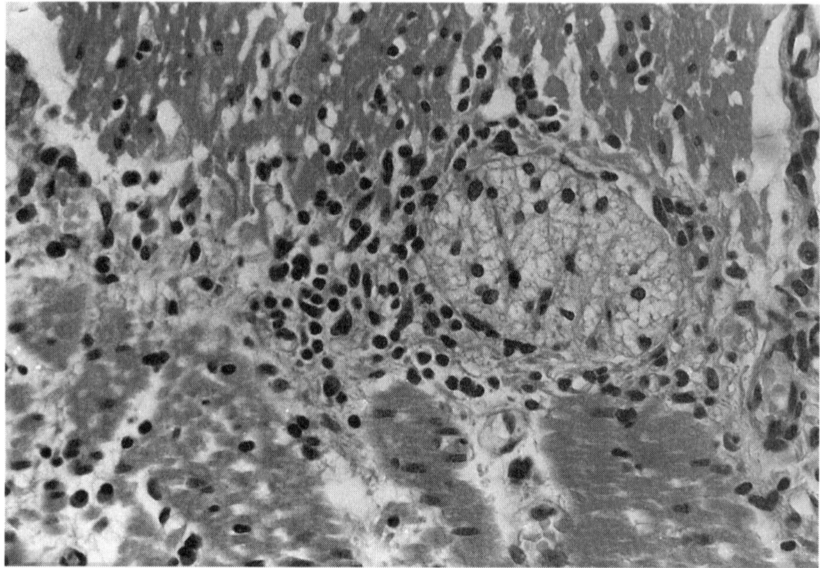

Figure 4 Lymphocytic neuritis of the myenteric plexus: sample obtained from an ileal section margin from a specimen with Crohn's disease (H&E, ×220)

identification of MHC Class II antigens. Routine microscopic analysis showed structural abnormalities of the myenteric plexus in 2/12 cases with CD. Immunohistochemistry confirmed the findings and showed additional alterations in all plexuses in 8 other patients. T lymphocytes were occasionally seen adjacent to ganglion cells and nerve fibres and glial MHC Class II expression was observed in all 10 patients. In samples from control patients no abnormalities were detected[39]. The possibility of a relationship between endoscopic recurrence and the presence of lymphocytic or other types of neuritis in section margins was further investigated in surgical specimens from 40 patients with CD. The findings were correlated with CD recurrence diagnosed endoscopically and histologically three months following surgery using standardized scores. Neural lesions were found in the ileal section margins in 22/40 CD cases, mainly in Auerbach's plexus (Figure 4). Twenty out of 32 patients with endoscopic recurrence had evidence of neuritis in the ileal section margins whereas only 2/8 patients without endoscopic recurrence at 3 months had similar lesions. These findings support the hypothesis that the neural network might present a pathway via which CD may spread and recur[40].

SUMMARY AND CONCLUSIONS

Routine microscopy and ultrastructural studies show that lesions of the ENS are common in Crohn's disease. Abnormalities are being detected in resection specimens in 50–90% of patients[14,40]. The lesions are, however, not specific. Lesions of the ENS are not confined to the grossly involved areas but occur equally at section margins, macroscopically not involved and covered by a normal-appearing mucosa. Plasma cells, macrophages, lymphocytes, mast cells and eosinophils are associated with the changes of the ENS both in grossly involved areas and in the section margins[20,40]. Mast cells and eosinophils may, however, be more common in lesions of the section margins. Immunohistochemical studies support the concept of the involvement of the ENS by showing expression of inflammation-associated markers[32].

These findings may be important for the natural history of CD. Mast cells are recruited by mediators such as IL-3, IL-4 and IL-10 and also by substance P and VIP. They can result in various products such as arachidonic acid metabolites and can modify the inflammatory reaction. The relationship between VIP and mast cells in CD is unclear and data on VIP in CD are conflicting, both increase and decrease being reported[12]. These conflicting data may, however, be the result of differences between early and chronic lesions. One could speculate that, in early lesions, VIP is increased, thus being capable of recruiting mast cells, while, in chronic lesions, a decrease occurs due to the damage to the ENS. This sequence might explain other phenomena observed in CD. In experimental studies, it has been shown that VIP has a region-specific antiproliferative effect on enteric smooth muscle[41]. Hypertrophy of the muscle layers (increase in size of the muscle cells) has been documented in CD and is accompanied by an increase in the number and size of VIPergic nerves and of the VIP and PACAP content of the gut wall[42,43]. In contrast, in CD, smooth muscle hyperplasia (increase in number) is limited and less common than hypertrophy. Hence, it can be suggested that VIP controls unlimited muscle hyperplasia, with subsequent hypertrophy resulting from this control.

Eosinophils also have a wide range of activity. They can produce neurotoxic substances, but also growth factors, proinflammatory substances and the main cytokines involved in the regulation of the immune response, such as IL-4, IL-2 and interferon-γ[44]. The production of neurotoxic substances by activated eosinophils might be responsible for the widespread axonal damage reported to occur in CD. The fact that eosinophils are also seen in conditions such as UC would explain why this axonal damage is not specific. The occurrence of eosinophils has been reported in mucosal biopsies from early recurrent lesions in the neoileum[45]. Their presence is furthermore associated with an enhancement of IL-5 synthesis[46]. A study of mucosal biopsies from early recurrent ileal lesions has also shown a significant increase of IL-4 and suggested that early lesions are associated with a Th-2-type reaction pattern while chronic lesions are rather associated with a Th-1 pattern[47]. Substantial spontaneous secretion of interferon-γ and IL-4 can already be found in duodenal biopsies with no inflammation of the mucosa[48]. In early CD, a difference from control biopsies is, however, noted[47]. Furthermore, eosinophils are more common in early CD. Our findings on the microscopic differences in the composition of the cellular infiltrate when comparing lesions of the ENS in the section margins and the chronic lesions point in the same direction and show that the inflammatory changes observed in the ENS in the section margins are closer to early recurrent mucosal lesions. They may therefore represent another form of early lesions. Plasma cells and lymphocytes are clearly involved in inflammation-associated tissue damage. While these cell types can be seen in early nervous lesions, they seem, however, to be more common in well-established lesions.

Taking all these data together, it seems thus that the ENS is involved in CD and might play a more active role than hitherto accepted, possibly in spreading the disease.

References

1. Gershon MD, Rothman TP. Enteric glia. Glia. 1991;4:195–204.
2. Armati PJ, Pollard JD, Gatenby P. Rat and human Schwann cells in vitro can synthesize and express MHC molecules. Muscle Nerve. 1990;13:106–16.
3. Hirata I, Berrebi G, Austin LL, Keren DF, Dobbins WO. Immunohistochemical characterization of intraepithelial and lamina propria lymphocytes in control ileum and colon in inflammatory bowel disease. Dig Dis Sci. 1986;31:593–603.
4. Samuels NM, Mirsky R, Grange JM, Jessen KR. Expression of major histocompatibility complex Class I and Class II antigens in human Schwann cell cultures and effects of infection with Mycobacterium leprae. Clin Exp Immunol. 1987;68:500–9.
5. Jenkins D, Balsitis M, Gallivan S et al. Guidelines for the initial biopsy diagnosis of suspected chronic idiopathic inflammatory bowel disease. The British Society of Gastroenterology Initiative. J Clin Pathol. 1997;50:93–105.
6. Smith VV, Milla PJ. Histological phenotypes of enteric smooth muscle disease causing functional intestinal obstruction in childhood. Histopathology. 1997;31:112–22.
7. El-Asrar A, Geboes K, Al-Kharashi SA, Tabbara KF, Missotten L. Collagen content and types in trachomatous conjunctivitis. Eye. 1998;12:735–9.
8. Graham M, Diegelman R, Elson C et al. Collagen content and types in the intestinal strictures of Crohn's disease. Gastroenterology. 1988;94:257–65.
9. Debinski HS, Kamm MA, Talbot IC, Khan G, Kangro HO, Jeffries DJ. DNA viruses in the pathogenesis of sporadic chronic idiopathic intestinal pseudo-obstruction. Gut. 1997;41:100–6.
10. Crohn BB, Oppenheimer GD. Regional ileitis: a pathologic and clinical entity. J Am Med Assoc. 1932;99:1323–9.
11. Mottet NK. Histopathologic spectrum of regional enteritis and ulcerative colitis. In: Bennington JL, ed. Major Problems in Pathology. Vol II. Philadelphia: WB Saunders Company; 1976:77–86.
12. Geboes K, Collins S. Structural abnormalities of the nervous system in Crohn's disease and ulcerative colitis. Neurogastroenterol Mot. 1998;10:189–202.
13. Storsten KA, Kernohan JW, Bargen JA. The myenteric plexus in chronic ulcerative colitis. Surg Gynecol Obstet. 1953;97:335–43.
14. Cook MG, Dixon MF. An analysis of the reliability of detection and diagnostic value of various pathological features in Crohn's disease and ulcerative colitis. Gut. 1973;14:255–62.
15. Nadorra R, Landing BH, Wells TR. Intestinal plexuses in Crohn's disease and ulcerative colitis in children: pathologic and microdissection studies. Pediatr Pathol. 1986;6:267–87.
16. Strobach RS, Ross A, Markin RS, Zetterman RK, Linder J. Neural patterns in inflammatory bowel disease: an immunohistochemical survey. Modern Pathol. 1990;3:488–93.
17. Von Herbay A, Castrucci M, Otten U, Otto HF. Coexpression of nerve growth factor receptor and cytokine receptor CD27 in enteric neurons and immune cells in ulcerative colitis and Crohn's disease. Gastroenterology. 1993;104:A797.
18. Dvorak AM, Silen W. Differentiation between Crohn's disease and other inflammatory conditions by electron-microscopy. Ann Surg. 1985;201:53–63.
19. Brewer DB, Thompson H, Haynes IG, Alexander-Williams J. Axonal damage in Crohn's disease is frequent but not specific. J Pathol. 1990;161:301–11.
20. Dvorak AM. Ultrastructural pathology of Crohn's disease. In: Goebell H, Peskar BM, Malchow H, eds. Inflammatory Bowel Diseases – Basic Research and Clinical Implications. Falk symposium 46. Lancaster: MTP Press Limited; 1988:3–42.
21. Geboes K, Rutgeerts P, Ectors N et al. Major histocompatibility class II expression on the small intestinal nervous system in Crohn's disease. Gastroenterology. 1992;103:439–47.
22. Koretz K, Momburg F, Otto HF, Moller P. Sequential induction of MHC antigens on autochthonous cells of ileum affected by Crohn's disease. Am J Pathol. 1987;129:493–502.

23. Peeters TL, Van Assche G, Tack J, Depoortere I, Janssens J. Neuropeptide mediated regulation of gastrointestinal motility in the inflamed gut. NeuroGastroenterologia. 1997;3:50–60.
24. Bishop AE, Polak JM, Bryant MG, Bloom SR, Hamilton S. Abnormalities of vasoactive intestinal polypeptide containing nerves in Crohn's disease. Gastroenterology. 1980;79:853–60.
25. Annese V, Bassotti G, Napolitano G et al. Most patients with inactive Crohn's disease have gastrointestinal motility disorders. Gastroenterology. 1993;104:A470.
26. Mourelle M, Casellas F, Guarnar F et al. Induction of nitric oxide synthase in colonic smooth muscle from patients with toxic megacolon. Gastroenterology. 1995;109:1497–502.
27. Geboes K, Mebis J, Rutgeerts P, Ectors N, Vantrappen G. Demonstration of nitric oxide positive neurons in Crohn's disease. Gastroenterology. 1993;104:A705.
28. Belai A, Boulos PB, Robson T, Burnstock G. Neurochemical coding in the small intestine of patients with Crohn's disease. Gut. 1997;40:767–74.
29. Rachmilewitz D, Stamler JS, Bachwich D, Karmeli F, Ackerman Z, Podolsky DK. Enhanced colonic nitric oxide generation and nitric oxide synthase activity in ulcerative colitis and Crohn's disease. Gut. 195;36:718–23.
30. Siemers PT, Dobbins W. The Meissner's plexus in Crohn's disease of the colon. Surg Gynecol Obstet. 1974;138:39–42.
31. Stead RH, Dixon MF, Bramwell NH, Riddell RH, Bienenstock J. Mast cells are closely apposed to nerves in the human gastrointestinal mucosa. Gastroenterology. 1989;97:575–85.
32. Geboes K, Rutgeerts P, Penninckx F, Desmet V, Vantrappen G. The destruction of the autonomous nervous system in Crohn's disease is due to immunologic effector cells. Gastroenterology. 1989;96:A168.
33. Antonius JL, Gump FE, Lattes R, Lepore M. A study of certain microscopic features in regional enteritis, and their possible prognostic significance. Gastroenterology. 1960;38:889–905.
34. Rutgeerts P, Geboes K, Vantrappen G, Kerremans R, Coenegrachts JL, Coremans G. Natural history of recurrent Crohn's disease at the ileocolonic anastomosis after curative surgery. Gut. 1984;25:665–72.
35. Geboes K, Rutgeerts P, Vantrappen G, Kerremans R. Early lesions in the neoterminal ileum after Crohn's resection do not originate from identifiable microscopic inflammation. Gastroenterology. 1986;90:1424.
36. Klein O, Colombel JF, Lescut D et al. Remaining small bowel endoscopic lesions at surgery have no influence on early anastomotic recurrence in Crohn's disease. Am J Gastroenterol. 1995;90:1949–52.
37. Wolff BG, Beart RW, Frydenberg HB, Weiland LH, Agrez MV, Ilstrup DM. The importance of disease-free margins in resections for Crohn's disease. Dis Colon Rectum. 1983;26:239–43.
38. Goldman H. Evaluation of resection margins in Crohn's disease. Surg Pathol. 1988;1:75–6.
39. Geboes K, Rutgeerts P, Ectors N, Mebis J, Desmet V, Vantrappen G. Are section margins useful for the prediction of recurrence of Crohn's disease after all? Gastroenterology. 1990;98:A171.
40. D'Haens G, Colpaert S, Peeters M et al. The presence and severity of neural inflammation predict postoperative recurrence of Crohn's disease. Gastroenterology. 1998;114:A964.
41. Van Assche G, Depoortere I, De Vos R et al. Region specific anti-proliferative effect of VIP and PACAP$_{38}$ on rabbit enteric smooth muscle. Am J Physiol. (submitted).
42. Bishop AE, Polak JM, Bryant MG, Bloom SR, Hamilton S. Abnormalities of vasoactive intestinal polypeptide-containing nerves in Crohn's disease. Gastroenterology. 1980;79:853–60.
43. O'Morain C, Bishop AE, McGregor GP et al. Vasoactive intestinal polypeptide concentrations and immunocytochemical studies in rectal biopsies from patients with inflammatory bowel disease. Gut. 1984;25:57–61.
44. Desreumaux P, Capron M. Eosinophils in allergic reactions. Curr Opin Immunol. 1996;8:790–5.
45. Rutgeerts P, Geboes K, Vantrappen G, Kerremans R, Coenegrachts JL, Coremans G. Natural history of recurrent Crohn's disease at the ileocolonic anastomosis after curative surgery. Gut. 1984;25:665–72.
46. Dubucquoi S, Janin A, Klein O et al. Activated eosinophils and interleukin 5 expression in early recurrence of Crohn's disease. Gut. 1995;37:242–6.
47. Desreumaux P, Brandt E, Gambiez L et al. Distinct cytokine patterns in early and chronic ileal lesions of Crohn's disease. Gastroenterology. 1997;113:118–26.
48. Carol M, Lambrechts A, Van Gossum A, Libin M, Goldman M, Mascart-Lemoine F. Spontaneous secretion of interferon gamma and interleukin 4 by human intraepithelial and lamina propria gut lymphocytes. Gut. 1998;42:643–9.

7
The infectious track in inflammatory bowel diseases

J.-F. COLOMBEL, P. BULOIS, E. LEDERMAN,
P. DESREUMAUX, A. DARFEUILLE-MICHAUD,
H. J. VAN KRUININGEN and A. CORTOT

Since its definition in 1932, it has been recognized that CD contains elements that are often the result of microbial processes in the gut[1–3]. These include evidence of onset in the Peyer's patches and in the lymphoid aggregates of the colon (where many agents find entrance), ulcerations, microabscesses, fissures, fistulas, granulomas and lymphangitis. Fujimura *et al.*, using magnifying colonoscopy, electron microscopy and immunohistochemistry, recently confirmed that ulcerations in colonic Crohn's disease originate in the follicle-associated epithelium of colonic lymphoid nodules[4]. Aphthoid ulcers represent the earliest lesions and these we know to occur in viral and bacterial infections (rotavirus, astrovirus, torovirus, adenovirus, measles virus, *Salmonella, Shigella, Yersinia* and *Escherichia coli*). The lesions of CD occur in segments that suggest the distribution of Peyer's patches. When the age-related incidence of CD is plotted, the greatest case frequency occurs between 15 and 25 years which parallels a similar peak representing the number of Peyer's patches as a function of age[5]. Recent studies in animal models have led to the widespread belief that microbial constituents provide the antigenic stimulus in IBD and, at present, the most admitted hypothesis is that chronic inflammation results from an abnormal host immune response to normal luminal flora. Although present data do not convincingly incriminate a single persistent pathogen as a universal cause of IBD, this hypothesis should not be abandoned. Our current understanding of the complexity of the intestinal flora is very limited and it is quite possible that one or more aetiological agents for IBD exist but have not been detected[6]. Several epidemiological studies have suggested a causal role of infectious factors in CD[7].

We will review in this paper the infectious agents which have been implicated in the aetiology of IBD over the last few years.

MYCOBACTERIA

The aetiological role of mycobacteria in CD has been a controversial issue for some time. In 1984, Chiodini *et al.* recovered slow-growing *Mycobacterium paratuberculosis* from tissues of three patients with CD[8]. It was encouraging when other laboratories also recovered this organism, albeit rarely. Now, 15 years later, the data do not strongly support this hypothesis since:

1. Six separate immunocytochemistry studies on varied groups of patients have failed to find *M. paratuberculosis* in the diseased tissues.

2. Numerous serological studies have failed to document elevated titres or changes in titre related to disease activity.

3. With the exception of a paper from Italy by Prantera *et al.*[9], controlled trials with antibiotics directed against mycobacteria have failed to make patients well – and the improvement in Prantera's patients may reflect a broad-spectrum antibiotic effect on secondary invaders (Table 1). A recent 5-year follow-up study of patients receiving rifampicin, isoniazid and ethambutol for up to two years was unable to show any benefit in treated patients[19]. When antibiotics other than those specific for mycobacteria were given to patients, as single broad-spectrum drugs or as combinations, several groups reported remission or significant clinical improvement. Clarithromycin alone[16], rifabutin with clarithromycin or azithromycin[17] and rifabutin with clarithromycin and clofazimine[18] were effective in a proportion of patients. However, these workers failed to show that they were treating infection with mycobacteria.

4. Dairy cattle with Johne's disease shed great numbers of *M. paratuberculosis* into the environment and it has been reported that *M. paratuberculosis* strains isolated from patients with CD had a common clonal origin with strains isolated from cows with Johne's disease[20]. However, there has never been a recorded case of CD occurring in farm help or farm families (including children) associated with these herds (although no epidemiological study could be found that specifically examined whether this association exists).

5. Studies involving the use of PCR techniques to amplify the IS900 insertion sequence, specific for *M. paratuberculosis*, have given controversial results (Table 2). Sanderson *et al.* reported that 65% of CD, 4% of ulcerative colitis (UC), and 13% of control tissues had detectable DNA[21]. This observation was confirmed by Dell'Isola *et al.* who detected IS900 sequences in intestinal tissues of 72% of children with CD but also 20% of UC and 29% of diseased controls, suggesting contamination[22]. Other groups reported much lower detection rates and we failed to detect any IS900 sequences in mesenteric lymph nodes from 19 patients operated on for CD[31]. Very recently, using the same technique, no association between *M. paratuberculosis* and oral lesions of CD was found[32].

At the present time, the possibility remains that only a specifically susceptible subset of CD patients might have a mycobacterial aetiology. Along this line, in the study by Fidler *et al.*, CD specimens containing granulomas were more likely to have positive PCR results than specimens without granulomas[24].

Table 1 Therapeutic trials with antimycobacterial drugs in Crohn's disease

Year	First author	No. of patients	Drugs	Duration	Results
1982	Elliott[10]*	51	Sulphadoxine, pyrimethamine	12 months	No CDAI improvement
1984	Shaffer[11]*	27 (cross over)	Rifampicin, ethambutol	12 months	No CDAI improvement
1989	Hampson[12]	20	Rifampicin, ethambutol, isoniazid, pyrazinamide	9 months	CDAI improvement: 50% Steroid requirement: 10/20 before treatment 1/20 after treatment
1991	Afdhal[13]*	49	Clofazimine	8 months	Disease remission (CDAI): Active treatment: 16/25 Placebo: 12/24 (NS)
1992	Rutgeerts[14]	16	Rifabutin, ethambutol	6 months	No endoscopic improvement No significant CDAI improvement
1994	Prantera[9]*	40	Rifampicin, ethambutol, clofazimine, dapsone	9 months	Clinical relapse: Active treatment: 3/19 Placebo: 11/17 ($p = 0.03$)
1994	Swift[15]*	126	Rifampicin, ethambutol, isoniazid	≥2 years	No significant differences in: CDAI, prednisolone requirement, surgery requirement, haematological measurements
1995	Graham[16]*	15 (cross over)	Clarithromycin	3 months	CDAI improvement
1997	Gui[17]	52	Rifabutin, clarithromycin or azithromycin	6–35 months	CDAI improvement at 6 and 24 months ($p<0.001$)
1998	Borody[18]	12	Rifabutin, clarithromycin, clafazimine	8–12 months	Harvey–Bradshaw index improvement ($p<0.0001$)

* Controlled trials

Table 2 Evidence for *Mycobacterium paratuberculosis* DNA (IS900) in Crohn's disease tissue

Year	First author (reference)	Country	CD*	UC*	Controls*
1992	Sanderson[21]	UK	26/40	1/23	5/40
1994	Dell'Isola[22]	France	13/18	1/5	7/24
1994	Lisby[23]	Denmark	11/24	2/10	3/28
1994	Fidler[24]	UK	4/31	0/10	0/20
1994	Yokoyama[25]	Japan	4/10	—	—
1995	Rowbotham[26]	UK	0/68	0/49	1/26
1995	Suenaga[27]	Japan	10/10	11/18	14/16
1996	Franck[28]	USA	0/23	—	—
1996	Dumonceau[29]	Belgium	17/36	6/13	13/23
1997	Al-Shamali[30]	Kuwait	0/10	0/6	0/21
1998	Bulois[31]	France	0/19	—	—

*, Positives/number tested; CD, Crohn's disease; UC, ulcerative colitis

VASCULITIS AND THE MEASLES VIRUS

A more recent thrust at discovery has been the work of Wakefield *et al.* from London, first put forward 8 years ago, when it was proposed that microvascular occlusion constitutes the earliest lesion and basis of CD. Arterial perfusion–fixation and immunostaining of vascular units in resected intestine from patients with CD demonstrated a widespread vasculitic process which may give rise to multifocal gastrointestinal infarction. Granulomatous and lymphocytic damage to intramural blood vessels, even in macroscopically normal areas, was observed. Possible mechanisms were proposed by which a chronic ischaemic process may explain some of the characteristics of CD, including skip lesions, transmural inflammation, aphthoid ulcerations, anastomotic recurrence and the prominence of ulcerations along the mesenteric border (reviewed in Reference 33).

A further step in the work from this group was the proposal that CD may be a persistent measles virus-induced granulomatous vasculitis. Paramyxovirus-like structures were recognized in the vascular endothelium of Crohn's patients[34]. Measles virus antigen and mRNA were localized to granulomas and endothelial cells by *in-situ* hybridization[34], immunofluorescence[35] and immunogold electron microscopy[36,37]. Antimeasles antibody was reported to be elevated in CD patients[38]. Epidemiological arguments support the hypothesis. Early exposure to measles virus was associated with an increased risk of CD[39] and live-attenuated measles vaccination was also implicated[40]. More recently, Ekbom *et al.* reported an apparently strong association between prenatal exposure to measles and CD later in life[41].

However, the interpretation of studies implicating measles virus in CD has been challenged (Table 3). Over the past few years, it has been shown by us and others that blood vascular units are not primary sites of CD[42,43] and attention has been refocused on lymphatic vasculature, the obstruction of which leads to chronic oedema, fibrosis, contracture and ulceration of a segment of intestine[42,44]. The presence of measles virus in the tissues has not been confirmed by independent investigators[45] and measles viral genomic sequences could not be

Table 3 Implication of measles virus in Crohn's disease?

Pros	*Cons*
Excess number of CD patients in those born up to 3 months after measles epidemic in Sweden[39]	No association between the development of CD and exposure to a measles epidemic in England[51]
Increased risk of IBD in individuals given live attenuated measles vaccine in early childhood[40]	Rise in the incidence of CD in England, Wales and Scotland antedated the introduction of measles vaccination[52]
	Several methodological biases put forward in the measles vaccine study
	No association between measles vaccination in a case–control study in UK[53]
3/4 babies whose mothers had measles infection during pregnancy subsequently developed severe CD[41]	No case of IBD in a large cohort of individuals exposed to viral infections during gestation[54]
	No case of CD among offspring of 25 women who had measles in pregnancy in a Danish hospital[55]
Antimeasles antibody elevated in CD patients[38]	No increased IgM-specific measles virus antibody in French families with a high frequency of CD[50]
Measles virus antigen and mRNA localized to granulomas and endothelial cells in intestinal tissues of patients with CD using *in-situ* hybridization[34], immunofluorescence[35] and immunogold electron microscopy[36,37]	No immunolabelling with a specific anti-MV monoclonal antibody in the tissues of patients with CD[45]
	Using PCR, measles virus genomic sequence not detected in intestinal tissue from CD in 3 different studies[46–48]

detected in intestinal tissue from CD by PCR[46–48]. Iizuka *et al.* recently proposed that previous positive immunohistochemical reactivity can be accounted for by antigen mimicry between measles virus and an undefined host protein in the intestine of CD[49]. Using serological studies, we saw no titres that would suggest measles virus participation in families with a high frequency of CD[50]. Finally, three recent epidemiological studies of the association between measles and CD have failed to confirm the original association. A case–control study by Feeney *et al.* in 1997 compared measles vaccination rates in 140 patients with IBD (83 with CD) and matched controls and found no association[53]. Jones *et al.* reported a case–control study of a large cohort of individuals exposed to viral infections during gestation, including 47 people exposed to measles *in utero*. Follow-up data on 88% found no cases of IBD in the index cases, but two among the controls[54]. Nielsen *et al.* examined the health records of all possible cases of measles in pregnancy admitted to an infectious diseases hospital in the Copenhagen area between 1915–1966. The offspring of 25 women who had measles during pregnancy were identified; none had developed CD[55]. Thus, the theory of measles as a causative factor in the development of CD is difficult to uphold at present[56].

LISTERIA

There has been renewed interest in the transmittable-agent hypothesis after a report of CD occuring in multiple siblings of two French families within a short time period[57]. When a polyclonal antibody against *Listeria monocytogenes* was applied to the tissues of patients with CD, including those of these families, antigen was demonstrated in 75% but not in controls[45]. The labelling for *Listeria* ocurred in many important locales, such as macrophages in the lymphoid follicles of Peyer's patches, adjacent to new ulcers, along fistulas, around microabscesses and in granulomas. It is not clear, however, whether the labelling was specific for *L. monocytogenes* or recognized other *Listeria* spp. or any other crossreacting invasive bacterium. Serology demonstrated high (>1/800) anti-listeriolysin-O titres with a four-fold greater frequency in the French family patients than in age- and sex-matched controls[58]. *Listeria* are ubiquitous (in foods, animals and the environment), are known to invade via M cells in Peyer's patches, and to produce ileitis or colitis in several animal species. In a study of oral *Listeria* infection in HLA-B27 transgenic rats and their non-transgenic counterparts, those with the B27 susceptibility genes developed ulcerative disease of the distal GI tract and numerous microabscesses and granulomas of the liver and spleen[59]. *Listeria monocytogenes* has been recently incriminated in an outbreak of gastroenteritis and fever in the US[60]. Given the intracellular growth capabilities of *Listeria*, it would seem unlikely that they never sequester and cause chronic disease. More studies are now needed but there are several data that mitigate against the hypothesis that *Listeria* are important in CD: *Listeria* have never been cultivated from CD intestinal tissues and there is no association in the literature between the occurrence of CD and *Listeria* meningoencephalitis or abortion.

HELICOBACTER HEPATICUS

Since the discovery of *H. pylori*, interest in other *Helicobacter* species has increased. *H. hepaticus* is a murine pathogen which can induce colitis and hepatitis in immunodeficient mice and in germ-free monoinfected mice[61]. *Scid* mice reconstituted with CD4+ T cells develop severe colitis when maintained in conventional conditions. In this model, the combination of *H. hepaticus* infection and CD45RB-high CD4+ T cells reconstitution resulted in severe disease expression[62]. A group of *Helicobacter* species has also been identified from the lower gastrointestinal tract of humans and, in the case of two species, *H. cinaedi* and *H. fenelliae*, human infection has been associated with colitis and proctitis in homosexual men[63,64]. However, the presence of *H. hepaticus* has no effect on the development of PF-induced colitis in IL-10-deficient mice[65]. *H. hepaticus* does not appear to influence chronic intestinal inflammation in mice with functioning T lymphocytes, and no *Helicobacter* species has been isolated so far from faeces or mucosal samples of patients with IBD.

YEASTS

Systemic antibodies to various dietary and bacterial antigens have been reported in sera from patients with CD and UC. Using ELISA which employs whole killed yeasts cells as antigens, elevated anti-*Saccharomyces cerevisiae* IgA and IgG levels were reported in the sera from patients with CD but not from patients with UC[66–68]. In 1996, we showed that this serological response recognizes mannose sequences in the cell wall mannan of a *S. cerevisiae* strain Su1 (formerly *S. uvarum* 1, a species now classified within *S. cerevisiae*)[69]. Using the crude mannan from this strain as an antigen in ELISA, we found that testing for the presence of anti-*S. cerevisiae* mannan antibodies (designated as ASCA) was 64% sensitive and 77% specific for discriminating CD from UC and 89% specific for distinguishing CD from controls[70]. Furthermore, the presence of ASCA in 20% of healthy relatives of patients with CD suggested that these antibodies could be a subclinical marker of CD[71]. Different hypotheses concerning the origin of ASCA can be proposed[69]. The first is that ASCA may originate from immunization by yeasts. A clinical study suggested that inclusion or exclusion of baker's yeast from the diet may influence the activity of CD[72]. Investigations concerning an antigenic stimulation from yeasts that colonize the digestive tract have been limited. An absence of specific serological reactivity against *Candida albicans* has been documented in CD. However, strains used as antigens belonged to the *C. albicans* serotype A, which accounts for only 60–80% of human *C. albicans* isolates. A second hypothesis worth testing is that yeast mannan oligomannosides could correspond to epitopes shared by other micro-organisms. Finally, the ubiquitous character of mannose residue sequences raised a third hypothesis: some *S. cerevisiae* oligomannosides could share structural homologies with oligomannosides expressed on human glycoconjugates as autoantigens or neoautoantigens.

ENDOGENOUS BACTERIA

Abundant experimental and clinical data incriminate normal luminal bacteria or bacterial products in the initiation and perpetuation of chronic intestinal inflammation[1–3]. The most convincing evidence of the potential role of bacteria comes from genetically engineered rodent models that develop intestinal inflammation as a result of disrupted cytokine genes or due to the expression of human HLA-B27/β_2-microglobulin. In these models, inflammation is absent or attenuated when animals are kept under germ-free conditions[73–75]. In humans, there is evidence from bacteriological culture, serology, immunohistochemistry and pathology that bacteria are involved, at least as secondary invaders, in the pathogenesis of CD[3]. Bacterial flora may also play a primary role. Endoscopic studies after surgery have suggested that bacteria are important in recurrence: diverting ileostomy prevents postoperative recurrence, which rapidly occurs after reanastomosis[76–78]. We have recently shown that, in this situation, the neoterminal ileum is heavily colonized by a colonic-like bacterial flora with prominent species being *Bacteroides*, *Clostridium* and *Escherichia coli*[79].

All bacterial species may not have equal activity in inducing inflammation. Defined flora studies showed that *Bacteroides* spp. preferentially induce colitis in

HLA-B27 transgenic rats[80]. In the study by D'Haens *et al.*[77], the ileal effluent which triggered postoperative recurrence of CD contained 6×10^4/ml *Bacteroides* spp. Among the numerous bacteria of the intestinal flora, *E. coli* has also been thought to be involved. Tabaqchali *et al.* showed that *E. coli* antibody titres were higher in patients with CD than in controls[81]. When bacteriological sampling was undertaken at surgery for CD, before opening of the bowel, *E. coli* were recovered from 18–31% of mesenteric lymph nodes[82,83]. Using immunocytochemistry, Cartun *et al.* observed *E. coli* antigen in 69% of 16 diseased intestinal resection specimens[84]. In a follow-up study of resected tissues from the two French families with a high frequency of CD and from patients in Connecticut, Liu *et al.* found *E. coli* antigen in 57%[45]. *E. coli* is the predominant aerobic Gram-negative species of the normal intestinal flora but is also involved in intestinal disease. Diarrhoeagenic *E. coli* differ from those normally resident in the colon in possessing distinct virulence properties, such as the production of enterotoxins and cytotoxins, tissue invasion and adherence to enterocytes[85,86]. In poultry, mucoid strains of *E. coli* are believed to be the cause of Hjarre's disease, an intestinal disease characterized by tuberculosis-like granulomas of the intestine and liver[87]. A granulomatous colitis that resembles malakoplakia (the latter associated with *E. coli* 075) occurs in dogs of the Boxer breed. Immunocytochemistry has demonstrated that the macrophages that characterize this disease are rich in *E. coli* antigen[88].

We recently characterized several *E. coli* isolates that were recovered from ileal mucosa of patients with CD[89]. Our findings first indicate that *E. coli* strains associated with the ileal mucosa of patients with CD adhere preferentially to differentiated Caco-2 cells, corresponding to mature intestinal cells. The preferential adhesion to differentiated Caco-2 cells may explain the discrepancy in published results concerning the adherence ability of *E. coli* isolated from patients with CD[90–93]. Most of the studies were performed with strains isolated from faeces or rectal biopsies and the adhesion tests were mostly performed with buccal epithelial cells or the Hep-2 cell line, which would appear to us to be less relevant than Caco-2 cells. The adhesion that we observed was mannose resistant and *E. coli* strains associated with the ileum of patients with CD harboured adhesins different from those of *E. coli* that occur in acute infections of the gastrointestinal tract of humans and animals and in infections of the urinary tract in humans (for a review, see Reference 94). The identification of the adhesins involved was performed by PCR experiments with several sets of primers specific to the structural genes encoding known adhesins. Of the 30 strains isolated from patients with CD that adhered to differentiated intestinal cells, 22 strains (73%) harboured an adhesin that was not identified by the use of molecular techniques using the different DNA probes or primers for the *E. coli* adhesins described so far. In order to identify additional virulence factors of the *E. coli* strains that are associated with CD, hybridization tests or PCR experiments with various DNA probes or primers for the different virulence factors encoding genes of *E. coli* strains involved in acute gastrointestinal tract diseases were performed. None of the *E. coli* strains isolated from biopsies of patients with CD possess any of the virulence genes harboured by enterotoxinogenic, enteroinvasive, enterohaemorrhagic, enteroaggregative or enteropathogenic *E. coli* strains. It was recently reported that enterohaemorragic *E. coli* O157:H7 infection can mimic CD[95] but none of the *E. coli* strains we recovered harboured any of the virulence factors of *E. coli* O157:H7. A cytotoxic effect in cultured intestinal cells was observed after a 3-h incubation with these new *E. coli* strains. DNA hybridization experiments with the various probes corresponding to known cytotoxin-encoding genes revealed a positive hybridization with the α-haemolysin probe for 21.8% of the stains. The *E. coli* α-haemolysin has been shown to represent a potent stimulus for the release of inflammatory mediators like O_2^-, β-glucuronidase and leukotriene from human polymorphonuclear granulocytes or histamine from human lymphocyte/monocyte basophil cells[96]. The combination of adhesive ability and synthesis of a cytotoxin would allow the bacteria to colonize intestinal epithelium, damage intestinal cells and participate in the inflammatory disease.

References

1. Sartor RB. Microbial factors in the pathogenesis of Crohn's disease, ulcerative colitis and experimental intestinal inflammation. In: Kirsner JB, Shorter RG, editors. Inflammatory Bowel Disease, 4th edn. Baltimore: Williams & Wilkins; 1995:96–124.
2. Sartor RB. Enteric microflora in IBD: pathogens or commensals? Inflam Bowel Dis. 1997;3:230–5.
3. Van Kruiningen HJ. On the use of antibiotics in Crohn's disease. J Clin Gastroenterol. 1995;20:310–16.
4. Fujimura Y, Kamoi R, Iida M *et al.* Pathogenesis of aphthoid ulcers in Crohn's disease: correlative findings by magnifying colonoscopy, electron microscopy, and immunohistochemistry. Gut. 1996;38:724–32.
5. Van Kruiningen HJ, Ganley L, Freda BJ. The role of Peyer's patches in the age-related incidence of Crohn's disease. J Clin Gastroenterol. 1997;24:470–5.
6. Blaser MJ. Microbial causation of the chronic idiopathic inflammatory bowel diseases. Inflam Bowel Dis. 1997;3:225–9.
7. Colombel JF, Louvet B, Müller-Allouf H, Desreumaux P. Recent advances in the etiology of Crohn's disease. Environment and genetics. In: Galmiche JP, Gournay J, editors. Recent Advances in the Pathophysiology of Gastro-Intestinal and Liver Diseases. Paris: John Libbey Eurotext; 1997:109–31.
8. Chiodini RJ, Van Kruiningen HJ, Thayer Jr. WR, Merkal RS, Coutu JA. Possible role of mycobacteria in inflammatory bowel disease. I. An unclassified *Mycobacterium* species isolated from patients with Crohn's disease. Dig Dis Sci. 1984;29:1073–9.
9. Prantera C, Kohn A, Mangiarotti R, Andreoli A, Luzi C. Antimycobacterial therapy in Crohn's disease: results of a controlled, double-blind trial with multiple antibiotic regimen. Am J Gastroenterol. 1994;89:513–18.
10. Elliott PR, Burnham WR, Berghouse LM, Lennard-Jones JE, Langman MJS. Sulphadoxine–pyrimethamine therapy in Crohn's disease. Digestion. 1983;23:132–4.
11. Shaffer JL, Hughes S, Linaker BD *et al.* Controlled trial of rifampicin and ethambutol in Crohn's disease. Gut. 1984;25:203–5.
12. Hampson SJ, Parker MC, Saverymuttu SH *et al.* Quadruple antimycobacterial chemotherapy in Crohn's disease: results at 9 months of a pilot study in 20 patients. Aliment Pharmacol Ther. 1989;3:343–52.
13. Afdhal NH, Long A, Lennon J *et al.* Controlled trial of antimycobacterial therapy in Crohn's disease. Dig Dis Sci. 1991;36:449–53.
14. Rutgeerts P, Geboes K, Vantrappen G *et al.* Rifabutin and ethambutol do not help recurrent Crohn's disease in the neoterminal ileum. J. Clin Gastroenterol. 1992;15:24–8.
15. Swift GL, Srivastava ED, Stone R *et al.* Controlled trial of anti-tuberculous chemotherapy for two years in Crohn's disease. Gut. 1994;35:363–8.
16. Graham DY, Al Assi MT, Robinson M. Prolonged remission in Crohn's disease following therapy for *Mycobacterium paratuberculosis*. Gastroenterology. 1995;108:A826.
17. Gui GP, Thomas PR, Tizzard ML *et al.* Two years outcome analysis of Crohn's disease treated with rifabutin and macrolides antibiotics. J Antimicrobiol Chemother. 1997;39:393–400.
18. Borody TJ, Pearce L, Bampton PA, Leis S. Treatment of severe Crohn's disease using rifabutin–macrolide–clofazimine combination: interim report. Gastroenterology. 1998;114:A938.

19. Thomas GAO, Swift GL, Green JT *et al.* Controlled trial of antituberculous chemotherapy in Crohn's disease: a five year follow up study. Gut. 1998;42:497–500.

20. Francois B, Krishnamoorthy R, Elion J. Comparative study of *Mycobacterium paratuberculosis* strains isolated from Crohn's disease and Johne's disease using restriction fragment length polymorphism and arbitrarily primed PCR. Epidemiol Infect. 1997;118:227–33.

21. Sanderson JD, Moss MT, Tizard MLV, Hermon-Taylor J. *Mycobacterium paratuberculosis* DNA in Crohn's disease tissue. Gut. 1992;33:890–6.

22. Dell'Isola B, Poyart C, Goulet O *et al.* Detection of *Mycobacterium paratuberculosis* by polymerase chain reaction in children with Crohn's disease. J Infect Dis. 1994;169:449–51.

23. Lisby G, Andersen J, Engbaek K, Binder V. *Mycobacterium paratuberculosis* in intestinal tissue from patients with Crohn's disease demonstrated by nested primer polymerase chain reaction. Scand J Gastroenterol. 1994;29:923–9.

24. Fidler HM, Thurrel W, McIJohnson N, Rook GAW, McFadden JJ. Specific detection of *Mycobacterium paratuberculosis* DNA associated with granulomatous tissue in Crohn's disease. Gut. 1994;35:506–10.

25. Yokoyama Y, Kino J, Okazaki K, Yamamoto Y. Mycobacteria in the human intestine. Gut. 1994;35:715–16.

26. Rowbotham DS, Mapstone NP, Treijdosiewicz LK, Howdle PD, Quirke P. *Mycobacterium paratuberculosis* DNA not detected in Crohn's disease tissue by fluorescent polymerase chain reaction. Gut. 1995;37:660–7.

27. Suenaga K, Yokoyama Y, Okazaki K, Yamamoto Y. Mycobacteria in the intestine of Japanese patients with inflammatory bowel disease. Am J Gastroenterol. 1995;90:76–80.

28. Franck TS, Cook SM. Analysis of paraffin sections of Crohn's disease for *Mycobacterium paratuberculosis* using polymerase chain reaction. Mod Pathol. 1996;9:32–5.

29. Dumonceau JM, Van Gossum A, Adler M *et al.* No *Mycobacterium paratuberculosis* found in Crohn's disease using the polymerase chain reaction. Dig Dis Sci. 1996;41:421–6.

30. Al-Shamali M, Khan I, Al-Nakib B, Al-Hassan F, Mustafa AS. A multiplex polymerase chain reaction assay for detection of *Mycobacterium paratuberculosis* DNA in Crohn's disease tissue. Scand J Gastroenterol. 1997;32:819–23.

31. Bulois P, Poyart C, Desreumaux P *et al.* Absence de détection par PCR de bactérie dans les ganglions mésentériques de patients opérés pour maladie de Crohn. Gastroenterol Clin Biol. 1998;22:A11.

32. Riggio MP, Gibson J, Lennon A *et al.* Search for *Mycobacterium paratuberculosis* DNA in orofacial granuloma and oral Crohn's disease tissue by PCR. Gut. 1997;41:646–50.

33. Wakefield AJ, Ekbom A, Dhillon AP, Pittilo RM, Pounder RE. Crohn's disease: pathogenesis and persistent measles virus infection. Gastroenterology. 1995;108:911–16.

34. Wakefield AJ, Pittilo RM, Sim R *et al.* Evidence of persistent measles virus infection in Crohn's disease. J Med Virol. 1993;39:345–53.

35. Miyamoto H, Tanaka T, Kitamoto N, Fukada Y, Takashi S. Detection of immunoreactive antigen with monoclonal antibody to measles virus in tissue from patients with Crohn's disease. J Gastroenterol. 1995;30:28–33.

36. Lewin J, Dhillon AP, Sim R, Mazure G, Pounder RE, Wakefield AJ. Persistent measles virus infection of the intestine: confirmation by immunogold electronmicroscopy. Gut. 1995;36:564–9.

37. Daszak P, Purcell M, Lewin J *et al.* Detection and comparative analysis of persistent measles virus infection in Crohn's disease by immunogold electron microscopy. J Clin Pathol. 1997;50:299–304.

38. Balzola F, Castellino F, Colombatto P *et al.* IgM antibody against measles virus in patients with inflammatory bowel disease: a marker of virus related disease? Eur J Gastroenterol Hepatol. 1997;9:660–3.

39. Ekbom A, Wakefield AJ, Zack M, Adami HO. Perinatal measles infection and subsequent Crohn's disease. Lancet. 1994;344:508–10.

40. Thompson N, Montgomery S, Pounder RE, Wakefield AJ. Is measles vaccination a risk factor for Crohn's disease? Lancet. 1995;345:1071–4.

41. Ekbom A, Daszak P, Kraaz W, Wakefield AJ. Crohn's disease after in-utero measles virus exposure. Lancet. 1996;348:515–17.

42. Talbot IC, Kamm MA, Leaker BR. Pathogenesis of Crohn's disease. Lancet. 1992;340:315–16.

43. Matson AP, Van Kruinigen HJ, West AB, Cartun RW, Colombel JF, Cortot A. The relationship of granulomas to blood vessels in intestinal Crohn's disease. Modern Pathol. 1995;8:680–5.

44. Mooney EE, Walter J, Hourihane DO'B. Relation of granulomas to lymphatic vessels in Crohn's disease. J Clin Pathol. 1995;48:335–8.

45. Liu Y, Van Kruiningen HJ, West AB, Cartun RW, Cortot A, Colombel JF. Immunocytochemical evidence of *Listeria, Escherichia coli* and *Streptococcus* antigens in Crohn's disease. Gastroenterology. 1995;108:1396–404.

46. Haga Y, Funakoshi O, Kuroe K *et al.* Absence of measles viral genomic sequence in intestinal tissues from Crohn's disease by nested polymerase chain reaction. Gut. 1996;38:211–15.

47. Iizuka M, Nakagomi O, Chiba M *et al.* Absence of measles virus in Crohn's disease. Lancet. 1995;345:199.

48. Armitage E, Afzal M, Minor P *et al.* Absence of measles virus genome in tissue and peripheral blood lymphocytes from patients with Crohn's disease. Gastroenterology. 1998;114:A922.

49. Iizuka M, Masamune O. Measles vaccination and inflammatory bowel disease. Lancet. 1997;350:1775.

50. Touze Y, Dubucquoi, Cortot A, Van Kruiningen HJ, Colombel JF. IgM-specific measles-virus antibody in families with a high frequency of Crohn's disease. Lancet. 1995;346:967.

51. Hermon-Taylor J, Ford J, Sumar N, Millar D, Doran T, Tizard M. Measles virus and Crohn's disease. Lancet. 1995;345:922–3.

52. Thompson NP, Pounder RE, Wakefield A. Perinatal and childhood risk factors for inflamatory bowel disease: a case-control study. Eur J Gastroenterol Hepatol. 1995;7:385–90.

53. Feeney M, Clegg A, Winwood P, Snook J. A case control study of measles vaccination in inflammatory bowel disease. Lancet. 1997;350:764–6.

54. Jones P, Fine P, Piracha S. Crohn's disease and measles. Lancet. 1997;349:473.

55. Nielsen LLW, Nielsen LM, Melbye M, Sodermann M, Jacobsen M, Aaby P. Exposure to measles in utero and Crohn's disease: a Danish register study. Br Med J. 1998;316:515–17.

56. Metcalf J. Is measles infection associated with Crohn's disease? Br Med J. 1998;316:166.

57. Van Kruiningen HJ, Colombel JF, Cartun RW *et al.* An in-depth study of Crohn's disease in two French families. Gastroenterology. 1993;104:351–60.

58. Van Kruiningen HJ, Colombel JF, Cortot A. La piste infectieuse au cours des maladies inflammatoires de l'intestin. Res Clin Forums. 1995;17:37–44.

59. Warner T, Madsen J, Starling J, Wagner RD, Taurog JD, Balish E. Human HLA-B27 gene enhances susceptibility of rats to oral infection by *Listeria monocytogenes*. Am J Pathol. 1996;149:1737–43.

60. Dalton CB, Austin CC, Sobel J *et al.* An outbreak of gastroenteritis and fever due to *Listeria monocytogenes* in milk. N Engl J Med. 1997;336:100–5.

61. Fox JG, Yan L, Shames B, Campbell J, Murphy JC, Li X. Persistent hepatitis and enterocolitis in germfree mice infected with *Helicobacter hepaticus*. Infect Immun. 1996;64:3673–81.

62. Cahill R, Foltz CJ, Fox JG, Dangler CA, Powrie F, Schauer DB. Inflammatory bowel disease: an immunity-mediated condition triggered by bacterial infection with *Helicobacter hepaticus*. Infect Immun. 1997;65:3126–31.

63. Fenell CL, Totten PA, Quinn TC, Patton DL, Holmes KK, Stamm WE. Characteristization of Campylobacter-like organisms isolated from homosexual men. J Infect Dis. 1984;149:58–66.

64. Totten PA, Fennel CL, Tenover FC *et al. Campylobacter cinaedi* (sp. nov) and *Campylobacter fennelliae* (sp. now): two new *Campylobacter* species associated with enteric disease in homosexual men. J Infect Dis. 1985;151:131–9.

65. Dieleman LA, Tonkonogy SL, Sellon RK, Sartor RB. Helicobacter hepaticus does not potentiate colitis in interleukin-10 deficient mice. Gastroenterology. 1998;114:965A.

66. Main J, McKenzie H, Yeaman GR *et al.* Antibody to *Saccharomyces cerevisiae* (baker's yeast) in Crohn's disease. Br Med J. 1988;297:1105–6.

67. Barnes RMR, Allan S, Taylor-Robinson CH, Finn R, Johnson PM. Serum antibodies reactive with *Saccharomyces cerevisiae* in inflammatory bowel disease. Is IgA antibody a marker for Crohn's disease? Int Arch Allergy Appl Immunol. 1990;92:9–15.

68. Giaffer MH, Clark A, Holdsworth CD. Antibodies to *Saccharomyces cerevisiae* in patients with Crohn's disease and their possible pathogenic importance. Gut. 1992;33:1071–5.

69. Sendid B, Colombel JF, Jacquinot PM *et al.* Specific antibody response to oligomannosidic epitopes in Crohn's disease. Clin Diag Lab Immunol. 1996;3:219–26.

70. Quinton JF, Sendid B, Reumaux D *et al.* Anti-*Saccharomyces cerevisiae* mannan combined with antineutrophil antibodies in inflammatory bowel disease: prevalence and diagnostic role. Gut. 1998;42:788–91.

71. Sendid B, Quinton JF, Charrier G *et al.* Anti-*Saccharomyces cerevisiae* mannan antibodies in familial Crohn's disease. Am J Gastroenterol. 1998;93:1306–10.

72. Barclay GRH, McKenzie J, Pennington D, Paratt D, Pennington CR. The effect of dietary yeast on the activity of stable chronic Crohn's disease. Scand J Gastroenterol. 1992;27:196–200.
73. Taurog JD, Richardson JA, Croft JT *et al.* The germfree state prevents development of gut and joint inflammatory disease in HLA-B27 transgenic rats. J Exp Med. 1994;180:2359–64.
74. Sellon R, Tonkogony S, Schultz M, Sartor RB. Absence of gastritis and colitis in germ-free IL-10 knockout mice. Gastroenterology. 1997;112:A1088.
75. Schultz M, Sellon RK, Tonkogony SL, Balish E, Sartor RB. IL-2 deficient mice raised under germfree conditions develop delayed mild focal intestinal inflammation and progressive loss of B cells. Gastroenterology. 1997;112:A1086.
76. Rutgeerts P, Goboes K, Peeters M *et al.* Effect of faecal stream diversion on recurrence of Crohn's disease in the neoterminal ileum. Lancet. 1991;338:771–4.
77. D'Haens G, Geboes K, Peeters M, Baert F, Penninckx F, Rutgeerts P. Early lesions of recurrent Crohn's disease caused by infusion of intestinal contents in excluded ileum. Gastroenterology. 1998;14:262–7.
78. Sartor RB. Postoperative recurrence of Crohn's disease: the enemy is within the faecal stream. Gastroenterology. 1998;114:398–407.
79. Lederman E, Neut C, Desreumaux P *et al.* Bacterial overgrowth in the neoterminal ileum after ileocolonic resection for Crohn's disease. Gastroenterology. 1997;112:A1023.
80. Rath HC, Herfarth HH, Ikeda JS *et al.* Normal luminal bacteria, especially Bacteroides species, mediate chronic colitis, gastritis, and arthritis in HLA-B27/human β2 microglobulin transgenic rats. J Clin Invest. 1996;98:945–53.
81. Tabaqchali S, O'Donoghue DP, Bettelheim KA. *Escherichia coli* antibodies in patients with inflammatory bowel disease. Gut. 1978;19:108–13.
82. Ambrose NS, Johnson M, Burdon DW, Keighley RB. Incidence of pathogenic bacteria from mesenteric lymphnodes and ileal serosa during Crohn's disease surgery. Br J Surg. 1984;71:623–5.
83. Laffineur G, Lescut D, Vincent P, Quandalle P, Wurtz A, Colombel JF. Translocation bactérienne dans la maladie de Crohn. Gastroenterol Clin Biol. 1992;16:777–81.
84. Cartun RW, Van Kruiningen HJ, Pedersen CA, Berman MM. An immunocytochemical search for infectious agents in Crohn's disease. Modern Pathol. 1993;6:212–19.
85. Levine MM. *Escherichia coli* that cause diarrhea: enterotoxigenic, enteropathogenic, enteroinvasive, enterohemorrhagic and enteroadherent. J Infect Dis. 1987;155:377–89.
86. Jallat C, Livrelli V, Darfeuille-Michaud A, Rich C, Joly B. *Escherichia coli* strains involved in diarrhea in France: high prevalence and heterogeneity of diffusely adhering strains. J Clin Microbiol. 1993;31:2031–7.
87. Hjärre A, Wramby G. Undersökningar över en med specifika granulom förlöpande hönssjukdom orsakad av mukoida kolibakterier (Koli-granulom). Skandinavish Veterinärtidskrijt. 1945;35:449–505.
88. Van Kruiningen HJ. Gastrointestinal system. In: McGavin MD, Carlton WW, editors, Special Veterinary Pathology, 2nd edn. St-Louis: Mosby; 1995;1–80.
89. Darfeuille-Michaud A, Neut C, Barnich N *et al.* Presence of adherent *Escherichia coli* strains in ileal mucosa of patients with Crohn's disease. Gastroenterology. 1998;115:1–10.
90. Burke DA, Axon ATR. Adhesive *Escherichia coli* inflammatory bowel disease and infective diarrhoea. Br Med J. 1988;297:102–4.
91. Giaffer MH, Holdsworth CD, Duerden BI. Virulence properties of *Escherichia coli* strains isolated from patients with inflammatory bowel disease. Gut. 1992;33:646–50.
92. Shen W, Steinrück H, Ljungh A. Expression of binding of plasminogen, thrombospondin, vitronectin, and fibrinogen, and adhesive properties by *Escherichia coli* strains isolated from patients with colonic diseases. Gut. 1995;36:401–6.
93. Schultsz C, Moussa M, van Ketel R, Tytgat GNJ, Dankert J. Frequency of pathogenic and enteroadherent *Escherichia coli* in patients with inflammatory bowel disease and controls. J Clin Pathol. 1997;50:573–9.
94. Krogfelt KA. Bacterial adhesion: genetics, biogenesis, and role in pathogenesis of fimbrial adhesins of *Escherichia coli*. Rev Infect Dis. 1991;13:721–35.
95. Ilnyckyi A, Greenberg H, Bernstein CN. *Escherichia coli* O157:H7 infection mimicking Crohn's disease. Gastroenterology. 1997;112:995–9.
96. König B, Ludwig A, Goebel W, König W. Pore formation by the *Escherichia coli* alpha-hemolysin: role for mediator release from human inflammatory cells. Infect Immun. 1994;62:4611–17.

8
The role of nutrition in the pathogenesis of inflammatory bowel disease

M. A. GASSULL and E. CABRÉ

INTRODUCTION

Although many factors may be involved in the pathogenesis of inflammatory bowel disease (IBD), data supporting a role of intestinal environment in triggering or perpetuating the inflammatory response of the intestine are more and more frequently reported. This is the case for intestinal bacteria and their metabolic products, such as endotoxin, bacterial peptides (formyl methyl leucine peptide or FMLP) and products of the bacterial metabolism of dietary substrates, such as phenolic substances. In addition, nutrients are important components of the intestinal milieu and it has been suggested that they may also play an important pathogenic role as modulators of the inflammatory events occurring in the intestine, not only through their bacterial metabolism, as already mentioned, but also through their role in the biochemical pathways of the intestinal epithelium and immune cells. In fact, treatments based on eliminating specific foodstuffs from the diet or substituting free amino acids for proteins in enteral formula diets have been attempted, especially in Crohn's disease (CD), with success in some instances[1,2]. However, this has been rarely and, in most cases, unsuccessfully tried in ulcerative colitis (UC).

In this chapter, some of the data and the hypothesis supporting a role for nutrients in the pathogenesis of IBD will be analysed.

DIETARY FIBRE, OTHER MALABSORBED CARBOHYDRATES, SHORT-CHAIN FATTY ACIDS AND SULPHATE-CONTAINING COMPOUNDS

It is well known that, in an individual with normal intestinal absorption, once dietary fibre and other malabsorbed carbohydrates reach the colon, they become a preferred substrate for anaerobic bacteria. The main metabolic products of such bacterial fermentation are short-chain fatty acids (SCFA), acetate, propionate and butyrate, and some gases (CO_2, H_2). Some of these gases are used to synthesize methane (CH_4) and some of the hydrogen formed is used by the sulphate-reducing bacteria to produce SH_2.

The role of SCFA has been highlighted in the last 10 years since it has been demonstrated, especially for butyrate, that it is the main fuel for the energy metabolism of colonocytes and a differentiating agent during colonic cell growth[3-6]. Butyrate oxidation in the colonocyte produces acetyl-CoA, which is involved in many metabolic processes, including detoxification of xenobiotics, mucus production, lipid synthesis and regulation of sodium and water absorption in the colon. In addition to its role providing energy to the colonic epithelia, butyrate also suppresses chemotaxis of PMN cells and stimulates DNA synthesis in lymphocytes.

Butyrate enemas have been successfully used in the therapy of diversion colitis as well as in distal UC[7-9]. These data suggest that, in both diversion and UC, there may be an energy deficit in the colonic epithelium. In the former, the lack of nutrients reaching the diverted colonic segment renders nutrient fermentation impossible; thus SCFA cannot be synthesized. In UC, there might be an intrinsic defect in the colonic cells preventing butyrate synthesis or utilization.

In this sense, it has been shown that faecal butyrate content is diminished in active UC compared with healthy individuals and patients with colonic CD. Also patients with inactive UC show reduced butyrate oxidation. However, colonic epithelial cells maintain the oxidative capacity for glucose and glutamine[10], suggesting that there must be a mechanism other that the oxidative capacity of the colonocyte to explain the diminished butyrate oxidation in UC. In addition, when looking at the activity of the enzymes involved in butyrate oxidation in the colonic mucosa of patients with UC, it was observed that they were in all instances normal[11]. Why then should butyrate oxidation be impaired?

In recent years, evidence has been presented for a potential role of sulphide in the pathogenesis of UC. Sulphide is produced in the human colon by sulphate-reducing bacteria[12-14]. These are strictly anaerobic organisms which use sulphate as a terminal electron acceptor in the oxidation of organic material, which is known as sulphate reduction[15]. In faeces of patients with UC, sulphate-reducing bacteria are almost always present. This is not so in healthy individuals[16]. In addition, faecal concentrations of sulphide are higher in patients with UC than in healthy controls[16]. In animals, experimental UC can be induced by feeding sulphated polysaccharides, such as carageenan of dextran sulphate sodium[17]. The end-product of sulphate reduction, sulphide, is a highly local cytotoxic compound, without systemic effects[18].

Roediger *et al.* have found evidence that sulphide is involved in the pathogenesis of UC[19-21] and that there is a relationship between sulphate-reducing flora, sulphide production and butyrate oxidation impairment.

How are sulphide and butyrate related in the pathogenesis of UC?

When human colonocytes were cultured *in vitro* in three different media, butyrate, butyrate plus sodium sulphide and the latter plus a sulphide blocker (S-aMet), it was demonstrated that, while sulphide inhibited butyrate oxidation (as measured by $^{14}CO_2$ formation), sulphide blockade resulted in amounts of $^{14}CO_2$ similar to those in the control culture.

It is thought that sulphide inhibits the action of butyryl-CoA-dehydrogenase, a key enzyme in the butyrate oxidative process. It is possible that a high concentration of butyrate, administered as enema to a given colonic segment, may overcome the sulphide-blocking action and hence explain its therapeutic effect. It may also be possible that butyrate exerts an antagonistic effect on sulphide metabolism in the cell[22].

Interestingly enough, in a recent report[23], Roediger's group argue against their own hypothesis because they failed to demonstrate high levels of sulphide in a group of 13 patients with inactive and 6 patients with active UC, compared with healthy controls. However, in this study, neither simultaneous levels of faecal butyrate nor dietary habits were studied. Moreover, the estimation of colonic exposure to sulphide based on faecal measurements is complicated due to the ability of sulphide to exist in the ionized or protonated forms at physiological faecal pH. The highly volatile SH_2 rapidly leaves the faeces and is either absorbed by the mucosa or passed as flatus. Levine *et al.*[24] showed that faeces of 25 patients with UC incubated in 4-L containers produced 3–4 times more SH_2 than those of healthy controls.

What are the potential therapeutic implications of a better knowledge of nutritional involvement in the pathogenesis of UC?

Answering this question may lead to extensive speculation. The presence in the colonic lumen of increased amounts of S-containing compounds from proteins which have escaped digestion and absorption in the small bowel, may occur when high-protein diets or enteral formula diets[25] or even, in some cases, drinking water[26] are administered. This, together with the tendency to decrease fibre intake (the main source of butyrate) for fear of damaging the colonic mucosa or inducing diarrhoea, may produce an optimal situation favouring disease flare-up.

Few studies have attempted to increase butyrate production in the colon in patients with UC by increasing the intake of dietary fibre. In a randomized controlled trial, Fernández-Bañares *et al.* compared the effect of feeding *Plantago ovata* seeds with feeding mesalazine and the combination of both treatments in preventing relapse in patients with inactive UC. The probability of maintaining remission for one year was similar with all treatments[27]. However, these results should be confirmed in larger series of patients.

Future studies are necessary to ascertain the role of nutrients in the pathogenesis of UC and the possible therapeutic implications of dietary manipulations. Emphasis should be placed on the complex colonic lumenal environment, especially the nutrient–bacteria relationship, the exact role of sulphide, the existence or not of a defective butyrate oxidation, the effect of butyrate in the immunocompetent cells and its possible effect on cytokine production by regulating transcription factors, such as NFkB[28,29].

ARGININE

Although it is not an essential amino acid, L-arginine may be considered essential in certain circumstances since it is required for development and growth and in metabolic stress (because of its immunostimulatory properties)[30–32]. In addition, L-arginine is the substrate for nitric oxide (NO) synthesis by NO synthases (NOS). There are at least three forms of NOS[33,34]. Constitutive forms of NOS (cNOS) rapidly release small amounts of short-lasting NO in response to increases in intracellular calcium. They are associated with neuronal elements and vascular endothelium and the NO released has a wide range of biological effects. Inducible NOS (iNOS) is produced in much larger quantities over many hours by cells after stimulation by cytokines or endotoxin. This sustained production of NO by iNOS depends on the presence of extracellular L-arginine[35,36]. Excessive calcium-independent synthesis of NO has been reported to be a key factor in the pathogenesis of UC, suggesting the presence of iNOS in the inflamed colon[37,38]. Supporting this idea is the fact that, in experimental models, the administration of NOS blockers ameliorates the intestinal damage[39,40].

On the other hand, arginine may be metabolized by arginase to ornithine. This, in turn, may be further metabolized to polyamines and L-proline[41,42] and both pathways may contribute to tissue repair. Experiments on the temporal expression of these two pathways in wound healing and glomerulonephritis, demonstrate an early phase of high NOS activity followed some days afterwards by an increase in arginase activity[43,44]. These data fit very well with the orderly progression from the early inflammatory response, with high NOS activity, to a later phase with tissue repair where high arginase activity may produce L-ornithine necessary for polyamine and proline synthesis. Increased arginase activity has been demonstrated recently in the colonic mucosa of UC patients[45,46].

Since both arginine metabolic pathways seem to be activated in patients with IBD, it may be possible that arginine administration may influence both the inflammatory and healing phases of the disease by increasing the inflammatory damage and fibrosis. In fact, it is possible that diets with low or no arginine content may be of therapeutic use in IBD, as has been found in experimental models of glomerulonephritis[47].

GLUTAMINE

Glutamine is a non-essential amino acid but it is a preferred fuel for tissues with high cell turnover, such as intestinal epithelium and immunocompetent cells[48–51]. Multiple beneficial effects have been documented in animals after glutamine supplementation. These include:

1. Maintenance of glutamine levels in muscle;
2. Increase in nitrogen retention and protein synthesis;
3. Improved trophism and immune function in the intestine during parenteral nutrition;
4. Decrease of pancreatic atrophy and liver steatosis associated to total parenteral nutrition or elemental diet administration;
5. Decrease in intestinal damage, bacteraemia and mortality in chemotherapy, radiation and sepsis models;
6. Maintenance of glutathion levels in these situations;
7. Increase in water and sodium transport in normal and inflamed bowel; and
8. Increased healing of NSAID-induced gastric damage[48–51].

In spite of all these potential beneficial effects, little work has been done on the effects of administering glutamine in IBD. In fact, there are only three studies of experimental colitis with controversial results[52–54]. There is no clinical trial on its possible role in human IBD. This is probably because glutamine is not stable in parenteral amino acid solutions and elemental formula diets. It is conceivable that after the introduction of glutamine-containing dipeptides to amino acid solutions for parenteral nutrition, studies will be performed looking specifically at this issue.

IRON

Together with copper, iron is a cofactor in oxygen free radical generation, facilitating the formation of hydroxyl radicals. Since patients with IBD often receive oral treatment with iron, unabsorbed iron in the intestinal lumen may contribute to the maintenance of oxidative stress in the inflamed intestine. This fact is seldom taken into account when treating these patients; oral iron should only be given in ferropenic states to these patients.

DIETARY FAT

Usually lipids in nutrition are regarded as energy donors. However, lipids have many biological functions as well as being oxidized to provide energy. Fatty acids (FA) are incorporated into cell membranes and, depending on their degree of unsaturation, influence the membrane physicochemical properties. Hence, FA membrane composition regulates the function of membrane receptors, enzymes and transport systems. In addition, some FA are precursors of second messengers, such as eicosanoids inositol-phosphate, diacylglycerol, PAF, etc.[55,56]. There are four families of FA relevant in the organism: n-3, n-6, n-9 and n-7. The precursors of these families are, respectively, α-linolenic, linoleic, oleic and palmitoleic acids. α-Linolenic and linoleic acids are essential fatty acids (EFA) whereas oleic and palmitoleic acids can be endogenously synthesized. EFA produce long-chain derivatives (PUFA) by sequential desaturation and elongation reactions. The main n-3 and n-6 long-chain PUFA are eicosapentaenoic (EPA) and arachidonic (ARA) acids, respectively. It is important to emphasize that the different FA families are not interconvertible *in vivo*. That is, n-3 long-chain PUFA will never be synthesized from the n-6 precursor and *vice versa*. This implies that the FA composition of the cell membranes could be changed by manipulating the FA composition of the diet. The most abundant eicosanoids are those resulting from the oxidation of ARA, some of them (PGE_2, TxA_2, and LTB_4) are important mediators of the inflammatory processes. In contrast, EPA-derived eicosanoids (PGE_3, TxA_3 and LTB_5) have very much attenuated inflammatory properties. This is the rationale for using n-3 PUFA-rich marine oils in the treatment of inflammatory conditions, including IBD[57,58].

Fish oil has been administered in the treatment of both active and inactive UC in at least 7 trials with disappointing results[59–65]. Recently, two large placebo-controlled trials using n-3 FA in the maintenance treatment of inactive

CD have been published with divergent results[66,67]. While, in the Belluzzi *et al.* study[66], the relapse rate was significantly lower in the therapeutic group, Lorenz-Meyer *et al.*[67] failed to reproduce this beneficial effect. The main differences between the two trials were:

1. In Belluzzi's study, fish oil was administered as enteric-coated free FA whereas Lorenz-Meyer *et al.* used FA-ethyl-esters which it is known are not optimally absorbed;
2. The predominant disease location was not comparable in both studies, exclusive small bowel involvement predominating in Belluzzi´s trial; and
3. The time elapsed since achieving remission with steroids greatly differed between both studies, being 3–23 months in Belluzzi's study whereas Lorenz-Meyer's patients were included immediately after going into remission with steroids.

All these facts may account for the different outcomes in these studies.

One fact seldom taken into account when explaining divergent results in trials evaluating the use of dietary supplements is the composition of the basic diet eaten by patients in different countries. This may be an additional factor accounting for the opposite results of the above-mentioned trials. The Beluzzi *et al.* study was performed in Italy whereas the Lorenz-Meyer *et al.* trial was performed in Germany. There are many differences between the diets in these two countries, one of them being the main sources of fat, olive oil being predominant in Italy, compared with butter and seed oils in Germany.

Oleic acid, the predominant FA in olive oil, only produces long-chain PUFA in the setting of EFA deficiency, which very seldom occurs in CD patients. In addition, oleic acid does not produce eicosanoids. Moreover, olive oil has been described to have other immunosuppressant effects in humans, both *in vitro* and *in vivo*[68,69]. Thus, the positive effect of n-3 PUFA in the Italian study may well be due to a synergistic effect with olive oil contained in the diet.

Supporting this hypothesis is the fact that, in all studies comparing the effects of chemically defined formula diets with steroids in active CD, only those diets with either very low fat contents (elemental) or those with high contents of oleic acid, were as effective as corticosteroids in achieving disease remission[70].

FINAL REMARKS

All of the above leads us to think that UC and CD behave in different ways as far as therapeutic dietary manipulations are concerned. In contrast to CD, where qualitative changes in dietary lipids may be of therapeutic benefit, UC seems to respond poorly to dietary manipulations aiming to modify eicosanoid release, and would be more sensitive to changes involving nutrient handling by the colonic flora.

References

1. Riordan AM, Hunter JO, Cowan RE *et al.* Treatment of active Crohn's disease by exclusion diet: East Anglian multicentre controlled trial. Lancet. 1993;342:1131–4.
2. O'Moráin C, Segal AW, Levi AJ. Elemental diet as primary treatment of acute Crohn's disease: a controlled trial. Br Med J. 1984;288:1859–62.

3. Rombeau JL, Kripke SA. Metabolic and intestinal effects of short-chain fatty acids. JPEN. 1990;14(Suppl):181S–5S.

4. Royall D, Wolever TMS, Jeejeebhoy KN. Clinical significance of colonic fermentation. Am J Gastroenterol. 1990;85:1307–12.

5. Reilly KJ, Rombeau JL. Metabolism and potential clinical applications of short-chain fatty acids. Clin Nutr. 1993;12(Suppl 1):S97–105.

6. Scheppach W. Effects of short chain fatty acids on gut morphology and function. Gut. 1994;35:S35–8.

7. Harig JM, Soergel KH, Komorowsky RA, Wood CM. Treatment of diversion colitis with short-chain fatty acid irrigation. N Engl J Med. 1989;320:23–6.

8. Scheppach W, Bartram HP, Richter F *et al.* Treatment of distal ulcerative colitis with short-chain fatty acid enemas – A placebo-controlled trial. Dig Dis Sci. 1996;41:2254–9.

9. Vernia P, Cittadini M, Caprilli R, Torsoli A. Topical treatment of refractory distal ulcerative colitis with 5-ASA and sodium butyrate. Dig Dis Sci. 1995;40:305–7.

10. Chapman MAS, Grahn MF, Boyle MA, Hutton M, Rogers J, Williams NS. Butyrate oxidation is impaired in the colonic mucosa of sufferers of quiescent ulcerative colitis. Gut. 1994;35:73–6.

11. Allan ES, Winter S, Light AM, Allan A. Mucosal enzyme activity for butyrate oxidation; no defect in patients with ulcerative colitis. Gut. 1996;38:886–93.

12. Beerens H, Romond C. Sulfate reducing anaerobic bacteria in human feces. Am J Clin Nutr. 1977;30:1770–9.

13. Gibson GR, Macfarlane GT, Cummings JH. Occurrence of sulphate reducing bacteria in human feces and the relationship of dissimilatory sulphate reduction to methanogenesis in the large gut. J Appl Bacteriol. 1988;65:103–11.

14. Gibson GR, Macfarlane S, Macfarlane GT. Metabolic interactions involving sulphate reducing and methanogenic bacteria in the large intestine. FEMS Microbiol Ecol. 1993;12:117–23.

15. Postgate JR. The Sulphate Reducing Bacteria, 2nd edn. Cambridge, UK: Cambridge University Press; 1984.

16. Gibson GR, Cummings JH, Macfarlane GT. Growth and activities of sulphate reducing bacteria in gut contents of healthy subjects and patients with ulcerative colitis. FEMS Microbiol Ecol. 1991;86:103–12.

17. Marcus R, Watt J. Seaweeds and ulcerative colitis in laboratory animals. Lancet. 1969;2:489.

18. Weiseger RA, Pinkus LM, Jacoby WB. Thiol S-methyltransferase: Suggested role in detoxication of intestinal hydrogen sulfide. Biochem Pharmacol. 1980;29:2885–7.

19. Roediger WEW, Duncan A, Kapanidis O, Millard S. Reducing sulfur compounds of the colon impair colonocyte nutrition: Implications for ulcerative colitis. Gastroenterology. 1993;104:802–9.

20. Roediger WEW, Duncan A, Kapanidis O, Millard S. Sulphide impairment of butyrate oxidation in rat colonocytes: A biochemical basis for ulcerative colitis? Clin Sci. 1993;85:623–7.

21. Roediger WEW. Utilization of nutrients by isolated cells of the rat colon. Gastroenterology. 1982;83:424–9.

22. Christl SU, Eisner HD, Dusel G, Kasper H, Scheppach W. Antagonistic effects of sulfide and butyrate on proliferation of colonic mucosa. A potential role of these agents in the pathogenesis of ulcerative colitis. Dig Dis Sci. 1996;41:2477–81.

23. Moore J, Babidge W, Millard S, Roediger W. Colonic luminal hydrogen sulfide is not elevated in ulcerative colitis. Dig Dis Sci. 1998;43:162–5.

24. Levine J, Ellis CJ, Furne JK, Springfield J, Levitt MD. Fecal hydrogen sulfide production in ulcerative colitis. Am J Gastroenterol. 1998;93:83–7.

25. Geypens B, Claus D, Evenpoel P *et al.* Influence of dietary protein supplements on the formation of bacterial metabolites in the colon. Gut. 1997;41:70–6.

26. Heizer WD, Sandler RS, Seal E *et al.* Intestinal effects of sulfate in drinking water on normal human subjects. Dig Dis Sci. 1997; 42:1055–61.

27. Fernández Bañares F, Hinojosa J, Sánchez Lombraña JL *et al.* Randomised clinical trial of Plantago ovata efficacy as compared to mesalazine in maintaining remission in ulcerative colitis. Gastroenterology. 1997;112:A971(Abstract).

28. Segain JP, Boureille A, Galmiche JP, Blottière HM. Butyrate modulates the production of TNF-α in Crohn's disease. Gut. 1997;41(Suppl 3):A226(Abstract).

29. Wu GD, Huang N, Wen XM, Yang H. Induction of IkB expression by sodium butyrate inhibits transcriptional activation of the interleukin 8 gene. Gastroenterology. 1997;112:A1121(Abstract).

30. Barbul A. Arginine: biochemistry, physiology and therapeutic implications. JPEN. 1986;10:227–38.
31. Barbul A. Arginine and immune function. Nutrition. 1990;6:53–8.
32. Park KGM, Hayles PD, Garlick PJ, Sewell H, Eremin O. Stimulation of lymphocyte natural cytotoxicity by L-arginine. Lancet. 1991;337:645–6.
33. Knowles RG, Moncada S. Nitric oxide synthases in mammals. Biochem J. 1994;298:249–58.
34. Southan GJ, Szabo C. Selective pharmacological inhibition of distinct nitric oxide synthase isoforms. Biochem Pharmacol. 1996;51:383–94.
35. Bogle RG, Baydoun AR, Parson JD, Moncada S, Mann GE. L-Arginine transport is increased in macrophages generating nitric oxide. Biochem J. 1992;284:15–18.
36. Granger DL, Hibbs JB, Perfect JR, Durack DT. Metabolic fate of L-arginine in relation to micro-biostatic capability of murine macrophages. J Clin Invest. 1990;85:264–73.
37. Boughton-Smith NK, Evans SM, Hawkey CJ *et al*. Nitric oxide synthase activity in ulcerative colitis and Crohn's disease. Lancet. 1993;342:338–40.
38. Rachmilewitz D, Stamler JS, Bachwich D *et al*. Enhanced colonic nitric oxide generation and stimulated nitric oxide synthase activity in experimental colitis and in active inflammatory bowel disease. Gut. 1995;36:718–23.
39. Miller MJS, Sadowska-Krowicka H, Chotanaruemol S, Kakkis JL, Clark DA. Amelioration of chronic ileitis by nitric oxide synthase inhibition. J Pharmacol Exp Ther. 1993;264:11–16.
40. Rachmilewitz D, Karmeli F, Okon E, Bursztyn M. Experimental colitis is ameliorated by inhibition of nitric oxide synthase activity. Gut. 1995;37:247–55.
41. McCormack SA, Johnson LR. Role of polyamines in gastrointestinal mucosal growth. Am J Physiol. 1991;260:G795–806.
42. Cynober L. Can arginine and ornithine support gut functions? Gut. 1994;35:S42–5.
43. Albina JE, Mills CD, Henry WL, Cladwell MD. Temporal expression of different pathways of L-arginine metabolism in healing wounds. J Immunol. 1990;144:3877–80.
44. Cook HT, Jansen A, Lewis S *et al*. Arginine metabolism in experimental glomerulonephritis: Interaction between nitric oxide synthase and arginase. Am J Physiol. 1994;267:F646–53.
45. Fric P, Zavoral M, Kocna P, Pelech T, Benesová A, Zadorová Z. Arginase activity of normal and diseased colorectal mucosa. Gut. 1994;35 (Suppl 4):A62–3(Abstract).
46. Kocna P, Fric P, Zavoral M, Pelech T. Arginase activity determination: A marker of large bowel mucosa proliferation. Eur J Clin Chem Clin Biochem. 1996;34:619–23.
47. Narita I, Border WA, Ketteler M, Ruoslahti E, Noble NA. L-Arginine may mediate the therapeutic effect of low protein diets. Proc Natl Acad Sci USA. 1995;92:4552–6.
48. Ziegler TR, Smith RJ, Byrne TA, Wilmore DW. Potential role of glutamine supplementation in nutrition support. Clin Nutr. 1993;12(Suppl 1):82–90.
49. Calder PC. Glutamine and the immune system. Clin Nutr. 1994;13:2–8.
50. Payne James JJ, Grimble GK. The present status of glutamine. Curr Opin Gastroenterol. 1995;11:161–7.
51. Hall JC, Heel K, McCauley R. Glutamine. Br J Surg. 1996;83:305–12.
52. Fujita T, Sakurai K. Efficacy of glutamine-enriched enteral nutrition in an experimental model of mucosal ulcerative colitis. Br J Surg. 1995;82:749–51.
53. Ameho CK, Adjei AA, Harrison EK *et al*. Prophylactic effect of dietary glutamine supplementation on interleukine 8 and tumour necrosis factor alpha production in trinitrobenzene sulphonic acid induced colitis. Gut. 1997;41:487–93.
54. Shinozaki M, Saito H, Muto T. Excess glutamine exacerbates trinitrobenzenesulphonic acid-induced colitis in rats. Dis Colon Rectum. 1997;40:S59–63.
55. Kinsella JE. Lipids, membrane receptors, and enzymes: Effects of dietary fatty acids. JPEN. 1990;14:200S–17S.
56. Kinsella JE, Lokesh B, Broughton S, Whelan J. Dietary polyunsaturated fatty acids and eicosanoids: Potential effects on the modulation of inflammatory and immune cells: An overview. Nutrition. 1990;6:24–44.
57. Katz DP, Schwartz S, Askanazi J. Biochemical and cellular basis for potential therapeutic value of n-3 fatty acids derived from fish oil. Nutrition. 1993;9:113–18.
58. Endres S. Messengers and mediators: Interactions among lipids, eicosanoids, and cytokines. Am J Clin Nutr. 1993;57(Suppl):798S–800S.
59. Aslan A. Fish oil fatty acid supplementation in active ulcerative colitis: A double-blind, placebo-controlled, crossover study. Am J Gastroenterol. 1992;87:432–7.

60. Hawthorne AB. Treatment of ulcerative colitis with fish oil supplementation: A prospective 12 month randomised controlled trial. Gut. 1992;33:922–8.
61. Stenson WF. Dietary supplementation with fish oil in ulcerative colitis. Ann Intern Med. 1992;116:609–14.
62. Greenfield SM. A randomized controlled study of evening primrose oil and fish oil in ulcerative colitis. Aliment Pharmacol Ther. 1993;7:159–66.
63. Loeschke K, Ueberschaer B, Pietsch A *et al.* n-3 Fatty acids only delay early relapse of ulcerative colitis in remission. Dig Dis. 1996;41:2087–94.
64. Lorenz R, Weber PC, Szimnau P, Heldwein W, Strasser T, Loeschke K. Supplementation with n-3 fatty acids from fish oil in chronic inflammatory bowel disease: a randomized, placebo-controlled, double-blind cross-over trial. J Intern Med Suppl. 1989;225:225–32.
65. Salomon P, Kornbluth AA, Janowitz HD. Treatment of ulcerative colitis with fish oil n-3-omega-fatty acid: an open trial. J Clin Gastroenterol. 1990;12:157–61.
66. Belluzzi A, Brignola C, Campieri M, Pera A, Boschi S, Miglioli M. Effect of an enteric-coated fish-oil preparation on relapses in Crohn's disease. N Engl J Med. 1996;334:1557–60.
67. Lorenz-Meyer H, Bauer P, Nicolay C *et al.* Omega-3 fatty acids and low carbohydrate diet for maintenance of remission in Crohn's disease – A randomized controlled multicenter trial. Scand J Gastroenterol. 1996;31:778–85.
68. Karsten S, Schäfer G, Schauder P. Cytokine production and DNA synthesis by human peripheral lymphocytes in response to palmitic, stearic, oleic, and linoleic acid. J Cell Physiol. 1994;161:15–22.
69. Yaqoob P, Knapper JA, Webb DH, Williams CM, Newsholme EA, Calder PC. Effect of olive oil on immune function in middle-aged men. Am J Clin Nutr. 1998;67:129–35
70. Fernández Bañares F, Cabré E, González-Huix F, Gassull MA. Enteral nutrition as primary therapy in Crohn's disease. Gut. 1994;35:S55–9.

9
Role of nutritional therapy in IBD

D. B. A. SILK

INTRODUCTION

Nutritional support can be administered via the parenteral or enteral route. There are two possible roles of nutritional support in inflammatory bowel disease (IBD): as adjunctive therapy to correct and maintain nutritional status and as primary therapy. This chapter examines the role of parenteral and enteral nutrition in the management of patients with acute exacerbations of ulcerative colitis and Crohn's disease.

Nutritional status of patients with IBD

Any patients with ulcerative colitis or Crohn's disease can become severely wasted during an acute unremitting attack of the disease. Chronic undernourishment, however, probably occurs more commonly in Crohn's disease than

Table 1 Causes of malnutrition in patients with IBD

Poor oral intake
  Disease-induced
  Restrictive diet/iatrogenic

Malabsorption
  Decreased absorptive surface (disease, surgical resection)
  Bile salt deficiency
  Bacterial overgrowth

Increased gut losses
  Protein-losing enteropathy
  Blood loss
  Electrolytes, minerals, trace elements (e.g. vis fistula)

Increased requirements
  Sepsis, fever
  Increased cell turnover

Drug–nutrient interactions
  Corticosteroids (calcium, protein)
  Cholestyramine (fat, vitamins)
  Sulphasalazinc (folate)

in ulcerative colitis[1-3]. Several factors can lead to protein-energy malnutrition (Table 1). These include a poor nutritional intake, malabsorption (due to active disease, previous resection or bypass) and protein losses through the colon or small bowel[4]. Rates of body protein synthesis and breakdown have both been found to increase in direct proportion to disease activity[5,6]. It is of interest that many of the complications of severe inflammatory bowel disease, e.g. poor wound healing, muscle wasting, depressed tumour and cellular immunity and increased susceptibility to infection, commonly occur in undernourished patients with other conditions. It seems reasonable to speculate, therefore, that nutritional depletion *per se* may be a major cause of these features, particularly in patients with IBD, since many can remit with nutritional therapy[7].

The manifestations of protein-energy malnutrition in IBD

A common clinical manifestation of protein-energy malnutrition in inflammatory bowel disease is weight loss. Anthropometrically, this has been shown to occur as muscle bulk[9]. Although clinicians will see individual exceptions, weight loss is more common in patients with Crohn's disease than in those with ulcerative colitis: thus, when Harries *et al.*[1] surveyed a group of outpatients with ulcerative colitis, they found no significant difference in their anthropometry compared with controls. Weight loss frequently occurs, however, in patients requiring hospital admission on account of acute exacerbations[8,10], weight loss occurring in up to 62% of the patients in the latter series[10].

Early studies documented weight loss in 70–80% of patients with Crohn's disease[11-13]. In contrast to ulcerative colitis, weight loss has been documented in patients with Crohn's disease receiving treatment as outpatients[14,19]. Weight loss can be particularly marked in hospitalized patients with acute exacerbations of Crohn's disease, particularly in those with diffuse disease[15].

Finally, in children with Crohn's disease, protein-energy malnutrition may present with stunted growth and delayed linear growth[16-20].

Protein metabolism

In some patients with IBD, nitrogen intake and faecal losses are the major determinants of N metabolism. With regard to N intake, this may be slightly diminished in outpatients with 'inflammatory bowel disease'. However, food intake in severely ill patients with IBD, for example those with acute colitis, subacute obstruction, sepsis or fistulas, may be severely compromised or absent. Faecal losses of N in IBD are variable, ranging from normal to low in mild disease to about 6.5 g/24 h in severe colitis[8]. In some patients, N balance is not determined by differences between intake and faecal loss of N, for example intra-abdominal abscess formation can be associated with large urinary losses of N^{21}. Moreover, increases in whole-body protein synthesis and breakdown correlate with disease activity[5]. These latter findings have illustrated how changes in whole-body protein turnover in IBD are not due to local tissue changes but to a more generalized effect, probably on several tissues within the body[8].

Fat absorption

Steatorrhoea is found in Crohn's disease but not ulcerative colitis, and, in the former patients, the overall incidence is about 30%[15,22]. Bile acid metabolism may be disturbed in extensive Crohn's disease as well as in patients who have had intestinal resection, and this may result in lumen concentrations of bile acid below the critical micelle concentration with resultant steatorrhoea. The extent and severity of small bowel disease may determine the degree of steatorrhoea in Crohn's disease, and the extent of any surgical small bowel resection will also influence the degree of steatorrhoea.

Haematinic deficiency

Of patients with Crohn's disease, 25–50% have iron deficiency[23] and up to two thirds of patients with ulcerative colitis have iron deficiency[24]. Folic acid depletion probably occurs in about one third of patients with IBD and usually varies with active disease[1,23]. Diminished vitamin B_{12} absorption occurs in half to two thirds of patients with Crohn's disease and may be due to different factors[9]. Deficiency is present, however, in only about one third of untreated patients with active disease[9].

Mineral and vitamin deficiencies

Recent research has highlighted the importance of magnesium deficiency, particularly in Crohn's disease[25]. Zinc deficiency also occurs in association with Crohn's disease in up to 40% of patients[26–28]. Various deficiency states affecting both water-soluble and fat-soluble vitamins have been reported in patients with Crohn's disease[29]. The relevance to the clinical condition has not been well documented.

The need for nutritional therapy

It is clear from the previous discussion that malnutrition is common in patients with active IBD, especially Crohn's disease, and a wide range of nutritional disturbances can be identified, particularly in patients with Crohn's disease. Early recognition of deficiency is appropriate so that replacement therapy can be prescribed. It is important to appreciate that nutritional defects may have important subtle effects. Thus, Fe and Zn deficiency can be associated with impaired immune competence[30], and specific nutrients like Zn[26] and potassium and calcium deficiencies will influence protein metabolism. The case for focussing attention on nutritional deficiencies in IBD is thus a clear one. If nutritional deficiencies cannot be corrected by increasing the intake of normal food or by administration of oral dietary supplements, then nutritional support should be administered wherever possible via the enteral route. The ensuing text develops a hypothesis that, in some situations, enteral nutrition may actually constitute primary therapy in IBD, the general indications for parenteral nutrition being restricted to patients with intestinal obstruction or gastrointestinal fistula and as a means of postoperative nutritional support in sick patients.

PARENTERAL NUTRITION AS PRIMARY THERAPY

Ulcerative colitis

In two carefully designed prospective randomized controlled trials, patients with acute exacerbations of ulcerative colitis, all of whom were being treated with corticosteroids, received either bowel rest and TPN or a standard ward diet[31,32]. TPN and bowel rest did not influence the outcome of disease; therefore, it can be concluded that TPN has no primary therapeutic effect in the treatment of acute exacerbations of ulcerative colitis.

Crohn's disease

Well-designed prospective randomized controlled trials of any medical treatment for Crohn's disease are difficult to perform, and trials of nutritional support as primary therapy are no exception. The heterogeneity of patients in terms of the extent and activity of disease, the presence or absence of complications such as fistulas, the duration of nutritional therapy and the use of different associated treatments, as well as the fact that trials have included different numbers of patients and have applied different criteria for remission and relapse, make objective analysis very difficult.

In the early 1970s, it was found that TPN obviated the need for surgical intervention in some patients with IBD[33,34] and it was postulated that 'bowel rest', achieved by the administration of TPN, might be of primary importance in the treatment of IBD[33,34]. Many trials over the following 15 years examined this theory but the results were difficult to interpret because of major methodological flaws. Some trials included both patients with Crohn's disease and patients with ulcerative colitis, some were uncontrolled or non-randomized, some were retrospective, most involved small numbers of patients, and definitions of the success or failure of treatment were often inadequate. In 1988, however, Greenberg *et al.*[35] conducted a prospective, controlled trial to compare directly the efficacy of TPN with total enteral nutrition as a primary therapeutic modality in patients with Crohn's disease; they found similar short-term remission rates and long-term outcomes. This trial dispelled the belief that bowel rest and TPN were of primary importance in the treatment of active Crohn's disease[36].

ENTERAL NUTRITION AS PRIMARY THERAPY

In addition to the methodological problems discussed above that make it difficult to compare the findings of the different clinical trials of nutritional support in Crohn's disease, an added problem exists with the trials of enteral nutrition because of the heterogeneity of the formulations of enteral diets used in the different trials.

The initial categorization of enteral diets into elemental, oligomeric and polymeric diets was based more on the composition of the nitrogen source than other components. Thus chemically defined so-called elemental diets were those containing free L-amino acids as the nitrogen source, partial enzymic hydrolysates of starch as the carbohydrate component of the energy source and low amounts of fat (usually long-chain triglycerides; LCTs).

Oligomeric diets were those containing partial hydrolysates of whole protein with varying peptide chain length profiles as the nitrogen source, partial enzymic hydrolysates of starch as the carbohydrate component of the energy source and rather larger amounts of fat (10–35% total calorics in the form of LTCs and medium chain triglycerides [MCTs]). Polymeric diets were those containing whole protein as the nitrogen source, partial enzymic hydrolysates of starch as the carbohydrate component of the energy source and the highest proportion of fat (30–40% of total calories) in the form of LCT and MCT.

Such a categorization of enteral diets seemed to be an appropriate tool to use when we initially analysed the different trials of enteral nutrition in IBD[37]. This was particularly so because, at the time, the pathogenesis of IBD was, at least in part, thought to be related to a possible role of luminal antigens in triggering acute attacks[38].

Such antigens were thought to act by inducing an anomalous or exaggerated immunological response, causing the release of inflammatory mediators, which, in turn, were considered responsible for the clinical and histological manifestations of the disease. In this regard, the polymeric and oligomeric diets were thought to be 'allergenic' whereas the elemental diets were not.

Ulcerative colitis

There are no prospective randomized controlled trials examining the effects of enteral nutrition as primary therapy in ulcerative colitis. One retrospective analysis suggested that enteral nutrition improved some aspects of nutritional status and reduced the need for albumin infusion compared with those patients who received normal ward diet alone[39].

Crohn's disease

In our initial analysis, we considered that the randomized controlled trials that had examined the role of enteral feeding as a primary therapeutic option in patients with Crohn's disease could be divided as follows (see Tables 2 and 3):

1. Elemental diet compared with standard medical therapy[38,40–43]
2. Oligomeric diet compared with standard medical therapy[44–47]
3. Polymeric diet compared with standard medical therapy[48]
4. Elemental diet compared with oligomeric diet[49–51]
5. Elemental diet compared with polymeric diet[52–55]

In group 1, Okada et al.[40] found a remission rate of 80% at 6 weeks in those receiving an elemental diet compared with a rate of only 11% in those receiving steroids, but the steroid group had more severe disease at the start of the trial. The other four trials[38,41–43], however, all showed similar benefit in the two groups in terms of remission rates.

In group 2, the largest study was the European Cooperative Trial[44], in which 107 patients were randomly assigned to either an oligomeric diet or a decreasing dose of methylprednisolone (from 48 to 12 mg/day over 6 weeks) plus salazopyrine. The steroid group had a higher remission rate at 6 weeks (79%) than the diet group (53%). In this study, 44% of those receiving the oligomeric diet showed no change at all in their Crohn's Disease Activity Index. The authors

Table 2 Controlled trials comparing enteral diets with standard medical treatment in the primary treatment of active Crohn's disease

Study reference	Number of patients	Duration of treatment	Treatment group	Control group	Follow-up	Remission rate [n (%)] Control	Remission rate [n (%)] Treatment	Nutrition non-compliance (%)
Elemental diet vs. standard medical therapy								
40	20	6 weeks	Elemental 40–60 kcal/kg/day	Prednisolone 0.7 mg/kg/day for 1/52, then reducing by 5 mg each week	6 weeks	3/10 (30)	8/10 (80)**	NR
38	21	4 weeks	Vivonex 40–60 kcal/kg/day	Prednisolone 0.75 mg/kg/day for 2/52, then reducing as appropriate	4 weeks / 12 weeks	8/10 (80) / 7/10 (70)	9/11 (82) / 8/11 (73)	18
41	19	3 weeks	Vivonex 50–80 kcal/kg/day	Prednisolone 1 mg/kg/day to max. of 45 mg for 3/52	3 weeks / 6 weeks	6/9 (67) / 9/9 (100)	8/10 (80) / 6/10 (60)	0
42	37	10 days	Vivonex 1800–2400 ml/day plus framycetin, colistin, nystatin	Prednisolone 0.75 mg/kg/day	10 days	16/16 (100)	15/21 (71)	24
43	42	4 weeks	Vivonex 2 L/day	Prednisolone 0.75 mg/kg/day, then as appropriate	4 weeks / 1 year	DAI 3.1 / 6/19 (32)	DAI 3.1 / 1/11 (9)*	41
Oligomeric diet vs. standard medical therapy								
44	107	6 weeks	Peptisorb 35 kcal/kg IBW/day	6-Methylprednisolone 45 mg/day for 1/52, then reducing by increments to 12 mg by week 6 plus salazopyrine 3 g/day	6 weeks	41/52 (79)	29/55 (53)**	13
45	17	6 weeks	Flexical RDA energy/day	ACTH 2 IU/kg/day for 5 days, then prednisolone 2 mg/kg/day to max. 30 mg/day reducing as appropriate after 3/52 plus salazopyrine 50 mg/kg/day	6 weeks	6/7 (86)	7/8 (88)	13
46	95	6 weeks	Survimed 25 kcal/kg	6-Methylprednisolone 48 mg/day for 1/52, then reducing by increments to 12 mg by week 6 plus salazopyrine 3 g/day	6 weeks	32/44 (73)	21/51 (41)*	39
47	27	4 weeks	Vital HN 40 kcal/kg orally	Prednisolone 0.75 mg/kg/day	4 weeks	7/10 (70)	3/9 (33)	44
Polymeric diet vs. standard medical therapy								
48	32	4 weeks	Edanec HN 2800 kcal/day	Prednisolone 1 mg/kg/day. Dose slowly withdrawn over 9 weeks	4 weeks / 1 year	15/17 (88) / 5/15 (33)	12/15 (80) / 7/12 (58)	20

* $p<0.05$: ** $p<0.01$. IBW, ideal body weight; DAI, disease activity index; NR, not recorded; RDA, recommended daily amount

94

Table 3 Controlled trials of enteral diets in the primary treatment of active Crohn's disease

Study	Number of patients	Duration of treatment	Formula		Follow-up	Remission rate [in (%)]	
			Elemental	Oligo/polymeric		Elemental	Oligo/polymeric
Elemental vs. oligomeric diets							
49	29	2 weeks	EO28	Pepdite 2	2 weeks	11/11 (100)	11/12 (92)
50	40	3 weeks	Vivonex	Peptamen	3 weeks	16/19 (84)	15/20 (75)
					1 year	6/19 (32)	8/20 (40)
51	44	4 weeks	EO28	Pepti-2000 LF	4 weeks	8/22 (36)	8/22 (36)
Elemental vs. polymeric diets							
52	30	4 weeks	Vivonex	Fortison	4 weeks	12/16 (75)	5/14 (36)*
53	14	4 weeks	EO28	Eneral 400	4 weeks	2/7 (29)	5/7 (71)
					1 year	0/7 (29)	2/6 (33)
54	30	4–6 weeks	Vivonex HN	Realmentyl	4 weeks	10/15 (67)	11/15 (73)
					1 year	3/15 (20)	4/15 (27)
55	24	3 weeks	EO28	Trisorbon	3 weeks	9/13 (69)	8/11 (73)

* $p < 0.05$

Table 4 Issues arising from clinical studies of enteral nutrition in acute Crohn's disease

- Objective evidence of efficacy?
- Does the site of disease affect chances of obtaining remission?
- Short-term or long-term remission?
- Mode of action of enteral diets
  - Nutritional status
  - Bowel rest
  - Nitrogen source
  - Lipid source

concluded that standard medical therapy was superior to the oligomeric diet in the treatment of active Crohn's disease. Malchow *et al.*[46] and Lindor *et al.*[47] found a similarly disappointing response to oligomeric diets.

In group 3, Gonzalez-Huix *et al.*[48] found no difference between the efficacy of a polymeric diet and that of standard medical therapy, and, in group 4, Middleton *et al.*[49], Royall *et al.*[50] and Mansfield *et al.*[51] all demonstrated that elemental and polymeric diets had similarly beneficial effects. In group 5, Giaffer *et al.*[52] showed that an elemental diet was superior to a polymeric diet, but, on close inspection of the data, it is apparent that those receiving the polymeric diet had more advanced disease. The other three trials in this group all showed similar remission rates for patients given elemental and polymeric diets[53–55].

At first sight, these seem encouraging results, with a definite trend suggesting that enteral nutrition and, in particular, the use of chemically defined elemental diets may be at least as good as corticosteroids in inducing a remission in patients with acute Crohn's disease. On close scrutiny, however, the results do raise more questions than answers. Table 4 summarizes some of these.

As outlined by Teahon and colleagues[56], scepticism about the use of enteral nutrition as primary treatment in Crohn's disease has been flawed by the lack of objective evidence about how this form of treatment works. In fact, there is a good deal of work with the chemically defined elemental diets that shows how these reduce gastrointestinal protein losses[57], improve intestinal permeability[56,58] and, importantly, cause a reduction in intestinal inflammation[56].

Given that there is objective evidence that enteral nutrition has primary therapeutic efficacy in acute Crohn's disease, is there any evidence that the site of disease affects the chances of obtaining a remission? The numbers of patients included in most of the prospective randomized trials are too small to allow statistical comparisons to be made. However, in a retrospective analysis of 113 patients with acute Crohn's disease treated with an elemental diet, the site of disease did not appreciably affect the chances of obtaining a remission[59] (Figure 1).

In most of the controlled trials of enteral nutrition in acute Crohn's disease, patients were treated for 4–6 weeks and, at the end of this time, were treated with a normal diet or reducing dose of corticosteroid therapy. One of the important issues is whether the mode of inducing a remission significantly affects the probability of relapse, and, if so, is this influenced in any way by the site of the disease?

In one prospective controlled trial in which patients were followed up for one year[43], the probability of maintaining remission was significantly greater in

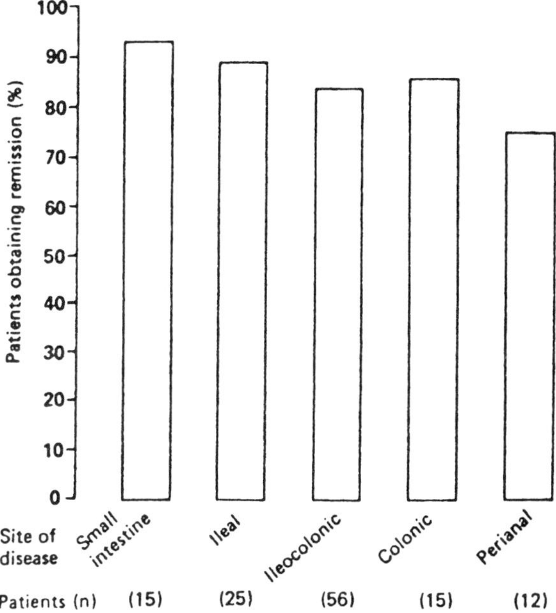

Figure 1 The success rate of obtaining remission vs. site of disease in patients treated for active Crohn's disease with elemental diet. After Teahon *et al.*[59] with permission

patients in whom remission was achieved with prednisolone than with an elemental diet.

In one of the other trials, however[48], the probability of maintaining remission at one year was similar whether remission had been induced by corticosteroids or with a polymeric diet. It was of interest that, in this trial[43], there was a trend for patients with small intestinal disease, treated with an elemental diet, to remain in remission longer (mean 29 weeks) than those with colonic disease (mean 13 weeks). In the respective analysis of patients with acute Crohn's disease in whom remission was induced with an elemental diet, there was a trend for patients with ileocolonic and colonic disease to relapse earlier[59], a finding that has been confirmed in a separate study[60] which showed that the duration of remission was longer in patients with small bowel disease than in those with colonic involvement ($p < 0.01$).

MODE AND ACTION OF ENTERAL NUTRITION IN ACUTE CROHN'S DISEASE

There has been much speculation as to how enteral nutrition achieves its efficacy in inducing remission in acute Crohn's disease. Firstly, it does not appear that elemental diets exert their effects by improving nutritional status alone[61], and, in one of the prospective randomized trials, patients were stratified for nutritional status prior to being randomized to receive corticosteroids or elemental diet to induce remission[43].

It has been widely believed that enteral nutrition is effective in Crohn's disease by achieving 'bowel rest'. Absorption of the minimal residue diets is virtually completed in the upper small intestine, so it is assumed that the distal small intestine and colon are 'medically bypassed'. All the diets used, however, including the elemental diets, provide a powerful stimulus to pancreaticobiliary secretions[62,63] to which inflamed ulcerated gut is then exposed. Moreover, following a study that failed to show superiority of intravenous nutrition over polymeric feeding or oral food with parenteral supplementation, it is now apparent that complete bowel rest is not a prerequisite for achieving remission in acute Crohn's disease with nutritional treatment[35].

It has been suggested that, in active Crohn's disease, dietary protein might gain access to the gut wall via ulcerated mucosa and cause secondary immune-mediated tissue damage[38]. A unique property of elemental diet, which might account for its effectiveness in acute Crohn's disease, is its hypoallergenic nature. The absence of whole protein or peptides in elemental diets effectively removes dietary antigenic stimuli, which might otherwise provoke immune-mediated damage on exposure to ulcerated gut mucosa. This may explain why two trials by the European Cooperative Crohn's Disease Group[41,64], both using a protein hydrolysate diet containing oligopeptides rather than solely free amino acids, have shown that enteral feeding is inferior to drug treatment with corticosteroids and sulphasalazine.

This theory, however, cannot explain the equal efficacy of elemental and polymeric diets in inducing remission in acute Crohn's disease[54,55], nor can it explain how, in one trial, the use of a polymeric diet was as efficacious as standard medical treatment in inducing remission in acute Crohn's disease[48].

In pursuing further the explanation of how nutritional therapy has a beneficial effect in inducing remission in acute Crohn's disease, Gassull and colleagues shave turned their attention to the fat component of enteral diets and have examined the influence of this on outcome[65,66]. They noted that the use of diets with a very low fat content has been associated with a good outcome. The use of diets containing higher quantities of fat was associated overall with a less favourable outcome and, in particular, when large amounts of linoleic acid were present, the outcome seemed to be particularly poor[65,66].

This fatty acid is the precursor of arachidonic acid, which in turn is the substrate for the synthesis of the eicosanoids with the highest proinflammatory activity (leukotriene B_4, thromboxane A_2, prostaglandin E_2). The outcome of patients treated with diets containing intermediate or large amounts of fat but containing large proportions of monounsaturated fatty acids was, however, more favourable[53,54].

These findings suggest the possibility that clinical remission achieved with elemental diets might be related to the administration of insufficient substrate for n-6-derived eicosanoid synthesis. In support of this, there are experimental data available showing that low-fat diets[67] or diets with low essential fatty acid contents[68] have an immunomodulatory effect in animal studies. Furthermore, essential fatty acid efficiency is known to diminish acute inflammation[69] and, in other studies, to improve experimental colitis in the rat[70]. Further controlled clinical trials are clearly required to test the hypothesis that it may be the serendipitous manipulation of the fat source of enteral diets that has exerted an anti-inflammatory effect in acute Crohn's disease which in turn has been the factor responsible for inducing remission.

The importance of identifying the mode of action of nutritional therapy in Crohn's disease is, of course, related to the potential that exists for applying the concepts to long-term dietary treatment in the hope that more success can be gained in maintaining remission in patients with Crohn's disease.

References

1. Harries AD, Baird A, Rhodes J. Non-smoking: a feature of ulcerative colitis. Br Med J. 1982;284:706.
2. Harries AD, Jones LA, Heatley RV, Rhodes J. Malnutrition in inflammatory bowel disease: anthropometric study. Hum Nutr Clin Nutr. 1982;36C:307–13.
3. Harries AD, Jones L, Heatley RV, Rhodes J, Fitzsimmons E. Mid-arm circumference as simple means of identifying malnutrition in Crohn's disease. Br Med J. 1982;285:1317–18.
4. Beeken WL, Busch HJ, Sylvester DL. Intestinal protein loss in Crohn's disease. Gastroenterology. 1972;62:207–15.
5. Powell-Tuck J, Fern EB, Garlick PJ, Waterlow JC. The effect of surgical trauma and insulin on whole-body protein turnover in parenterally-fed undernourished patients. Hum Nutr Clin Nutr. 1984;38:11–22.
6. Powell-Tuck J, Garlick PJ, Lennard-Jones JE, Waterlow JC. Rates of whole body protein synthesis and breakdown increase with the severity of inflammatory bowel disease. Gut. 1984;25:460–4.
7. Harries AD, Jones LA, Danis V. Controlled trial of supplemented oral nutrition in Crohn's disease. Lancet. 1984;1:887–90.
8. Powell-Tuck J. Protein metabolism in inflammatory bowel disease. Gut. 1986;27,Suppl.1:67–71.
9. Heatley RV. Assessing nutritional state in inflammatory bowel disease. Gut. 1986;27,Suppl.1:61–6.
10. Goligher JC, deDombal FT, McKwatts J, Watkinson JG. Ulcerative Colitis. London: Bailliere Tindall Cassell; 1968.
11. Van Patter WN, Bargen JA, Dockerty MB, Feldman WH, Mayo CW, Waugh JM. Regional enteritis. Gastroenterology. 1954;26:347–50.
12. Dyer NH, Dawson AM. Malnutrition and malabsorption in Crohn's disease with reference to the effect of surgery. Br J Surg. 1973;60:134–40.
13. Mekhjian HS, Switz DN, Meunyk CS, Rankin GB, Brooks RK. Clinical features and natural history of Crohn's disease. Gastroenterology. 1979;77:898–906.
14. Lanfranchi GA, Brignola C, Campieri M. Assessment of nutritional status in Crohn's disease in remission or low activity. Hepatogastroenterology. 1984;31:129–32.
15. Dyer NH. Studies on Crohn's Disease. Thesis, University of Cambridge; 1970.
16. McCaffery TD, Nasr K, Lawrence AM, Kirsner JB. Severe growth retardation in children with inflammatory bowel disease. Pediatrics. 1970;45:386–93.
17. Burbige EJ, Huang S, Bayless TM. Clinical manifestations of Crohn's disease in children and adolescents. Pediatrics. 1975;55:866–71.
18. Layden T, Rosenberg J, Nemchausky B, Elson C, Rosenberg I. Reversal of growth arrest in adolescents with Crohn's disease after parenteral alimentation. Gastroenterology. 1976;70:1017–21.
19. Grand RJ, Shen G, Werlin SL, Kelts DG, Boehme C. Reversal of growth arrest in Crohn's disease (CD). A new approach. Ped Res. 1977;11:44 Abstr.
20. Kelts DG, Grand R, Shen G, Watkins JB, Werlin SL, Boehme C. Nutritional basis of growth failure in children and adolescents with Crohn's disease. Gastroenterology. 1979;76:720–7.
21. Clark RG, Lauder MN. Undernutrition and surgery in regional ileitis. Br J Surg. 1969;56:736–8.
22. Smith AN, Balfour TW. Malabsorption in Crohn's disease. Clin Gastroenterol. 1972:433–48.
23. Hoffbrand AV, Stewart JS, Both CC, Mollin DL. Folate deficiency in Crohn's disease: incidence, pathogenesis, and treatment. Br Med J. 1968;2(597):71–5.

24. Driscoll RH, Rosenberg IH. Total parenteral nutrition in inflammatory bowel disease. Med Clin N Am. 1978;62:185–201.
25. Hessov I, Hasselblad C, Fasth S, Hulten L. Abstract book: world congresses. Scand J Gastroenterol. 1982;17,Suppl.78:A1973.
26. McClain C, Soutor C, Zieve L. Zinc deficiency: a complication of Crohn's disease. Gastroenterology. 1980;78:272–9.
27. Sturniolo GC, Molokhia MM, Shields R, Turnberg LA. Zinc absorption in Crohn's disease. Gut. 1980;21:387–91.
28. Fleming CR, Huizenga KA, McCall JR, Gildea J, Dennis R. Zinc nutrition in Crohn's disease. Dig Dis Sci. 1981;26:865–70.
29. Harries AD, Heatley RV. Nutritional disturbances in Crohn's disease. Postgrad Med J. 1983;59:690–7.
30. Dowd PS, Heatley RV. The influence of undernutrition on immunity. Clin Sci. 1984;66:241–8.
31. Mackintyre PB, Powell-Tuck J, Wood SR et al. Controlled trial of bowel rest in the treatment of severe acute colitis. Gut. 1986;27:481–5.
32. Dickinson RJ, Ashton MR, Axon ATR, Smith RC, Yeung CK, Hill GL. Controlled trial of intravenous hyperalimentation and total bowel rest as an adjunct to the routine therapy of acute colitis. Gastroenterology. 1980;79:1199–204.
33. Vogel CM, Corwin TR, Baue AE. Intravenous hyperalimentation in the treatment of inflammatory diseases of the bowel. Arch Surg. 1974;108:460–7.
34. Fischer JE, Foster GS, Abel RM, Abbott WM, Ryan JA. Hyperalimentation as primary therapy for inflammatory bowel disease. Am J Surg. 1973;125:165–73.
35. Greenberg GR, Fleming CR, Jeejeebhoy KN, Rosenberg IH, Sales D, Tremaine WJ. Controlled trial of bowel rest and nutritional support in the management of Crohn's disease. Gut. 1988;29:1309–15.
36. Payne-James JJ, Silk DBA. Total parenteral nutrition as primary treatment in Crohn's disease – RIP? Gut. 1988;29:1304–8.
37. Bowling TE. Inflammatory bowel disease. Eur J Gastroenterol Hepatol. 1995;7:521–7.
38. O'Morain C, Segal AW, Levi AJ. Elemental diet as primary treatment of acute Crohn's disease: a controlled trial. Br Med J. 1984;288:1859–62.
39. Abad A, Cabre E, Giue JJ et al. Total enteral nutrition in hospitalized patients with inflammatory disease. J Clin Nutr Gastroenterol. 1986;1:1–8.
40. Okada M, Yao T, Yamamoto T et al. Controlled trial comparing elemental diet with prednisolone in the treatment of active Crohn's disease. Hepatogastroenterology. 1990;37:72–80.
41. Seidman EG, Bouthillier L, Weber AM, Roy CC, Morin CL. Elemental diet versus prednisolone as primary treatment of Crohn's disease [abstract]. Gastroenterology. 1986;90:1625a.
42. Saverymuttu S, Hodgson HJF, Chadwick VS. Controlled trial comparing prednisolone with an elemental diet plus non-absorbable antibiotics in active Crohn's disease. Gut. 1985;26:994–8.
43. Gorard DA, Hunt JB, Payne-James JJ et al. Initial response and subsequent course of Crohn's disease treated with elemental diet or prednisolone. Gut. 1993;34:1198–202.
44. Lochs H, Steinhardt HJ, Klaus-Wentz B et al. Comparison of enteral nutrition and drug treatment in active Crohn's disease. Results of the European Cooperative Crohn's disease Study IV. Gastroenterology. 1991;101:881–8.
45. Sanderson IR, Udeen S, Davies PSW, Savage MO, Walker-Smith JA. Remission induced by an elemental diet in small bowel Crohn's disease. Arch Dis Child. 1987;61:123–7.
46. Malchow H, Steinhardt HJ, Lorenz-Meyer H et al. Feasibility and effectiveness of a defined-formula diet regimen in treating active Crohn's disease. Scand J Gastroenterol. 1990;25:235–44.
47. Lindor KD, Fleming CR, Burnes JU, Nelson JK, Ilstrup DM. A randomized prospective trial comparing a defined formula diet, corticosteriods, and a defined formula diet plus corticosteroids in active Crohn's disease. Mayo Clin Proc. 1992;328:328–33.
48. Gonzalez-Huix F, de Leon R, Fernandez-Banares F et al. Polymeric enteral diets as primary treatment of active Crohn's disease: a prospective steroid controlled trial. Gut. 1993;34:778–82.
49. Middleton SJ, Riodan AM, Hunter JO. Peptide based diet: an alternative to elemental diet in the treatment of acute Crohn's disease [abstract]. Gut. 1991;32:A578.
50. Royall D, Jeejeebhoy KN, Baker JP et al. Comparison of amino acid versus peptide-based enteral diets in active Crohn's disease: clinical and nutritional outcome. Gut. 1994;35:783–7.
51. Mansfield JC, Giaffer MH, Holdsworth CD. Controlled trial of oligopeptide versus amino acid diet in treatment of active Crohn's disease. Gut. 1995;36:60–6.

52. Giaffer MH, North G, Holsworth CD. Controlled trial of polymeric versus elemental diet in treatment of active Crohn's disease. Lancet. 1990;335:816–19.

53. Park RHR, Galloway A, Danesh BSZ, Russel RI. Double blind controlled trial of elemental and polymeric diets as primary therapy in active Crohn's disease. Eur J Gastroenterol Hepatol. 1991;3:483–90.

54. Rigaud D, Cosnes J, Le Quintrec Y, Gendre JP, Mignon M. Control-led trial comparing two types of enteral nutrition in treatment of active Crohn's disease: elemental versus polymeric diet. Gut. 1991;32:1492–7.

55. Raouf AH, Hildrey V, Daniel J *et al.* Enteral feeding as sole treatment for Crohn's disease: controlled trial of whole protein versus amino acid based feed and a case study of dietary challenge. Gut. 1991;32:702–7.

56. Teahon K, Smethurst P, Pearson M, Levi AJ, Bjarnason I. The effect of elemental diet on intestinal permeability and inflammation in Crohn's disease. Gastroenterology. 1991;101:84–9.

57. Logan RFA, Gillon J, Ferrington C, Ferguson A. Reduction of gastrointestinal protein loss by elemental diet in Crohn's disease of the small bowel. Gut. 1981;22:383–7.

58. Sanderson IR, Boulton P, Menzies I, Walker-Smith JA. Improvement of abnormal lactulose/rhamnose permeability in active Crohn's disease of the small bowel by an elemental diet. Gut. 1987;28:1073–6.

59. Teahon K, Bjarnson I, Pearson M, Levi AJ. Ten years' experience with an elemental diet in the management of Crohn's disease. Gut. 1990;31:1133–7.

60. Giaffer MH, Cann P, Holdsworth CD. Long-term effects of elemental and exclusion diets for Crohn's disease. Aliment Pharmacol Ther. 1991;5:115–25.

61. Teahon K, Pearson M, Levi AJ, Smith T, Bjarnason I. Improved nutrition is not an important mechanism by which elemental diets work in acute Crohn's disease. Gut. 1990;31:A624.

62. Go VLW, Hofman AF, Summerskill WHJ. Pancreozymin bioassay in man based on pancreatic enzyme secretion: potency of specific amino acids and other digestive products. J Clin Invest. 1970;49:1558–64.

63. Hopman WPM, de Jong AJL, Rosenbusch G, Jansen JBMJ, Lamers CBHW. Elemental diet stimulates gallbladder contraction and secretion of cholecystokinin and pancreatic polypeptide in man. Dig Dis Sci. 1987;32:45–9.

64. Malchow H, Steinhardt HJ, Lorenz-Meyer H *et al.* Feasibility and effectiveness of a defined-formula diet regimen in treating active Crohn's disease: European Cooperative Crohn's Disease Study III. Scand J Gastroenterol. 1990;25:235–44.

65. Fernández-Bañares F, Cabré E, González-Huix F *et al.* Enteral nutrition as primary therapy in Crohn's disease. Gut. 1994;35(Suppl 1):S55–9.

66. Fernández-Bañares F, Cabré E, Esteve-Comas M, Gassul MA. How effective is enteral nutrition in inducing clinical remission in active Crohn's disease? A meta-analysis of the randomized clinical trials. JPEN. 1995;19.5:356–62.

67. Morrow WJW, Homsy J, Swanson CA, Ohashi Y, Estes J, Levy JA. Dietary fat influences the expression of autoimmune disease in MLR. Immunology. 1986;59:439–43.

68. Schreiner GF, Flye W, Brunt E, Korber K, Lefkowith JB. Essential fatty acid depletion of renal allografts and prevention of rejection. Science. 1988;240:1032–3.

69. Denko CW. Modification of adjuvant inflammation in rats deficient in essential fatty acids. Agents Actions. 1976;65:636–41.

70. Lohoues MJ, Russo P, Gurbindo C *et al.* Essential fatty acid deficiency improves the course of experimental colitis in the rat: possible role of dietary immunomodulation. Gastroenterology. 1992;102:A655.

Section III
Immunological basis of IBD

10
Animal models of IBD: impact on understanding immunologically mediated intestinal inflammation

R. B. SARTOR

INTRODUCTION

Recent advances in rodent models of chronic intestinal inflammation have provided important insights into mechanisms of immunologically mediated tissue injury which are directly relevant to human IBD[1-3]. Identification of macrophage and T lymphocyte-driven responses in animal models have led to new hypotheses which can be explored in human IBD and to novel therapeutic approaches. In addition, new pharmacological compounds and molecular techniques of delivery are first tested for efficacy and toxicity in laboratory models of enterocolitis before undergoing human phase one studies. Animal models of intestinal inflammation can be broadly categorized into spontaneous and induced groups (Table 1). Recent advances have been made in genetically engineered rodents employing transgenic overexpression and targeted deletion (knockout) of selected immunoregulatory and structural genes and in the identification of new inbred mouse strains[4,5] that are presumably the result of spontaneous mutations of yet to be identified genes. These models share many clinical and histopathological features with human IBD, including extraintestinal manifestations and colonic adenocarcinoma[3]. Although no animal model completely recapitulates human ulcerative colitis or Crohn's disease, broad mechanisms of inflammation and tissue injury have emerged that have profoundly affected our

Table 1 Categories of animal models of intestinal inflammation

Spontaneous	*Induced*
Cotton-top tamarin	Infections
Inbred mice	Toxins
Transgenic rats and mice	Bacterial products
Knockout mice	T cell subsets → immunodeficient mice
Infections	Bone marrow transplant → CD_3 E_{26} transgenic mice

understanding of the pathophysiology of IBD. This chapter will succinctly review recent advances in mechanisms of immunologically mediated inflammation in animal models. Readers are referred to more extensive reviews for detailed analysis of microbial and genetic influences in experimental enterocolitis and for in-depth descriptions of individual models[1–3,6,7].

INSIGHTS INTO IMMUNOPATHOGENESIS

Chronic enterocolitis is immunologically mediated

Most animal models display a characteristic profile of cytokine expression in inflamed intestinal tissues, indicating activation of mucosal macrophages and T lymphocytes (Table 2). This pattern is remarkably similar to that seen in ulcerative colitis and Crohn's disease in regard to monokine activation, with upregulation of interleukin 1 (IL-1), IL-1 receptor antagonist, IL-6, chemokines and TNFα[3]. The vast majority of chronic T-lymphocyte-mediated models display activation of Th-1 lymphocytes (interferon-γ and IL-12) similar to human Crohn's disease. The exception to this rule is T-cell receptor (TCR-α)-deficient mice which have a dominant Th-2 profile (IL-4, IL-5, and IL-10 but low interferon-γ)[8] analogous to human ulcerative colitis.

Mucosal macrophages are important regulators of experimental enterocolitis. In all models studied to date, tissue macrophages are increased in number and have an activated phenotype with increased tissue concentrations of monokines. Furthermore, blockade of IL-1 and TNF-α attenuates inflammation[9–11] whereas blockade of IL-1 receptor antagonist exacerbates disease[12,13] indicating important immunoregulatory effects of these endogenous molecules. Moreover, administration of recombinant IL-10, which down regulates macrophages and Th-1 function, prevents but does not treat established inflammation[14]. These results strongly implicate mucosal macrophages in the pathogenesis of acute and chronic phases of intestinal inflammation.

Table 2 Tissue cytokine profile in experimental colitis and human IBD

Cytokine	Experimental colitis	Crohn's disease	UC
IL-1	↑	↑	↑
IL-1RA	↑	↑	↑
IL-6	↑	↑	↑
Chemokines	↑(MIP-2)	↑(IL-8)	↑(IL-8)
TNFα	↑	↑	N
IFNγ	↑*	↑	N (?)
IL-4	N*	N	↑(?)
IL-5	N*	N	↑
IL-12	↑*	↑	N

*exception: TCR-α-deficient mice have ↑ IL-4 and IL-5, normal IFNγ and IL-12; ↑ = increased; N = normal, not increased; ? = inconsistent results

Table 3 T-lymphocyte regulation of chronic experimental colitis and IBD

	Experimental colitis	*Crohn's disease*	*UC*
Activated T cell	Yes	Yes	Yes
Cytokine profile	Th-1*	Th-1	Th-2 (?)
Cyclosporin response	Yes	Yes	Yes
Response to ↓ T cells	Yes	Yes	?
Response to blockade of IFNγ, IL-12	Yes	?	?
Response to IL-10	Yes	Yes	?
Disease transferred by CD4+ lymphocytes	Yes	?	?
Disease altered by bone marrow transplant	Yes	Yes	Yes

* TCR-α knockout mice have a Th-2 lymphokine profile

Compelling evidence has accumulated to indicate that chronic intestinal inflammation is mediated by T lymphocytes (Table 3). All models of chronic intestinal inflammation studied to date display activated T cells by FACS analysis and lymphokine levels[15]. As mentioned above, with one exception (TCR knockout), chronic models display Th-1 lymphokine profiles[11,14,16–18]. Chronic enterocolitis and extraintestinal disease is completely blocked by cyclosporin or FK506 administration and chronic intestinal inflammation fails to occur in T-cell-deficient hosts, including nude rats and Rag2-deficient mice[19–22]. However, chronic intestinal inflammation is not altered by the absence of B lymphocytes[21,22] consistent with the concept that Th-1 lymphocytes mediate chronic intestinal inflammation. Furthermore, disease can be blocked by neutralization of endogenous interferon-γ or IL-12 and responds to recombinant IL-10[11,14,16,23]. Additional proof of this theory is provided by transfer of disease by CD4+ lymphocytes from diseased rodents to immunodeficient hosts[16,24,25]. Finally, disease can be transferred or prevented by bone marrow transplant from HLA B27 transgenic rats or non-transgenic donors, respectively[26]. Taken together, these studies conclusively demonstrate that chronic experimental intestinal inflammation in a wide variety of models is mediated by activated macrophages and T lymphocytes and provide a strong experimental background to support therapeutic blockade of regulatory cytokines and T lymphocyte subsets in human IBD.

Defective immunoregulation, especially of immune suppression, leads to intestinal inflammation

In the intestine, there is a delicate balance of proinflammatory and anti-inflammatory molecules. Each proinflammatory molecule has a counterbalancing immunosuppressive molecule which appropriately down regulates the inflammatory response to prevent chronic uncontrolled inflammation. For example, IL-1 is competitively inhibited by IL-1 receptor antagonist (IL-1RA), which binds to the type IL-1 receptor with no agonist activity. Compensatory anti-inflammatory molecules are found, not only for proinflammatory cytokines, but also for lymphokines, arachidonic acid metabolites and neuropeptides (Table 4). Important immunoregulatory activities of these endogenous immunosuppressive molecules are confirmed by exacerbation of disease when these anti-inflammatory molecules are blocked or deleted. For example, IL-10 and TGFβ

Table 4 Opposing effects of immunoregulatory molecules

Proinflammatory	*Anti-inflammatory*
IL-1, TNFα, IL-18	IL-1RA, TNF-BP, IL-11
IL-8, gro, MIP-2	TGFβ
IL-12, IFNγ (Th-1)	IL-4, IL-10 (Th-2)
TxA$_2$, LTB$_4$	PGE$_2$, PGI$_2$
Sub P, TSH, CRH	VIP, cortisol

knockout mice spontaneously develop aggressive colitis[16,27]. Similarly, pharmacological blockade of prostaglandin synthesis by indomethacin induces enterocolitis[28]. Targeted deletion of IL-1RA and cyclo-oxygenase 1 and 2 does not lead to spontaneous colitis but dramatically potentiates dextran sodium sulphate (DSS)-induced colitis[13,29]. Similarly, immunoneutralization of IL-1RA and TGFβ potentiates colitis induced by immune complexes and CD45RB high T cells, respectively[12,30]. Consistent with the protective effects of these endogenous inhibitory molecules, administration of recombinant IL-1RA, IL-10, IL-11, TGFβ and PGE$_2$ attenuates experimental colitis[9,10,14,31,32]. In addition to endogenous immunosuppressive molecules, regulatory elements in proinflammatory genes can inhibit transcription of aggressive proteins. For example, targeted deletion of the inhibitory 3-AU-rich region of the TNFα gene leads to constitutive TNFα production and ileocolitis in mice[33]. These results strongly suggest that the balance of proinflammatory versus suppressive molecules determines inflammation versus homeostasis and progression versus resolution of inflammation.

Similarly, animal model experiments elegantly illustrate an important role for endogenous lymphocyte subsets in suppressing intestinal inflammation. Transfer of the CD45RB high subset of CD4 lymphocytes derived from normal hosts induces colitis in immunodeficient recipients[34,35]. The reciprocal CD45RB low population not only does not transfer disease, but inhibits colitis in immunodeficient hosts when cotransferred with the CD45RB high population, indicating that normal hosts have endogenous T-cell subsets capable of down regulating inflammation. Similarly, deletion of endogenous T cells in hosts prior to transplant with HLA B27 transgenic rat bone marrow exacerbates disease[24]. These studies indicate that active immunosuppression mediated by inhibitory cytokines, T cell subsets, arachidonic acid metabolites and neuropeptides is necessary to maintain mucosal homeostasis. Clinical implications of these observations are that ineffective immunosuppression could cause IBD and, conversely, stimulation of endogenous inhibitory pathways should be a non-toxic approach to therapy of chronic intestinal inflammation.

A variety of immunoregulatory mutations can induce identical phenotypes of intestinal inflammation

A striking feature of most of the genetically engineered rodent models of spontaneous colitis is that the clinical and histopathological features of each model bear a striking resemblance to each other, even though the specific genetic alterations are quite divergent. For example, overexpression of HLA B27/human β_2 microglobulin in rats and targeted deletion of IL-2, IL-2 receptor, IL-10, TCRα

Antigenic drive	Mucosal barrier	Immunoregulation	Intestinal response
	↗ unbroken	→ normal	→ no reaction
	↗ unbroken	→ abnormal	→ IBD
Ubiquitous luminal contents	→ transiently broken	→ normal	→ self-limited inflammation
	↘ transiently broken	→ abnormal	→ IBD
	↘ dysfunctional	→ normal	→ IBD

Figure 1 Progression or resolution of intestinal inflammation stimulated by normal resident luminal bacteria in hosts with genetically regulated normal or defective immunoregulation and epithelial healing. Reproduced with permission from Reference 38

and Gi2α all lead to mucosal hyperplasia, infiltration of the lamina propria by predominantly mononuclear cells, diarrhoea and a wasting syndrome[8,16,24,36,37]. These results indicate that different genetic alterations result in similar disease phenotypes with identical cytokine profiles. Based on these results in animal models, it is likely that ulcerative colitis and Crohn's disease are probably genetically heterogeneous groups of diseases with a final common immunological pathway of cytokine activation and intestinal injury.

CONCLUSIONS

These results in animal models support the hypothesis that chronic intestinal inflammation and related systemic manifestations are due to an overly aggressive immune response to resident luminal bacterial constituents, mediated by Th-1 lymphocytes and macrophages. Predisposing factors are genetic dysregulation of immune response and barrier function, with onset triggered by environmental stimuli. The importance of endogenous immunoregulatory molecules is illustrated in Figure 1, which outlines the different consequences of exposure to environmental stimuli by genetically susceptible versus resistant hosts. Susceptible hosts with defective immunoregulation or barrier function/healing lack the ability to appropriately down regulate inflammatory responses to endogenous luminal bacteria, leading to the development of chronic intestinal inflammation and its local and systemic complications. Both the older induced and newer genetically engineered animal models of chronic intestinal inflammation are ideally suited to pursue studies to better understand mechanisms of disease induction, perpetuation and resolution which will profoundly impact our ability to develop novel therapeutic approaches that fundamentally alter the natural history of human IBD.

Acknowledgements

Original research presented in this review was supported by NIH grants DK 40249 and DK 34989 and the Crohn's and Colitis Foundation of America. The author thanks Beverly Vought for excellent editorial support.

References

1. Elson CO, Sartor RB, Tennyson GS, Riddell RH. Experimental models of inflammatory bowel disease. Gastroenterology. 1995;109:1344–67.
2. Sartor RB. Insights into the pathogenesis of inflammatory bowel diseases provided by new rodent models of spontaneous colitis. Inflamm Bowel Dis. 1995;1:64–75.
3. Sartor RB. Review article: How relevant to human inflammatory bowel disease are current animal models of intestinal inflammation. Aliment Pharmacol Ther. 1997;11:89–96.
4. Sundberg JP, Elson CO, Bedigian H, Birkenmeier EH. Spontaneous, heritable colitis in a new substrain of C3H/HeJ mice. Gastroenterology. 1994;107:1726–35.
5. Kosiewicz MM, Shah M, Bentz M, Nast C, Matsumoto S, Cominelli F. Characterization of a new spontaneous murine model of inflammatory bowel disease. Gastroenterology. 1998;114:1012A.
6. Strober W, Ludviksson BR, Fuss IJ. The pathogenesis of mucosal inflammation in murine models of inflammatory bowel disease and Crohn disease. Ann Intern Med. 1998;128:848–56.
7. Sartor RB. Microbial factors in the pathogenesis of Crohn's disease, ulcerative colitis and experimental intestinal inflammation. In: Kirsner JB, editor. Inflammatory Bowel Diseases. 5th edition. Orlando, FL: WB Saunders, 1998:(in press).
8. Mizoguchi A, Mizoguchi E, Chiba C et al. Cytokine imbalance and autoantibody production in T cell receptor-alpha mutant mice with inflammatory bowel disease. J Exp Med. 1996;183:847–56.
9. Cominelli F, Nast CC, Duchini A, Lee M. Recombinant interleukin-1 receptor antagonist blocks the proinflammatory activity of endogenous interleukin-1 in rabbit immune colitis. Gastroenterology. 1992;103:65–71.
10. McCall RD, Haskill S, Zimmermann EM, Lund PK, Thompson RC, Sartor RB. Tissue interleukin 1 and interleukin-1 receptor antagonist expression in enterocolitis in resistant and susceptible rats. Gastroenterology. 1994;106:960–72.
11. Powrie F, Leach MW, Mauze S, Menon S, Caddle LB, Coffman RL. Inhibition of Th1 responses prevents inflammatory bowel disease in scid mice reconstituted with CD45RBhi CD4+ T cells. Immunity. 1994;1:553–62.
12. Ferretti M, Casini-Raggi V, Pizarro TT, Eisenberg SP, Nast CC, Cominelli F. Neutralization of endogenous IL-1 receptor antagonist exacerbates and prolongs inflammation in rabbit immune colitis. J Clin Invest. 1994;94:449–53.
13. Melani L, Hirsch E, Gaunzon M, Pizarro TT, Hirsh D, Cominelli F. Deletion of the IL-1 receptor antagonist (IL-1 ra) gene increases susceptibility to experimental colitis in mice. Gastroenterology. 1997;112:1040A.
14. Herfarth HH, Mohanty SP, Rath HC, Tonkonogy S, Sartor, RB. Interleukin 10 suppresses experimental chronic, granulomatous inflammation induced by bacterial cell wall polymers. Gut. 1996;39:836–45.
15. Tonkongy SL, Sartor RB. Immune system activation in C_3H/HeJ Bir mice exhibiting spontaneous perianal ulceration. Inflamm Bowel Dis. 1997;3:10–19.
16. Berg DJ, Davidson N, Kuhn R et al. Enterocolitis and colon cancer in interleukin-10-deficient mice are associated with aberrant cytokine production and CD4(+) TH1-like responses. J. Clin. Invest. 1996;98:1010–20.
17. Sellon RK, Tonkonogy SL, Schultz M. Normal enteric flora are necessary for the development of spontaneous colitis and immune system activation in IL-10 deficient mice. Infect Immun. 1998; (in press).
18. Cong Y, Brandwein SL, McCabe RP. CD4+ T cells reactive to enteric bacterial antigens in spontaneously colitic C3H/HeJBir mice: increased T helper cell type 1 response and ability to transfer disease. J Exp Med. 1998;187:855–64.
19. Aiko S, Conner EM, Fuseler JA, Grisham MB. Effects of cyclosporine or FK506 in chronic colitis. J. Pharmacol Exp Ther. 1997;280:1075–84.
20. Sartor RB, Bender DE, Allen JB et al. Chronic experimental enterocolitis and extraintestinal inflammation are T lymphocyte dependent. Gastroenterology. 1993;104:775A.
21. Ma A, Datta M, Margosian E, Chen J, Horak I. T cells, but not B cells, are required for bowel inflammation in interleukin 2-deficient mice. J Exp Med. 1995;182:1567–72.
22. Davidson NJ, Leach MW, Fort MM et al. T helper cell 1-type CD4+ T cells, but not B cells, mediate colitis in interleukin 10-deficient mice. J Exp Med. 1996;184:241–51.

23. Neurath MF, Fuss I, Kelsall BL, Stuber E, Strober W. Antibodies to interleukin 12 abrogate established experimental colitis in mice. J. Exp Med. 1995;182:1281–90.

24. Breban M, Fernandez-Sueiro JL, Richardson JA *et al.* T cells, but not thymic exposure to HLA-B27, are required for the inflammatory disease of HLA-B27 transgenic rats. J Immunol. 1996;156:794–803.

25. Hollander GA, Simpson SJ, Mizoguchi E *et al.* Severe colitis in mice with aberrant thymic selection. Immunity. 1995;3:27–38.

26. Breban M, Hammer RE, Richardson JA, Taurog JD. Transfer of the inflammatory disease of HLA-B27 transgenic rats by bone marrow engraftment. J Exp Med. 1993;178:1607–16.

27. Boivin GP, O'Toole BA, Orsmby IE. Onset and progression of pathological lesions in transforming growth factor-beta 1-deficient mice. Am J. Pathol. 1995;146:276–88.

28. Yamada T, Deitch E, Specian RD, Perry MA, Sartor RB, Grisham MB. Mechanisms of acute and chronic intestinal inflammation induced by indomethacin. Inflammation. 1993;17:641–62.

29. Morteau O, Morham S, Sellon RD, Boroviov J, Smithies O, Sartor RB. Genetic deficiency in cyclooxygenase-2 but not in cyclooxygenase-1 exacerbates DSS-induced acute colitis in mice. Gastroenterology. 1997;112:1046A.

30. Powrie F, Carlino J, Leach MW, Mauze S, Coffman RL. A critical role for transforming growth factor-beta but not interleukin 4 in the suppression of T helper type 1-mediated colitis by CD45RB(low) CD4+ T cells. J Exp Med. 1996;183:2669–74.

31. Qiu BS, Pfeiffer CJ, Keith JC Jr. Protection by recombinant human interleukin-11 against experimental TNB-induced colitis in rats. Dig Dis Sci. 1996;41:1625–30.

32. Allgayer H, Deschryver K, Stenson WF. Treatment with 16,16'-dimethyl prostaglandin E2 before and after induction of colitis with trinitrobenzenesulfonic acid in rats decreases inflammation. Gastroenterology. 1989;96:1290–300.

33. Cominelli F, Kontoyannis D, Pizarro TT, Kollias G. Mice carrying an endogenous deletion of the 3'-AU-rich region of the TNFα gene develop a Crohn's disease-like phenotype: a key role of TNFα in the pathogenesis of chronic intestinal inflammation. Gastroenterology. 1998;114:954A.

34. Morrissey PJ, Charrier K, Braddy S, Liggitt D, Watson, JD. CD4+ T cells that express high levels of CD45RB induce wasting disease when transferred into congenic severe combined immunodeficient mice. Disease development is prevented by cotransfer of purified CD4+ T cells. J Exp Med 1993;178:237–44.

35. Powrie F, Leach MW, Mauze S, Caddle LB, Coffman RL. Phenotypically distinct subsets of CD4+ T cells induce or protect from chronic intestinal inflammation in C. B-17 scid mice. Int Immunol. 1993;5:1461–71.

36. Sadlack B, Merz H, Schorle H, Schimpl A, Feller AC, Horak I. Ulcerative colitis-like disease in mice with a disrupted interleukin-2 gene. Cell. 1993;75:253–61.

37. Hornquist CE, Lu X, Rogers-Fani PM *et al.* G(alpha)i2-deficient mice with colitis exhibit a local increase in memory CD4+ T cells and proinflammatory Th1-type cytokines. J. Immunol. 1997;158:1068–77.

38. Schultz M, Sartor SB. Abberant host responses to luminal bacteria in the pathogenesis of chronic intestinal inflammation. In: Ernst PB, Michetti P, Smith PD, editors. The Immunobiology of *H. pylori* – From Pathogenesis to Prevention. New York: Raven Press; 1997:16–82.

11
The role of IFN-γ in inflammation and immunopathology

A. BILLIAU, P. MATTHYS, K. VERMEIRE and H. HEREMANS

Interferon-γ (IFN-γ) owes its name to its ability to interfere with virus replication in cultured cells. By virtue of this antiviral potential, IFN-γ contributes to host defence against virus infections. However, IFN-γ has an equally, or perhaps more, important role to play in host defence against bacterial infections and cancer, and in the pathogenesis of allergy and autoimmune disease. The basis of this role is its ability to:

(1) Enable phagocytes to effectively kill ingested bacteria,
(2) Regulate, in concert with other cytokines, the intensity and components of inflammation, and
(3) Regulate, also in concert with other cytokines, the intensity and type of antigen-specific immune responses mounted against micro-organisms, allergens and auto-antigens. This discussion will be limited to items (2) and (3).

REGULATORY EFFECTS IN INFLAMMATION

One approach to analysis of the role of IFN-γ in inflammation has consisted of describing the nature of its effects on cells known to be involved in inflammation. In view of the complexity of the inflammatory reaction, this approach allows the definition of the nature of possible underlying mechanisms but not their relative importance in the *in-vivo* situation. A second more holistic approach consists of using animal models of inflammation.

Underlying cellular mechanisms

The main cellular mechanisms underlying the *in-vivo* pro- and anti-inflammatory activities of IFN-γ are: (1) generation of reactive oxygen and nitrogen, (2) augmentation of endothelial adhesiveness, (3) induction of chemokines, and (4) synergy with other cytokines.

Table 1 Influence of IFN-γ on chemokine production

Cells tested	Inducer	Chemokine	Effect	Comment	References
CC-chemokines					
Human fibroblastoid synoviocytes	IFN-γ (+ TNF-α)	MCP-1	Induction	Synergy with TNF-α	66
Human leukocytes	LPS + IFN-γ	MIP-1α, -1β, (IL-8)	Early inhibition; later enhancement	IFN-γ by itself inactive; anti-TNF abrogates enhancement	67
Human umbilical vein endothelial cells	TNF-α + IFN-γ	RANTES	Enhancement	Single cytokines inactive; IFN-γ pretreatment sensitizes; IL-4 and IL-13 inhibit; IL-10 has no effect	68
Human fibroblasts; HEP-2 and MG-63 tumour cells	IFN-γ	MCP-1, MCP-2	Induction	MCP-2 more responsive to IFN-γ; synergy with IL-1β	69–71
Human monocytes	β-Amyloid peptide + IFN-γ	MCP-1	Induction and enhancement		72
CXC-chemokines					
Human monocytes	IL-2 + IFN-γ	IL-8	Inhibition	IFN-γ by itself inactive	73
Murine peritoneal cells	LPS + IFN-γ	KC/GRO/MGSA JE γIP-10	Inhibition Inhibition No effect	Cell-specific effect (not in endothelial or 3T3 cells)	74

Exposure of mononuclear phagocytes to IFN-γ augments their potential to mount a respiratory burst response to exogenous stimuli such as LPS. Reactive oxygen formed as part of this response is necessary for effective microbicidal activity but can also cause tissue damage and hence contribute to inflammatory changes. The same holds true for nitrogen oxide (NO) which is generated by inducible NO synthase, the synthesis of which is induced by IFN-γ in various cell types (for a review, see Reference 1).

Vascular endothelial cells are a more important element in inflammation as they form the barrier to be transgressed by fluid and leukocytes to generate the inflammatory infiltrate. IFN-γ augments expression of the adhesion molecule ICAM-1 on cultured endothelial cells of extracerebral[2] as well as cerebral origin[3], resulting in increased adhesiveness for leukocytes expressing the integrin LFA-1[4].

As soon as leukocytes have transgressed the endothelial barrier, they encounter chemokines which control their further movement to the target and cause them to release proteases and other granular contents which, aside from fulfilling useful tasks, can also cause tissue damage. CC-chemokines are typically chemotactic for monocytes, whereas CXC-chemokines attract neutrophils. IFN-γ exerts control over the production of certain chemokines as well as the expression of certain chemokine receptors. Most studies have been performed using human cells (Table 1). In non-immune cells (fibroblasts, synoviocytes, endothelial cells, tumour cell lines), IFN-γ can by itself induce CC-chemokines or it can sensitize cells for increased production after stimulation by TNF-α or IL-1β. In leukocyte cultures, IFN-γ has been shown to exert a biphasic effect: early inhibition of LPS-induced chemokine production is followed by a later augmented production, which can, however, be accounted for by extra TNF-α generated in the system. The induction of CXC-chemokines in mouse and human cells is inhibited by IFN-γ. Thus, IFN-γ tends to promote monocyte attraction and downregulate neutrophil attraction. However, IFN-γ has been shown to also downregulate the CC-chemokine receptor CCR2 on monocytes[5], leaving other chemokine receptors unaffected. This inhibitory effect may serve as a means of retaining phagocytes at the site of inflammation.

IFN-γ is reputed to synergize with TNF which, by itself, exerts effects on endothelial cells and mononuclear phagocytes leading to inflammation. In particular, TNF causes release of procoagulant, prostaglandins, proteases, cytokines and chemokines.

In-vivo effect: animal models

In vivo, NK and T cells are the main producers of IFN-γ. Production is initiated following stimulation by a ligand of the NK or the T cell receptor, respectively. Optimal production requires 'priming' by cytokines, namely TNF, IL-12 and IL-18 generated by other cells, as well as 'co-stimulation' by cell–cell interaction through several ligand systems, e.g. the CD40/CD40L system.

In vitro, the production rate of IFN-γ by a population of lymphocytes reaches a maximum about 24–48 h following exposure to a stimulus. Thereafter, the production rate rapidly returns almost to zero. *In vivo*, a bolus stimulation also results in a short-lived burst of systemic IFN-γ production. Little information is available on production rates during situations of sustained immune stimulation; conceivably, continuous recruitment of fresh, activated lymphocytes results in sustained base-line IFN-γ production.

It should be noted that any IFN-γ which reaches the blood stream is quickly cleared. Rapid clearance is most probably due to adsorption to receptors which occur on virtually all cells of the body, followed by internalization and degradation of the cytokine. Therefore, except in very severe acute inflammatory reactions, IFN-γ remains undetectable in the circulation. Local production of IFN-γ in organs is also difficult to detect: the cytokine is not stored in producing cells and does not remain bound to membranes for a sufficiently long time to be readily detectable by immunostaining. In many studies, investigators have relied on *ex-vivo* methodology: lymphoid cells taken from the body at particular stages in a disease process are cultured and observed for spontaneous or induced production of IFN-γ. Producing cells can be enumerated by the ELISPOT technique. Alternatively, treatment of the lymphocytes with brefeldin, resulting in accumulation of IFN-γ, allows cytoplasmic immunostaining.

Application of these methods has documented production of IFN-γ in lymphoid organs and in local sites of inflammation, e.g. in the central nervous system during experimental autoimmune encephalomyelitis (reviewed in Reference 6). However, most of our current understanding of the role of IFN-γ in inflammation stems from experiments employing monoclonal antibodies to neutralize IFN-γ *in vivo*, and from experiments involving the use of IFN-γ or IFN-γR knock-out mice, the former being unable to produce IFN-γ and the latter being unable to respond to it.

Very little documentation is available on the role of IFN-γ in strictly local inflammatory reactions. We have studied the local Shwartzman reaction elicited by a single injection of endotoxin in the mouse footpad[7]. Pretreatment of the mice with monoclonal antibody to IFN-γ resulted in the modification of the footpad swelling reaction: the early oedema was reduced, whereas the later phase, consisting of cellular infiltration and intravascular thrombosis, remained largely unchanged. This result indicates that IFN-γ which is produced subsequent to the inflammatory stimulus, exerts a local pro-inflammatory effect. However, it is unclear whether this IFN-γ came from a local source (sporadic NK or T cells in the footpad) or had its origin in the spleen or lymph nodes. The local endotoxin injection most probably sufficed to induce a generalized cytokine response, as it was found to prime for a generalized Shwartzman reaction induced by a second systemic endotoxin injection[8]. Remarkably, pretreatment of the mice with exogenous IFN-γ, instead of augmenting the local reaction, also inhibited it. A possible interpretation is that the effect of IFN-γ differs depending on whether it hits the local site prior to or subsequent to application of endotoxin. Opposing effects of IFN-γ depending on time of entry into the system are a recurrent theme in studies with animal models.

This example illustrates the difficulty of distinguishing local from generalized pathogenetic inflammatory events. Model systems for generalized acute inflammation have been extremely popular in IFN-γ studies. One of the first to be studied was the generalized lethal effect of endotoxin. Pretreatment of mice with anti-IFN-γ antibody was found to make mice completely resistant to the generalized Shwartzman reaction. This resistance seemed to be related to a reduced systemic production of TNF[8]. As already mentioned, IFN-γ and TNF synergize, at the levels of both production and action. These early results from treatment with anti-IFN-γ antibody have subsequently been reinforced by studies of knock-out mice[9,10].

Other models of acute inflammation in which the antibody approach led to evidence for a pro-inflammatory effect of IFN-γ are the superantigen-induced shock syndrome[11], the anti-CD3 antibody-induced syndrome[12], tumour-associated cachexia[13,14] and the ConA-induced lethal hepatitis syndrome[15]. In each of these instances, pretreatment with anti-IFN-γ antibody protected the animals against the toxic manifestations of the inflammatory reaction.

Of special note is the anti-CD3 syndrome because the results and conclusions from antibody-mediated ablation of IFN-γ were contradicted by the results of experiments with knock-out mice. The CD3 membrane molecule is present on all T cells. Injection of the antibody initiates a response of all T cells, resulting in massive production of several cytokines, including not only IFN-γ, but also IL-2, IL-4, TNF and several others. The result is a shock-like syndrome characterized by hypomotility and piloerection, hypothermia and hypoglycaemia. Depending on inherent sensitivity of the mice and on the dose of antibody, the syndrome may be self-contained or lethal. Mouse strains which are good IFN-γ producers, e.g. Balb/c mice, were found to be more sensitive than others. Pretreatment of the mice with anti-IFN-γ antibody prior to injection of the anti-CD3 antibody was found to provide near complete protection against the disease manifestations[12], indicating that IFN-γ, produced as a result of the anti-CD3 challenge, contributes to the severity of the syndrome. Studies with IFN-γR knock-out mice, however, yielded data that led to a different conclusion[16]. These studies were performed using mice of the 129 background. Wild-type 129 mice are poorly sensitive to the anti-CD3 syndrome; the IFN-γR knock-out mice, however, turned out to be more sensitive, indicating that, in that situation, an IFN-γ-dependent protective pathway is operational. Obviously, IFN-γ generates more than one pathway in the pathogenesis of the syndrome; some pathways make the syndrome worse, others rather provide protection. The obvious question is why the protective pathway prevails in one case and the disease-promoting pathway in the other. An obvious difference between blockage with anti-IFN-γ antibody and blockage by knocking out the IFN-γ receptor, is that the former affects only IFN-γ formed after anti-CD3 challenge, while the latter affects all IFN-γ, including any that is formed prior to the anti-CD3 challenge. IFN-γ produced in the animal's life time before exposure to the challenge with anti-CD3 antibody may be important for the protective pathway to be available; IFN-γ produced as a result of the anti-CD3 challenge may be critical for full-blown disease to develop. Again, as was the case in the localized Shwartzman reaction, the effect of IFN-γ seems to differ depending on the time of its entry into the system.

REGULATORY EFFECTS IN THE IMMUNE RESPONSE

Immunoregulatory effects of IFN-γ result mainly from effects on antigen-presenting cells and on T lymphocytes.

Antigen presentation and activation of T lymphocytes

Antigen-specific immune responses critically rely on antigen presentation to B and T lymphocytes via MHC molecules on antigen-presenting cells. IFN-γ has long been recognized to be able to enhance expression of MHC Class II molecules by professional antigen-presenting cells and to convert certain non-immune-competent tissue cells into non-professional antigen presenters by inducing *ab ovo* expression of MHC Class II molecules. However, the reaction of lymphocytes to presented antigen may be positive (activation) or negative (tolerance or anergy) depending on the presence or absence of 'priming' signals from specific cytokines and of 'co-stimulatory' signals from cell–cell interaction.

Interestingly, IFN-γ itself can affect the expression of ligands and receptors involved in costimulation. Thus, it induces expression of the B7 (CD80/86) antigen, whose ligand on T cells is the CD28 molecule[17]. The presence of B7 on antigen-presenting cells is necessary for them to avoid delivering an anergizing signal[18]. On the other hand, IFN-γ inhibits expression of CD40 ligand (CD40L or gp39) by activated CD4+ lymphocytes[19]. The CD40/CD40L system is important for mutual full activation of T cells and APCs[20]. Clearly, these direct and indirect effects of IFN-γ on antigen presentation allow for overall immunostimulatory as well as immunosuppressive effects.

For instance, studies involving addition of IFN-γ or anti-IFN-γ antibody to primary one-way MLR have yielded opposing results in different laboratories[1,21]. An important confounding variable may be the quality of costimulatory signals. In the absence of accessory cells, IFN-γ has been found to cause apoptosis, which does not occur in the presence of such cells[22]. This is a theme which recurs in *in-vivo* studies (*vide infra*).

Graft-versus-host disease (GVH), a major complication of bone marrow transplantation, is associated with suppression of cellular immune responses, as evident from reduced proliferative responses of lymphocytes to mitogens. Addition of monoclonal antibodies against IFN-γ has been shown to relieve suppression, implying that endogenous IFN-γ is involved[23]. The target cell for IFN-γ in this system is believed to be a so-called natural suppressor cell[24].

IFN-γ-dependent suppressive circuits in particular have been observed to occur in models of modulation of the immune response by infectious agents. A macrophage-like suppressor cell which inhibits mitogen-induced lymphocyte proliferation occurs in mice infected with *Myobacterium lepraemurium*[25] or *Myobacterium avium* complex[26]. Induction of these cells *in vivo* is independent of IFN-γ, but their suppressive action *in vitro* does require IFN-γ. Another example is infection with *Trypanosoma brucei*[27]; a murine macrophage hybridoma, upon interacting with *T. brucei*, was found to acquire the ability to suppress mitogenic responses of T lymphocytes[28]. This suppressive activity was accompanied by decreased expression of IL-2 receptors but increased production of IFN-γ. Addition of anti-IFN-γ antibody to the system prevented suppression of the mitogenic responses and of IL-2R expression, implying that IFN-γ was instrumental in bringing about the suppressive activity.

A possible mechanism of IFN-γ-dependent suppression through mononuclear phagocytes is generation of H_2O_2 and prostaglandins, since both catalase and indomethacin can alleviate suppression[29]. Boraschi *et al.*[30], on the other hand, found that IFN-γ reduces rather than stimulates murine macrophage suppressive activity by inhibiting prostaglandin E_2 release and inducing IL-1. Another pathway used by suppressor macrophages, which can be activated by IFN-γ, is the generation of nitric oxide[31,32]. IFN-γ also enhances release by mononuclear phagocytes of TGF-β[33], which is generally known as an anti-inflammatory cytokine.

IFN-γ in the Th-1/Th-2 system

A parallel line of speculation concerning the immuno-regulatory action of IFN-γ is canvassed on the Th-1/Th-2 concept, which focusses on the ability of CD4+ lymphocytes to tune their reaction towards antigens by developing different profiles of helper activity for other T cells, B cells and mononuclear phagocytes. The extreme Th-1 profile is characterized by production of mainly IL-2 and IFN-γ, as opposed to the extreme Th-2 profile which is characterized by production of mainly IL-4, IL-5 and IL-10. Whether an immune response chooses the Th-1, the Th-2 or an intermediate track is believed to depend on the cytokine environment during the initial stages of the response. Early production of IL-12 (e.g. by mononuclear phagocytes) is believed to prepare CD4+ cells for taking the Th-1 direction. Early production of IL-4 (e.g. by mastocytes) would prepare the system for choosing the Th-2 direction. The effector mechanisms triggered by a Th-1-type response are tuned to mobilize and activate mononuclear phagocytes to kill ingested micro-organisms, e.g. mycobacteria. The effector mechanisms of Th-2-type responses are more adapted for defence against non-phagocytable organisms, e.g. nematodes. The inflammatory reactions which accompany Th-1- and Th-2-type antimicrobial actions differ in nature, the first being of the cell-mediated delayed-hypersensitivity type, the second being of the IgE-mediated immediate-hypersensitivity type.

In this Th-1/Th-2 dualism, IFN-γ is believed to fulfil both effector and regulator functions. Its effector functions coincide with those that it fulfils in aspecific inflammation (*vide supra*), i.e. to provide activating signals for phagocytes and endothelial cells, enabling them to exert microbicidal effects and recruit additional leukocytes. As to the regulator function of IFN-γ in Th-1/Th-2 balance,

Table 2 Animal model systems of immunopathology in which IFN-γ acts as an immunosuppressant

Model	Description	Observation	References
DTH reaction	Haptene-specific suppressor cells lose *in-vivo* suppressor activity upon prolonged culture	Addition of IFN-γ restores suppressive activity	38
Skin or heart allograft	Rejection prolonged by blockage of CD40–CD40L or B7–CD28 pathways	Rejection not prolonged in IFN-γ knock-out mice	21,40
Experimental autoimmune encephalomyelitis (EAE)	Immunization with CNS antigens causes CNS inflammation and demyelination	Anti-IFN-γ antibody enhances disease	75–78
		Exogenous IFN-γ alleviates disease	75
		IFN-γ-ligand and/or -receptor knock-out mice are more sensitive	41,42
Experimental autoimmune uveitis (EAU)	Immunization with bovine retinal antigen	Anti-IFN-γ antibody enhances disease	79
		Exogenous IFN-γ inhibits disease	80

in-vitro studies have indicated that IFN-γ promotes the differentiation of CD4+ T cells to Th-1 cells, and downregulates Th-2 cells[34–37]. In studies using murine T cell clones, it was found that IFN-γ exerts a slight suppressive effect on IL-2- and IL-4-mediated proliferation of Th-2 but not Th-1 clones[34,37]. However, *in-vivo* studies (*vide infra*) are not always in line with a Th-1-promoting effect of IFN-γ.

In-vivo modulation of immune pathology by IFN-γ

In various animal model systems, IFN-γ has been found to protect against immune pathology (Table 2). For instance, IFN-γ seems to be able to induce suppressor cells for DTH reactions. Splenic adherent cells incubated with haptene and then injected into mice were found to suppress DTH and induce appearance of haptene-specific suppressor cells, demonstrable by transfer into mice that were subsequently tested for DTH responsiveness. On prolonged culture, the splenic cells lost their ability to induce suppression, but addition of IFN-γ could restore this ability[38].

Treatment of skin-allograft-recipient mice with anti-IFN-γ antibody has been found to prolong rejection if the graft is MHC Class II antigen incompatible, but not if it is only MHC Class I incompatible[39], suggesting that, if endogenous IFN-γ contributes to the rejection of a skin allograft, it does so because it induces Class II expression on keratinocytes. More recent evidence from allograft rejection studies is rather indicative of a suppressive effect of endogenous IFN-γ. The rejection rate of cardiac transplants was found to be similar in IFN-γ gene knock-out mice and in wild types[21]. However, in the knock-out mice, and also in wild-type mice treated with neutralizing anti-IFN-γ antibody, it proved impossible to prolong graft survival by blockage of the B7–CD28 or the CD40–CD40L pathways, as was possible in the control wild types[40]. Thus, it appears that endogenous IFN-γ mediates a suppressive circuit when costimulation is inadequate.

Experimental autoimmune encephalomyelytis (EAE) and experimental autoimmune uveitis (EAU) in mice are two examples in which the net effect of endogenous IFN-γ, produced in the course of the immune process, is immunosuppression. In several variant models of the disease, treatment of the mice with neutralizing antibody against IFN-γ was found to result in augmented symptoms and mortality (reviewed in Reference 1). Furthermore, both IFN-γ and IFN-γ receptor knock-out mice were found to be more sensitive to induction of EAE than their wild-type counterparts[41,42].

Examples of models in which IFN-γ accelerates or intensifies autoimmune disease are autoimmune diabetes and lupus-like disease in NZB/W mice and inflammatory bowel disease (Table 3). Reports on the role of IFN-γ in autoimmune diabetes models are controversial. Streptozotocin-induced diabetes, as assessed by hyperglycaemia and body weight loss, was found to be more severe in mice that also received IFN-γ injections[43]. Anti-IFN-γ antibody pretreatment was found to reduce the incidence and severity of diabetes in non-obese diabetic (NOD/Wehi) mice in which occurrence of diabetes is boosted by cyclophosphamide[44,45]. Counter to expectation, administration of IFN-γ in this mouse model of diabetes did not affect blood glucose profiles. In fact, in combination

Table 3 Animal model systems of immunopathology in which IFN-γ acts as an immunopotentiator

Model	Description	Observation	References
Autoimmune diabetes	Streptozotocin-induced	Exogenous IFN-γ aggravates disease	43
	Spontaneous or cyclophosphamide-boosted diabetes in NOD mice	Anti-IFN-γ antibody alleviates disease	44,45
		IFN-γ receptor knock-out mice are protected	47
Lupus-like disease	Female (NZB × NZW) F1 mice	Anti-IFN-γ antibody or soluble IFN-γ receptors alleviate disease	48, 49
		IFN-γ receptor knock-out mice are protected	50
Inflammatory bowel disease	IL-10 knock-out mice	Anti-IFN-γ antibody prevents disease	52,53
	SCID mice reconstituted with CD45Rb[hi] CD4+ T cells	Anti-IFN-γ antibody prevents disease	51
	IL-12-induced enteropathy	IFN-γ knock-out mice are insensitive; exogenous IFN-γ induces enteropathy	54
Experimental autoimmune neuritis	Immunization with peripheral nerve antigen	Anti-IFN-γ antibody alleviates disease	81–83

with TNF-α, IFN-γ treatment was associated with a reduction in severity of islet inflammation, although this treatment caused moderate to severe pancreatitis and several other pathological changes[46]. Breeding of a null mutation of the IFN-γ receptor into the NOD mice resulted in a drastic reduction of insulitis and diabetes[47]. Thus, the weight of the evidence favours the view that endogenous IFN-γ stimulates autoimmune diabetes. The underlying mechanisms are considered to be: (1) upregulation of MHC Class I molecules, which could augment targeting of cytotoxic T cells to the islet cells, and (2) increased production of aspecific inflammatory mediators, e.g. NO.

Female (NZB×NZW)F1 mice spontaneously develop a lupus-like syndrome, which has long been considered a prototype autoantibody-mediated autoimmune disease. This view is reinforced by the cytokine production profile in these mice which is of the Th-2 type. Moreover, interventions which interfere with Th-2-type cytokines, e.g. administration of anti-IL-10 antibodies, have been found to alleviate disease. Endogenous or exogenous IFN-γ would therefore be expected to also play a disease-alleviating role. However, the experiments demonstrated the opposite result. Treatment with neutralizing anti-IFN-γ antibody[48] or soluble IFN-γ receptor[49] were found to prevent disease. These observations were recently reinforced by the report that IFN-γ receptor-deficient (NZB×NZW)F1 mice are insensitive to the disease[50]. The difference in sensitivity between the wild-type and mutant mice can be explained entirely by the different levels of autoantibody, indicating that IFN-γ accelerates disease via this pathway. An obvious implication is that the Th-1/Th-2 concept fails to provide a suitable framework to explain the role of IFN-γ in the NZB/NZW lupus model.

Inflammatory bowel diseases are now considered to be disturbances in the delicate balance between immune reactivity and anergy towards microbial antigens and toxins present in the gut lumen. Few studies have been performed on the role of IFN-γ in models of IBD (see Table 3). The weight of evidence is in favour of a disease-promoting role for endogenous IFN-γ. Intestinal mucosal involvement in mice with GVH disease (*vide infra*), in SCID mice reconstituted with CD45Rb[hi] CD4+ T cells and in IL-10 knock-out mice was found to be alleviated by treatment with anti-IFN-γ antibody[51–53]. Also, IFN-γ knock-out mice were found to be resistant to IL-12-induced small bowel enteropathy, and exogenous IFN-γ was found to be able, by itself, to cause mucosal epithelial damage[54], indicating that IFN-γ, produced by intraepithelial lymphocytes, has direct cytotoxic effects on epithelial cells. Thus, in IBD, IFN-γ seems to act more through its inflammatory than its immunoregulatory potential.

Table 3 reviews evidence for mixed immunosuppressive and immunostimulatory effects of IFN-γ in a number of animal models. GVH disease develops in irradiated mice reconstituted with allogeneic bone marrow. In several independent studies[55,56], the contribution of this IFN-γ to the disease manifestations has been assessed by the use of neutralizing anti-IFN-γ antibodies. These studies are unanimous in observing that blockage of IFN-γ inhibits disease development, in particular lesions in the gut mucosa. On the other hand, as an apparent paradox, it has been reported that systemic administration of IFN-γ inhibits disease development in much the same way as anti-IFN-γ

Table 4 Animal models of immunopathology in which IFN-γ exerts mixed immunosuppressive and immunostimulatory effects

Model	Description	Observation	References
GVH disease	Reconstitution of irradiated mice with allogeneic bone marrow	Both IFN-γ and anti-IFN-γ antibody alleviate disease	55,56
	Allogeneic lymphocytes in neonatal mice cause Th-2-associated SLE-like pathology	Exogenous IFN-γ prevents disease, restores Th-1 responsiveness	57
Collagen-induced arthritis (CIA)	Immunization with chicken collagen causes joint inflammation and deformity	Early anti-IFN-γ antibody reduces severity; late antibody aggravates	58
		Anti-IFN-γ antibody aggravates disease	59–61
		IFN-γ receptor knock-out mice are more sensitive	60
Experimental autoimmune thyroiditis (EAT)	Immunization with thyroglobulin induces mononuclear infiltrate thyroiditis; transferrable by spleen cells	*In-vivo* anti-IFN-γ inhibits actively induced disease; anti-IFN-γ-treated splenocytes are more pathogenic in the transfer model	64,65
		IFN-γ-deficient mice develop more severe disease with eosinophilic infiltration; disease unmodified in IFN-γ receptor knock-out mice	63,84

antibody does. This inhibition was associated with reduced numbers of IFN-γ-producing cells[55].

Another model of GVH disease consists of inoculating semiallogeneic lymphocytes into neonatal mice, which allows for the persistence of donor cells in the host. These cells differentiate into Th-2-like cells as evident from the predominance of IL-4 production over that of IL-2 and IFN-γ. As an apparent consequence, donor B cells differentiate to produce large quantities of IgE and IgG_1 autoantibodies, resulting in immune deposits and SLE-like pathology. In this model, exogenous IFN-γ was found to prevent the disease, apparently by restoring the ability of the lymphocytes to produce IL-2 and IFN-γ[57].

In collagen-induced arthritis, treatment with anti-IFN-γ antibody has been reported to either inhibit or enhance disease, depending on the time of administration[58]. However, more recent studies have provided evidence for a uniform disease-aggravating effect, as evident from accelerated occurrence of symptoms and a higher cumulative incidence[59–61]. Moreover, IFN-γ receptor knock-out mice were found to be more sensitive than corresponding wild types[60]. Remarkably, both EAE and CIA were found to be completely inhibited by treatment with anti-IL-12 antibody, indicating that, in these models, IL-12 acts independently from, and in the opposite direction to, IFN-γ[42,62]. On the basis of cytokine production profiles, EAE and CIA are both considered to result from Th-1-type activity of autoreactive T cells. These observations are therefore at variance with the tenet, based on *in-vitro* observations, that endogenous IFN-γ participates in upregulating Th-1-type reactivity.

In experimental autoimmune thyroiditis (EAT), a model which is operationally similar to EAE, EAU and CIA, the role of endogenous IFN-γ varies with the genetic background and experimental conditions (Table 4). Deletion of the IFN-γ receptor gene in $H2^k$-haplotype mice has been reported to have little effect[63] but deletion of the IFN-γ ligand gene in $H2^q$-haplotype mice resulted in more severe thyroiditis with granulomatous lesions and eosinophil infiltrations[64]. On the other hand, treatment with anti-IFN-γ antibody was found to inhibit actively induced disease[65] but to enhance disease if used to treat donor splenocytes in a transfer model[64].

CONCLUSIONS

IFN-γ has long been recognized to have a strong impact on inflammation and on immune reactions. The underlying molecular and cellular mechanisms are increasingly well understood. Unfortunately, however, it has remained impossible to establish the ground rules by which to fully explain and, even less, to predict the effects of IFN-γ in complex systems, such as mixed mononuclear cell populations or whole-animal model systems. It is clear that the effect of IFN-γ in such systems varies from pro- to anti-inflammatory and from immunostimulatory to immunosuppressive, depending on various other determinants of the immunological environment. Some progress is being made in defining which factors codetermine the effects of IFN-γ. One such factor is the presence or absence of costimulatory signals, such as those delivered through the CD40/CD40L or the B7/CD28 systems. Another possible factor is the time point at which IFN-γ enters into the inflammatory cascade or into the ontogenesis of immune response. A distinction needs to be made between 'physiological' IFN-γ, produced and acting before stimuli hit the system, and IFN-γ produced as a result of the stimuli. Further study of the time component is much needed to fully understand the role of IFN-γ.

Acknowledgements

Studies in the authors' laboratory are supported by the Fund for Scientific Research of Flanders (FWO), the Regional Government of Flanders (GOA initiative) and the Federal Government of Belgium (IUAP initiative).

References

1. Billiau A. Inteferon-γ: biology and role in pathogenesis. In: Dixon FJ, editor. Advances in Immunology Vol. 26. San Diego, California: Academic Press; 1996:61–130.
2. Dustin ML, Rothlein R, Bhan AK, Dinarello CE, Springer TA. Tissue distribution, biochemistry and function of a natural adherence molecule (ICAM-1). Induction by IL-1α and interferon-γ. J Immunol. 1993;137:245–54.
3. McCarron RM, Wang L, Racke MK, McFarlin DE, Spatz M. Cytokine-regulated adhesion between encephalitogenic T lymphocytes and cerebrovascular endothelial cells. J Neuroimmunol. 1993;43:23–30.
4. Yu CL, Haskard DO, Cavender D, Johnson A, Ziff M. Human γ interferon increases the binding of T lymphocytes to endothelial cells. Clin Exp Immunol. 1985;62:554–60.
5. Penton-Rol G, Polentarutti N, Luini W et al. Selective inhibition of expression of the chemokine receptor CCR2 in human monocytes by IFN-γ. J Immunol. 1998;160:3869–73.
6. Heremans H, Billiau A. The effects of interferons and other cytokines on experimental autoimmune encephalomyelitis. In: Reder AT, editor. Interferon therapy of multiple sclerosis. New York: Marcel Dekker, Inc.; 1997:215–44.
7. Heremans H, Dijkmans R, Sobis H, Vandekerckhove F, Billiau A. Regulation by interferons of the local inflammatory response to bacterial lipopolysaccharide. J Immunol. 1987;138:4175–9.
8. Heremans H, Van Damme J, Dillen C, Dijkmans R, Biliau A. Interferon-γ, a mediator of lethal lipopolysaccharide-induced Shwartzman-like shock reactions in mice. J Exp Med. 1990;171:1853–69.
9. Kamijo R, Le J, Shapiro D et al. Mice that lack the interferon-γ receptor have profoundly altered responses to infection with bacillus Calmette-Guérin and subsequent challenge with lipopolysaccharide. J Exp Med. 1993;178:1435–40.
10. Car BD, Eng VM, Schnyder B et al. Interferon γ receptor deficient mice are resistant to endotoxic shock. J Exp Med. 1994;179:1437–44.
11. Matthys P, Mitera T, Heremans H, Van Damme J, Billiau A. Anti-IFN-γ and anti-IL-6 antibodies affect staphylococcal enterotoxin B-induced weight loss, hypoglycemia and cytokine release in D-galactosamine-sensitized and unsensitized mice. Infect Immun. 1995;63:1158–64.
12. Matthys P, Dillen C, Proost P, Heremans H, Van Damme J, Billiau A. Modification of the anti-CD3-induced cytokine release syndrome by anti-interferon-γ or anti-interleukin-6 antibody treatment: protective effects and biphasic changes in blood cytokine levels. Eur J Immunol. 1993;23:2209–16.
13. Matthys P, Heremans H, Opdenakker G, Billiau A. Anti-interferon-γ-antibody treatment, growth of Lewis lung tumors in mice and tumor-associated cachexia. Eur J Cancer. 1991;27:182–7.
14. Matthys P, Dijkmans R, Proost P et al. Severe cachexia in mice inoculated with interferon-γ-producing tumor cells. Int J Cancer. 1991;49:77–82.
15. Tagawa Y, Sekikawa K, Iwakura Y. Suppression of concanavalin A-induced hepatitis in IFN-γ−/− mice, but not in TNF-α−/− mice. J Immunol. 1997;159:1418–28.
16. Matthys P, Froyen G, Huang S et al. Interferon-γ receptor-deficient mice are hypersensitive to the anti-CD3-induced cytokine release syndrome and thymocyte apoptosis: Protective role of endogenous nitric oxide. J Immunol. 1995;155:3823–9.

17. Freedman AS, Freeman GJ, Rhynhart K, Nadler LM. Selective induction of B7/BB-1 on interferon-γ stimulated monocytes: a potential mechanism for amplification of T cell activation through the CD28 pathway. Cell Immunol. 1991;137:429–37.
18. Harding FA, McArthur JG, Gross JA, Raulet DH, Allison JP. CD28-mediated signaling costimulates murine T cells and prevents induction of anergy in T-cell clones. Nature. 1992;356:607–9.
19. Roy M, Waldschmidt T, Aruffo A, Ledbetter J, Noelle RJ. The regulation of the expression of gp39, the CD40 ligand, on normal cloned CD4+ cells. J Immunol. 1993;2497–510.
20. Grewal IS, Flavell RA. A central role of CD40 ligand in the regulation of CD4+ T-cell responses. Immunol Today. 1996;17:410–14.
21. Konieczny BT, Dai Z, Elwood ET *et al.* IFN-γ is critical for long-term allograft survival induced by blocking the CD28 and CD40 ligand T cell costimulation pathways. J Immunol. 1998;160:2059–64.
22. Liu Y, Janeway CAJ. Interferon γ plays a critical role in induced cell death of effector T cell: a possible third mechanism of self-tolerance. J Exp Med. 1990;172:1735–9.
23. Wall DA, Hamberg SD, Burakoff SJ, Reynolds DS, Abbas AK, Ferrara LM. Immunodeficiency in graft-versus-host disease. I. Mechanism of immune suppression. J Immunol. 1988;140:2970–6.
24. Huchet R, Bruley-Rosset M, Mathiot C, Grandjon D, Halle-Pannenko O. Involvement of IFN-γ and transforming growth factor-β in graft-vs-host reaction-associated immunosuppression. J Immunol. 1993;150:2517–24.
25. Gosselin D, Turcotte R, Lemieux S. Cellular target of in vitro-induced suppressor cells derived from the spleen of *Mycobacterium lepraemurium*-infected mice and role of IFN-γ in their development. J Leuk Biol. 1995;57:122–8.
26. Tomioka H, Sato K, Maw WW, Saito H. The role of tumor necrosis factor, interferon-γ, transforming growth factor β, and nitric oxide in the expression of immunosuppressive functions of splenic macrophages induced by *Mycobacterium avium* complex infection. J Leuk Biol. 1995;58:704–12.
27. Sileghen M, Hamers R, De Baetselier P. Experimental Trypanosoma brucei infections selectively suppress both interleukin 2 production and interleukin 2 receptor expression. Eur J Immunol. 1987;17:1417–21.
28. Darji A, Sileghem M, Heremans H, Brys L, Billiau A, De Baetselier P. Inhibition of T-cell responsiveness during experimental infections with Trypanosoma brucei: active participation of endogenous γ interferon. Infect Immun. 1993;61:3098–102.
29. Metzger Z, Hoffeld JT, Oppenheim JJ. Macrophage-mediated suppression. I. Evidence for participation of both hydrogen peroxide and prostaglandin in suppression of murine lymphocyte proliferation. J Immunol. 1980;124:983–8.
30. Boraschi D, Censini S, Tagliabue A. Interferon-γ reduces macrophage-suppressive activity by inhibiting prostaglandin E2 release and inducing interleukin 1 production. J Immunol. 1984;133:764–8.
31. Albina JE, Abate JA, Henry WLJ. Nitric oxide production is required for murine resident peritoneal macrophages to suppress mitogen-stimulated T cell proliferation. Role of IFN-γ in the induction of nitric oxide-synthesizing pathway. J Immunol. 1991;147:144–8.
32. Mills CD. Molecular basis of suppressor macrophages. Arginine metabolism via the nitric oxide synthetase pathway. J Immunol. 1991;146:2719–23.
33. Twardzik DR, Mikovits JA, Ranchalis JE, Purchio AF, Ellingsworth L, Ruscetti FW. c-Interferon-induced activation of latent transforming growth-factor-β by human monocytes. Ann NY Acad Sci. 1990;593:276–84.
34. Fernandez-Botran R, Sanders VM, Mosmann TR, Vitetta ES. Lymphokine-mediated regulation of the proliferative response of clones of T helper 1 and T helper 2 cells. J Exp Med. 1988;168:543–58.
35. Gajewski TF, Fitch FW. Anti-proliferative effect of IFN-γ in immune regulation. III. Differential selection of Th1 and Th2 murine helper T lymphocyte clones using recombinant IL-2 and recombinant IFN-γ. J Immunol. 1989;143:15–22.
36. Bradley LM, Dalton DK, Croft M. A direct role for interferon-γ in regulation of Th1 cell development. J Immunol. 1996;157:1350–8.
37. Gajewski TF, Fitch FW. Anti-proliferative effect of IFN-γ in immune regulation. I. IFN-γ inhibits the proliferation of Th2 but not Th1 murine helper T lymphocyte clones. J Immunol. 1988;140:4252.

38. Noma T, Dorf ME. Modulation of suppressor T cell induction with γ-interferon. J Immunol. 1985;135:3655–60.

39. Rosenberg AS, Finbloom DS, Maniero TG, Van der Meide PH, Singer A. Specific prolongation of MHC Class II disparate skin allografts by *in vivo* administration of anti-IFN-γ monoclonal antibody. J Immunol. 1990;144:4648–50.

40. Saleem S, Konieczny BT, Lowry SF, Baddoura FK, Lakkis FG. Acute rejection of vascularized heart allografts in the absence of IFN. Transplantation. 1996;62:1908(Abstract).

41. Ferber IA, Brocke S, Taylor-Edwards C *et al.* Mice with a disrupted IFN-γ gene are susceptible to the induction of experimental autoimmune encephalomyelitis (EAE). J Immunol. 1996;156:5–7.

42. Heremans H, Dillen C, Role of IFN-γ and IL-12 in a model of chronic relapsing EAE in Biozzi mice. Eur Cytokine Network. 1996;7:458 (Abstract).

43. Campbell IL, Oxbrow L, Koulmanda M, Harrison LC. IFN-γ induces islet MHC antigens and enhances autoimmune, streptozotocin-induced diabetes in the mouse. J Immunol. 1988;140:1111–16.

44. Campbell IL, Kay TWH, Oxbrow L, Harrison LC. Essential role for interferon-γ and interleukin-6 in autoimmune insulin-dependent diabetes in NOD/Wehi mice. J Clin Invest. 1991;87:739–42.

45. Debraye-Sachs M, Carnaud C, Boitard C *et al.* Prevention of diabetes in NOD mice treated with antibody to murine IFNγ. J Autoimmun. 1991;4:237–48.

46. Campbell IL, Oxbrow L, Harrison LC. Reduction in insulitis following administration of IFN-γ and TNF-α in the NOD mouse. J Autoimmun. 1991;4:249–62.

47. Wang B, André I, Gonzalez A *et al.* Interferon-γ impacts at multiple points during the progression of autoimmune diabetes. Proc Natl Acad Sci USA. 1997;94:13844–9.

48. Jacob CO, Van der Meide PH, McDevitt HO. *In vivo* treatment of (NZBxNZW)F1 mice with monoclonal antibody to γ interferon. J Exp Med. 1987;166:798.

49. Ozmen L, Roman D, Fountoulakis M, Schmid G, Ryffel B, Garotta G. Experimental therapy of systemic lupus erythematosus: the treatment of NZB/W mice with soluble interferon-γ receptor inhibits the onset of glomerulonephritis. Eur J Immunol. 1995;25:6.

50. Haas C, Ryffel B, Le-Hir M. IFN-γ receptor deletion prevents autoantibody production and glomerulonephritis in lupus-prone (NZBxNZW)F1 mice. J Immunol. 1998;160:3713–18.

51. Powrie E, Leach MW, Mauze S, Menon S, Caddle LB, Coffman RL. Inhibition of Th1 responses prevents inflammatory bowel disease in SCID mice with CD45RB^{hi} CD4+ cells. Immunity. 1994;1:553–62.

52. Berg DJ, Davidson N, Kühn R *et al.* Enterocolitis and colon cancer in interleukin-10-deficient mice are associated with aberrant cytokine production and CD4$^+$ TH1-like responses. J Clin Invest. 1996;98:1010–20.

53. Rennick DM, Fort MM, Davidson NJ. Studies with IL-10$^{-/-}$ mice: an overview. J Leuk Biol. 1997;61:39–96.

54. Guy-Grand D, DiSanto JP, Henchoz P, Malassis-Séris M, Vassalli P. Small bowel enteropathy: role of intraepithelial lymphocytes and of cytokines (IL-12, IFN-γ, TNF) in the induction of epithelial cell death and renewal. Eur J Immunol. 1998;28:730–44.

55. Brok HPM, Heidt PJ, Van der Meide PH, Zurcher C, Vossen J. Interferon-γ prevents graft versus host disease after allogeneic bone marrow transplantation in mice. J Immunol. 1993;151:6451–9.

56. Mowat AMI. Antibodies to IFN-γ prevent immunologically mediated intestinal damage in murine graft-versus-host reaction. Immunology. 1989;68:18–23.

57. Donckier V, Abramowicz D, Bruyns C *et al.* IFN-γ prevents TH2 cell-mediated pathology after neonatal injection of semiallogenic spleen cells in mice. J Immunol. 1994;153:2361–8.

58. Boissier M-C, Chiocchia G, Bessis N *et al.* Biphasic effect of interferon-γ in murine collagen-induced arthritis. Eur J Immunol. 1995;25:1184–90.

59. Vermeire K, Heremans H, Vandeputte M, Huang J, Billiau A, Matthys P. Accelerated collagen-induced arthritis in interferon-γ receptor-deficient mice. J Immunol. 1997;158:5507–13.

60. Manoury-Schwarz B, Chiocchia G *et al.* High susceptibility to collagen-induced arthritis in mice lacking IFN-γ receptors. J Immunol. 1997;158:5501–6.

61. Williams RO, Williams DG, Feldmann M, Maini RN. Increased limb involvement in murine collagen-induced arthritis following treatment with anti-interferon-γ. Clin Exp Immunol. 1993;92:323–7.

62. Matthys P, Vermeire K, Mitera T, Heremans H, Huang S, Billiau A. Anti-IL-12 antibody prevents the development and progression of collagen-induced arthritis in IFN-γ receptor-deficient mice. Eur J Immunol. 1998;28:2143–51.

63. Alimi E, Huang S, Brazillet MP, Charreire J. Experimental autoimmune thyroiditis (EAT) in mice lacking the IFN-γ receptor gene. Eur J Immunol. 1998;28:201–8.

64. Stull SJ, Sharp GC, Kyriakos M, Bickel JT, Braley-Mullen H. Induction of granulomatous experimental autoimmune thyroiditis in mice with in vitro activated effector T cells and anti-IFN-γ antibody. J Immunol. 1992;149:2219.

65. Tang H, Mignon-Godefroy K, Meroni PL, Garotta G, Charreire J, Nicoletti F. The effects of a monoclonal antibody to interferon-γ on experimental autoimmune thyroiditis (EAT): Prevention of disease and decrease of EAT-specific T cells. Eur J Immunol. 1993;23:275–8.

66. Hachicha M, Rathanaswami P, Schall TJ, McColl SR. Production of monocyte chemotactic protein-1 in human type B synoviocytes: synergistic effect of tumor necrosis factor α and interferon-γ. Arthritis Rheum. 1993;36:26–34.

67. Kasama T, Strieter RM, Lukacs NW, Lincoln PM, Burdick MD, Kunkel SL. Interferon γ modulates the expression of neutrophil-derived chemokines. J Invest Med. 1995;43:58–67.

68. Marfaing-Koka A, Devergne O, Gorgone G et al. Regulation of the production of the RANTES chemokine by endothelial cells: Synergistic induction by IFN-γ plus TNF-α and inhibition by IL-4 and IL-13. J Immunol. 1995;154:1870–8.

69. Struyf S, Van Coillie E, Paemen L et al. Synergistic induction of MCP-1 and -2 by IL-1β and interferons in fibroblasts and epithelial cells. J Leuk Biol. 1998;63:364–72.

70. Van Damme J, Proost P, Put W et al. Induction of monocyte chemotactic proteins MCP-1 and MCP-2 in human fibroblasts and leukocytes by cytokines and cytokine inducers. Chemical synthesis of MCP-2 and development of a specific RIA. J Immunol. 1994;152:5495–502.

71. Van Collie E, Froyen G, Nomiyama H et al. Human monocyte chemotactic protein-2: cDNA cloning and regulated expression of mRNA in mesenchymal cells. Biochem Biophys Res Commun. 1997;231:726–30.

72. Meda L, Bernasconi S, Bonaiuto C et al. β-Amyloid (25–35) peptide and IFN-γ synergistically induce the production of the chemotactic cytokine MCP-1/JE in monocytes and microglial cells. J Immunol. 1996;157:1213–18.

73. Gusella GL, Musso T, Bosco MC, Espinoza-Delgado I, Matsushima K, Varesio L. IL-2 upegulates but IFN-γ suppresses IL-8 expression in human monocytes. J Immunol. 1993;151:2725–32.

74. Ohmori Y, Hamilton TA. IFN-γ selectively inhibits lipopolysaccharide-inducible JE/monocyte chemoattractant protein-1 and KC/GRO/melanoma growth-stimulating activity gene expression in mouse peritoneal macrophages. J Immunol. 1994;153:2204–12.

75. Billiau A, Heremans H, Vandekerckhove F et al. Enhancement of experimental allergic encephalomyelitis in mice by antibodies against IFN-γ. J Immunol. 1988;140:1506–10.

76. Heremans H, Dillen C, Groenen M, Martens E, Billiau A. Chronic relapsing experimental autoimmune encephalomyelitis (CREAE) in mice: enhancement by monoclonal antibodies against IFN-γ. Eur J Immunol. 1996;26:2393–8.

77. Duong TT, St Louis J, Gilbert JJ, Finkelman FD, Strejan GH. Effect of anti-interferon-γ and anti-interleukin-2 monoclonal antibody treatment on the development of actively and passively induced experimental allergic encephalomyelitis in the SJL/J mouse. J Neuroimmunol. 1992;36:105–15.

78. Duong TT, Finkelman FD, Singh B, Strejan GH. Effect of anti-interferon-γ monoclonal antibody treatment on the development of experimental allergic encephalomyelitis in resistant mouse strains. J Neuroimmunol. 1994;53:101–7.

79. Caspi RR, Chan C-C, Grubbs BG et al. Endogenous systemic IFN-γ has a protective role against ocular autoimmunity in mice. J Immunol. 1994;152:890–9.

80. Caspi RR, Chan C-C, Grubbs BG, Silver PB, Wiggert B, Heremans H. Interferon-γ at the systemic level protects mice against experimental autoimmune uveoretinitis. Reg Immunol. 1994;6:153–5.

81. Hartung H-P, Schäfer B, Van der Meide PH, Fierz W, Heininger K, Toyka KV. The role of interferon-γ in the pathogenesis of experimental autoimmune disease of the peripheral nervous system. Ann Neurol. 1990;27:247–57.

82. Strigard K, Holmdahl R, Van der Meide PH, Klareskog L, Olsson T. In vivo treatment of rats with monoclonal antibodies against γ interferon: effects on experimental allergic neuritis. Acta Neurol Scand. 1989;80:201–7.

83. Tsai CP, Polard JD, Armati PJ. Interferon-γ inhibition suppresses experimental allergic neuritis: modulation of major histocompatibility complex expression on Schwann cells in vitro. J Neuroimmunol. 1991;31:133–45.
84. Tang H, Sharp GC, Peterson KP, Braley-Mullen H. IFN-γ-deficient mice develop severe granulomatous experimental autoimmune thyroiditis with eosinophil infiltration in thyroids. J Immunol. 1998;160:5105–12.

12
The role of interleukin-12 in inflammatory bowel disease

F. PALLONE, G. MONTELEONE, R. MARASCO, L. BIANCONE
and T. PARRELLO

Crohn's disease (CD) and ulcerative colitis (UC) are examples of chronic inflammatory processes involving the human intestine. The aetiology of CD and UC is unknown but immune phenomena are believed to play a key role in the pathogenesis of tissue damage in both disorders[1,2]. Although some of the immunological perturbations seem to be shared by CD and UC, there are important distinguishing features, possibly reflecting different pathways of immune-mediated intestinal inflammation. A hypersensitivity reaction mediated by the local release of antibodies takes place in UC whereas both histological and immunological observations indicate that cell-mediated immunity and T-cell activation are key features of CD. Moreover, substantial evidence supports the concept that an imbalance of immunoregulatory factors may lead to uncontrolled T-cell activation within the mucosal compartment and that macrophage and T-cell-derived cytokines mediate mucosal inflammation in both disorders[3]. However, no aberrant cytokine secretion has been documented in inflammatory bowel disease (IBD) and no convincing evidence has been as yet provided that cytokine changes occur as a result of disease-specific immune activation. A number of quantitative changes in the secretion and/or activity of both proinflammatory and regulatory cytokines have been reported in CD and UC. Based on variation in the magnitude of these changes, different cytokine profiles seem to evolve into which the inflammatory process may fall during the course of the disease. Studies from experimental models support the concept that two major T-lymphocyte subsets may be defined according to their respective cytokine secretion profiles: Th-1 lymphocytes, which produce interleukin (IL)-2 and interferon-γ (IFN-γ), and Th-2 lymphocytes, which produce IL-4, IL-5 and IL-10. Taken together, all available data from both human and experimental studies suggest that, in CD, the local immune response tends to be predominantly Th-1 in type while, in UC, Th-2-mediated phenomena tend to predominate[4–8]. It has been suggested that this may not be the case in early lesions of CD where an enhanced accumulation of Th-2 cytokines (e.g. IL-4) may be documented[9]. Evidence has also been accumulated to indicate that, within inflamed tissues, locally released cytokines may contribute to preferential differentiation of helper T cells toward defined cytokine patterns[10,11]. The recent demonstration of an enhanced expression of IL-12 in CD mucosal tissue supports this view[12].

IL-12 is a heterodimeric cytokine, consisting of two covalently linked polypeptide subunits (p35 and p40) encoded by two separate genes, produced mainly by activated monocytes/macrophages[13–16]. Two different pathways of IL-12 synthesis are known: one involving the interaction monocyte/macrophage-T mediated by the CD40 molecule, another involving direct cell stimulation by bacteria, bacterial products or components[15,16]. IL-12 plays a pivotal role in promoting IFN-α synthesis and Th-1 cell differentiation[17,18]. IL-12 manifests its biological functions through interaction with specific cell-surface IL-12 receptors (IL-12R). Two cDNA encoding different IL-12R subunits have been cloned. Although each IL-12R chain is capable of binding IL-12, the presence of both subunits is required for generating a functional high-affinity IL-12 receptor[19]. Stimulation of T and natural killer cells by IL-12 induces tyrosine phosphorylation of the janus family tyrosine kinases JAK2 and Tyk2 with consequent activation of a specific transcription factor: the STAT-4 molecule[20,21]. As result of its ability to modulate T-cell polarization, IL-12 has been used as an effective treatment of experimental diseases exhibiting a Th-2 cytokine profile, whereas anti-IL-12 Abs proved to prevent development of Th-1-mediated disorders[22,23].

Functionally active IL-12 has been found in mucosal samples from CD patients[12]. Transcripts for both IL-12 subunits (p40 and p35) have been detected in CD lamina propria mononuclear cells (LPMC)[12], and immunohistochemical analysis data have shown that, in human intestine, IL-12 production is restricted to macrophages[24]. By contrast, no p40 transcript has been detected in unstimulated autologous CD peripheral blood mononuclear cells (PBMC), although these cells are fully capable of expressing p40 and releasing IL-12 after appropriate stimulation. Data seem therefore to suggest that spontaneous IL-12 expression and release is compartmentalized in CD as seen in other disease states[25]. The IL-12 expression and release by LPMC in CD do not seem to be dependent on the cell sampling site. LPMC from either ileal or colonic mucosa are equally capable of expressing and releasing IL-12 (Table 1), suggesting that neither mucosal microenvironment nor variation in the luminal content is involved. Moreover, in CD, IL-12 is expressed and released by LPMC from spared intestinal samples, from either ileum or colon (Table 1), indicating that IL-12 production may not be an epiphenomenon of active inflammation and suggesting that IL-12 upregulation occurs as a result of disease-specific stimuli.

Table 1 Spontaneous IL-12 release in 24-h culture supernatants of CD LPMC

	Involved area (pg/ml)	*Spared area (pg/ml)*
Ileal	10 ± 1.2	9.0 ± 2.5
Colonic	12.5 ± 2.4	10.2 ± 1.5

Numbers indicate mean values of IL-12 produced by LPMC isolated from either involved (ileal and colonic) or spared (ileal and colonic) areas of 6 surgical samples

IL-12 is also measurable in sera of most patients with CD at concentrations significantly higher than those found in UC patients and healthy controls (personal unpublished observation). Circulating IL-12 levels seem to correlate with disease activity and current treatment.

IL-12 released by CD LPMC is biologically active as indicated by the marked IFN-α-inducing effect in PBMC cultures and by the ability of an anti-IL-12 polyclonal antibody to inhibit the effect in a dose-dependent fashion. In addition, anti-IL-12 Abs proved to inhibit the development of IFN-γ-producing T cells in CD gut specimen cultures[24]. Both unstimulated and PHA-activated T-lamina propria lymphocytes (LPL) isolated from normal mucosal samples are capable of synthesizing IFN-γ after exposure to recombinant human IL-12[26]. The ability of IL-12 to induce IFN-γ is not dependent on endogenous IL-2 and may be enhanced by T-LPL stimulation via CD2 or CD28 pathways[26]. Moreover, the IL-12 induced T-LPL IFN-γ synthesis may be enhanced by other cytokines, such as IL-7, IL-15 and IL-18 (Reference 26 and personal unpublished observations) produced by human intestinal cells[27,28]. Upon IL-12 driving, these cytokines may thus promote type 1 cell expansion and contribute to the breakdown of tolerance to the resident luminal antigens described in both human and experimental colitis[29,30].

In CD, lipopolysaccharide (LPS), pokeweed mitogen (PWM) or staphylococcal enterotoxin B(SEB) may significantly enhance LPMC IL-12 release. This is in agreement with other studies showing that macrophages in the intestinal inflammatory infiltrates undergo further *in-situ* activation and upregulation of their capacity to release cytokines[31–33]. SEB is more potent than other stimuli in enhancing CD LPMC IL-12 release, suggesting that SEB-induced mediators, including IFN-γ, may potentiate *in-situ* macrophage activation and IL-12 release[34]. The demonstration that IFN-γ-neutralizing antiserum decreases both spontaneous and LPS-stimulated CD LPMC IL-12 release (personal unpublished observations) would support the hypothesis that IL-12-induced IFN-γ acts in a positive feedback loop capable of amplifying the Th-1 inflammatory response in CD tissues.

In contrast to CD, IL-12 is hardly detected in normal intestinal mucosa or in the unstimulated LPMC from either UC patients or normal controls[12,24]. However, these cells are fully capable of producing IL-12 after appropriate stimuli (e.g. SEB)[12] suggesting, therefore, that in the normal human intestinal mucosa, IL-12 synthesis is a downregulated function. This is also supported by the demonstration that human intestinal epithelial cell lines do not express IL-12/p40 mRNA in response to bacterial stimulation[35].

A critical question is what induces IL-12 production in CD. No data have been provided to show whether CD LPMC IL-12 production occurs as result of a disease-specific stimulus or whether it reflects macrophage activation by T-cell derived cytokines and/or luminal bacteria. In addition, it is unclear what are the molecular mechanisms regulating IL-12 release. At the intestinal mucosal level, where luminal (dietary, bacterial and viral) antigens are continuously interacting with immune cells, multiple and complex mechanisms operate in promoting local tolerance. In particular, counterbalancing molecules seem to determine the promotion or blocking of chronic mucosal inflammation[11]. Preliminary data from our own laboratory show that IFN-γ and PGE$_2$ have opposing effects on LPS-stimulated LPMC IL-12 production: whereas IFN-γ facilitates IL-12 release by both unfractioned and adherence-separated LPMC exposed to LPS in a dose-dependent manner, PGE_2 is essential in preventing IL-12 synthesis (personal unpublished observations).

Taken together, all available data suggest that IL-12 may account for part of the Th-1 predominance in CD and that inhibiting or blocking its biological effects may be a promising way to control the CD mucosal inflammatory process. This is further supported by the demonstration that an experimental colitis, mediated by a delayed hypersensitivity reaction and exhibiting a Th-1 type cytokine profile, may be successfully treated with antibodies to IL-12, even after the lesion is established[36].

References

1. Podolsky DK. Inflammatory bowel disease (first of two pats). N Engl J Med. 1991;324:928–37.
2. MacDermott RP, Stenson WF. Alterations of the immune system in ulcerative colitis and Crohn's disease. Adv Immunol. 1988;42:285–328.
3. Sartor RB. Cytokines in intestinal inflammation: pathophysiologic and clinical considerations. Gastroenterology. 1994;106:533–9.
4. Niessner M, Volk BA. Altered Th1/Th2 cytokine profiles in the intestinal mucosa of patients with inflammatory bowel disease as assessed by quantitative reversed transcribed polymerase chain reaction (RT-PCR). Clin Exp Immunol. 1995;101:428–35.
5. Pallone F, Fais S, Boirivant M. The interferon system in inflammatory bowel disease. In: Claudio Fiocchi, ed. Cytokines in Inflammatory Bowel Disease. Austin, Texas: RG Landes Company; 1995:57–67.
6. Fais S, Capobianchi MR, Pallone F et al. Spontaneous release of interferon gamma by intestinal lamina propria lymphocytes in Crohn's disease. Kinetics of *in vitro* response to interferon gamma inducers. Gut. 1991;32:403–7.
7. Fais S, Capobianchi MR, Silvestri M, Mercuri F, Dianzani F, Pallone F. Interferon expression in Crohn's disease patients: increased interferon-gamma and -alpha mRNA in the intestinal lamina propria mononuclear cells. J Interferon Res. 1994;14:235–8.
8. Fuss IJ, Neureth M, Boirivant M et al. Disparate CD4+ lamina propria (LP) lymphokine secretion profiles in inflammatory bowel disease. Crohn's disease LP cells manifest increased secretion of IFN-α, whereas ulcerative colitis LP cells manifest increased secretion of IL-5. J Immunol. 1996;157:1261–70.
9. Desreumaux P, Brandt E, Gambiez L et al. Distinct cytokine pattern in early and chronic ileal lesions of Crohn's disease. Gastroenterology. 1997;113:118–26.
10. Elson CO, Sartor RB, Tennyson GS, Riddell RH. Experimental models of inflammatory bowel disease. Gastroenterology. 1995;109:1344–67.
11. Strober W, Kelsall B, Fuss I et al. Reciprocal IFN-γ and TGF-β responses regulate the occurrence of mucosal inflammation. Immunol Today. 1997;18:61–4.
12. Monteleone G, Biancone L, Marasco R et al. Interleukin 12 is expressed and actively released by Crohn's disease intestinal lamina propria mononuclear cells. Gastroenterology. 1997;112:1169–78.
13. Wolf SF, Temple PA, Kobayashi M et al. Cloning of cDNA for natural killer cell stimulatory factor, a heterodimeric cytokine with multiple biologic effects on T and natural killer cells. J Immunol. 1991;146:3074–82.
14. Gubler U, Chua AO, Schoenhaut DS et al. Coexpression of two distinct genes is required to generate secreted bioactive cytotoxic lymphocyte maturation factor. Proc Natl Acad Sci USA. 1991;88:4143–7.
15. Trinchieri G. Interleukin-12: a cytokine produced by antigen-presenting cells with immunoregulatory functions in the generation of T-helper cells type 1 and cytotoxic lymphocytes. Blood. 1994;84:4006–27.
16. D'Andrea A, Rengaraju M. Valiante NM et al. Production of natural killer cell stimulatory factor (interleukin 12) by peripheral blood mononuclear cells. J Exp Med. 1992;176:1387–98.
17. Germann T, Gately MK, Schoenhaut DS et al. Interleukin-12/T cell stimulating factor, a cytokine with multiple effects on T helper type 1 (Th1) but not on Th2 cells. Eur J Immunol. 1993;23:1762–70.

18. Manetti R, Parronchi P, Giudizi MG *et al.* Natural killer cell stimulatory factor (interleukin 12) induces T helper type (Th1)-specific immune response and inhibits the development of IL-4 producing Th cells. J Exp Med. 1993;177:1199–204.
19. Presky DH, Yang H, Minetti LJ *et al.* A functional interleukin 12 receptor complex is composed of two β-type cytokine receptor subunits. Proc Natl Acad Sci. 1996;93:14002–7.
20. Zou J, Presky DH, Wu C-Y, Gubler U. Differential associations between the cytoplasmic regions of the interleukin-12 receptor subunits β_1 and β_2 and JAK kinases. J Biol Chem. 1997;272:6073–7.
21. Bacon CM, Petricon EF, Ortaldo JR *et al.* Interleukin 12 induces tyrosine phosphorylation and activation of STAT4 in human lymphocytes. Proc Natl Acad Sci. 1995;92:7307–11.
22. Murray HW, Hariprashad J. Interleukin 12 is effective treatment for an established systemic intracellular infection: experimental visceral leishmaniasis. J Exp Med. 1995;181:387–91.
23. Leonard JP, Walburger KE, Goldman SJ. Prevention of experimental autoimmune encephalomyelitis by antibodies against interleukin 12. J Exp Med. 1995;181:381–6.
24. Parronchi P, Romagnani P, Annunziato F *et al.* Type 1 T-helper cell predominance and interleukin-12 expression in the gut of patients with Crohn's disease. Am J Pathol. 1997;150:823–32.
25. Zhang M, Gately MK, Wang E *et al.* Interleukin 12 at the site of disease in tuberculosis. J Clin Invest. 1994;93:1733–9.
26. Monteleone G, Parrello T, Luzza F, Pallone F. Response of human intestinal lamina propria T lymphocytes to interleukin-12: additive effects of IL-15 and IL-7. Gut. 1998;(in press).
27. Watanabe M, Ueno Y, Yajima T *et al.* Interleukin 7 is produced by human intestinal epithelial cells and regulates the proliferation of intestinal mucosal lymphocytes. J Clin Invest. 1995;95:2945–53.
28. Reinecker H-C, MacDermott RP, Mirau S, Dignass A, Podolsky DK. Intestinal epithelial cells both express and respond to interleukin 15. Gastroenterology. 1996;111:1706–13.
29. Duchmann R, Kaiser I, Hermann E, Mayet W, Ewe K, Meyer Zum Buschenfelde K-H. Tolerance exists towards resident intestinal flora but is broken in active inflammatory bowel disease (IBD). Clin Exp Immunol. 1995;102:448–55.
30. Duchmann R, Schmitt E, Knolle P, Meyer Zum Buschenfelde K-H, Neurath M. Tolerance towards resident intestinal flora in mice is abrogated in experimental colitis and restored by treatment with interleukin-10 or antibodies to interleukin-12. Eur J Immunol. 1996;26:934–8.
31. Mahida YR, Wu K, Patel S, Jewell DP. Interleukin 2 receptor expression by macrophages in inflammatory bowel disease. Clin Exp Immunol. 1988;74:382–6.
32. Mahida YR, Wu K, Jewell DP. Respiratory burst activity of intestinal macrophages in normal and inflammatory bowel disease. Gut. 1989;30:1362–4.
33. Burgio VL, Fais S, Boirivant M, Perrone A, Pallone F. Peripheral monocyte and naive T-cell recruitment and activation in Crohn's disease. Gastroenterology. 1995;109:1029–38.
34. Ma X, Chow JM, Cri G *et al.* The interleukin 12 p40 gene promoter is primed by interferon γ in monocytic cells. J Exp Med. 1996;183:147–57.
35. Jung HC, Eckmann L, Yang S-K *et al.* A distinct array of proinflammatory cytokines is expressed in human colon epithelial cells in response to bacterial invasion. J Clin Invest. 1995;95:55–65.
36. Neurath MF, Fuss I, Kelsall BL, Stuber E, Strober W. Antibodies to interleukin 12 abrogate established experimental colitis in mice. J Exp Med. 1995;182:1281–90.

13
Cytokines and inflammatory bowel disease

P. C. F. STOKKERS and S. J. H. VAN DEVENTER

INTRODUCTION

The development, differentiation and maintenance of immunity is dependent on processes that balance immune cell proliferation and cell death, immune cell activation and tolerance. Exogenous factors, such as bacteria, viruses and other non-self components, and numerous endogenous factors influence these processes. Among these endogenous factors, the cytokines tumour necrosis factor-α and interleukin-10 are of particular interest because of their pivotal role in regulating immune responses. Moreover, modulation of these cytokines has been demonstrated to alter the severity of T-lymphocyte-dependent experimental colitis, and both cytokines are therapeutic targets in Crohn's disease. In this paper, we discuss briefly the functions of interleukin-10 and tumour necrosis factor in the immune response, and their role in inflammatory bowel disease (IBD) will be discussed.

TUMOUR NECROSIS FACTOR-α

Tumor necrosis factor-α (TNF-α) is a member of an expanding family of molecules that includes the Fas-ligand, CD40-ligand and lymphotoxin-α and -β. These molecules have pleiotropic actions on immune cells, including proliferation, activation and death of immune cells and cytotoxicity to a range of other cells. TNF-α is mainly produced by monocytes and macrophages but production by other cell types, such as lymphocytes, mast cells, neurtrophils, keratinocytes, Paneth cells and smooth muscle cells, has been reported[1,2]. TNF-α activates target cells through binding to two specific receptors that are widely expressed[3]. TNF-α is expressed as a 26-kDa cell-associated prepeptide, which is cleaved by a highly specific cell-surface-associated matrix-metalloproteinase, named TNF-α-converting enzyme (TACE)[4] and released as a 17-kDa mature protein. Both the soluble and the membrane-associated form spontaneously trimerize to form the biologically active cytokine[2]. The soluble form exerts proinflammatory actions in a paracrine, autocrine and endocrine way, and its biological effects include up-regulation of adhesion molecules on endothelium and leukocytes, cell-mediated cytotoxicity, induction of proinflammatory cytokines and procoagulant activity[2]. Membrane-bound TNF is involved in cytotoxic action and serves as a cellular store that can be rapidly released[2,5,6].

TNF receptors

TNF is able to bind two different receptors, the 55-kDa TNF-receptor I and the 75-kDa TNF receptor II. Interestingly, although these two receptors have very different intracellular signalling domains, their biological actions overlap[7]. TNFRI shares significant homology with Fas, the membrane-bound receptor that induces apoptosis upon binding of its ligand[8]. Like Fas, the intracellular part of TNFRI contains a so-called death domain and binding of lymphotoxin or TNF-α can induce apoptosis in specific target cells[9]. However, only TNF-α is able to also induce NF-kβ activation, which in turn leads to expression of survival genes[10]. Therefore, the apoptotic signal transmitted by TNFRI is generally weaker than the one transmitted by Fas[8], Fas- and TNFRI-induced apoptosis may modulate the immune response in several ways (see below).

TNFRII lacks the intracellular death domain but, nonetheless, it is capable of inducing apoptosis, although its effect is less pronounced than TNFRI-mediated signals. In contrast to TNFRI, which is constitutively expressed on many cells, TNFRII is restricted to fewer cell types, including T lymphocytes, and its expression can be modulated[7]. TNFRII binds TNF with a higher affinity but also with a higher dissociation rate. Thus, regulated expression of TNFRII may influence binding of TNF to TNFRI: First, TNF-α is captured by the high-affinity TNFRII and subsequently handed over to TNFRI[7]. Both TNF receptors can be shed from the cell membrane and may thus function as an antagonist of TNF activity[11].

Biological activities of TNF-α

As early as 1893, the surgeon William Coley showed that administration of bacterial extract induced tumour regression in terminally ill cancer patients. The mechanism of action of this therapy remains uncertain but may have been related to necrosis of tumour-feeding vessels as a consequence of localized TNF-induced expression of tissue factor, or to a direct cytolytic action. The subsequent characterization of a serum-transferable factor that induced necrosis of tumours in BCG-sensitized mice led to the identification of TNF-α (and hence its name)[12]. Through an independent line of research, TNF-α was identified as a protein causing cachexia (cachectin) in chronic infectious disease[13,14]. In the course of time, the pleiotropic actions of TNF-α have become evident and the list of its physiological and pathological activities is ever expanding[15,16]. The most prominent functions of TNF-α under physiological circumstances are modulation of immune responses (including innate immunity and inflammation), haematopoiesis and reproduction[17].

TNF and the immune response

Many effects of TNF-α as a proinflammatory mediator can be attributed to its ability to stimulate neutrophils and the endothelium[15]. Upon stimulation with TNF-α, the endothelial cells express E-selectin[18], which enables rolling and adhesion of the neutrophils to the endothelium[19]. In addition, TNF-α increases endothelial cell production of platelet-activating factor (PFA) and the chemokine interleukin-8, resulting in ICAM-1-dependent transmigration of neutrophils through the vessel wall[20]. Stimulation of neutrophils with TNF-α results in enhanced phagocytosis, degranulation respiratory burst activity and upregulation of CD11b/CD18 expression on the cell membranes[20–22]. The latter molecule is a ligand for ICAM-1 involved in tight adhesion of the neutrophils and other leukocytes to the endothelium[19]. In addition, other immune and non-immune cells, such as monocytes, macrophages and fibroblasts, are stimulated by TNF-α to produce several secondary inflammatory mediators, such as interleukin-1, prostaglandin E_2, granulocyte-macrophage colony-stimulating factor and interleukin-6[17]. Experiments in lethal endotoxin-induced shock in mice showed that soluble TNF-α can exert all the proinflammatory actions mentioned above: lethal shock was prevented by treatment with an enzyme inhibitor that prevented the matrix-metalloproteinase from cleaving TNF from the cell membrane[23].

Recently, a role for TNF in the regulation of peripheral T lymphocyte homeostasis by means of activation-induced apoptosis has become apparent[24,25]. Activation-induced apoptosis is important for immune function in two different ways. First, this process leads to clonal deletion of immune cells that are self-reactive. Second, following an immune response, which involves expansion of antigen reactive clones, activation-induced apoptosis can re-establish the immune repertoire[26]. It has now become clear that activation of the CD4 complex on T lymphocytes leads to increased susceptibility to apoptosis that is mediated through FasL and TNF[27]. Interestingly, a role for interleukin-10 activation-induced apoptosis has also been suggested (see below).

Several lines of evidence suggest an important role for TNF in the inflammatory reaction in IBD[28]. TNF levels are increased in the mucosa and stools of IBD, particularly in CD patients with active inflammation[29–31]. In parallel with the histopathological findings, TNF-producing cells in CD patients are found throughout the mucosa whereas, in UC patients, only subepithelial macrophages produce TNF[30]. Moreover, the T-helper 1 response that defines the immunopathology in CD is characterized by an enhanced production of TNF-α[32]. Importantly, although the precise mechanism of action is unknown, the administration of anti-TNF antibodies was effective in animal models for intestinal inflammation. Indeed, infusion of a human–mouse chimeric antibody was successfully applied as a treatment for therapy-resistant Crohn's disease[28,33].

TNF and disease susceptibility

The tumour necrosis factor-α gene is located in between the MHC Class III and Class I genes[34–37]. The TNF genes have been implicated in the pathogenesis of many immune-mediated diseases and stable interindividual differences in TNF production have been reported[38,39]. Thus, it appears that certain levels of TNF production are associated with certain HLA phenotypes, and, although the autoimmune haplotype A1-B8-DR3 has been related to higher production levels[40], it remains unclear which genes are responsible. Obviously, the issue was raised whether HLA associations with disease and the differences in TNF production can be attributed to sequence variants in the TNF genes. Several polymorphisms in the TNF gene region have been described[41–50] (Figure 1) and

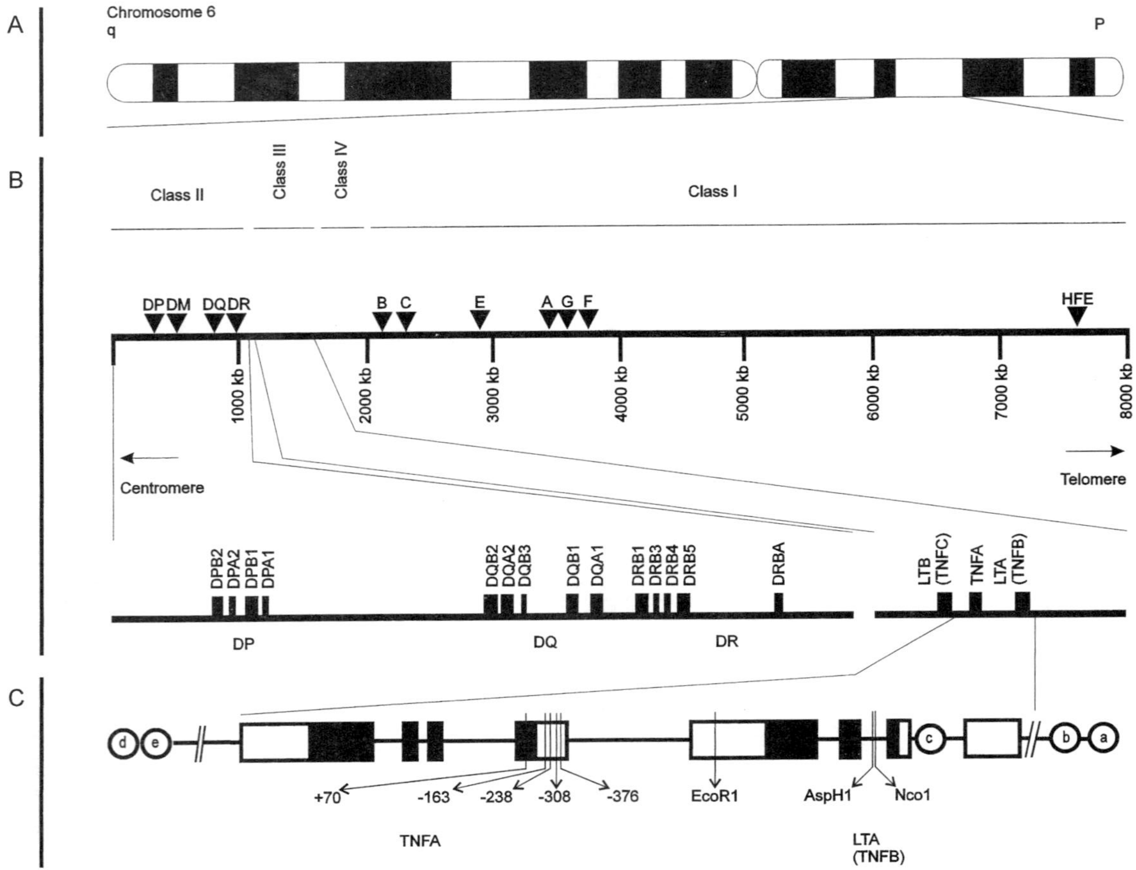

Figure 1 Chromosomal localization and polymorphisms in the TNF genes. The TNF genes are located on the short arm of chromosome 6 (**A**), in the MHC class III region of the Major Histocompatibility Complex (**B**). Five microsatellites, designated a, b, c, d and e, have been found (circles). Three restriction fragment length polymorphisms (RFLP) have been found in LTA (arrows): One rare EcoR1 RFLP and two RFLPs in intron 1 of this gene (AspH1 and Nco1). In TNFA four RFLPs at positions −163, −238, −308 and −376 of the promoter region and one RFLP at position +70 have been reported (**C**).

138

two of them appear to be related to the observed differences in the TNF production. An Nco1 RFLP in the TNF-β gene was associated with higher levels of TNF-β[51] and TNF-α[52,53], and the infrequent allele of a RFLP at position −308 in the promoter region of the TNF-α gene was related to higher TNF-α levels[54,55]. In addition, this latter polymorphism is in strong linkage disequilibrium with the A1-B8-DR3 haplotype[56]. However, functional analyses of the promotor region of TNF-α have not resulted in unequivocal evidence for a functional role of the −308 RFLP in gene transcription[57–59]. Others have argued that the stimulatory effect of LPS on TNF production is due to influences on mRNA translation, by blocking the translation-repressive TTATTTAT element in the 3′ untranslated region, rather than to enhancement of the gene transcription[60,61]. To date, no polymorphisms in the 3′ untranslated region have been identified.

A few studies have investigated polymorphisms in the TNF genes in relation to IBD[62–64] but no associations were found. One study found a significant association between CD and a TNF haplotype defined as TNFa2b1c2d4e1, which is in linkage disequilibrium with the CD-associated haplotype DR1-DQ5[65]. Interestingly, in a group of CD patients with per-anal fistulas, a lower frequency of HLA DR3 was reported with a normal frequency of the linked −308 A allele[66]. This could indicate that, in this group of CD patients, recombination between DR3 and the TNF −308 allele may play a role. Crossing-over events with adverse effects fit well with the observation of ancestral haplotypes on the MHC.

INTERLEUKIN-10

Interleukin-10 (IL-10) is a 35-kDa non-covalently linked homodimeric cytokine which is produced by T lymphocytes, B cells, keratinocytes, monocytes and mast cells. It can be described as a potent immunosuppressive agent, as is illustrated by the fact that it down regulates the production of proinflammatory cytokines, chemokines and immune-related growth factors. On the other hand, interleukin-10 is a costimulator of B cells, mast cells and thymocytes. A suppressive effect of IL-10 on bone formation has been described and this effect is probably due to blockade of TGF-β synthesis. Blockade of TGF-β synthesis could also explain the enhanced growth of haematopoietic progenitor cells induced by IL-10. The deleterious effect of interleukin-10 is illustrated by the fact that it appears to have considerable importance in the development of human cancer. IL-10 levels are often elevated in patients with tumours, inhibiting anti-tumour activity of the immune system, and the source may be the tumour cells themselves[67].

Interleukin-10 receptor

The ligand-binding subunit of the interleukin-10 receptor (IL-10R1) belongs to the Class II cytokine receptor family, which includes tissue factor, the two subunits forming the interferon-γ receptor and the subunits of the interferon-α receptor[68]. Recently, another member of this family, cytokine receptor family 2–4 (CRF2–4) was identified as the second subunit of the interleukin-10 receptor, designated IL-10R2[69,70]. Interleukin-10 signal transduction is similar to signal transduction induced by the proinflammatory cytokine interferon-γ. Both ligands are structurally related homodimers[71], which bind to the ligand-binding subunits (the R1). Another subunit (the R2 chains) is required for subsequent signal transduction via the JAK/STAT (Janus tyrosine kinases/signal transducers and activators of transcription) pathway[70].

Interleukin-10 and the immune response

IL-10 inhibits the expression of major histocompatibility complex Class II molecules (involved in antigen presentation) and intracellular adhesion molecule-1 (ICAM) involved in leukocyte transmigration). Moreover, IL-10 inhibits the expression of B7, which binds to CD28 on the surface of T lymphocytes and is essential for optimal T-lymphocyte activation. Antigen presentation to T lymphocytes in the absence of B7 inhibits cytokine production and proliferation of the T lymphocyte, and results in an irreversible non-responsive state (tolerance induction). IL-10 inhibits the cellular immune response also by preventing macrophage activation and blocking cytokine production of these cells[72].

Interleukin-10 may play an important role in the immunopathology of IBD. Mice with a disrupted interleukin-10 gene were shown to develop spontaneous chronic bowel inflammation[73]. Development of colitis in these mice was linked to the uncontrolled production of proinflammatory cytokines by macrophages and T-helper 1 cells, due to a lack of suppression by IL-10[74]. Recently, interleukin-10 in combination with antigenic stimulation (ovalbumin) was shown to induce CD4+ T-lymphocyte clones, which mainly produced high levels of interleukin-10. Interestingly, this novel subset of CD4+ T lymphocytes (designated T-regulatory cells, Tr1) was able to suppress the proliferation of CD4+ T-lymphocytes in response to antigen and prevented colitis in a mouse model for T lymphocyte-subset-mediated intestinal inflammation[75]. A negative regulatory role for CD4+ interleukin-10-producing T lymphocytes was also reported in another model for autoimmunity and this effect may be mainly due to a suppression of the production of the proinflammatory cytokine interleukin-12[76]. Other studies have suggested that the regulatory interleukin-10-producing cells are anergic T lymphocytes, which emerge when antigenic stimulation without co-stimulation by accessory molecules takes place[77,78]. A study of lymphocytes of patients with SLE showed that interleukin-10 triggers Fas-mediated activation induced cell death and this may constitute another regulatory mechanism[79].

In IBD patients, T-lymphocyte subsets comparable with those found in animal models for colitis may be important mediators of the immunopathology[80,81]. Treatment with interleukin-10 was effective in some of these models[75,82–84]. A dose-finding study of treatment of CD patients with doses of recombinant interleukin-10 showed encouraging results[85].

Interleukin-10 and disease susceptibility

The interleukin-10 gene maps to chromosome 1q in an area that also contains other immune-related genes, such as the genes for the Fc-γ receptors and components of the complement system[86]. Recently, interleukin-10 production was shown to be under genetic control: a promotor region polymorphism at position −1082 controls interleukin-10 synthesis *in vitro*[87] and both CD patients and UC patients were found to carry more often the low-producing genotype[88]. However, others did not find this association in larger groups of patients[89,90].

CONCLUSIONS

Tumour necrosis factor-α and interleukin-10 are two cytokines with pleiotropic actions. Grossly, TNF-α potentiates the cellular immune response, whereas interleukin-10 plays an inhibitory role. Genetic polymorphisms for both genes have been described but no role in genetic susceptibility to IBD has been established so far. Nonetheless, treatment with anti-TNF antibodies was shown to be successful in Crohn's disease and treatment by means of interleukin-10 may be effective. Both treatments affect T-lymphocyte function and may have long-term immunomodulating effects.

References

1. Vassalli P. The pathophysiology of tumor necrosis factors. Annu Rev Immunol. 1992;10:411–52.
2. Hill CM, Lunec J. The TNF-ligand and receptor superfamilies: controllers of immunity and the Trojan horses of autoimmune disease? Mol Asp Med. 1996;17(5):455–509.
3. Armitage RJ. Tumor necrosis factor receptor superfamily members and their ligands. Curr Opin Immunol. 1994;6(3):407–13.
4. Gearing AJ, Beckett P, Christodoulou M *et al.* Processing of tumour necrosis factor-alpha precursor by metalloproteinases. Nature. 1994;370(6490):555–7.
5. Kriegler M, Perez C, DeFay K, Albert I, Lu SD. A novel form of TNF/cachectin is a cell surface cytotoxic transmembrane protein: ramifications for the complex physiology of TNF. Cell. 1988;53(1):45–53.
6. Grell M, Douni E, Wajant H *et al.* The transmembrane form of tumor necrosis factor is the prime activating ligand of the 80 kDa tumor necrosis factor receptor. Cell. 1995;83(5):793–802.
7. Vandenabeele P, Declercq W, Beyaert R, Fiers W. Two tumour necrosis factor receptors: structure and function. Trends Cell Biol. 1995;5:392–9.
8. Nagata S. Apoptosis by death factor. Cell. 1997;88(3):355–65.
9. Tartaglia LA, Ayres TM, Wong GH, Goeddel DV. A novel domain within the 55 kD TNF receptor signals cell death. Cell. 1993;74(5):845–53.
10. Liu Z-G, Hsu H, Goeddel DV., Karin M. Dissection of TNF receptor 1 effector functions: INK activation is not linked to apoptosis while NF-kappa B activation prevents cell death. Cell. 1996;87:565–76.
11. Engelmann H, Aderka D, Rubinstein M, Rotman D, Wallach D. A tumor necrosis factor-binding protein purified to homogeneity from human urine protects cells from tumor necrosis factor toxicity. J Biol Chem. 1989;264(20):11974–80.
12. Carswell EA, Old LJ, Kassel RL, Green S, Fiore N, Williamson B. An endotoxin-induced serum factor that causes necrosis of tumors. Proc Natl Acad Sci USA. 1975;72(9):3666–70.
13. Beutler B, Mahoney J, Le Trang N, Pekala P, Cerami A. Purification of cachectin, a lipoprotein lipase-suppressing hormone secreted by endotoxin-induced RAW 264.7 cells. J Exp Med. 1985;161(5):984–95.
14. Beutler B, Greenwald D, Hulmes JD *et al.* Identity of tumour necrosis factor and the macrophage-secreted factor cachectin. Nature. 1985;316(6028):552–4.
15. Barbara JA, Van Ostade X, Lopez A. Tumour necrosis factor-alpha (TNF-alpha): the good, the bad and potentially very effective. Immunol Cell Biol. 1996;74(5):434–43.
16. Korner H, Sedgwick JD. Tumour necrosis factor and lymphotoxin: molecular aspects and role in tissue-specific autoimmunity. Immunol Cell Biol. 1996;74(5):465–72.
17. Aggarwal BB, Natarajan K. Tumor necrosis factors: developments during the last decade. Eur Cytokine Netw. 1996;7(2):93–124.
18. Bevilacqua MP, Stengelin S, Gimbrone MA Jr, Seed B. Endothelial leukocyte adhesion molecule 1: an inducible receptor for neutrophils related to complement regulatory proteins and lectins. Science. 1989;243(4895):1160–5.
19. Carlos TM, Harlan JM. Leukocyte–endothelial adhesion molecules. Blood. 1994;84(7):2068–101.
20. Kuijpers TW, Hakkert BC, Hart MH, Roos D. Neutrophil migration across monolayers of cytokine-prestimulated endothelial cells: a role for platelet-activating factor and IL-8. J Cell Biol. 1992;117(3):565–72.

21. Klebanoff SJ, Vadas MA, Harlan JM *et al.* Stimulation of neutrophils by tumor necrosis factor. J Immunol. 1986;136(110):4220–5.
22. Smart SJ, Casale TB. TNF-alpha-induced transendothelial neutrophil migration is IL-8 dependent. Am J Physiol. 1994;266(3 Pt 1):L238–45.
23. Mohler KM, Sleath PR, Fitzner JN *et al.* Protection against a lethal dose of endotoxin by an inhibitor of tumour necrosis factor processing. Nature. 1994;370(6486):218–20.
24. Smith CA, Farrah T, Goodwin RG. The TNF receptor superfamily of cellular and viral proteins: activation, costimulation, and death. Cell. 1994;76(6):959–62.
25. Penninger JM, Mak TW. Signal transduction, mitotic catastrophes, and death in T-cell development. Immunol Rev. 1994;142:231–72.
26. Green DR, Scott DW. Activation-induced apoptosis in lymphocytes. Curr Opin Immunol. 1994;6(3):476–87.
27. Algeciras A, Dockrell DH, Lynch DH, Paya CV. CD4 regulates susceptibility to Fas ligand- and tumor necrosis factor-mediated apoptosis. J Exp Med. 1998;187(5):711–20.
28. Van Deventer SJ. Tumour necrosis factor and Crohn's disease. Gut. 1997;40(4):443–8.
29. Breese EJ, Michie CA, Nicholls SW *et al.* Tumor necrosis factor alpha-producing cells in the intestinal mucosa of children with inflammatory bowel disease. Gastroenterology. 1994;106(6):1455–66.
30. Murch SH, Braegger CP, Walker-Smith JA, MacDonald TT. Location of tumour necrosis factor alpha by immunohistochemistry in chronic inflammatory bowel disease. Gut. 1993;34(12):1705–9.
31. Reinecker HC, Steffen M, Witthoeft T *et al.* Enhanced secretion of tumour necrosis factor-alpha, IL-6, and IL-1 beta by isolated lamina propria mononuclear cells from patients with ulcerative colitis and Crohn's disease. Clin Exp Immunol. 1993;94(1):174–81.
32. Mosmann TR, Sad S. The expanding universe of T-cell subsets: Th1, Th2 and more. Immunol Today. 1996;17(3):138–46.
33. Targan SR, Hanauer SB, van Deventer SJ *et al.* A short-term study of chimeric monoclonal antibody cA2 to tumor necrosis factor alpha for Crohn's disease. Crohn's Disease cA2 Study Group. N Engl J Med. 1997;337(15):1029–35.
34. Carroll MC, Katzman P, Alicot EM *et al.* Linkage map of the human major histocompatibility complex including the tumor necrosis factor genes. Proc Natl Acad Sci USA. 1987;84(23):8535–9.
35. Dunham I, Sargent CA, Trowsdale J, Campbell RD. Molecular mapping of the human major histocompatibility complex by pulsed-field gel electrophoresis. Proc Natl Acad Sci USA. 1987;84(20):7237–41.
36. Spies T, Morton CC, Nedospasov SA, Fiers W, Pious D, Strominger JL. Genes for the tumor necrosis factors alpha and beta are linked to the human major histocompatibility complex. Proc Natl Acad Sci USA. 1986;83(22):8699–702.
37. Nedospasov SA, Shakhov AN, Turetskaya RL *et al.* Tandem arrangement of genes coding for tumor necrosis factor (TNF-alpha) and lymphotoxin (TNF-beta) in the human genome. Cold Spring Harbor Symp Quant Biol. 1986;51 Pt 1:611–24.
38. Jacob CO, Fronek Z, Lewis GD, Koo M, Hansen JA, McDevitt HO. Heritable major histocompatibility complex class II-associated differences in production of tumor necrosis factor alpha: relevance to genetic predisposition to systemic lupus erythematosus. Proc Natl Acad Sci USA. 1990;87(3):1233–7.
39. Derkx BHF, Bruin KF, Jongeneel V *et al.* Familial differences in endotoxin-induced NF release in whole blood and peripheral blood mononuclear cells *in vitro*: relationship to HLA-haplotype and TNF gene polymorphism. J Endotoxin Res. 1995;2:19–25.
40. Abraham LJ, French MA, Dawkins RL. Polymorphic MHC ancestral haplotypes affect the activity of tumour necrosis factor-alpha. Clin Exp Immunol. 1993;92(1):14–18.
41. Partanen J, Koskimies S. Low degree of DNA polymorphism in the HLA-linked lymphotoxin (tumour necrosis factor beta) gene. Scand J Immunol. 1988;28(3):313–16.
42. Fugger L, Morling N, Ryder LP *et al.* Ncol restriction fragment length polymorphism (RFLP) of the tumour necrosis factor (TNF alpha) region in primary biliary cirrhosis and in healthy Danes. Scand J Immunol. 1989;30(2):185–9.
43. Webb GC, Chaplin DD. Genetic variability at the human tumor necrosis factor loci. J Immunol. 1990;145(4):1278–85.
44. Jongeneel CV, Briant L, Udalova IA, Sevin A, Nedospasov SA, Cambon-Thomsen A. Extensive genetic polymorphism in the human tumor necrosis factor region and relation to extended HLA haplotypes. Proc Natl Acad Sci USA. 1991;88(21):9717–21.

45. Nedospasov SA, Udalova IA, Kuprash DV, Turetskaya RL. DNA sequence polymorphism at the human tumor necrosis factor (TNF) locus. Numerous TNF/lymphotoxin alleles tagged by two closely linked microsatellites in the upstream region of the lymphotoxin (TNF-beta) gene. J Immunol. 1991;147(3):1053–9.

46. Pociot F, D'Alfonso S, Compasso S, Scorza R, Richiardi PM. Functional analysis of a new polymorphism in the human TNF alpha gene promoter. Scand J Immunol. 1995;42(4):501–4.

47. D'Alfonso S, Richiardi PM. An intragenic polymorphism in the human tumor necrosis factor alpha (TFA) chain-encoding gene. Immunogenetics. 1996;44(4):321–2.

48. Brinkamn BM, Kaijzel EL, Huizinga TW, Giphart MJ, Breedveld FC, Verweij CL. Detection of a C-insertion polymorphism within the human tumor necrosis factor alpha (TNFA) gene. Hum Genet. 1995;96(4):493.

49. Hamann A, Mantzoros C, Vidal-Puig A, Flier JS. Genetic variability in the TNF-alpha promoter is not associated with type II diabetes mellitus (NIDDM). Biochem Biophys Res Commun. 1995;211(3)833–9.

50. Wilson AG, di Giovine FS, Blakenove AI, Duff GW. Single base polymorphism in the human tumour necrosis factor alpha (TNF alpha) gene detectable by NcoI restriction of PCR product. Hum Mol Genet. 1992;1:353.

51. Messer G, Spengler U, Jung MC et al. Polymorphic structure of the tumor necrosis factor (TNF) locus: an Ncol polymorphism in the first intron of the human TNF-beta gene correlates with a variant amino acid in position 26 and a reduced level of TNF-beta production. J Exp Med. 1991;173(1):209–19.

52. Pociot F, Molvig J, Wogensen L et al. A tumour necrosis factor beta gene polymorphism in relation to monokine secretion and insulin-dependent diabetes mellitus. Scand J Immunol. 1991;33(1):37–49.

53. Fugger L, Bendtzen K, Morling N, Ryder L, Svejgaard A. Possible correlation of TNF alpha-production with RFLP in humans. Eur J Haematol. 1989;43(3):255–6.

54. Pociot F, Briant L, Jongeneel CV et al. Association of tumor necrosis factor (TNF) and class II major histocompatibility complex alleles with the secretion of TNF-alpha and TNF-beta by human mononuclear cells: a possible link to insulin-dependent diabetes mellitus. Eur J Immunol. 1993;23(1):224–31.

55. Bouma G, Crusius JB, Oudkerk Pool M et al. Secretion of tumour necrosis factor alpha and lymphotoxin alpha in relation to polymorphisms in the TNF genes and HLA-Dr alleles. Relevance for inflammatory bowel disease. Scand J Immunol. 1996;43(4):456–63.

56. Wilson AG, de Vries N, Pociot F, di Giovine FS, van der Putte LB, Duff GW. An allelic polymorphism within the human tumor necrosis factor alpha promoter region is strongly associated with HLA A1, B8, and DR3 alleles. J Exp Med. 1993;177(2):557–60.

57. Wilson AG, Symons JA, McDowell TL, McDevitt HO, Duff GW. Effects of a polymorphism in the human tumor necrosis factor alpha promoter on transcriptional activation. Proc Natl Acad Sci USA. 1997;94(7)3195–9.

58. Brinkman BM, Huizinga TW, Breedveld FC, Verweij CL. Allele-specific quantification of TNFA transcripts in rheumatoid arthritis. Hum Genet. 1996;97(6):813–18.

59. Fong CL, Siddiqui AH, Mark DF. Identification and characterization of a novel repressor site in the human tumor necrosis factor alpha gene. Nucl Acids Res. 1994;22(6):1108–14.

60. Han J, Brown T, Beutler B. Endotoxin-response sequences control cachectin/tumor necrosis factor biosynthesis at the translational level [published erratum appears in J Exp Med. 1990;171(3):971–2]. J Exp Med. 1990;171(2):465–75.

61. Kroeger KM, Carville KS, Abraham LJ. The −308 tumor necrosis factor-alpha promoter polymorphism effects transcription. Mol Immunol. 1997;34(5):391–9.

62. Bouma G, Xia B, Crusius JB et al. Distribution of four polymorphisms in the tumour necrosis factor (TNF) genes in patients with inflammatory bowel disease (IBD). Clin Exp Immunol. 1996;103(3):391–6.

63. Louis E, Satsangi J, Roussomoustakaki M et al. Cytokine gene polymorphisms in inflammatory bowel disease. Gut. 1996;39(5):705–10.

64. Mansfield JC, Holden H, Tarlow JK et al. Novel genetic association between ulcerative colitis and the anti-inflammatory cytokine interleukin-1 receptor antagonist. Gastroenterology. 1994;106(3)637–42.

65. Plevy SE, Targan SR, Yang H, Fernandez D, Rotter JI, Toyoda H. Tumor necrosis factor microsatellites define a Crohn's disease-associated haplotype on chromosome 6. Gastroenterology. 1996;110(4):1053–60.

66. Bouma G, Poen AC, Garcia-Gonzalez MA *et al.* HLA-DRB1*03, but not the TNFA −308 promoter gene polymorphism, confers protection against fistulising Crohn's disease. Immunogenetics. 1998;47(6):451–5.
67. Fortis C, Foppoli M, Gianotti L *et al.* Increased interleukin-10 serum levels in patients with solid tumours. Cancer Lett. 1996;104(1):1–5.
68. Bazan JF. Structural design and molecular evolution of a cytokine receptor superfamily. Proc Natl Acad Sci USA. 1990;87(18):6934–8.
69. Spencer SD, Di Marco F, Hooley J *et al.* The orphan receptor CRF2-4 is an essential subunit of the interleukin 10 receptor. J Exp Med. 1998;187(4):571–8.
70. Kotenko SV, Krause CD, Izotova LS, Pollack BP, Wu W, Pestka S. Identification and functional characterization of a second chain of the interleukin-10 receptor complex. EMBO J. 1997;16(19):5894–903.
71. Walter MR, Nagabhushan TL. Crystal structure of interleukin 10 reveals an interferon gamma-like fold. Biochemistry. 1995;34(38):12118–25.
72. Fiorentino DF, Zlotnik A, Mosmann TR, Howard M, O'Garra A. IL-10 inhibits cytokine production by activated macrophages. J Immunol. 1991;147(11):3815–22.
73. Kuhn R, Lohler J, Rennick D, Rajewsky K, Muller W. Interleukin-10-deficient mice develop chronic enterocolitis. Cell. 1993;75(2):263–74.
74. Berg DJ, Davidson N, Kuhn R *et al.* Enterocolitis and colon cancer in interleukin-10-deficient mice are associated with aberrant cytokine production and CD4(+) TH1-like responses. J Clin Invest. 1996;98(4):1010–20.
75. Groux H, O'Garra A, Bigler M *et al.* A CD4+ T-cell subset inhibits antigen-specific T-cell responses and prevents colitis. Nature. 1997;389(6652):737–42.
76. Segal BM, Dwyer BK, Shevach EM. An interleukin (IL)-10/IL-12 immunoregulatory circuit controls susceptibility to autoimmune disease. J Exp Med. 1998;187(4):537–46.
77. Sundstedt A, Hoiden I, Rosendahl A, Kalland T, van Rooijen N, Dohlsten M. Immunoregulatory role of IL-10 during superantigen-induced hyporesponsiveness *in vivo*. J Immunol. 1997;158(1):180–6.
78. Buer J, Lanoue A, Franzke A, Garcia C, von Boehmer H, Sarukhan A. Interleukin 10 secretion and impaired effector function of major histocompatibility complex class II-restricted T cells anergized *in vivo*. J Exp Med. 1998;187(2):177–83.
79. Georgescu L, Vakkalanka RK, Elkon KB, Crow MK. Interleukin-10 promotes activation-induced cell death of SLE lymphocytes mediated by Fas ligand. J Clin Invest. 1997;100(10)2622–33.
80. Elson CO, Sartor RB, Tennyson GS, Riddell RH. Experimental models of inflammatory bowel disease. Gastroenterology. 1995;109(4):1344–67.
81. Romagnani P, Annunziato F, Baccari MC, Parronchi P. T cells and cytokines in Crohn's disease. Curr Opin Immunol. 1997;9:793–9.
82. Duchmann R, Schmitt E, Knolle P, Meyer zum Buschenfelde KH, Neurath M. Tolerance towards resident intestinal flora in mice is abrogated in experimental colitis and restored by treatment with interleukin-10 or antibodies to interleukin-12. Eur J Immunol. 1996;26(4):934–8.
83. Grool TA, Van Dullemen H, Meenan J *et al.* Anti-inflammatory effect of interleukin-10 in rabbit immune complex-induced colitis. Scand J Gastroenterol. 1998;33:754–8.
84. Ribbons KA, Thompson JH, Liu X, Pennline K, Clark DA, Miller MJ. Anti-inflammatory properties of interleukin-10 administration in hapten-induced colitis. Eur J Pharmacol. 1997;323(2–3):245–54.
85. van Deventer SJ, Elson CO, Fedorak N. Multiple doses of intravenous interleukin 10 in steroid-refractory Crohn's disease. Crohn's Disease Study Group. Gastroenterology. 1997;113(2):383–9.
86. Eskdale J, Kube D, Tesch H, Gallagher G. Mapping of the human IL10 gene and further characterization of the 5′ flanking sequence. Immunogenetics. 1997;46(2):120–8.
87. Turner DM, Williams DM, Sankaran D, Lazarus M, Sinnott PJ, Hutchinson IV. An investigation of polymorphism in the interleukin-10 gene promoter. Eur J Immunogenet. 1997;24(1):1–8.
88. Tagore A, Gonsalkorale WM, Whorwell PJ. Interleukin-10 genotype and susceptibility to inflammatory bowel disease. Gastroenterology. 1998;114(4):A1097.
89. Crusius BA, Perez Centeno CM, Keijsers V *et al.* Interleukin-10 gene polymorphisms in ulcerative colitis and Crohn's disease. Gastroenterology. 1998;114(4):A957.
90. Aithal PG, Grove J, Daly AK *et al.* Polymorphism in the interleukin-10 (IL-10) gene in patients with inflammatory bowel disease. Gastroenterology. 1998;114(4):A918.

14
Immunomodulation therapy in inflammatory bowel diseases: cytokines and anti-cytokines

L. C. KARP and S. R. TARGAN

INTRODUCTION

Crohn's disease and ulcerative colitis are gastrointestinal syndromes characterized by chronic uncontrolled inflammation of the intestinal mucosa. Elevated levels of a large variety of inflammatory mediators, including lipid mediators, neuropeptides, oxygen metabolites and cytokines, have been measured in mucosal tissue samples from patients with these diseases[1]. Given the current state of technology, the precise role played by any of these mediators can be determined only by selective inhibition of their expression and/or activity. This chapter reviews the available body of knowledge regarding the immunopathogenic mechanisms of two soluble mediators, the cytokines tumour necrosis factor-alpha (TNF-α) and interleukin (IL-10). The clinical experience to date, with cytokine and anti-cytokine therapy, using TNF-α and IL-10 respectively, is summarized. Progress in investigation of the therapeutic potential of cytokines and monoclonal antibodies to cytokines in non-human experimental systems is reviewed. Finally, future directions for investigations are considered within a hypothetical context.

CYTOKINES AND MUCOSAL INFLAMMATION

Normal mucosa is in a state of perpetually controlled or orchestrated inflammation, characterized by an intricate balance of immune mediators in response to various antigenic stimuli in a genetically regulated environment[2]. Failure of regulatory mechanisms, and perhaps persistent antigen presence, may result in a lack of downregulation of inflammation. Inflammatory bowel disease pathogenesis may be the result of an abnormal immune response to a common antigen or may represent a failure to suppress the 'normal' immune response.

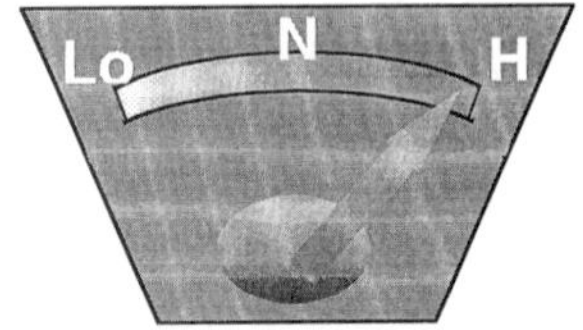
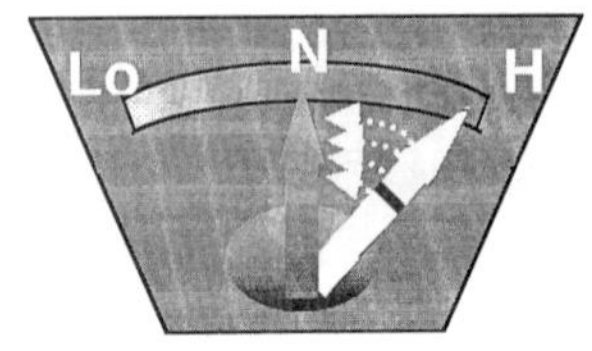
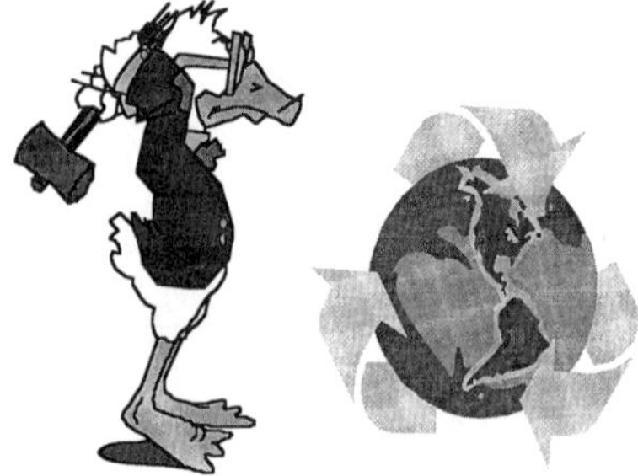

Figure 1 Exogenously administered cytokines and anticytokines may serve to re-regulate the exaggerated immune process to baseline levels, and the 'normal' state of mucosal inflammation.

Th-1 cells and macrophages help to promote inflammation by producing pro-inflammatory cytokines, including IL-1, IL-6, IL-8, IL-12, TNF-α and gamma-interferon (IFN-γ), all of which incite inflammation[3,4]. Production of Th-1-type cytokines is stimulated by TNF-α[5–7]. Th-2 cells and macrophages produce anti-inflammatory cytokines, which include IL-4, IL-10, transforming growth factor-beta (TGF-β), and IL-1 receptor antagonist (IL-1RA).

THE 'IMMUNOSTAT' HYPOTHESIS (FIGURE 1)

It is feasible that the therapeutic effect of cytokines in the regulation of immune responses may be to reset the immune response to a 'normal' level of balanced Th-1 and Th-1 cytokine secretion. The 'immunostat' properties of cytokines may persist beyond the point where the therapeutic cytokine can be measured in the case of cytokine therapy, or the absence thereof detected, as with the use of anti-cytokines. Therefore, alteration of the basic mechanism of inflammation can result in long-term regulation.

THE ROLE OF TNF-α IN MUCOSAL INFLAMMATION AND INFLAMMATORY BOWEL DISEASE PATHOGENESIS

Several studies have detected increased TNF-α protein and mRNA levels in the mucosal biopsies from patients with Crohn's disease[8,9], while other studies have generated confounding conclusions[10,11]. Several recent trials of intravenously administered anti-TNF-α monoclonal antibody therapy have shown dramatic responses in Crohn's disease[12,13]. These results demonstrate a primary role for TNF-α in the mediation of altered mucosal immune function and inflammation in this disease. The extended duration of clinical responses (up to one year) in patients treated with a single infusion of anti-TNF-α implicates the elimination of soluble TNF-α and/or blockage of transmembrane TNF-α function, or the elimination of a cell(s) expressing transmembrane TNF-α, in induction of prolonged periods of remission. Thus, the removal of TNF-α for a relatively short period of time by anti-TNF-α antibodies results in a prolonged and sustained downregulation of the hyperactive inflammatory state. Anti-TNF-α therapy in human Crohn's disease has been shown to retain its effect long after elimination of the antibodies. This finding suggests that the most important effect of blocking TNF-α is a protracted adjustment of the level of immune response(s) within the mucosa.

The mechanism by which TNF-α regulates inflammation in the gut of Crohn's disease patients is likely to be complex and multifactorial. To determine this mechanism, a series of *in-vitro* experiments were performed using specimens from patients participating in clinical trials of anti-TNF-α[14,15]. The role of TNF-α in induction of the hyperactive T cell state known to be present in Crohn's mucosa was evaluated in a study of 10 patients with steroid-resistant disease[15]. In this small study, 9 of 10 patients were evaluated at baseline and 4 weeks after administration of a single infusion of anti-TNF-α monoclonal antibody. Nine attained clinical and endoscopic remission, and 6 of the 9 patients maintained remission for 8 weeks. The leukocyte chemoattractant, RANTES, derived from activated T cells, was detectable in biopsy specimens taken at baseline but not in samples taken 4 weeks after the infusion[14]. These results demonstrate that anti-TNF-α downregulates the number, or activation state, of mucosal T cells and suggest that TNF-α is critical for maintenance of the hyperactive T cell state in Crohn's disease.

We examined the lengthy duration of response to one infusion of anti-TNF-α monoclonal antibody in another series of *in-vitro* studies performed in conjunction with an open-label trial. Among patients' responses to treatment with anti-TNF-α, sequential downregulation of TNF-α and IFN-γ production in the mucosa has been demonstrated. Th-1 T cells were not eliminated, rather their function was reduced in inflamed mucosa to a level comparable with that seen in uninflamed mucosa. This reduction in Th-1 cytokines suggests that TNF-α-augmented Th-1 function, not simply Th-1 function, is critical for disease pathogenesis. This decrease in Th-1 cell function persisted through the entire duration of the clinical response[15].

Both studies demonstrate that anti-TNF-α therapy has a profound effect on the level and function of activated T cells within the mucosa and confirm that the hyperactive T cell state and Th-1 cytokine enhancement are central to Crohn's disease pathogenesis. The presence of soluble or transmembrane TNF-α in the mucosa plays a critical role in the maintenance of this heightened and shifted T-cell response. Finally, the data suggest that the prolonged clinical benefit seen with anti-TNF-α therapy may indeed be effected through partial reversal of these altered processes.

Monocytes[16], macrophages and T cells[16] are the major producers of TNF-α. Increased TNF-α levels are associated with sequential increases in IL-1, IL-6 and IL-8[17], and *vice versa*. The correlative response suggests that TNF-α functions early in the inflammatory cascade.

TNF-α appears to have an important role in regulation of the inflammation that characterizes Crohn's disease[15,18–23]. Patients with IBD have greater numbers of mucosal TNF-α-producing cells[23–25] and higher levels of mucosa TNF-α[19–23] than healthy individuals.

THE ROLE OF INTERLEUKIN-10 IN MUCOSAL INFLAMMATION AND INFLAMMATORY BOWEL DISEASE PATHOGENESIS

The primary function of the cytokine IL-10 is as an inhibitor of immune effector functions. IL-10 is produced by T cells, B cells, macrophages, IFN-γ, IL-2, IL-1, IL-6, IL-8, TNF-α and granulocyte-macrophage colony stimulating factor. IL-10 is an important anti-inflammatory cytokine that is involved in regulation of pro-inflammatory cytokines and T-cell responses, including inhibition of TNF-α. IL-10 also has effects on various other cell types of haematopoietic origin, such as β cells, neutrophils, and most importantly T cells[26].

The increased IL-10 mRNA expression at sites of active disease in both Crohn's disease and ulcerative colitis suggests that IL-10 is an important regulatory component involved in the control of the inflammatory response that characterizes the inflammatory bowel diseases[27].

IL-10 is elevated in serum of patients with active Crohn's disease and ulcerative colitis, suggesting that IL-10 acts as a naturally occurring damper in the acute phases of inflammatory bowel diseases[28].

IL-10 seems to play an important antagonistic role in the G-CSF regulation of PMN apoptosis. Because of the importance of apoptosis in the downregulation of inflammatory reactions, the IL-10 regulatory effect may be an important mechanism in the initiation of inflammation[29].

EXPERIMENTAL MODELS OF CYTOKINE REGULATION OF MUCOSAL INFLAMMATION

Several rodent models of mucosal inflammation have been refined using cellular and molecular manipulations of mucosal T-cell regulation. The vast majority of these experimental models develop colitis that is marked by overproduction of T-helper-1 (Th-1) type cytokines, particularly IFN-γ and TNF-α. More recently, a rodent model of mucosal inflammation that is characterized by increased numbers and activity of Th-2 cytokine production (IL-4) has been generated by deletion of the T-cell receptor-alpha (TCRα) gene in mice[30].

In Th-1-type models, inhibition of specific cytokines responsible for initiation of a T-cell response (e.g. anti-IFN-γ, anti-TNF-α or anti-IL-12) either eliminates or ameliorates the development of mucosal inflammation. Treatment of these models with the Th-1 downregulatory cytokine, IL-10, and/or stimulation of local TGF-β production also inhibited inflammatory responses in these models[30]. The roles played by any one or a combination of cytokines and anti-cytokines developed to counteract their effects in human disease can only be determined by clinical trials in populations of patients with inflammatory bowel diseases.

TNF-α

Several studies in rodent models have defined TNF-α as a critical factor in mucosal inflammation. The first model to indicate such a role for TNF-α was the CD4+ CD45RB[high] T-cell transfer to congenic or semisyngeneic scid mouse. The resultant inflammation was more severe in the large intestine, and pathogenesis was characterized by the overproduction of Th-1-type cytokines (IFN-γ)[31,32]. This model system is similar to at least two thirds of Crohn's disease patients in whom cytokine secretion undergoes a shift to a Th-1 phenotype[31,32]. Production and synthesis of Th-1 cytokines appear to be important for disease pathogenesis in this model since treatment with either recombinant IL-10, anti-IFN-γ or anti-TNF-α monoclonal antibodies (inhibitors of Th-1 development/function) attenuate or completely eliminate the colitis[32]. Using a mouse model of TNBS-induced colitis, several studies have highlighted the importance of TNF-α in mucosal inflammation. In this model, colitis has been shown to be Th-1 dependent by the successful elimination of disease with administration of anti-IFN-γ, anti-TNF-α or anti-IL-2 monoclonal antibodies[33,34]. A predominant role of TNF-α in the pathogenesis of the TNBS-induced colitis has been shown by a series of investigations. Mice with chronic colitis were treated by intraperitoneal injection of antibodies to TNF-α that resulted in a marked improvement of both clinical and histopathological signs of disease[33,34]. LPMC from mice treated with anti-TNF-α produced much less IL-1, IL-6 and particularly IFN-γ. The predominant role of TNF-α in colitis was further demonstrated by the finding that much more severe, indeed lethal, disease could be induced in TNF-α mice with TNBS-induced colitis[34]. No significant colitis could be induced in mice in whom the TNF-α gene had been inactivated by homogeneous recombination. Complementation of TNF-α function in TNF-/- mice by expression of a mouse TNF-α transgene was sufficient to reverse this effect[33]. These studies, therefore, have provided direct evidence of a predominant role for TNF-α in mouse models of Th-1-mediated chronic intestinal inflammation. Other studies using the TNBS model have demonstrated a dominant pathogenic role of Th-1 T-cell-derived cytokines, suggesting that TNF-α may regulate inflammation by modulation of IFN-γ production[33,34]. Determination of the mechanism by which TNF-α regulates Th-1 cytokines may lend great insight into a component of the critical regulatory processes that initiate and/or perpetuate chronic intestinal inflammation.

Interleukin-10

IL-10-deficient mice (IL-10 knockout mice) spontaneously develop enteritis in several parts of the digestive tract. Administration of IL-10 has been shown to improve or even to prevent the enteritis in these mice. One of the functions of IL-10 is to inhibit TNF-α production[35].

C3H/HeJBir and IL-10 deficiency develop an earlier onset and more severe colitis than B6 Kos. The marked differences in susceptibility should allow the mapping of the background susceptibility genes involved[36].

T cells from IL-10-deficient mice tend to be autoreactive while IL-10 can inhibit autoreactive T cells that are induced in response to stimulation with microbial antigens. These data suggest that IL-10 plays a protective role in maintaining self tolerance[37].

Exogenous IL-10 can inhibit experimental granulomatous inflammatory responses and suggests that IL-10 treatment could be an effective new therapeutic approach in human disorders such as Crohn's disease, rheumatoid arthritis and sarcoidosis[38].

There is now increasing evidence that hyperresponsiveness to intestinal flora is a crucial event in the pathogenesis of inflammatory bowel disease. Our data suggest that tolerance to BsA is an important protective mechanism and that restoration of tolerance to intestinal flora by IL-10 and antibodies to IL-12 may be of potential therapeutic utility in patients with inflammatory bowel disease[39].

CLINICAL UTILITY OF CYTOKINE AND ANTI-CYTOKINE THERAPY: ANTI-TNF-α AND IL-10

Monoclonal antibodies to TNF-α

Recent clinical trials[12,13,40,41], in which patients were treated successfully with intravenous infusions of anti-TNF-α, highlight the importance of TNF-α in the inflammatory process of the majority of patients with Crohn's disease. Approximately two thirds of patients responded to treatment, as measured by changes in the Crohn's disease activity index (CDAI) and/or closure of fistulae. Differences among types of mucosal inflammation may account for the disparity in response among the studied populations. Parallel laboratory investigations found enhanced levels of Th-1-type cytokines in mucosal samples from the group of responsive patients.

By contrast downregulation of Th-1 activity by treatment with IL-10 has not been as successful, with responses from one study measured in approximately 30% of treated study participants. Again, it is hypothesized that the disparity in response may be due to differences in types of inflammation with features that perhaps can only be differentiated subclinically.

Because TNF plays a central role in the inflammation present in inflammatory bowel disease, other anti-TNF therapies have been proposed and are in the early stages of development[42]. These include recombinant TNF receptors (designed to bind TNF and prevent its subsequent effects) and the humanized IgG$_4$ antibody CDP571. CDP571 demonstrated promising results in a short-term (2-week) efficacy trial conducted in 31 patients with Crohn's disease[43]; however, its long-term efficacy and safety have not yet been established.

An initial open-labelled study of 10 patients with steroid-resistant active Crohn's disease assessed clinical benefit of a single infusion of anti-TNF-α. Eight of 10 patients showed improvement, as measured by CDAI and endoscopy, at 2 weeks and achieved clinical remission by week 4[12].

In a multicentre double-blind placebo-controlled 12-week trial of anti-TNFα in medically resistant moderate-to-severe Crohn's disease[13], 81% of patients treated with a single infusion of 5 mg/kg were significantly improved compared with placebo at the end of 4 weeks. In the same trial, 64% of patients treated with 20 mg/kg anti-TNF-α also demonstrated significant clinical improvement at week 4. Thirty-three per cent of trial participants achieved remission.

Multiple infusions of anti-TNF-α were studied in 73 patients who initially responded to a single anti-TNF-α infusion[41]. These patients received 4 infusions of anti-TNF-α at a dose of 10 mg/kg or placebo at 8 week intervals, starting at 12 weeks following the initial anti-TNF-α infusion. At the end of 44 weeks, 66% of patients maintained a clinical response to anti-TNF-α, and 51% ($p < 0.05$) were maintained in remission, compared with 35% and 21%, respectively, of patients treated with placebo. There was also an additional increase (10%) in the number of patients who went into remission over the 12–44-week treatment period. These encouraging results support the use of multiple infusions of anti-TNF-α to maintain disease response and remission following initial treatment with anti-TNF-α.

Anti-TNF-α has also been studied for the treatment of fistulae[40] in a 14-week trial of 94 patients with active fistulizing Crohn's disease. Patients were administered 3 infusions of anti-TNF-α at 5 mg/kg or 10 mg/kg, or placebo. Sixty-eight per cent and 56% of fistulae were 50% closed, respectively, versus only 26% of those treated with placebo. A statistically significant 55% and 38% of fistulae treated with 5 mg/kg or 10 mg/kg per day respectively, of anti-TNF-α completely resolved by the end of the study. Improvement in fistulae was often observed within 2 weeks of treatment and lasted a median of at least 3 months. These results show that anti-TNF-γ may be a rapid and effective treatment for fistulizing Crohn's disease and a promising alternative for those who do not respond to standard therapy.

Interleukin-10

A double-blind randomized multicentre trial was designed to evaluate the safety, tolerance and pharmacokinetics of IL-10 in Crohn's disease. Forty-six patients with active steroid-resistant Crohn's disease were treated with one of five doses of recombinant human IL-10 (0.5, 1, 5, 10 or 25 μg/kg) or placebo administered once daily by intravenous bolus injection on 7 consecutive days. Treatment was safe and well tolerated, and no evidence for IL-10 accumulation was observed at the end of the treatment period. At the end of the study, the mean CDAI scores were 179 in IL-10-treated patients and 226 in patients receiving placebo. The proportion of patients experiencing complete remission at any time in the 3-week follow-up period was 50% in the IL-10 group and 23% in placebo-treated patients[44].

A multicentre randomized double-blind placebo-controlled dose-finding study was conducted in patients with chronic active Crohn's disease. Patients were randomly assigned to receive rHuIL-10 (1, 4, 8 or 20 μg/kg) or placebo administered once daily for 28 days. Results from this large placebo-controlled trial indicated that rHuIL-10 administration in Crohn's disease was well tolerated with clinical benefit[45].

As part of two randomized double-blind multicentre trials, 10 patients with Crohn's disease and 7 patients with ulcerative colitis received daily doses (5, 10 or 20 mg/kg) of rHuIL-10 or placebo by subcutaneous injection for 4 weeks. The results indicate that rHuIL-10 treatment is associated with little change in lymphocyte subpopulations and downregulation of T-cell activity markers, such as HLA-DR and CD25. The transient increase of CD71 is thought to result from concomitant anaemia. In contrast to T cells and to *in-vitro* studies, rHuIL-10 does not affect HLA-DR expression on monocytes. CD54 (ICAM-1) regulation on monocytes and neutrophils is mild and inconsistent. The prominent effect of rHuIL-10 on the upregulation of FcgRI on both monocytes and neutrophils may point to previously underestimated immunoactivating properties of rHuIL-10 treatment in inflammatory bowel disease[46].

A multicentre randomized double-blind rising-dose placebo-controlled study was conducted in patients with active Crohn's disease (CDA >200 and <350). Four dose levels of IL-10 were used (1, 5, 10, 20 μg/kg per day) or placebo. Ninety-five patients were treated (n = 72 for IL-10; n = 23 for placebo). Complete remission of disease was achieved in 29% of patients at the 5 μg/kg per day dose[47].

Ulcerative colitis

A multicentre randomized double-bind placebo-controlled escalating dose study was conducted in patients with mild-to-moderate ulcerative colitis. Patients received rHuIL-10 (1, 5, 10, 20 μg/kg) or placebo administered s.c. once daily for 28 days. This study was the first trial assessing the safety of rHuIL-10 in ulcerative colitis. rHuIL-10 has been shown to be safe and well tolerated. Disease activity was not significantly improved in the treatment groups compared with placebo[48].

THE FUTURE OF CYTOKINE AND ANTI-CYTOKINES IN THE TREATMENT OF INFLAMMATORY BOWEL DISEASES

As described in the sections above, cytokine and anti-cytokines show great promise for the treatment of inflammatory bowel disease. Both anti-TNF-α and IL-10 have been demonstrated to be beneficial, albeit for varying percentages of the affected populations. Data from laboratory science investigations performed in parallel with the clinical trials indicate that it may be possible to determine which patients will respond to a particular modality (ANCA). Furthermore, the magnitude and duration of the response may be predictable as well (ANCA). At present, a panel of tests to detect the presence of specific serum immune markers associated with ulcerative colitides and Crohn's diseases are being evaluated for their usefulness in this regard.

While the evidence for the use of cytokines and anti-cytokines individually is encouraging, perhaps their greatest potential will be realized in combination or sequential administration. Additional laboratory and clinical investigation will help to define the appropriate combination and identify the patients most likely to respond to the therapy. Table 1 presents potential cytokine/anti-cytokine combinations which, based on their effects on the immune system, may prove to be highly beneficial.

Combinations and sequences may be based on the 'immunostat' hypothesis described above (Figure 1). Anti-TNF-α may be used to re-set the immunoregulatory functions of the gut, while another less-potent immunomodulator can then

Table 1 Potential sequences and combinations for future cytokine and anti-cytokine therapy of inflammatory bowel diseases

Modality	Sequential/combination	Modality
Anti-TNF-α	$\rightarrow$	6MP
Anti-TNF-α	$\rightarrow$	Anti-IL-12, anti-IL-18
Anti-TNF-α	$\rightarrow$	Antigen manipulation
Anti-TNF-α	+	IL-10
Anti-TNF-α	+	Downregulatory cells/TR3 (IL-10)
Anti-sense-cytokine specific		
Induction of antigen-specific regulatory cells		

be used to maintain it. Alternatively, based on the cytokine profile of an individual patient, a combination of cytokines/anti-cytokines may be indicated. Once antigen culprits have been further identified, disease may be brought under control by cytokines/anti-cytokines and then maintained by antigen manipulation. Alternatively, an agent, such as anti-TNF-α, may be used to downregulate Th-1 function and then IL-10 employed, perhaps with increased success, for its potent anti-inflammatory effects on induction of selectively down-regulated T-cell populations.

Serological markers, in combination with genetic and immunological profiles, will allow specific characterization of patients and indicate certain therapeutics. For example, a patient who is shown to produce limited IFN-γ is likely not to respond to anti-TNF-α or other agents targeted at manipulation of this inflammatory cytokine. As more characteristics are defined, the available therapeutic armamentarium will increase and rely more heavily on combination therapy.

References

1. McAlindon ME, Mahida YR. Pro-inflammatory cytokines in inflammatory bowel disease. Aliment Pharmacol Ther. 1996;10(suppl 2):72–4.
2. Stenson WF. Inflammatory Bowel Disease. In: Yamada T, ed. Textbook of Gastroenterology. 2nd edn. Philadelphia, PA: JB Lippincott Company; 1995:1748–806.
3. Mosmann TR, Coffman RL. Th1 and Th2 cells: different patterns of lymphokine secretion lead to different functional properties. Annu Rev Immunol. 1989;7:145–73.
4. Powrie F, Coffman RL. Cytokine regulation of T-cell function: potential for therapeutic intervention. Immunol Today. 1993;14:270–4.
5. Flesh IEA, Hess JH, Huang S et al. Early interleukin 12 production by macrophages in response to mycobacterial infection depends on interferon G and tumor necrosis factor α. J Exp Med. 1995;181:1615.
6. Hernandez-Pando R, Rook GAW. The role of TNF-α in T-cell mediated inflammation depends on the Th1/Th2 cytokine balance. Immunology. 1994;82:591–5.
7. Halpern MD, Kurlander RJ, Pisetsky DS. Bacterial DNA induces murine interferon-G production by stimulation of interleukin-12 and tumor necrosis factor-α. J Immunol. 1996;167:72–8.
8. MacDonald TT, Hutchings P, Choy M-Y, Murch S, Cooke A. Tumor necrosis factor-alpha and interferon-gamma production measured at the single cell level in normal and inflamed human intestine. Clin Exp Immunol. 1990;81:301–5.
9. Murch SH, Braegger CP, Walter-Smith JA, MacDonald TT. Location of tumour necrosis factor α by immunohistochemistry in chronic inflammatory bowel disease. Gut. 1993;34:1705–9.
10. Isaacs KL, Sartor RB, Haskill S. Cytokine messenger RNA profiles in inflammatory bowel disease mucosa detected by polymerase chain reaction amplification. Gastroenterology. 1992;103:1587–95.
11. Stevens C, Walz G, Singaram C et al. Tumor necrosis factor-α, interleukin-1β, and interleukin-6 expression in inflammatory bowel disease. Dig Dis Sci. 1992;37:818–26.

12. van Dulleman HM, van Deventer SJH, Hommes DW *et al.* Treatment of Crohn's disease with anti-tumor necrosis factor chimeric monoclonal antibody (cA2). Gastroenterology. 1995;109:129–35.

13. Targan SR, Hanauer SB, van Deventer SJ *et al.* A short-term study of chimeric monoclonal antibody cA2 to tumor necrosis factor-alpha for Crohn's disease. Crohn's Disease cA2 Study Group. N Engl J Med. 1997;337(15):1029–35.

14. Radema SA, van Dullemen HM, Mevissen M, Tytgat GNJ, van Deventer SJH. Anti-tumor necrosis factor therapy decreases production of the chemokines rantes, MCP, and MIP-2 in patients with Crohn's disease. Gastroenterology. 1995;108:A898.

15. Plevy SE, Landers CJ, Prehn J *et al.* A role for TNF-α and mucosal T helper-1 cytokines in the pathogenesis of Crohn's disease. J Immunol. 1997;159:6276–82.

16. Vassalli P. The pathophysiology of tumor necrosis factors. Annu Rev Immunol. 1992;10:411–52.

17. Feldman M, Elliott MJ, Woody JN, Maini RN. Anti-tumor necrosis factor-α therapy of rheumatoid arthritis. Adv Immunol. 1997;64:283–350.

18. van Deventer SJH. Tumour necrosis factor and Crohn's disease. Gut. 1997;40:443–8.

19. Murch SH, Braegger CP, Walter-Smith JA, MacDonald TT. Distribution and density of TNF immunoreactivity in chronic inflammatory bowel disease. Adv Exp Med Biol. 1995;371B:1327–30.

20. MacDonald TT, Hutchings P, Choy M-Y, Murch S, Cooke A. tumour necrosis factor-alpha and interferon-gamma production measured at the single cell level in normal and inflamed human intestine. Clin Exp Immunol. 1990;81:301–5.

21. Reimund J-M, Wittersheim C, Dumont S *et al.* Mucosal inflammatory cytokine production by intestinal biopsies in patients with ulcerative colitis and Crohn's disease. J Clin Immunol. 1996;16:144–50.

22. Reimund J-M, Dumont S, Muller CD *et al.* Increased production of tumour necrosis factor-α, interleukin-1β, and interleukin-6 by morphologically normal intestinal biopsies from patients with Crohn's disease. Gut. 1996;39:684–9.

23. Reinecker H-C, Steffen M, Witthoeft T *et al.* Enhanced secretion of tumour necrosis factor-alpha, IL-6, and IL-1β by isolated lamina propria mononuclear cells from patients with ulcerative colitis and Crohn's disease. Clin Exp Immunol. 1993;94:174–81.

24. Breese EJ, Michie CA, Nicholls SW *et al.* Tumor necrosis factor α-producing cells in the intestinal mucosa of children with inflammatory bowel disease. Gastroenterology. 1994;106:1455–66.

25. Braegger CP, Nicholls S, Murch SH, Stephens S, MacDonald TT. Tumour necrosis factor alpha in stool as a marker of intestinal inflammation. Lancet. 1992;339:89–91.

26. Narula SK, Cutler D, Grint P. Immunomodulation of Crohn's disease by interleukin-10. Agents Actions Suppl. 1998;49:57–65.

27. Niessner M, Volk BA. Altered Th1/Th2 cytokine profiles in the intestinal mucosa of patients with inflammatory bowel disease as assessed by quantitative reversed transcribed polymerase chain reaction (RT-PCR). Clin Exp Immunol. 1995;101(3):428–35.

28. Kucharzik T, Stoll R, Lugering N, Domschke W. Circulating antiinflammatory cytokine IL-10 in patients with inflammatory bowel disease (IBD). Clin Exp Immunol. 1995;100(3):452–6.

29. Kuhbacher T, Ebert B, Lochs H, Schreiber S. Antagonistic regulation of PMN apoptosis by G-CSF and IL-10/IL-4. Gastroenterology. 1998;114:4158.

30. Mizoguchi E, Mizoguchi A, Bhan AK. Role of cytokines in the early stages of chronic colitis in TCR alpha-mutant mice. Lab Invest. 1997;76(3):385–97.

31. Powrie F, Correa-Oliveira R, Mauze S, Coffman RL. Regulatory interactions between CD45RBhigh and CD45RBlow CD4+ cells are important for the balance between protective and pathogenic cell-mediated immunity. J Exp Med. 1994;179:589–600.

32. Powrie F, Leach MW, Mauze S, Menon S, Caddle LB, Coffman RL. Inhibition of Th1 responses prevents inflammatory bowel disease in scid mice reconstituted with CD45RB[hi] CD4+ T-cells. Immunity. 1994;1:553–62.

33. Neurath MF, Fuss I, Pasparakis M *et al.* Predominant pathogenic role of tumor necrosis factor in experimental colitis in mice. Eur J Immunol. 1997;27(7):1743–50.

34. Strober W, Kelsall B, Fuss I *et al.* Reciprocal IFN-gamma and TGF-beta responses regulate the occurrence of mucosal inflammation. Immunol Today. 1997;18(2):61–4.

35. van Hogezand RA, Verspaget HW. New therapies for inflammatory bowel disease: an update on chimeric anti-TNF alpha antibodies and IL-10 therapy. Scand J Gastroenterol Suppl. 1997;223:105–7.

36. Bristol IJ, Mahler M, Sundberg JP, Leiter EH, Cong Y, Elson CO. Severe, early colitis in C3H/HeJBir-IL-10-deficient mice. Gastroenterology. 1998;114(4):3865.

37. Ito K, Ernst PB. IL-10 regulates autoreactive T-cell activity in colitis prone mice. Gastroenterology. 1998;114(4):4108.
38. Herfarth HH, Mohanty SP, Rath HC, Tonkonogy S, Sartor RB. Interleukin 10 suppresses experimental chronic, granulomatous inflammation induced by bacterial cell wall polymers. Gut. 1996;39(96):836–45.
39. Duchmann R, Schmitt E, Knolle P, Meyer zum Buschenfelde KH, Neurath M. Tolerance towards resident intestinal flora in mice is abrogated in experimental colitis and restored by treatment with interleukin-10 or antibodies to interleukin-12. Eur J Immunol. 1996;26(4):934–8.
40. Present D, D'Haens G, van Deventer SGH *et al.* Anti-TNF-alpha chimeric antibody (cA2) is effective in the treatment of the fistulae of Crohn's disease: A multicenter, randomized, double-blind, placebo-controlled study. Gastroenterology. 1997;92:648A.
41. Rutgeerts P, Present D, Mayer L *et al.* Retreatment with anti-TNF-α chimeric antibody (cA2) effectively maintains cA2- induced remission in Crohn's disease. Gastroenterology. 1997;92:A1078.
42. Sands BE. Biologic therapy for inflammatory bowel disease. Inflamm Bowel Dis. 1997;3:95–113.
43. Stack WA, Mann SD, Roy AJ *et al.* Randomized controlled trial of CDP571 antibody to tumour necrosis factor-α in Crohn's disease. Lancet. 1997;349:521–4.
44. van Deventer SJ, Elson CO, Fedorak RN. Multiple doses of intravenous interleukin 10 in steroid-refractory Crohn's disease. Crohn's Disease Study Group. Gastroenterology. 1997;113(2):383–9.
45. Schreiber S, Fedorak RN, Nielsen OH *et al.* Safety and efficacy study of recombinant human interleukin-10 (rHuIL-10) treatment in 329 patients with chronic active Crohn's disease. Gastroenterology. 1998;114(4):4423.
46. Dejaco C, Lichtenberger C, Reinisch W, Kuhn I, Tilg H, Gaschev C. *In vivo* changes of lymphocyte subpopulations and leukocyte surface markers by multiple doses of recombinant human interleukin-10 in inflammatory bowel disease. Gastroenterology. 1998;114(4):3939.
47. Fedorak RN, Gangl A, Elson CO *et al.* and the IL-10 IBD Cooperative Study Group. Safety, tolerance and efficacy of multiple doses of subcutaneous interleukin-10 in mild to moderate active Crohn's disease. Gastroenterology. 1998;114(4):3993.
48. Schreiber S, Fedorak RN, Wild G *et al.* Safety and tolerance of rHuIL-10 treatment in patients with mild/moderate active ulcerative colitis. Gastroenterology. 1998;114(4):4424.

Section IV
Cancer in IBD

15
Risk factors for development of colorectal cancer in inflammatory bowel disease

T. A. BRENTNALL

Patients with inflammatory bowel disease (IBD) have an increased risk of colorectal cancer. Important observations made over the past thirty years demonstrate that the natural history of ulcerative-colitis-associated cancer differs from that of sporadic colon cancer. Neoplasia develops in ulcerative colitis (UC) at a younger age and may be multifocal. Furthermore, dysplasia in UC may be widespread and is often present in mucosa that *appears normal at colonoscopy*. In sporadic colon cancer, precancerous dysplasia is localized to a focal visible mass, the adenoma, and is absent in the surrounding normal-appearing mucosa.

The lack of an endoscopically visible mass or other lesion in UC tumorigenesis makes understanding risk factors for colorectal cancer all the more important. When UC patients undergo surveillance, the endoscopist must take numerous biopsies to detect histologically grossly invisible areas of dysplasia. Such surveillance is time consuming and costly and must be repeated for as long as the IBD patient has a colon. The clinical management of this cancer risk is controversial because annual colonoscopic surveillance with extensive biopsy discovers relatively few patients with neoplasia. A better knowledge of the risk factors in the process of IBD-associated tumorigenesis could be used to design more effective surveillance programmes to detect dysplasia.

DURATION AND EXTENT OF DISEASE, AND AGE AT ONSET

The risk of colon cancer is directly linked to duration of inflammatory bowel disease. However, the exact magnitude of this risk is controversial. Studies evaluating the risk can be difficult to interpret because they: a) used referral-centre populations which may have an increased risk of neoplasia; b) included patients with cancer at the time of referral; c) included patients who had undergone colectomy for intractable disease, whose cancer outcome will be forever undefined; and d) used numbers of patients too small to provide adequate power for statistical analysis. Controversy notwithstanding, most experts would agree that there is relatively low risk in the first 8–10 years of ulcerative colitis but that cancer risk escalates with each year thereafter[1–9].

A large well-designed population-based study from Sweden determined that the absolute risk of colorectal cancer is approximately 0.5–1% per year of pancolitis, escalating with each passing decade of disease[10]. Neoplastic transformation takes time, with an average duration of colitis of 20–25 years before cancer is diagnosed. Although cancer can occasionally occur early in the disease, it is a relatively rare event in the first decade of illness. These findings are the basis of recommendations that colonoscopic surveillance be started after 8–10 years of colitis.

Risk of colorectal cancer is greatest for those patients with pancolitis[1–3,10]. Patients with disease distal to the hepatic/splenic flexure (left-sided disease) also have an elevated risk of colorectal cancer, but lower than that for pancolitis[7]. Cancer risk in proctitis probably approaches that of the normal population. However, there are occasional reports of cancer developing in patients with disease confined to the rectosigmoid[10,11]. The Swedish population-based study of 3117 UC patients detected an increased relative risk of colon cancer of 14.8 for patients with pancolitis, 2.8 for those with left-sided disease, and 1.7 for those with ulcerative proctitis, as compared with the general population[10].

The age of disease onset may be a separate factor for colorectal cancer in the setting of pancolitis or left-sided colitis, *independent of disease duration*. Two studies found that UC patients with disease onset *before the age of 15 years* have an absolute risk of colorectal cancer of 40% after 35 years of *pancolitis* compared with 30% for patients with onset after 15 years of age[10,11]. While the younger cohort was more likely to develop cancer, many decades may be required to do so.

There may be genetic factors that predispose certain subsets of UC patients to colorectal cancer. Early age of onset appears to be associated with positive family history of IBD[12,13]. Furthermore, UC patients with a positive family history of colon cancer are twice as likely to develop colorectal cancer as are UC patients without a family history, matched for extent and duration of disease[14]. Whether the genes that predispose to familial IBD and early onset, also predispose to cancer, remains to be determined.

PRIMARY SCLEROSING CHOLANGITIS

Primary sclerosing cholangitis (PSC) is a chronic inflammatory disease of the biliary tract and is present in 1–6% of patients with ulcerative colitis. Conversely, nearly all patients with PSC have IBD[15]. PSC appears to be an important risk factor for the development of colorectal cancer in UC. Studies have reported that the risk of colorectal neoplasia approaches 50% for PSC patients who have had UC for 25 years[16,17,64]. The risk and natural history of colonic tumorigenesis in PSC/UC patients has been evaluated and compared with UC patients without PSC. The duration of disease, age of onset, and time course for progression to dysplasia is similar between the PSC/UC and UC patients; however, the PSC/UC patients are 5 times more likely to develop dysplasia[17]. Some hypothesize that altered bile acids associated with PSC may play a role in the elevated risk of colon carcinogenesis. In support of this theory, PSC/UC patients tend to have right-sided colon cancers, where bile acid concentrations are highest in the colon, compared with UC patients without PSC, who have mainly left-sided tumours[18]. Recent data suggest that liver transplantation is not a statistically significant additional risk in PSC patients[17,19]. Thus, PSC patients represent a subset of UC patients who are at markedly increased risk for colonic neoplasia and who need close colonoscopic surveillance with extensive biopsy sampling.

CROHN'S DISEASE

While it is well known that ulcerative colitis has an increased risk of colorectal cancer, the risk of colon cancer in Crohn's disease has been more controversial. Initial reports suggested that there is an increased risk of colon cancer among Crohn's patients. However, the studies were relatively small and were not applied to clinical practice[20–22]. Over the past 2 decades, an increasing number of reports have confirmed that Crohn's patients with colitis or ileocolitis are at increased risk for colorectal carcinoma, comparable to the risk seen in UC. Again, as with UC, risk of cancer is determined mainly by the extent and duration of disease and is small during the first 8–10 years of disease but rises steadily thereafter at approximately 0.5–1% per year[23–25]. Of note, the location of the cancers appears to be right sided, in contrast to the colon cancer seen in UC which occurs predominantly in the rectosigmoid. In addition, there have been reports of cancer occurring in endoscopically uninvolved colon in Crohn's colitis. One study showed that as many as a third of colon cancers arose in grossly unaffected areas distant from sites of active disease[26]. The latter finding has implications for surveillance protocols, suggesting that the entire colon should be surveyed, even if only part of the colon appears to be grossly affected. Colonic strictures are of especial concern in Crohn's colitis because up to 12% of them are malignant[27].

MOLECULAR MARKERS

Neoplasia associated with UC offers a unique and valuable model with which to study the molecular events in colorectal tumorigenesis. The histological progression in UC cancer appears to occur in a step-wise fashion (negative → indefinite for dysplasia → dysplasia → cancer). Unlike sporadic colon cancer, in which dysplasia is limited to the adenomas that precede cancer, the dysplastic epithelium in UC may cover extensive areas of mucosa. Foci of high-grade dysplasia and/or cancer are often surrounded by broader regions of mucosa that are less dysplastic. Thus, the cancer in UC often does not destroy its precursor lesion; the geographic distribution of the histological changes can therefore be mapped and correlated with the distribution of abnormalities in different tumour suppressor genes and oncogenes. These correlations can lead to insights into the mechanisms of neoplastic progression (Figure 1).

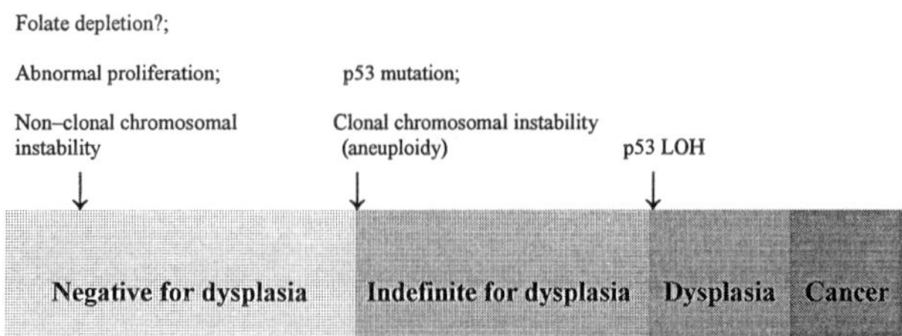

Figure 1   A model of molecular events in UC tumorigenesis

p53

The p53 tumour suppressor gene, located on chromosome 17p, exerts a pivotal influence on cell repair, proliferation and death. p53 acts as a cell-cycle checkpoint or guardian, delaying entry of genetically damaged cells into the cell cycle until the DNA damage can be repaired[28]. Inactivation or loss of one normal p53 allele and mutation within the remaining allele have been detected in many different tumours, including those from the gastrointestinal tract[29].

A relationship has been found between *p53 allelic loss* and histological progression and aneuploidy in UC-associated neoplasms: p53 allelic loss increases as the histological abnormality worsens. Occasionally, p53 allelic loss may be detected in epithelium that is histologically negative or indefinite for dysplasia, but it is more often a later event, found in areas of dysplasia and cancer[30].

The timing of *p53 mutation* differs in UC-associated colon cancers compared with sporadic colon cancer[30,31]. It is an early event in UC, and it can even be found in diploid histologically normal tissue on the periphery of a field of cancer or high-grade dysplasia. Further, the mutation can often be detected over relatively widespread areas of the UC colon in association with dysplastic change. Thus, p53 mutation is an example of the type of early biomarker that might potentially prove valuable in the prospective identification of UC patients at higher risk for neoplastic progression. The detection of p53 mutations in the stool of patients with ulcerative colitis has recently been demonstrated[32]. The use of p53 as a biomarker may prove to be useful in the future once screening for it becomes more technically feasible.

Aneuploidy

Aneuploidy, a measure of chromosomal instability, is frequently associated with dysplasia, cancer and surrounding non-dysplastic tissue in UC[33–35]. Aneuploidy is detected by flow cytometric analysis of colonic biopsies and it may be a more objective marker than histological interpretation of dysplasia, which is prone to observer variation. The abnormal DNA content correlates closely with dysplasia but appears to be an early event in UC tumorigenesis because it is also found in biopsies that are negative or indefinite for dysplasia. Aneuploidy can be a useful predictor of future progression to dysplasia and cancer. Prospective colonoscopic biopsy studies indicate that there is a tendency for aneuploid cells to persist and for additional new aneuploid populations of cells to develop and to expand to cover larger areas of mucosa over time. More than 75% of patients with aneuploidy and considered to be negative or indefinite for histology will progress to overt dysplasia within 1–10 years[36–38]. Use of aneuploidy as an adjunct to histology in the surveillance of patients who have negative or indefinite histology, may help determine which patients are most likely to progress, and thus warrant more frequent surveillance. However, aneuploidy requires expansion of a fairly large clone of cells for detection. The predictive value of aneuploidy is not 100%, as occasional cancers do develop in IBD with no evidence of aneuploidy. Other methods of measuring chromosomal instability, which do not require clonal expansion, may prove to be more sensitive markers in the future.

Sialosyl-Tn

Sialosyl-Tn is a mucin antigen expressed in IBD and sporadic colon cancers, not in normal mucosa. Antibody to sialosyl-Tn binds to 11% of all surveillance biopsy specimens in UC patients who are negative for dysplasia, but to more than 40% of surveillance biopsies in patients with high-grade dysplasia or cancer. Moreover, sialosyl-Tn may be expressed in negative biopsies from patients who later develop dysplasia[39,40].

MSH2

The human MSH2 gene on chromosome 2p appears to play an important role in DNA mismatch repair. Genetic studies have shown that hMSH2 is involved in the 'proofreading' of DNA, to ensure that mistakes are detected and repaired. MSH2 malfunction leads to accumulation of DNA mutations and loss of genomic stability[41]. Germline mutations in the hMSH2 gene are implicated in the pathogenesis of some colorectal cancers, including hereditary non-polyposis colorectal cancer (HNPCC)[41–43].

The MSH2 mismatch repair gene may be a potential genetic marker in UC[44]. A constitutional intronic T to C substitution is present within this gene in 24% of UC patients with neoplasia compared with 11% of UC patients without neoplasia and 9% of normal controls. UC patients who have this T to C substitution are 3 times more likely to develop neoplasia than UC patients who do not carry it.

Because this substitution is present in the normal population, the data suggest that the substitution does *not* confer a phenotypic effect (development of cancer) unless a second event takes place. It is possible that the substitution might be phenotypically silent (normal population) until the system is stressed (chronic colonic inflammation in UC patients). An alternative and equally plausible explanation is that the intronic substitution may be linked to another gene that is responsible for the elevated risk in cancer. Interestingly, this same mutation has been associated with an elevated risk of sporadic colorectal cancer in the general population. Twenty-seven per cent of patients with colorectal cancer carry the germline substitution compared with 10% of controls, yielding a 3.2-fold increased cancer risk[45]. While the MSH2 substitution is interesting from a basic science standpoint, it currently lacks sufficient predictive value to be clinically useful.

REDUCTION OF RISK FOR COLON CANCER IN INFLAMMATORY BOWEL DISEASE

Chemoprevention: use of folate

Folate deficiency is associated with a variety of malignancies, including colon cancer. Large case–control studies have found that an inverse relationship exists between dietary folic acid intake and sporadic colonic neoplasia[46–48]. Patients with UC may develop folate deficiency due to intestinal malabsorption, increased folate turnover or inadequate dietary intake, as well as competitive inhibition by sulphasalazine[49,50]. Red-cell folate is commonly depleted in blood from patients with UC-associated neoplasia. Moreover, neoplastic colonic epithelium from UC patients is folate depleted, while adjacent normal mucosa is not[51,52]. Folic acid supplementation may have a protective effect against neoplastic transformation in a dose-dependent manner. The relative risk of neoplasia is 0.76 for patients taking 0.4 mg of folate per day (one multivitamin) and 0.54 for patients taking 1 mg per day. While these data are not statistically significant ($p = 0.08$), they are supported by an earlier study showing that a lack of folate supplementation was associated with neoplastic progression in UC patients[53,54].

The mechanism of folate deficiency and neoplastic transformation is just beginning to be elucidated. Folate deficiency causes uracil misincorporation into DNA and can lead to chromosome strand-breaks[55]. Indeed, unrepaired DNA strand-breaks have been detected in the irradiated lymphocytes of UC patients compared with normal controls[56]. In addition, folate may play a role in proliferation of colonic epithelial cells. Ulcerative colitis patients treated with 15 mg of folate for 3 months were found to have a significant reduction in proliferating cells at the crypt surface, compared with controls[57]. Abnormal proliferation is the base in which neoplastic transformation can grow. Thus, regulation of colonic mucosa proliferation may be one of the first early steps to cancer prevention.

Surveillance

Several long-term studies have been undertaken to evaluate the effectiveness of biopsy surveillance programmes in patients with chronic IBD[58–60]. Surveillance programmes can be an effective aid in diagnosing precancerous conditions and identifying early colorectal cancer (Dukes A) that are amenable to surgical cure. In the final analysis, surveillance programmes have been demonstrated to significantly decrease mortality, extending life by 7–14 months compared with no surveillance. While this may not seem impressive, recall that yearly cervical Pap smears increase life expectancy by 3 months and annual faecal occult blood tests plus flexible sigmoidoscopy every 5 years increase life expectancy by only 1.5 months[61–63].

SUMMARY

The current standard practice is to perform life-long annual colonoscopy with extensive biopsy in all patients with extensive UC of 8 or more years duration. This approach is both time and cost intensive, and requires patient compliance, but it is life saving. Better understanding of neoplastic progression in UC may provide a basis for more efficient surveillance. Use of molecular biomarkers, as well as thorough identification of clinical risk factors, can help define those IBD patients who are at highest risk for neoplastic progression; surveillance efforts should be tailored to provide close scrutiny for those who warrant it. In addition, the development of new methods of screening may someday reduce the time, cost and effort now required to be confident of detecting dysplasia and early carcinoma when present. The role of chemoprevention is evolving and may prove important in the future.

References

1. Goligher JC, de Dombal FT, Watts JM *et al.* Course and prognosis. In: Ulcerative Colitis. Baltimore: Williams & Wilkins Co.; 1968:150–74.
2. Edwards FC, Truelove SC. The course and prognosis of ulcerative colitis. III. Complications. Gut. 1964;5:1–22.
3. Nugent FW, Haggitt RC, Colcher H, Kutteruf GC. Malignant potential of chronic ulcerative colitis. Preliminary report. Gastroenterology. 1979;76:1–5.
4. Nugent FW, Haggitt RC, Gilpin PA. Cancer surveillance in ulcerative colitis. Gastroenterology. 1991;100:1241–8.
5. Ransohoff DF. Colon cancer in ulcerative colitis. Gastroenterology. 1988;94:1089–91.
6. Lennard-Jones JE. Cancer risk in ulcerative colitis: Surveillance or surgery. Br J Surg. 1985;72(suppl):84–6.
7. Dawson IM, Pryse-Davies J. The development of carcinoma of the large intestine in ulcerative colitis. Br J Surg. 1959;47:113–28.
8. Morson BC, Pang LS. Rectal biopsy as an aid to cancer control in ulcerative colitis. Gut. 1967;8:423–34.
9. Sparberg M, Fennessy J, Kirsner JB. Ulcerative proctitis and mild ulcerative colitis: a study of 220 patients. Medicine (Baltimore). 1966;45:391–412.
10. Ekbom A, Helmick C, Zack M, Adami H-O. Ulcerative colitis and colorectal cancer. A population-based study. N Engl J Med. 1990;323:1228–33.
11. Devroede GJ, Taylor WF, Sauer W, Jackman RJ, Stickler GB. Cancer risk and life expectancy of children with ulcerative colitis. N Engl J Med. 1971;285:17–21.
12. Monsén U, Broström O, Nordenwall B, Sörstad J, Hellers G. Prevalence of inflammatory bowel disease among relatives of patients with ulcerative colitis. Scand J Gastroenterol. 1987;22:214–18.
13. Monsén U, Bernell O, Johansson C, Hellers G. Prevalence of inflammatory bowel disease among relatives of patients with Crohn's disease. Scand J Gastroenterol. 1991;26:302–6.
14. Nuako W, Ahlquist DA, Schaid DJ *et al.* Familial predisposition as a risk factor for colorectal cancer in chronic ulcerative colitis: A case–control study. Gastroenterology. 1996;110:A569.
15. Olsson R, Danielsson A, Jarnerot G *et al.* Prevalence of primary sclerosing cholangitis in patients with ulcerative colitis. Gastroenterology. 1991;100:1319–23.
16. Broome U, Lofberg R, Veress B, Eriksson LS. Primary sclerosing cholangitis and ulcerative colitis: evidence for increasing neoplastic potential. Hepatology. 1995;22:1404–8.
17. Brentnall TA, Haggitt RC, Rabinovitch RS *et al.* Risk and natural history of colonic neoplasia in patients with primary sclerosing cholangitits and ulcerative colitis. Gastroenterology. 1996;110:331–8.
18. Marchesa P, Lashner BA, Lavery IC *et al.* The risk of cancer and dysplasia among ulcerative colitis patients with primary sclerosing cholangitis. Am J Gastroenterol. 1997;92:1285–8.
19. Loftus EV Jr, Aguilar HI, Sandborn WJ *et al.* Risk of colorectal neoplasia in patients with primary sclerosing cholangitis and ulcerative colitis following orthotopic liver transplantation. Hepatology. 1998;27:685–90.
20. Weedon DD, Shorter RG, Ilstrup DM, Huizenga KA, Taylor WF. Crohn's disease and cancer. N Engl J Med. 1973;289:1099–102.
21. Gyde SN, Prior P, Macartney JG, Thompson H, Waterhouse JAH, Allan RN. Malignancy in Crohn's disease. Gut. 1980;21:1024 9.
22. Shorter RG. Risk of intestinal cancer in Crohn's disease. Dis Colon Rectum. 1983;26:686–90.

23. Sachar DB. Cancer in Crohn's disease: dispelling the myths. Gut. 1994;35:1507–8.
24. Gillen CD, Prior P, Andrews HA, Allan RN. Ulcerative colitis and Crohn's disease: a comparison of the colorectal cancer risk in extensive colitis. Gut. 1994;35:1590–2.
25. Ekbom A, Helmick C, Zack M, Adami H-O. Increased risk of large-bowel cancer in Crohn's disease with colonic involvement. Lancet. 1990;336:357–9.
26. Greenstein AJ, Sachar DB, Smith H, Janowitz HD, Aufses AH. A comparison of cancer risk in Crohn's disease and ulcerative colitis. Cancer. 1981;48:2742–5.
27. Yamazaki Y, Ribeiro MB, Sacher DB et al. Malignant colorectal strictures in Crohn's disease. Am J Gastroenterol. 1991;86:882–5.
28. Lane DP. p53, Guardian of the genome. Nature. 1992;358:15–26.
29. Harris CC, Hollstein M. Clinical implications of the p53 tumor-suppressor gene. N Engl J Med. 1993;329:1318–27.
30. Brentnall TA, Crispin DA, Rabinovitch PS et al. Mutations in the p53 gene: An early event in neoplastic progression in ulcerative colitis. Gastroenterology. 1994;107:369–78.
31. Baker SJ, Preisinger AC, Jessup M et al. p53 mutations occur in combination with 17p allelic deletions as late events in colorectal tumorigenesis. Cancer Res. 1990;50:7717–22.
32. Heinzlmann M, Fricke H, Loeschke K. K-ras and p53 gene mutations in colonic lavage and p53 antibodies in serum in long-standing inflammatory bowel disease. Gastroenterology. 1998;114:A1442.
33. Borkje B, Hostmark J, Skagen DW, Schrumpf E, Laerum OD. Flow cytometry of biopsy specimens from ulcerative colitis, colorectal adenomas, and carcinomas. Scand J Gastroenterol. 1987;22:1231–7.
34. Melville DM, Jass JR, Shepherd NA et al. Dysplasia and deoxyribonucleic acid aneuploidy in the assessment of precancerous changes in chronic ulcerative colitis. Observer variation and correlations. Gastroenterology. 1988;95:668–75.
35. Lofberg R, Brostrom O, Karlen P, Ost A, Tribukait B. DNA aneuploidy in ulcerative colitis. Reproducibility, topographic distribution, and relation to dysplasia. Gastroenterology. 1992;102:1149–54.
36. Rubin CE, Haggitt RC, Burmer GC et al. DNA aneuploidy in colonic biopsies predicts future development of dysplasia in ulcerative colitis. Gastroenterology. 1992;103:1611–20.
37. Befrits R, Hammarberg C, Rubio C, Jaramillo E, Tribukait B. DNA aneuploidy and histologic dysplasia in long-standing ulcerative colitis. A 10-year follow-up study. Dis Colon Rectum. 1994;37:313–19.
38. Lofberg R, Tribukait B, Ost A, Brostrom O, Reichard H. Flow cytometric DNA analysis in long-standing ulcerative colitis: a method of prediction of dysplasia and carcinoma development? Gut. 1987;28:1100–6.
39. Itzkowitz SH, Yaun M, Montgomery CK et al. Expression of Tn, sialosyl Tn, and T antigens in human colon cancer. Cancer Res. 1989;49:197–204.
40. Itzkowitz SH, Young E, DuBois D et al. Sialosyl-Tn antigen is prevalent and precedes dysplasia in ulcerative colitis: A retrospective case–control study. Gastroenterology. 1996;110:694–704.
41. Modrich P. Mismatch repair, genetic stability, and cancer. Science. 1994;266:1959–60.
42. Fishel R, Lescoe M, Rao M et al. The human mutator gene homolog MSH2 and its association with hereditary nonpolyposis colon cancer. Cell. 1993;75:1027–38.
43. Leach FS, Nicolaides NC, Papadopoulos N et al. Mutations of a mutS homolog in hereditary nonpolyposis colorectal cancer. Cell. 1993;75:229–53.
44. Brentnall TA, Rubin CE, Crispin DA et al. A germ-line substitution in the human MSH2 gene is associated with cancer and high-grade dysplasia in ulcerative colitis. Gastroenterology. 1995;109:151–5.
45. Goessl C, Plaschke J, Pistorius S et al. An intronic germline transition in the HNPCC gene hMSH2 is associated with sporadic colorectal cancer. 1997;33:1869–74.
46. Heimburger DC. Localized deficiencies of folic acid in aerodigestive tissues. Ann NY Acad Sci. 1992;669:87–95.
47. Freudenheim J, Graham S, Marshall J, Haughey B, Cholewinski S, Wilkinson F. Folate intake and carcinogenesis of the colon and rectum. Int J Epidemiol. 1991;20:368–74.
48. Meyer F, White E. Alcohol and nutrients in relation to colon cancer in middle-aged adults. Am J Epidemiol. 1993;138:225–36.
49. Franklin JL, Rosenberg IH. Impaired folic acid absorption in inflammatory bowel disease: effects of salicylazosulfapyridine. Gastroenterology. 1973;64:517–25.

50. Elsborg L, Larsen L. Folate deficiency in chronic inflammatory bowel disease. Scand J Gastroenterol. 1979;14:1019–24.
51. Lashner BA. Red blood cell folate is associated with the development of dysplasia and cancer in ulcerative colitis. J Cancer Res Clin Oncol. 1993;119:549–54.
52. Meenan J, Ohallinan E, Scott J, Weir DG. Epithelial cell folate depletion occurs in neoplastic but not adjacent normal colon mucosa. Gastroenterology. 1997;112:1163–8.
53. Lashner BA, Provencher KS, Seidner DL, Knesebeck A, Brzezinski A. The effect of folic acid supplementation on the risk for cancer or dysplasia in ulcerative colitis. Gastroenterology. 1997;112:29–32.
54. Lashner BA, Heidenreich PA, Su LG, Kane SV, Hanauer SB. Effect of folate supplementation on the incidence of dysplasia and cancer in chronic ulcerative colitis. A case–control study. Gastroenterology. 1989;97:255–9.
55. Blount BC, Mack MM, Wehr CM *et al*. Folate deficiency causes uracil misincorporation into human DNA and chromosome breakage: implications for cancer and neuronal damage. PNAS. 1997;94:3290–5.
56. Sandford KK, Price FM, Brodeur C, Makrauer FL, Parshad R. Deficient DNA repair in chronic ulcerative colitis. Cancer Detect Prev. 1997;21:540–5.
57. Biasco G, Sannoni U, Paganelli GM *et al*. Folic acid supplementation and cell kinetics of rectal mucosa in patients with ulcerative colitis. Cancer Epidemiol Biomarkers Prev. 1997;6:469–71.
58. Nugent FW, Haggitt RC, Gilpin PA. Cancer surveillance in ulcerative colitis. Gastroenterology. 1991;100:1241–8.
59. Rosenstock E, Farmer RG, Petras R, Sivak M Jr, Rankin G, Sullivan B. Surveillance for colonic ulcerative colitis. Gastroenterology. 1985;89:1342–6.
60. Lennard-Jones JE, Morson BC, Ritchie JK, Williams CB. Precancer and cancer in extensive ulcerative colitis: findings among 401 patients over 22 years. Gut. 1990;31:800–6.
61. Choi PM, Nugent FW, Schoetz DJ, Silverman ML, Haggitt RC. Colonoscopic surveillance reduces mortality from colorectal cancer in ulcerative colitis. Gastroenterology. 1993;105:418–24.
62. Provenzale D, Kowdley K, Arora S, Wong J. Prophylactic colectomy or surveillance for chronic ulcerative colitis? A decision analysis. Gastroenterology. 1995;109:1188–96.
63. Eddy DM. Screening for colorectal cancer. Ann Intern Med. 1990;113:373–84.

16
Early detection of cancer in inflammatory bowel disease: what should be done?

A. FORBES and D. ROWLANDS

COLORECTAL CANCER IN ULCERATIVE COLITIS

Colorectal carcinoma is widely recognized to be more common in those with long-standing extensive ulcerative colitis. The historically described risks of 5–10% at 20 years rising to 12–30% at 30 years are probably overestimates, however, and are not entirely consistent with 15–20-fold increased lifetime risks which have also been suggested. Given a lifetime frequency of around 1 in 30 for colorectal carcinoma in unselected Western populations, the latter figures would predict up to two thirds of patients with unresected extensive colitis going on to develop malignancy. Additionally, it was not clear whether young age at onset of colitis is an additional risk factor, nor if colitis-related tumours have a worse prognosis than sporadic cancers.

More recent data clarify these issues and prove less pessimistic. A Swedish population study yields a risk of colorectal carcinoma of only three times the background level[1], and the key Danish study shows no increase in the incidence of carcinoma even after 25 years follow up (probably linked to a relatively aggressive surgical policy)[2]. Disease confined to the rectum and sigmoid is confirmed to present no significant additional risk of neoplasia, while the patient with left-sided disease appears to be at intermediate risk[3], perhaps in part because of proximal extension of colitis, which can be expected to affect up to 20% of patients with the passage of time.

Colorectal carcinoma complicating ulcerative colitis shares many features with sporadic disease, but differences have been described, not least in the St Mark's review of 157 tumours in 120 patients[4]. The tumours were predominantly left-sided (56% rectosigmoid, 12% descending/splenic flexure), but 32% were proximal – a higher figure than in most sporadic series; 67.5% of all patients had a rectosigmoid tumour. The 5-year survival of 59.4%, however, is similar to UK data on sporadic tumours, and there were comparable data when stratified for Dukes' staging. The large case-controlled US study of colorectal carcinoma in military veterans[3] reached similar conclusions with generally more proximal tumours occurring a mean of 7 years earlier than in the general population.

COLORECTAL CARCINOMA IN CROHN'S DISEASE

There is controversy as to the risk of colorectal carcinoma: one population study showed an increased risk of colorectal cancer[5], while four population-based studies indicate no overall increase[6–9]. Amongst 373 patients reviewed in Copenhagen[10], the relative risk for any colorectal carcinoma was 1.1 (NS), and 1.7 for colonic cancer (NS). Studies performed in referral centres more consistently show increased frequencies of colorectal carcinoma, however, with relative risks between 3.0 and 20[11–17]. Only two such units reported an absence of increased risk[18,19]. The risk appears to be greatest in patients with extensive colitis of long duration[16,17] with a median of 15 years' disease prior to malignancy. It is difficult to reconcile these data with a recent Swedish paper reporting that 55% ($n = 22$) of all inflammatory bowel disease-associated colorectal carcinomas are in Crohn's colitis[20]. Misclassification of the nature of the colitis in patients from the 1950s can only partly explain the differences, but this serves to alert clinician, endoscopist and pathologist alike to the risk of neoplasia in the Crohn's colon. The clinical course of Crohn's-related colorectal carcinoma appears to be different from that in the general population. The median age at diagnosis is younger (around 50 years), and up to 40% of patients have right-sided lesions. The diagnosis still tends to be late, probably influenced by the attribution of symptoms to the Crohn's disease, and the predominance of right-sided lesions. The prognosis is accordingly poorer than for sporadic carcinomas, and a median 5-year survival of only 20% is typical, which may be even worse than would be predicted by these patients' more advanced Dukes' staging[11,13,15,18,21]. There is also concern that Crohn's disease patients may have a greater tendency to acquire multiple tumours[22]. Few centres offer routine colonoscopy to these patients at present.

Patients with Crohn's who appear to be at substantially higher risk of colorectal carcinoma include those with prolonged disease, disease onset before the age of 20, those with particularly extensive or stricturing disease, those with chronic fistulae, and those with bypassed segments of intestine. As in ulcerative colitis, the frequency will be substantially influenced by the prevailing surgical policy, and (for example) the 30% risk attributed to bypass operation may simply reflect the persistence of unresected chronic inflammation[13,15,16].

COLON CANCER SURVEILLANCE

Surveillance for colorectal carcinoma in inflammatory bowel disease is still a controversial topic. The reasons for this are clear, given that: cancer is an emotive issue, there are no controlled trials to document benefit, and the principal tool for surveillance is at best moderately invasive and expensive.

Patients and doctors see a clear advantage in regular assessment by gastrointestinal specialists[23]; re-investigation of clinical changes is then straightforward and, were the symptoms of inflammatory bowel disease not so similar to the symptoms of colonic neoplasms, this approach would generally permit their early diagnosis. Surveillance strategies have been developed to fill this 'gap'.

All cancer surveillance must satisfy a number of criteria to be warranted. It must be able to identify early-stage curable cancers, or treatable high-risk lesions that would otherwise progress to malignancy. The surveillance method must be safe and acceptable to the subjects to whom it is to be offered, and who must, in turn, be available to the surveyors. The ideal method with perfect sensitivity and specificity is unattainable, but, to minimize the medical, emotional and financial problems that arise from false positive and false negative results, the methodology should at least ensure an appropriate balance between missed cancers and prolonged and potentially hazardous investigation in those not at risk. Inflammatory bowel disease presents an identifiable and accessible high-risk population for colorectal carcinoma, and colonoscopy with histology offers a surveillance tool, but one that has obvious disadvantages. Even the experienced colonoscopist may miss early lesions hidden amongst the abnormalities of the inflammatory bowel disease, and may not take enough random biopsies for the detection of premalignant change (which is not usually macroscopically identifiable).

SURVEILLANCE IN ULCERATIVE COLITIS

Colonoscopic surveillance of long-standing ulcerative colitis has been performed in many centres for more than 20 years. The results have been disappointingly ambiguous, and the lack of controlled data at the time of its introduction is now greatly regretted. Axon's critical analysis in 1994[24] attracted much attention and had a negative influence on surveillance strategy in many units. Twelve programmes (1916 patients) which together yielded 92 cancers were reviewed. Only 52 of the cancers were Dukes' A or B lesions, and only 41 had a preoperative or antemortem diagnosis. Only 24 of these were sufficiently asymptomatic to satisfy Axon that the colonoscopies were performed entirely for surveillance reasons. By excluding a further 11 patients in whom tumours were found at the first 'screening' colonoscopy, he accepted only 13 cases as true surveillance finds. As he was then sceptical of the significance of low-grade dysplasia, 476 colonoscopies were required for each useful result. The likely benefit from random surveillance of a middle-aged European population looking for adenomatous polyps and early cancers would arguably be greater and Axon concluded that colonoscopic surveillance in ulcerative colitis was not justified.

The detection of dysplasia is admittedly an imperfect science, with problems of definition and between-observer variation[25]. The revised histological criteria reduce, but do not eliminate, these problems[26], and it is recognized that some patients develop malignancy apparently without previous dysplasia. In about 25% of colitis-related cancers, no dysplasia can be found at a site separate from the malignancy, even though the whole resected colon is available for examination[27,28]. In one of these studies, 18% had dysplasia neither at the site of malignancy nor on any previous surveillance biopsy[27]. It is possible that prior dysplasia was missed at the site of the subsequent tumours but this phenomenon is a limiting factor for the success of current surveillance protocols.

The finding of dysplasia is nevertheless a crucial observation. The revised criteria generally down-grade most historic borderline and low-grade cases. This increases the significance of those that retain a diagnosis of low- or high-grade dysplasia. Approximately half of those with high-grade dysplasia will develop frank malignancy within 5 years if earlier surgery is not performed[28,29]. Moreover, nearly one third of those with high-grade dysplasia are found to have otherwise unsuspected cancer in the resected colon even with prompt surgical intervention.

Low-grade dysplasia has less prognostic significance but undoubtedly progresses to high-grade dysplasia or cancer in some patients in all the centres that have addressed this issue[27–29]. The risk is at least 18%, and, in one series, was over 50% at 5 years[27]. Current practice at St Mark's Hospital is to advise colectomy for all patients with confirmed low-grade dysplasia, at a more mandatory level if identified on two occasions or at two separate sites on the same occasion.

The 1994 report on the St Mark's surveillance programme included 332 patients with macroscopically right-sided ulcerative colitis (to or above the hepatic flexure) of more than 10 years' duration[27]. The programme then required colonoscopy with multiple biopsies every two years, and a rigid sigmoidoscopy and rectal biopsy in the intervening years. The overall colorectal carcinoma rate was 6.0% ($n = 20$), occurring at a median age of 51 years in patients who had had colitis for a median of 21 years; 60% of the tumours were in the rectosigmoid. Only 11 of the tumours were detected by the surveillance programme (Dukes' stages 8 A; 1 B and 2 C). Nine of these were therefore 'useful' diagnoses. Surveillance missed 6 cancers, all of which were advanced at the time of diagnosis (4 Dukes' C, 2 disseminated), with an interval of 10–23 months from the most recent colonoscopy. These 6 patients were younger (median 38 years) but also had a median duration of disease of 21 years. Three cancers occurred in previously surveyed patients after they had left the programme for a variety of reasons. Surveillance detected dysplasia in 21 patients, 9 of whom had cancer. Twelve patients with dysplasia had no cancer at resection. The surveillance programme was considered to have benefited 9 patients with early cancers and a further 12 with dysplasia. This entailed a total of 1316 colonoscopies, and as one diagnosis was made by rigid sigmoidoscopy (in the alternate year between colonoscopies), 66 colonoscopies were required for each useful result, at a cost of about $40 000 per case detected. There were no important complications from colonoscopy in the series, and it was felt that surveillance colonoscopy (at St Mark's) was justifiable, but not mandatory.

The latest data from Sweden, which approach surveillance from an epidemiological standpoint, are also supportive[30]. The study base comprised all patients with ulcerative colitis for the Stockholm and Uppsala areas (for 1955–84 and 1965–83, respectively), representing 4664 cases in a population of about 3 million. Cases of fatal colorectal carcinoma occurring after 1975 were identified from cancer registry data (almost 100% inclusive), and were included if ulcerative colitis had been present for 5 years or more prior to death. Forty such patients were found, and 102 colitic controls matched for age, sex, disease duration, and disease extent, were selected. It was required that controls were alive at the time of death of the matching case, and had not undergone colectomy in the 5 years prior to the case's cancer diagnosis. Cases were then compared with controls for the utilization of surveillance colonoscopy. Colonoscopies performed for diagnosis, index examinations and those for clinical indications were excluded. These assessments were made retrospectively from clinical notes and may not be entirely free from error and/or bias. Although just failing to reach statistical significance, the results are nevertheless impressive. Only 2 of the 40 cancer patients had ever received a surveillance colonoscopy (5%) compared with 18 of the 102 controls (17.6%) (relative risk 0.29; 95% CI 0.06–1.31). Furthermore, 12 controls compared with only 1 case had received more than one surveillance procedure (RR 0.22; CI 0.03–1.74), indicating a 'dose-response'. This final observation is of potentially key importance as it generally proves difficult to maintain momentum and in most series the median number of colonoscopies performed is only 2 or 3.

MODELLING OF SURVEILLANCE STRATEGY IN ULCERATIVE COLITIS BASED ON EXISTING KNOWLEDGE

In 1995, Provenzale *et al.*[31] tried to determine the most cost-effective strategy against cancer based on the knowledge then current. A decision analytic model was employed and costings were based on those thought reasonable for a health maintenance organization (and which probably match those of European centres). Prophylactic colectomy after 10 years' extensive colitis was compared with a strategy of surveillance colonoscopy at 1–5 yearly intervals, with surgery subsequently performed for carcinoma or any grade of dysplasia, or only for carcinoma/high-grade dysplasia. Other than prophylactic colectomy, annual colonoscopy with colectomy for any dysplasia offered the most protection from malignancy, but this was also by far the most expensive option ($247 200 per life-year gained) and gained very little additional expected life compared with biennial colonoscopy, at $159 500 per life-year gained. Even 5-yearly colonoscopy (with colectomy with any dysplasia) appeared potentially highly effective and is cheaper than prophylactic colectomy ($40 700 vs. $60 400 per life-year gained), a cost not hugely dissimilar from that for the endoscopic screening of the general population now advocated for middle-aged North Americans and Germans.

RECENT (UNPUBLISHED) OBSERVATIONS FROM ST MARK'S HOSPITAL

A quinquennial review of neoplasia in ulcerative colitis and of the surveillance programme is in progress. Data are not yet finalized (and the study period runs until August 1998) but some interesting observations are emerging. There does not seem to have been any improvement in discovery of early cancers – the proportion of

Dukes' A and B tumours seems to have reached a plateau. There appears to have been an increase in detection rates of dysplasia and cancer (to greater than 1% per annum follow up once in the surveillance programme). Most striking of all, however, is the loss of the previous variance in distribution of the lesions from sporadic tumours. In only one case to date has a tumour been proximal to the splenic flexure, and the great majority of lesions now seem to be in the rectosigmoid. These observations, if confirmed, may be accounted for in part by the changing nature of our surveillance population, many of whom have been under colonoscopic follow-up for more than 15 years, and some of whom are now reaching an age at which sporadic colorectal carcinoma might be expected. The implication that some colonoscopies might safely be substituted by flexible sigmoidoscopy is to be tested.

CANCER SURVEILLANCE IN CROHN'S DISEASE

The problems associated with surveillance of ulcerative colitis are common also to Crohn's disease. However, the data are more sparse, and very few units have adopted a general colonoscopic surveillance policy in their Crohn's patients. Dysplasia does seem to be a predictor of future malignancy, probably of similar robustness to that in ulcerative colitis, with a frequency of 80% or more in published series once malignancy has supervened[21].

A biennial colonoscopy surveillance programme commencing at 8 years in those with total or segmental Crohn's colitis began in New York in 1988, and provisional data have been presented[32]. It seems that the index colonoscopy was included as well as the subsequent surveillance examinations. Dysplasia or frank malignancy was found in 6% of cases, and these patients were generally older, with disease for longer, and more likely to have had previous partial colectomy. The colonoscopies were technically demanding and, even with paediatric endoscopes, were incomplete in 11%. The authors advocate surveillance for those with long-standing total or segmental colitis. The arguments in favour of this approach must be considered weaker than for extensive ulcerative colitis, especially since 35% of patients appeared to enter the New York programme because of new symptoms and accordingly represent a selected cohort, probably at above-average risk of neoplasia. It is unfortunate that the acknowledged difficulties in interpreting ulcerative colitis surveillance programmes did not prompt a more controlled comparison of surveillance with normal clinical practice when Crohn's was considered.

HOW CAN SURVEILLANCE BE IMPROVED?

Colonoscopic surveillance is evidently imperfect, and should not be considered mandatory for patients with long-standing extensive ulcerative colitis, but it is unlikely that any major centre will now feel able to sanction a trial comparing surveillance with routine care. It is to be hoped that this can yet be done in Crohn's disease. Strategies intended to improve the performance of surveillance are, however, more readily open to controlled evaluation.

There is little potential for improvement in the colonoscopy itself, although doubtless it will become easier and more comfortable with improvements in endoscopic technology and training. A higher yield of tissue would help the pathologist but it is currently impractical to consider more than 15–20 biopsies per examination. Technical advances and/or the use of cytological brushing may help here, however. Performing the colonoscopies at greater frequency would probably improve the positive pick-up rate, and a switch to annual colonoscopy would at first sight appear to be a rational response to the failings of the St Mark's 1994 analysis. However, it is unlikely that all 5 of the tumours missed between 12 and 24 months would have been identified, and this strategy could not have influenced the detection of the tumour that presented at 10 months. Moreover, the doubling of procedure numbers (and therefore the cost of the programme) could lead to a reduction in quality (increased morbidity) and would probably reduce specificity. Alternative means to supplement existing data should therefore be sought, aiming to identify the patient at especially high risk who can be most aggressively targeted, and, conversely, to identify those at relatively low risk in whom efforts may legitimately be less (e.g. colonoscopy only every 5 years).

ADDITIONAL MARKERS OF MALIGNANCY AND PREMALIGNANCY

Work with sporadic colorectal carcinoma and other solid tumours demonstrates value from the detection of aneuploidy or of mutations of oncogenes (e.g. K-ras or c-myc), tumour suppressor genes (e.g. p53 or apc), or of mismatch repair genes (e.g. MLH-1). There is so far little reliable information on the place of these phenomena in inflammatory bowel disease-related tumours or in surveillance thereof.

Aneuploidy – a disturbance of the normal diploid state of cells – is often to be found in colonic biopsies from colitic patients with dysplasia and malignancy. On the whole, it seems that it precedes dysplasia, which itself precedes carcinoma[33], but some carcinomas are unassociated with either, and, in some cases, there is a transition from aneuploidy to carcinoma without dysplasia[34]. The detection of aneuploidy may have similar prognostic significance to that of low-grade dysplasia. Numbers are small and progression is not inevitable, but a high proportion of patients with aneuploidy seem likely to progress to malignancy relatively quickly (100% within 3 years in one study[33]). It is possible that an apparent high degree of protection (strong negative predictive value) in patients without aneuploidy on any biopsy may be even more valuable prognostically. It will be interesting to see if this is borne out in controlled prospective assessment.

Mutations of the p53 tumour suppressor gene are found in around 75% of most solid tumours, including sporadic colorectal carcinoma. It is still not resolved as to whether this frequency is different in colitis-related cases, nor whether such mutations can be expected to predate or supplement dysplasia usefully. A correlation of p53 mutations with the discovery of aneuploidy[35] suggests that gain is there to be had – especially if molecular techniques for mutation detection prove less complex and less costly than scanning for aneuploidy, again tentatively supported by provisional data demonstrating overexpression of p53 in 1.6% of 500 prior biopsies in patients who went on to develop high-grade dysplasia or carcinoma, compared with none in matched controls in whom no neoplasia developed[36]. Again, prospective trials are needed to clarify whether search for aberrant p53 expression is a cost-effective component of colitis surveillance. The approach under evaluation in Munich using colonic lavage to provide DNA for p53 (and K-ras) analysis is especially exciting as it offers the potential of reserving colonoscopy for the highest-risk patient[37].

Increased evidence of cell proliferation is a feature of inflammation but it is also possible that this could be of prognostic significance in cancer surveillance. The Ki-67 antigen and proliferating cell nuclear antigen (PCNA) have been examined in biopsies from patients with ulcerative colitis with and without dysplasia compared with normal controls[38]. Although there were strong trends and good statistics, there was insufficient discrimination for either marker used alone to be other than a further guide if dysplasia is the gold standard. It remains possible that (like aneuploidy) proliferation markers may provide partly independent warnings of future invasion.

The mucin-associated carbohydrate antigen, sialosyl-Tn (also linked with sporadic colorectal carcinoma) is found more often in patients with colitis-related cancers (44%) than in controls without carcinoma or dysplasia (11%)[39], having previously been identifiable up to 7 years earlier and before dysplasia or aneuploidy was found. A small prospective study supports this observation and its interpretations[40]. Sialosyl-Tn is also expressed in Crohn's disease, but when there are no complications, and at too frequent a rate to be useful in surveillance for neoplasia[41].

OTHER DETERMINANTS OF COLONOSCOPIC FREQUENCY IN CANCER SURVEILLANCE

Sporadic colorectal carcinoma is more common when there have previously been colonic adenomas and when there is a positive family history[42]. Until recently, these factors have not been addressed in colitis surveillance. The Mayo Clinic group has now begun to re-examine its own programme (203 colitis-related cancers) in case-control fashion[43]. Recall bias was apparently slight. Colorectal carcinoma affecting a first-degree relative was 2.4 times more common in colitis patients with neoplasia than in those without (95% CI 1.1–5.8), a difference unexplained by familial colitis, and similar in ratio to that in the general population for sporadic cancers. The family history should thus help to determine surveillance strategy, but the magnitude of its influence perhaps requires further analysis before changes are implemented.

It is probable that adenomas are associated with an increased risk of malignancy in colitis but there are no reliable data. Pascal has reviewed this topic[44].

Primary sclerosing cholangitis may be a marker of increased risk of colorectal carcinoma in colitis. The results from different centres are not concordant, however, and it is probably wise to discount the earliest reports on the grounds of inadequate numbers and selection bias. A careful retrospective analysis has now been performed by the Stockholm group[45], which has a series which is almost population based and yet in which both inflammatory bowel disease and sclerosing cholangitis are likely to have been identified and recorded. Eighty controls with colitis but without sclerosing cholangitis were paired with the 40 with both diseases, matching for age and for the extent and duration of colitis. During follow up, 16 patients with sclerosing cholangitis developed colonic dysplasia or carcinoma (40%) compared with only 10 in the controls (12.5%; $p<0.001$). The cumulative risk of colorectal neoplasia was 9% and 31%, at 10 and 20 years respectively, compared with only 2% and 5% in the controls without cholangitis. Interestingly, both colorectal and biliary neoplasia coincided in 7 cases. Brentnall *et al.*[46] have reported on a prospective series of 20 patients with extensive colitis and sclerosing cholangitis, and saw 9 patients with dysplasia (45%), compared with only 4 in 25 patients matched for colitis but without cholangitis (16%). At the Mayo Clinic, a retrospective review of 178 patients with sclerosing cholangitis led to almost opposite conclusions[47]. The relative risk for colorectal neoplasia (excluding dysplasia alone) was elevated to 10.3 times that of the general population of the USA but this was not influenced by the presence or absence of cholangitis. The relative risk for colorectal neoplasia was, however, numerically increased (though not significant) for patients with sclerosing cholangitis without colitis at 4.9, with confidence intervals between 0.1 and 27 times. Their subsequent analysis comparing cancer frequency in colitis patients with or without cholangitis also shows an absence of association (but there was a non-significant increased relative risk of 1.23 in those with sclerosing cholangitis)[48]. Reports from other centres support an increased risk of colorectal carcinoma in patients with sclerosing cholangitis but are subject to the same reservations. Major changes in surveillance strategy are not yet called for.

Groups at lower risk have not been identified with any confidence but our experience at St Mark's suggests that patients with inactive colitis, with persistently satisfactory endoscopic appearance and persistently quiescent histology, are under-represented amongst those with dysplasia and carcinomas[49]. A significant difference in the prior frequency of colonoscopic quiescence (78% vs. 58% in those going on to neoplasia; $p < 0.05$) and a non-significant difference in histological quiescence (58% vs. 48%) were demonstrated in a retrospective study. Complementary data approaching the question from the opposite direction came from Japan where a higher risk of neoplasia was associated with continued disease activity[50]. Although of interest, these differences are not of sufficient magnitude to permit, on their own, any amendment to the intensity of surveillance.

Non-steroidal anti-inflammatory drugs (NSAIDs) may play a protective role against colorectal carcinoma in general. Few data exist to support or refute this hypothesis in inflammatory bowel disease but, in the huge (and therefore remote) review of hospital discharges[51], history of a disease associated with the use of NSAIDs was protective in inflammatory bowel disease (odds ratio 0.84; CI 0.65–1.09), and a history of NSAID consumption was itself protective against colorectal carcinoma mortality (OR 0.68; CI 0.65–0.72) (see also aminosalicylates below). The expression of cyclo-oxygenase-2 in sporadic and colitis-related tumours, and in tissue adjacent to neoplasia, but *only* in ulcerative colitis patients[52] may provide a further clue.

Again prompted by work on colorectal carcinoma in general, there has been interest as to whether folic acid might be protective in inflammatory bowel disease patients. The data are as yet quite preliminary, but at least one retrospective study shows modest reduction in frequency of neoplasia in ulcerative colitics who have used folate supplements[53]. This might be expected to offer greater advantage in patients with Crohn's disease given the likelihood of subclinical or frank folate deficiency but this has not yet been assessed.

CANCERS OTHER THAN COLORECTAL CARCINOMA

Cholangiocarcinoma

Cholangiocarcinomas are substantially over-represented in patients with primary sclerosing cholangitis, affecting at least 5% of patients on a life-time basis[45,47], and is commoner in those with underlying inflammatory bowel disease than in those without[45,54]. Surgical resection is the only curative option but early diagnosis is difficult; clinicians must maintain a high index of suspicion. Identification of the progression to carcinoma is severely hampered by the similarity of the symptoms, signs and investigations to those of the cholangitis, but this should be suspected in the patient whose condition suddenly deteriorates or becomes progressive rather than episodic. There are no reliable laboratory markers, even tumour markers frequently proving positive in uncomplicated sclerosing cholangitis. Positive cytological brushings or biliary biopsies obtained at ERCP are conclusive but false negatives are frequent, in part because of the relatively fibrous nature of the tumours. Changes in the cholangiogram may sometimes help, especially when the axis of a strictured area of duct deviates from the general axis of the remainder of the duct; this strongly suggests neoplastic change. Conventional imaging with ultrasound and CT scanning has not proved sufficiently discriminatory, but endoscopic ultrasound (perhaps using intrabiliary probes) and MRCP may make an increasingly useful contribution through their ability to demonstrate small-mass lesions.

Small bowel cancer

Malignancy of the small bowel is over-represented in Crohn's disease but remains a rare condition. Although a relative risk of 50 compared with the general population ($p = 0.001$)[10] seems striking, it reflects only 2 patients, and there were no cases identified in the St Mark's series of 2500 patients[19]. The reported cumulative incidence of 0.6% is perhaps a more helpful statistic[18]. The small bowel cancers usually occur in those who have had Crohn's for 10 years or more; the diagnosis is usually delayed and rarely made preoperatively. The prognosis is very poor, with a median survival as short as 6 months. Genetic analysis of small bowel tumours in Crohn's disease suggests differences from sporadic tumours at this site (less K-ras mutation, more p53 overexpression)[5] but it is not clear that this could be diagnostically helpful nor contribute to a pre-invasive diagnosis. Crohn's disease patients at most risk seem to be those with proximal and/or chronic unremitting disease; males are also over-represented[13,18]. Clinicians and radiologists should be alert to this possible complication, but there are no data to suggest additional routes to early diagnosis.

Anal carcinoma

Carcinoma of the anal canal and of the transitional zone leading into the rectum is seen more often in Crohn's disease than in the general population, with at least a 6-fold increase in incidence (5 cases in 2500 patients; less than 1 expected[19]). These patients have typically suffered from severe and very chronic anorectal disease. Although multimodality non-surgical therapy is now yielding good results for late-stage anal carcinoma, in Crohn's disease, suspicious anorectal lesions that are not responding to medical therapy should always be biopsied. This will usually require general anaesthetic to achieve adequate analgesia.

Iatrogenic malignancy in inflammatory bowel disease?

The over-representation of malignancies in patients with inflammatory bowel disease is reasonably attributed to the disease process, but there have also been concerns that diagnostic and therapeutic interventions, particularly immunosuppressive drugs, may also play a role. Steroids and aminosalicylates are unlikely to influence cancer risk adversely. On the contrary, there is evidence that the latter may reduce the risk in ulcerative colitis[6]. This case-control study in a defined population compared the pharmacological records of ulcerative colitis patients with complicating carcinoma with those of matched controls with no malignancy. There was a significant protective effect in those treated for at least 3 months with an aminosalicylate preparation, the relative risk for neoplasia being only 0.38 (CI 0.20–0.69).

Azathioprine/mercaptopurine is implicated in non-Hodgkin's lymphoma, intestinal lymphoma, myeloma and the skin cancers seen in patients immunosuppressed for connective tissue diseases and after transplantation[57,58]. A number of case reports, and a review of 26 Crohn's patients with colorectal carcinoma, 2 of whom had previously taken azathioprine[9], suggested a greater than chance association in inflammatory bowel disease also. The much larger report of 723 inflammatory bowel disease patients treated with immunosuppressants, which demonstrated no excess risk, was therefore especially reassuring[60]. The influence of azathioprine on cancer risk in inflammatory bowel disease was further explored at St Mark's in a series of 755 patients followed prospectively for a median of 9 years from the time of introduction of the drug[61]. A small overall increase in malignancies was detected, there being 31 malignancies compared with the 24.3 predicted by national mortality rates for the same age and sex distribution. This difference did not, however, reach statistical significance ($p = 0.186$). There were no lymphomas, but a significant excess of colorectal and anal tumours was found. It was thought likely that the excess of colorectal and anal tumours (15 observed vs. 2.27 expected; $p > 0.00001$) represented an effect of the underlying disease rather than a complication of treatment, and was supported by a case-control analysis. It should also be noted that, although the period of follow up was substantial, the period of azathioprine usage was not, with a median of only 12.5 months; very long durations of immunosuppression may not be as safe. The apparent loss of benefit after more than 4 years' therapy also lends support to elective drug withdrawal at this time[62]. To date, only the New York group have suggested that 6-mercaptopurine might *reduce* the risk of colorectal carcinoma in Crohn's disease[63].

Cyclosporin may increase the incidence of lymphoproliferative disorders and skin cancers after transplantation[64,65] but few data particular to inflammatory bowel disease exist. Continued monitoring is indicated, especially in patients treated for longer periods. It is disturbing[66] that colorectal carcinoma has occurred in no less than 3 of 27 patients with ulcerative colitis (and retained colons) within the first 14 months after liver transplantation for primary sclerosing cholangitis. These patients were immunosuppressed (conventionally) with prednisolone, azathioprine and cyclosporin, and clearly represent a highly selected group, not least since sclerosing cholangitis may be a risk factor for colonic neoplasia. It seems wise to enter such patients into an accelerated colonoscopic screening programme, but whether the increased risk is primarily related to drug, transplant or disease remains unclear.

Methotrexate is probably not carcinogenic, since it neither reacts with, nor becomes incorporated into nucleic acid[67]. To date, no carcinogenic effect of the relatively low doses of methotrexate typically used for non-malignant indications has been demonstrated, background neoplasia rates remaining unaltered[68,69]. Again data specific to inflammatory bowel disease are lacking.

Diagnostic imaging and risk of neoplasia

Many patients with inflammatory bowel disease have repeated radiological examinations over many years, raising the possibility that medical exposure to ionizing radiation might contribute to their risk of neoplasia. Ultrasound and MRI appear to be exonerated, and both frequency and dose from scintigraphic imaging are reassuringly low, but conventional radiographic imaging and computed tomography deserve brief attention. The average total annual radiation exposure in Western nations is about 2.5 mSv per person[70], of which around 12% comes from medical sources[71]. Most of these examinations are of the chest or periphery, which expose the patient to a much lower 'effective dose equivalent' than a plain abdominal film at 1.14 mSv (10 mGy absorbed dose), a barium meal at 3.8 mSv, or a barium enema at 7.7 mSv[72]. The high dose from barium enema is a combined result of longer screening times, more full-sized abdominal films, and the greater energy required for lateral views. Accordingly, although barium enemas account for only 0.9% of all radiological procedures, they contribute 14% of the medical radiation dose in the UK[70].

Extrapolation from occupational exposure predicts a roughly linear relationship between increasing radiation exposure and increasing risk of malignancy[73], with no minimum radiation dose below which there is freedom from this increased risk. These assumptions lead to between 100 and 250 fatal cancers being attributed to medical radiation each year in the UK (1.8–4.5 per million population). The approximate life-time risk that a given procedure induces a fatal malignancy can be calculated to lie between 20 and 60 per million for abdominal radiography, 50 and 170 for barium meal, and 100 and 350 for barium enema, with the rather higher figure for abdominal CT scanning of around 500 per million[70,72]. It is not likely that this contributes to the increased risk of colorectal carcinoma in ulcerative colitis, as occupational and atomic bomb data indicate that the gastrointestinal mucosa is a 'protected' site[72,73]. However, even if all excess cancers resulting from radiological investigation of colitis were in the large bowel, then radiation would still account for only about 0.14% of colitis cancers – around 1.5% of the excess relative to the general population. The situation is less easily modelled in Crohn's disease but a larger number of radiographic studies of the small bowel and CT scans are typical. The relatively extreme case of a patient in whom 20 small bowel series, 2 barium enemas, and 10 CT scans had been performed, would be at an increased risk of fatal malignancy in the region of 7400 per million, but this is a life-time risk of nearly 1% and should not be ignored when considering the need for radiological investigation. Again, these excess malignancies can be expected to be extraintestinal.

CONCLUSIONS

Ulcerative colitis

The epidemiology of colorectal carcinoma surveillance in microscopically extensive ulcerative colitis indicates a risk of carcinoma or of high-grade dysplasia in the region of 0.5% per year of follow up after 10 years of disease. For every 100 patients in any given programme, one high-risk lesion or early cancer can be expected every 2 years (or approximately 1 per million population per year). A screening colonoscopy at 8–10 years is justified, whether or not subsequent surveillance is intended, to check the extent of colitis and because an important proportion of high-risk lesions are found at this index examination in most surveillance series. High-grade dysplasia, dysplasia-associated lesions and masses (DALMs), and confirmed low-grade dysplasia warrant colectomy; the minimum response to a finding of low-grade dysplasia is 6 monthly colonoscopy for the patient who refuses colectomy. Up to 25% of cancers will not be preceded (or detectable) by dysplasia. Tumours currently missed by surveillance are likely to be biologically different. Colonoscopic surveillance is expensive and of unproven value, indicating a need for better markers of high- and low-risk patients, but, if it is to be done, then it must be safe and proficiently performed to be well tolerated by patients. In the absence of controlled data or a clearly mandated decision based on clinical criteria, decisions are properly made on grounds of health economics. Colonoscopy every 2 years is thus a reasonable frequency for units planning to commence or continue surveillance outside a trial setting. It is less clear at what age surveillance should stop if commenced, and what, if anything, should be done for patients with less extensive disease; stopping at 75 years, and a rectal biopsy every 2 years from 10 years, respectively, are suggested. The modifications suggested are not rigorously tested but take a pragmatic view based on clinical, laboratory, epidemiological and economic criteria, with an emphasis on the former. The addition of NSAIDs or folate would be speculative.

Crohn's disease

In extensive Crohn's colitis of more than 8–10 years' duration, regular clinical assessment, especially of the anorectum, is warranted, with a high index of suspicion and a low threshold for examination and biopsy under anaesthetic if strictures are present. Those in whom the disease began in childhood or adolescence, those with chronic fistulae, and those with bypassed segments of intestine are probably those at greatest risk. There are, as yet, no data which firmly justify more than clinically prompted investigations, but the accumulating evidence suggests that the approach for the patient with extensive Crohn's colitis should be similar to that for extensive ulcerative colitis. A controlled trial of surveillance is certainly still justifiable. Folate supplementation may be particularly relevant.

Acknowledgements

Some of the data considered here have previously been reviewed in the first author's monograph, *Clinicians' Guide to Inflammatory Bowel Disease*, published in 1997 by Chapman & Hall, London. The authors thank Dr Kay Wilkinson for helping with the interpretation of the current status of the St Mark's surveillance database.

References

1. Ekbom A, Helmick CG, Zack M, Holmberg L, Adami HO. Survival and causes of death in patients with inflammatory bowel disease: a population-based study. Gastroenterology. 1992;103:954–60.
2. Langholz E, Munkholm P, Davidsen M, Binder V. Colorectal cancer risk and mortality in patients with ulcerative colitis. Gastroenterology. 1992;103:1444–51.
3. Nugent FW, Haggitt RC, Gilpin PA. Cancer surveillance in ulcerative colitis. Gastroenterology. 1991;100:1241–8.
4. Connell WR, Talbot IC, Harpaz N *et al*. Clinicopathological characteristics of colorectal carcinoma complicating ulcerative colitis. Gut. 1994;35:1419–23.
5. Ekbom A, Helmick C, Zack M, Adami HO. Increased risk of large bowel cancer in Crohn's disease with colonic involvement. Lancet. 1990;336:357–9.
6. Binder V, Hendriksen C, Kreiner S. Prognosis in Crohn's disease – based on results from a regional patient group from the county of Copenhagen. Gut. 1985;26:146–50.
7. Kvist N, Jacobsen O, Norgaard P *et al*. Malignancy in Crohn's disease. Scand J Gastroenterol. 1986;21:82–6.
8. Gollop JH, Phillips SF, Melton LJ, Zinsmeister AR. Epidemiological aspects of Crohn's disease: a population based study in Olmsted County, Minnesota, 1943–1982. Gut. 1988;29:49–56.
9. Fireman Z, Grossman A, Lilos P *et al*. Intestinal cancer in patients with Crohn's disease: a population study in central Israel. Scand J Gastroenterol. 1989;24:346–50.
10. Munkholm P, Langholz E, Davidsen M, Binder V. Intestinal cancer risk and mortality in patients with Crohn's disease. Gastroenterology. 1993;105:1716–23.
11. Korelitz BI. Carcinoma of the intestinal tract in Crohn's disease: results of a survey conducted by the National Foundation for Ileitis and Colitis. Am J Gastroenterol. 1983;78:44–6.
12. Weedon DD, Shorter RG, Ilstrup DM, Huizenga KA, Taylor WF. Crohn's disease and cancer. N Engl J Med. 1973;289:1099–103.

13. Greenstein AJ, Sachar DB, Smith H, Janowitz HD, Aufses AH. A comparison of cancer risk in Crohn's disease and ulcerative colitis. Cancer. 1981;48:2742–5.

14. Gyde SN, Prior P, Macartney JC, Thompson H, Waterhouse JAH, Allan RN. Malignancy in Crohn's disease. Gut. 1980;21:1024–9.

15. Stahl TJ, Schoetz DJ, Roberts PL *et al.* Crohn's disease and carcinoma: increasing justification for surveillance? Dis Colon Rectum. 1992;35:850–6.

16. Gillen CD, Walmsley RS, Prior P, Andrews HA, Allan RN. Ulcerative colitis and Crohn's disease: a comparison of the colorectal cancer risk in extensive colitis. Gut. 1994;35:1590–2.

17. Cohen RD, Gordon DW, Argo CK, Hanauer SB. Risk factors for adenocarcinoma in ulcerative colitis and Crohn's disease: a retrospective, matched case-control study. Gastroenterology. 1996;110:A505.

18. Michelassi F, Testa G, Pomidor WJ, Lashner BA, Block GE. Adenocarcinoma complicating Crohn's disease. Dis Colon Rectum. 1993;36:654–61.

19. Connell WR, Sheffield JP, Kamm MA, Ritchie JK, Hawley PR, Lennard-Jones JE. Lower gastrointestinal mallignancy in Crohn's disease. Gut. 1994;35:347–52.

20. Rubio CA, Befrits R. Colorectal adnocarcinoma in Crohn's disease: a retrospective histologic study. Dis Colon Rectum. 1998;40:1072–8.

21. Richards ME, Rickert RR, Nance FC. Crohn's disease-associated carcinoma. Ann Surg. 1989;209:764–73.

22. Artru P, Canedo S, Gendre JP *et al.* Intestinal cancer in patients with Crohn's disease – relation with duration of inflammatory disease. Gastroenterology. 1998;114:A559.

23. British Society of Gastroenterology. Guidelines in Gastroenterology 4: Inflammatory bowel disease. London: British Society of Gastroenterology; 1996.

24. Axon ATR. Cancer surveillance in ulcerative colitis – a time for reappraisal. Gut. 1994;35:587–9.

25. Dixon MF, Brown LJR, Gilmour HM *et al.* Observer variation in the assessment of dysplasia in ulcerative colitis. Histopathology. 1988;13:385–97.

26. Theodossi A, Spiegelhalter DJ, Jass J *et al.* Observer variation and discriminatory value of biopsy features in inflammatory bowel disease. Gut. 1994;35:961–8.

27. Connell WR, Lennard-Jones JE, Williams CB, Talbot IC, Price AB, Wilkinson KH. Factors influencing the outcome of endoscopic surveillance for cancer in ulcerative colitis. Gastroenterology. 1994;107:934–44.

28. Woolrich AJ, DaSilva MD, Korelitz BI. Surveillance in the routine management of ulcerative colitis: the predictive value of low grade dysplasia. Gastroenterology. 1992;103:431–8.

29. Bernstein CN, Shanahan F. Are we telling patients the truth about surveillance colonoscopy in ulcerative colitis? Lancet. 1994;343:71–4.

30. Karlén P, Kornfeld D, Broström O, Löfberg R, Persson P-G, Ekbom A. Is colonoscopic surveillance reducing colorectal cancer mortality in ulcerative colitis? A population based case control study. Gut. 1998;42:711–14.

31. Provenzale D, Kowdley KV, Arora S, Wong JB. Prophylactic colectomy or surveillance for chronic ulcerative colitis? A decision analysis. Gastroenterology. 1995;109:1188–96.

32. Rubin PH, Present DH, Chapman ML, Cortes JL, Harpaz N. Chronic Crohn's colitis: a 7 year experience with screening and surveillance colonoscopy in 113 patients. Gastroenterology. 1996;110:A1005.

33. Rubin CE, Haggitt RC, Burmer GC *et al.* DNA aneuploidy in colonic biopsies predicts future development of dysplasia in ulcerative colitis. Gastroenterology. 1992;103:1611–20.

34. Befrits R, Hammarberg C, Rubio C, Jaramillo E, Tribukait B. DNA aneuploidy and histologic dysplasia in long-standing ulcerative colitis. A 10-year follow-up study. Dis Colon Rectum. 1994;37:313–19.

35. Brentnall TA, Crispin DA, Rabinovitch PS *et al.* Mutations in the p53 gene: an early marker of neoplastic progression in ulcerative colitis. Gastroenterology. 1994;107:369–78.

36. Wang C, Cymes K, Young E, Meltzer SJ, Itzkowitz SH, Harpaz N. p53 overexpression in colonoscopic surveillance biopsies of patients with longstanding UC: a retrospective case-control study. Gastroenterology. 1996;110:A611.

37. Heinzlmann M, Stratakis DF, Lang SM *et al.* K-ras and p53 gene mutation in colonic lavage and p53 antibodies in serum in long-standing inflammatory bowel disease. Gastroenterology. 1998;114:A608.

38. Kullmann F, Fadaie M, Gross V *et al.* Expression of proliferating cell nuclear antigen (PCNA) and Ki-67 in dysplasia in inflammatory bowel disease. Eur J Gastroenterol Hepatol. 1996;8:371–9.

39. Itzkowitz SH, Young E, Dubois D *et al.* Sialosyl-Tn antigen is prevalent and precedes dysplasia in ulcerative colitis: a retrospective case-control study. Gastroenterology. 1996;110:694–704.
40. Karlén P, Broström O, Löfberg R *et al.* Chronology of sialosyl-Tn (STn) antigen expression and aneuploidy in prospective colonoscopic biopsies from patients with long-standing ulcerative colitis. Gastroenterology. 1996;110:A538.
41. Ta A, Harpaz N, Chen A, Bodian C, Itzkowitz S. Expression of the tumor-associated sialosyl-Tn antigen in Crohn's colitis. Gastroenterology. 1996;110:A599.
42. Rustgi AK. Hereditary gastrointestinal polyposis and nonpolyposis syndromes. N Engl J Med. 1994;331:1694–702.
43. Nuako KW, Ahlquist DA, Schaid DJ, Siems DM, Mahoney DW. Familial predisposition as a risk factor for colorectal cancer in chronic ulcerative colitis: a case-control study. Gastroenterology. 1996;110:A569.
44. Pascal RR. Dysplasia and early carcinoma in inflammatory bowel disease and colorectal adenomas. Hum Pathol. 1994;25:1160–71.
45. Broomé U, Löfberg R, Veress B, Eriksson LS. Primary sclerosing cholangitis and ulcerative colitis: evidence for increased neoplastic potential. Hepatology. 1995;22:1404–8.
46. Brentnall TA, Haggitt RC, Rabinovitch PS *et al.* Risk and natural history of colonic neoplasia in patients with primary sclerosing cholangitis and ulcerative colitis. Gastroenterology. 1996;110:331–8.
47. Loftus EV Jr, Sandborn WJ, Tremaine WJ *et al.* Risk of colorectal neoplasia in patients with primary sclerosing cholangitis. Gastroenterology. 1996;110:432–40.
48. Nuako KW, Ahlquist DA, Sandborn WJ, Mahoney DW, Siems DM, Zinsmeister AR. Primary sclerosing cholangitis and colorectal carcinoma in patients with chronic ulcerative colitis: a case-control study. Cancer. 1998;82:822–6.
49. Chiotakaou-Faliakou E, Ganesh S, Wilkinson K, Forbes A. Macroscopic and histologic inactivity in ulcerative colitis surveillance: a good prognostic sign? Gastroenterology. 1997;112:A948.
50. Shinozaki M, Muto T, Yokoyama T, Masaki T. Higher disease activity enhances cancer risk in ulcerative colitis. Gastroenterology. 1998;114:A679.
51. Bansal P, Sonnenberg A. Risk factors of colorectal cancer in inflammatory bowel disease. Am J Gastroenterol. 1996;91:44–8.
52. Weiss A, Harpaz N, Chen A *et al.* Immunoreactive cyclooxygenase-2 expression in ulcerative colitis-associated neoplasms. Gastroenterology. 1998;114:A702.
53. Burke A, Lichtenstein GR, Rombeau JL. Nutrition and ulcerative colitis. Baill Clin Gastroenterol. 1997;11:153–74.
54. Gurbuz AK, Giardiello FM, Bayless TM. Colorectal neoplasia in patients with ulcerative colitis and primary sclerosing cholangitis. Dis Colon Rectum. 1995;38:37–41.
55. Rashid A, Hamilton SR. Genetic alterations in sporadic and Crohn's-associated adenocarcinomas of the small intestine. Gastroenterology. 1997;113:127–35.
56. Pinczowski D, Ekbom A, Baron J, Yuen J, Adami HO. Risk factors for colorectal cancer in patients with ulcerative colitis: a case control study. Gastroenterology. 1994;107:117–20.
57. Kinlen LJ. Incidence of cancer in rheumatoid arthritis and other disorders after immunosuppressive treatment. Am J Med. 1985;78suppl:44–9.
58. Matteson EL, Hickey AR, Maguire L, Tilson HH, Urowitz MB. Occurrence of neoplasia in patients with rheumatoid arthritis enrolled in a DMARD registry. J Rheumatol. 1991;18:809–14.
59. Zelig MP, Choi PM. Azathioprine or 6-mercaptopurine therapy and colon carcinoma in Crohn's disease. Gastroenterology. 1992;102:1448(letter).
60. Present DH, Meltzer ST, Krumholz MP, Wolke A, Korelitz BI. 6-Mercaptopurine in the management of inflammatory bowel disease: short- and long-term toxicity. Ann Intern Med. 1989;111:641–9.
61. Connell WR, Kamm MA, Dickson M, Balkwill AM, Ritchie JK, Lennard-Jones JE. Long-term neoplasia risk after azathioprine treatment in inflammatory bowel disease. Lancet. 1994;343:1249–52.
62. Bouhnik Y, Lémann M, Mary J-Y *et al.* Long-term follow-up of patients with Crohn's disease treated with azathioprine or 6-mercaptopurine. Lancet. 1996;347:215–19.
63. Goldstein ES, Marion JF, Wheeler S, Present DH. 6-Mercaptopurine: does it increase or decrease the risks of colon cancer in Crohn's disease? Gastroenterology. 1998;114:A986.
64. Von Graffenried B. Sandimmun (ciclosporin) in autoimmune disease: overview on early clinical experience. Am J Nephrol. 1989;9:51–6.
65. Kurki PT. Safety aspects of long-term cyclosporin A therapy. Scand J Rheumatol. 1992;95:35–8.

66. Bleday R, Lee E, Jessurun J, Heine J, Wong WD. Increased risk of early colorectal neoplasms after hepatic transplant in patients with inflammatory bowel disease. Dis Colon Rectum. 1993;36;908–12.
67. Turnbull C, Roach M. Is methotrexate carcinogenic? Br Med J. 1980;281:808.
68. Tishler M, Caspi D, Yaron M. Long-term experience with low dose methotrexate in rheumatoid arthritis. Rheumatol Int. 1993;13:103–6.
69. Weinblatt ME. Methotrexate for chronic diseases in adults. N Engl J Med. 1995;332:330–1.
70. National Radiation Protection Board. Patient dose reduction in diagnostic radiology. Documents of the NRPB. London: HMSO; 1990.
71. Mettler FA, Davis M, Kelsey CA, Rosenberg R, Williams A. Analytical modeling of worldwide medical radiation use. Health Phys. 1987;52:133–41.
72. National Radiation Protection Board. A national survey of doses to patients undergoing a selection of routine X-ray examination in English hospitals. NRPB-R200. London: HMSO; 1986.
73. Sevc J, Kunz E, Tomasek L, Placek V, Horacek J. Cancer in man after exposure to Rn daughters. Health Phys. 1988;54:27–46.

17
Utility of IBD classification: is it helpful from a therapeutic standpoint?

D. B. SACHAR

If someone were to ask a haematologist to describe the proper treatment of anaemia, the probable response would be a quizzical look at best and a derisive laugh at worst. Obviously, in the modern world, 'anaemia' refers to such a heterogeneous set of disorders that a unitary approach to their aetiology and management is quite simply unthinkable. By the same token, clinical research in the late 20th century has advanced to the point where we can no longer regard 'inflammatory bowel disease' (IBD) as though it were a single entity either.

Indeed, even the traditional binary classification into 'Crohn's disease' and 'ulcerative colitis' is no longer sufficient to encompass our current understanding of these disorders. Proctocolitis alone is now recognized to comprise at least half a dozen categories ranging from infections through ischaemic syndromes to drug reactions. Each one of these categories, moreover, can be broken down into further subclassifications on the basis of distinct aetiologies, some recognized only recently, such as *Clostridia difficile*, *Campylobacter* or haemorrhagic *Escherichia coli 0157:H7*, to name just a few among the many bacterial infections affecting the colon. Similarly, ischaemic bowel disease is now subclassified according to vascular anatomy (arterial or venous), intestinal distribution (enteritis or colitis) and clinical behaviour (healing or non-healing).

Even when limiting our focus to chronic idiopathic ulcerative colitis, there appear to be several distinct clinical patterns. Extensive colitis follows a different natural history and is associated with an array of complications different from those occurring in cases of limited proctitis. This latter entity also may present in clinically different forms, with severe refractory proctitis behaving as though it were a disease altogether distinct from the typically mild treatment-responsive variety seen in the great majority of ambulatory patients[1].

At present, our clinical distinctions among different forms of ulcerative colitis are crude at best. Although we have recently acquired an impressive array of genetic and serological tests to apply to our colitis patients, revealing considerable heterogeneity in these profiles, we still cannot begin to fathom the significance of this genetic and serological heterogeneity without a fuller grasp of clinical heterogeneity. For example, it is known that some patients with ulcerative colitis bear the HLA haplotype DR3/DQ2, while others have DR103; these observations carry little importance for us, however, until they are linked with clinical associations, such as the former haplotype possibly marking for extensive colitis, or the latter signalling a higher frequency of extraintestinal manifestations and an increased need for surgery.

The situation is, if anything, even more complex for Crohn's disease, which is clinically more heterogeneous than ulcerative colitis. Indeed, even the simple anatomical classification into ileitis, colitis and ileocolitis, which today we take for granted, was not acknowledged by Burrill Crohn himself for 30 years. Furthermore, the common term 'ileitis' does not accurately describe other forms of small bowel Crohn's disease, such as segmental jejunitis or diffuse jejunoileitis, each of which may follow a different course and carry a different prognosis.

For these reasons, an international Working Team that issued its report in Rome in 1991 proposed a classification of patients with Crohn's disease into several subgroups based upon anatomical distribution, operative history, and predominant clinical 'behaviour', *viz.* inflammatory, fistulizing or stenotic[2]. Another international Working Group, commissioned for the 1998 World Congress of Gastroenterology in Vienna, is now refining this clinical phenotypic classification of Crohn's disease. These several classification schemes, rudimentary as they are, already have obvious therapeutic implications. For example, patients with chronically obstructing *stenotic* Crohn's disease should not be subjected to fruitless medical management, especially with steroids, but should instead undergo elective surgery. Conversely, the postoperative prognosis following resection for primarily *inflammatory* disease is notoriously poor[3] so every effort should be made to maintain such cases on long-term medical therapy. *Fistulizing* disease, on the other hand, might be best managed either by medical or surgical treatment depending upon the nature and severity of its complications[4].

Beyond these obvious therapeutic implications, however, there are three other areas of applicability for subgrouping inflammatory bowel disease patients. First is the design and interpretation of *clinical trials*. The results of clinical trials cannot be adequately interpreted without attention to the possible heterogeneity and stratification of the patient population. In one major study of postoperative prophylaxis, for example, the efficacy of the treatment appeared to differ between cases of ileitis and colitis[5]. Similarly, another recently completed postoperative trial of budesonide showed no overall therapeutic benefit but suggested the possibility of efficacy in the small subgroup with fistulizing as opposed to fibrostenotic disease.

A second implication of subclassifying patients relates to our understanding of the *natural history* of Crohn's disease. Separate analyses of the course of fistulizing and fibrostenotic cases have indicated that these may represent two distinct clinical forms that retain their identities postoperatively, with the former being more aggressive and requiring operation and reoperation significantly faster[6,7]. Other studies have confirmed different prognoses for different clinical patterns of Crohn's disease[8] and have even suggested a biological basis for the distinction[9]. It has also been shown that the length of the involved segment predicts the length of the segment of postoperative recurrence[10].

Third and perhaps most important are the fundamental implications of clinical classification for understanding *pathophysiology*. Besides clinical heterogeneity among patients with ulcerative colitis and Crohn's disease, there are distinctions based upon genotypes, serotypes, cytokine profiles and permeability patterns. Without clinical phenotyping, however, these various laboratory markers are operating in a vacuum. It has been noted, for example, that, in certain ulcerative colitis patients, pANCA-positive patients are more likely to be HLA haplotype DR3/DQ2, while pANCA-negativity correlates with DR6/DQ6. The question remains, though, whether these observations have anything to do with the colitis itself. After all, we may also observe that ulcerative colitis patients with blond hair tend to have blue eyes while patients with black hair tend to have brown eyes. Genetic heterogeneity and genetic associations, in other words, are simply facts of life. Before these phenomena become interesting to us in the study of IBD, however, we must determine that they have something to do with particular disease patterns or behaviours. Promising examples of this type of correlation are preliminary data linking the classical pANCA-negative ASCA-positive serotype profile of Crohn's disease to small bowel location, and the atypical pANCA-positive ASCA-negative profile to colonic involvement. Other proposed genotypic–phenotypic correlations include the findings of different pANCA patterns and different TNF-locus microsatellites among Crohn's disease patients who were either good responders or poor responders to anti-TNF therapy. Studies like these promise to bring basic pathophysiological observations back into the arena of therapeutics. In the final analysis, the key to the mysteries of IBD will depend upon our ability to find more links between newly emerging laboratory markers and freshly defined clinical phenotypes of disease[11].

References

1. Farmer RG, Easley KA, Rankin GB. Clinical patterns, natural history, and progression of ulcerative colitis: A long-term follow-up of 1116 patients. Dig Dis Sci. 1993;38:1137–46.
2. Sachar DB, Andrews HA, Farmer RG *et al.* Proposed classification of patient subgroups in Crohn's disease. Gastroenterol Int. 1992;5:141–54.
3. Griffiths AM, Wesson DE, Shandling B *et al.* Factors influencing postoperative recurrence of Crohn's disease in childhood. Gut. 1991;32:491–5.
4. Sachar DB. Classification of Crohn's disease: implications for management. In: McLeod RS, Martin F, Sutherland LR, Wallace JL, Williams CN, editors, Trends in Inflammatory Bowel Disease Therapy 1996, Chapter 12. Dordrecht: Kluwer Academic Publishers; 1997:93–8.
5. McLeod RS, Wolff BG, Steinhart AH *et al.* Prophylactic mesalamine treatment decreases post-operative recurrence of Crohn's disease. Gastroenterology. 1995;109:404–13.
6. Greenstein AJ, Lachman P, Sachar DB *et al.* Perforating and non-perforating indications for surgery in Crohn's disease: Evidence for two clinical forms. Gut. 1986;29:588–92.
7. Aeberhard P, Berchtold W, Riedtmann H-J *et al.* Surgical recurrence of perforating and nonperforating Crohn's disease: A study of 101 surgically treated patients. Dis Colon Rectum. 1996;39:80–7.
8. Perri F, Annese V, Napolitano G *et al.* Subgroups of patients with Crohn's disease have different clinical outcomes. Inflam Bowel Dis. 1996;2:1.
9. Gilberts ECAM, Greenstein AJ, Katsel P *et al.* Molecular evidence for two forms of Crohn's disease. Proc Natl Acad Sci USA. 1994;91:12721–4.
10. D'Haens GR, Gasparaitis AE, Hanauer SB. Duration of recurrent ileitis after ileocolonic resection correlates with presurgical extent of Crohn's disease. Gut. 1993;36:715–17.
11. Sachar DB. Crohn's disease: A family affair. Gastroenterology. 1996;111:573–4.

18
Aetiopathogenesis of IBD: where do we stand?

C. FIOCCHI

INTRODUCTION

Tracking down the culprits responsible for inflammatory bowel disease (IBD) remains one of the great challenges in the field of gastroenterology. Although investigation of the cause and mechanism of Crohn's disease (CD) and ulcerative colitis (UC) has been going on for about half a century, it has been only during the last 30 years that scientifically sound and modern methodology, due to developments in cell biology, immunology and molecular biology, has been applied to IBD research. During the last three decades, a large body of knowledge has been progressively amassed, but, during the same period of time, some of the paths to IBD pathogenesis have turned cold, some continued to be explored, while new 'hot' ones are discovered from time to time. Without any doubt, we are presently experiencing the most exciting and rewarding time in IBD research, both clinical and basic. This chapter will review developments which have occurred during the last 30 years of basic research in IBD. In doing so, we will attempt to follow a path that should lead us to understand IBD and describe, with as little personal bias as possible, what is no longer being pursued (a 'cold' path), what is still under study but seems to go nowhere or is struggling with problems of validity, consistency or interpretation (a 'warm' path), and what is a promising new lead (a 'hot' path). During this journey, a series of key questions will be asked to which we will reply based on state-of-the-art knowledge of the aetiology and pathogenesis of IBD[1]. At the end of this journey, we will hopefully be in a position to know where we stand and where we should go.

KEY QUESTIONS IN IBD PATHOGENESIS

Investigating IBD poses special problems related to the fact that this disorder occurs in a system with two absolutely unique features, both of which may mask the cause as well as the mediation of tissue damage. The first feature is the existence of 'physiological inflammation' in the healthy mucosa[2]. This background of abundant immune cell infiltration with a heightened state of activation may hide what could otherwise be clear-cut readily identifiable immune abnormalities in an organ normally free of lymphoid tissue. The second feature is the presence of a rich endogenous enteric flora which could easily conceal a pathogenic micro-organism responsible for CD or UC[3]. So determining are these two features that, in addition to asking how would IBD be in the absence of physiological inflammation and enteric flora, one is even tempted to ask whether IBD itself would exist without them.

Primary vs. secondary events

Dealing with the typical IBD patient almost invariably means dealing with an individual whose disease has been in existence for years, if not with symptoms, then with previously silent intestinal inflammation and damage. When did the disease start? It is currently impossible to answer that question because we cannot identify the cause or fully understand the mechanisms. A new approach in trying to answer that question is to study children with IBD and investigate whether, beyond the routine clinical manifestations, in a child with recent-onset disease, IBD is mechanistically different from IBD affecting adults. Ongoing investigations suggest so, since the immune response of children with the first attack of CD or UC seems to be far more malleable than that of adults. This is based on recent observations that mucosal T cells can be readily modulated in response to certain cytokines, a phenomenon no longer detectable in patients with late-stage IBD[4]. In comparing IBD in children and adults, we must learn whether the primary pathogenic events responsible for triggering inflammation and initiating tissue damage are still present during the chronic phase of IBD, or whether completely different unrelated secondary events become responsible for the perpetuation of gut inflammation.

Clinical presentation

Even at the clinical level, where the diversity and variability of clinical manifestations may challenge the most experienced gastroenterologist, there are several fundamental questions that remain unresolved. We still do not know what underlines the inflammatory vs. stenosing vs. fistulizing forms of CD. Similarly, we still do not have a good handle on how to define or separate pancolitis from left-sided colitis, proctosigmoiditis or proctitis. In addition, what really is indeterminate colitis? Is it a form of CD, as many believe, or does it represent an altogether different form of IBD? In other words, is all 'IBD' really IBD?

ENVIRONMENTAL FACTORS

Among a hopelessly long list of potentially important environmental factors, attention has concentrated on diet, smoking and the issue of intestinal permeability. Although diet has been shown to have an impact on the outcome of CD, but not UC, the reasons why this is so are obscure. Additional investigation of how diet affects IBD is still warranted, but little new is happening in this area (a cold path). The dramatic effect of smoking on UC and CD clinical activity and the apparent therapeutic effect of nicotine in UC are puzzling but totally open questions[5]. Clearly, something in tobacco has the capacity to impact oppositely on each form of IBD, and discovering what that might be could be extremely informative about the role of environmental agents in the pathogenesis of IBD. At the moment, no new clues have emerged and this path is only warm. By contrast, the issue of increased intestinal permeability in healthy first-degree relatives of CD, but not UC, patients continues to be pursued with great interest[6]. Currently, there is general agreement that the phenomenon is real and probably important (a hot path).

FAMILIAL AND GENETIC FACTORS

The current emphasis on the importance of genetic factors in IBD started with the observation of a higher-than-expected prevalence of CD or UC in first-degree relatives[7]. This has been widely confirmed, but simply studying frequency or the appearance of new cases of IBD in families is no longer a particularly productive approach (a warm path). In contrast, genetic studies and the phenomenon of genetic anticipation are considered current and are very hot topics of research[8,9]. Although several associations with MHC Class II antigens and linkages to specific chromosomes have been described and at times confirmed[10–12], as this investigation continues, lack of previously reported associations has been found in different populations[13], and new associations have been described[14]. This lack of consistency and controversial results raise the question of how many strong and relevant genetic associations exist or, in other words, how much genetic heterogeneity really exists among IBD patients. The greater the number of associations, the less useful this information will be to understand IBD, and the stronger the importance of environmental factors will become. This latter comparison raises the fundamental question of how genetic and environmental factors interact to cause IBD or, who is in charge: genes or the environment?

MICROBIAL AGENTS

A possible infectious cause for IBD has been sought since the initial reports describing CD and UC, but no putative microbial agent has withstood the test of time. Still, the idea that IBD may be an infectious disease cannot be dismissed. The investigation of *Mycobacterium paratuberculosis* as the specific cause of CD has yielded inconclusive data[15], and this path appears to be cold. The possibility that viral agents are involved has also been pursued, and investigation into the measles virus as the cause of a vasculitis responsible for the pathological and clinical manifestation of CD is still ongoing[16], but no new strong substantiating evidence has emerged (a warm path). Most of the current attention is being given to the normal enteric flora as an initiating or contributing factor to the pathogenesis of IBD, CD in particular (a hot path)[3]. This attention is justified by studies of animal models of IBD in which intestinal inflammation fails to develop when the animals are kept in a sterile environment[17], studies showing the crucial importance of bacterial flora in the development of pouchitis[18], and the early recurrence of inflammation upon establishing a contact between the faecal stream and the mucosa of CD patients[19]. Based on these observations, the key questions to be addressed by ongoing and future investigation are: whether the whole or only selected flora is involved; how faecal stasis triggers mucosal inflammation; and why flora from different segments of the bowel appears to induce gut inflammation when in contact with mucosa from different intestinal segments.

IMMUNE FACTORS

In the absence of an identified infectious agent or well-characterized predisposing factors, for the last 30 years immunology has dominated the field of IBD research[20]. In the 1970s and through the 1980s, studies were concentrated on classical humoral and cell-mediated immunity, prostaglandins, neuropeptides and cytokines. In the 1990s, some of these areas declined in interest, while others surged, including growth factors, reactive oxygen and nitrogen metabolites, adhesion molecules, non-immune cells and the extracellular matrix, and, lastly, the phenomenon of apoptosis. While all these topics opened new paths of investigation, at the same time, they revealed that intestinal inflammation is a process of unprecedented complexity[21]. It is fair to say that an enormous amount of progress has been made but many critical questions remain unanswered; these include whether either one of the forms of IBD is a true autoimmune disorder, whether CD and UC can be unmistakably distinguished on the basis of unique immune reactivities, and whether immune abnormalities specific for CD or UC really exist.

Humoral and cell-mediated immunity

The involvement of immune reactivity in IBD started with the demonstration of anticolon antibodies in the serum of UC patients[22]. This was followed by the detection of lymphocytotoxic antibodies, dietary and bacterial antibodies and immune complexes. None of them, however, appeared to translate immune events directly linked to IBD pathogenesis, but rather all seemed to represent secondary epiphenomena (cold paths). Several abnormalities of antibody production at the systemic and mucosal levels have also been reported but the remarkable elevation of IgA and IgG levels in either CD or UC almost certainly reflects mere alterations secondary to chronicity of the inflammation in IBD (cold paths). In the last few years, the high frequency of antinuclear cytoplasmic antibodies in the serum of UC patients was proposed as a possible immune marker with specificity for this form of IBD[23], a contention that appears to be supported by multiple studies (a hot path). Other serum and mucosal antibodies that are still of considerable interest are those against tropomyosin fraction 5, a potential epithelial cell autoantigen which may be relevant to UC[24].

Investigation of cell-mediated immunity in IBD has been pursued even more intensely than that of humoral immunity. Initially, almost all studies were carried out with circulating lymphocytes, and their behaviour could reflect abnormalities of systemic immunity in IBD. Various findings were reported, including cytotoxicity against colonocytes, the presence of activated leukocytes in the peripheral blood of CD and UC patients, as well as defects of lymphocyte proliferation, cytotoxicity, suppressor cell function, and mixed lymphocyte reactivity. None of these results helped to define specific and reproducible abnormalities and at present all these paths are cold. With the development of techniques to isolate and study the immune cells present in the inflamed gut and implicitly involved in the local inflammatory response, an additional series of studies were performed which led to the enumeration and classification of mucosal T cells in the normal and IBD mucosa, and identification of differential abnormalities of cytotoxic function between CD and UC T cells[1]. All this expanded our knowledge of mucosal immunity in IBD but failed to result in definitive clues to which aberrations are truly important for CD or UC. In the last few years, restriction in T-cell receptor $V\beta$ region utilization and the oligoclonality of the T-cell populations in IBD-involved mucosa (both being a reflection of an assumed selectivity of the immune response against specific antigens) have attracted considerable attention (warm or hot paths) but have yet to result in the identification of unique immune defects. The last of the very hot topics under investigation is whether defects in epithelial-cell or T-cell apoptosis exist in IBD. If detected, they could lead respectively to identification of mechanisms of epithelial damage or explain chronicity of inflammation because of an excessively prolonged survival of T cells in the inflamed mucosa, a phenomenon common to other autoimmune disorders[25].

Cytokines

Among the various components of the IBD inflammatory response, none has received as much attention as cytokines, soluble mediators pivotal to immune cell activation, growth, differentiation and effector function. Currently, a large body of information has been accumulated on the source, level and role of mucosal cytokines in IBD[26], a topic that continues to be quite hot. Among immunoregulatory cytokines, mostly products of T cells that dictate the outcome of an immune response, there is some contradiction on low or high levels of IL-2 and IFN-γ, while there is consensus on low IL-4 and high IL-10 production. These results tell us that various defects of immunoregulatory cytokines are present in IBD but they do not necessarily point to a unique defect responsible for IBD. However, when all available data are collected and examined, there is reason to believe that CD is more representative of a Th1-type, and UC of a Th2-type, of immune response[27]. Put very simply, cell-mediated immunity is more involved in the first, and humoral immunity in the latter, type of IBD.

The study of proinflammatory cytokines has yielded more consistent but predictable results since classical mediators, such as IL-1, IL-6, IL-8 and chemokines, are all elevated in the actively inflamed mucosa and, at times, even in the circulation of IBD patients. The results on TNF-α are more controversial since levels of this potent inflammatory molecule are not always elevated in IBD, which is not to say that TNF-α is not involved in its pathogenesis. An important concept derived from these studies is that the ratio between pro- and anti-inflammatory cytokines is probably more relevant than the absolute level of each cytokine, as exemplified by the imbalance found in both CD and UC between IL-1 receptor antagonist (a natural and specific anti-inflammatory molecule) and IL-1 (the prototypical inflammatory cytokine)[28].

When the global status of immunoregulatory and inflammatory cytokines is analysed objectively, various key questions remain unanswered. We still do not know whether any dominant cytokine abnormality exists in CD or UC, or how well polarized towards a Th1 or Th2 profile cytokines are in either form of IBD. With the continuous appearance of new cytokines displaying a multiplicity of overlapping activities, these questions may remain unanswered for the foreseeable future.

Growth factors, lipid mediators, neuropeptides and reactive metabolites

In addition to classical glycoprotein cytokines produced primarily by lymphoid cells, many other mediators also contribute to the pathogenesis of gut inflammation, and they represent warm or hot paths to IBD.

Growth factors participate in the process of mucosal protection, wound formation and healing, and their levels tend to be elevated in IBD, such as fibroblast growth factor, keratinocyte growth factor and trefoil peptide[29]. Whether some growth factors are involved in the phenomenon of excessive proliferation leading to cancer development in the chronically inflamed mucosa is still not clear[30].

Lipid mediators are products of the arachidonic acid metabolism, and include prostaglandins, thromboxanes and leukotrienes, all of which have been extensively studied in IBD[31]. At the moment, interest in simply measuring these molecules is no longer intense (a cold path) but their regulation is under intense scrutiny, in particular the role of cyclo-oxygenase 2 (COX-2), an inducible enzyme controlling the production of PGE_2, which is presently believed to mediate mucosal cytoprotection.

Neuropeptides represent another category of molecules involved in IBD pathogenesis. Neuropeptides, such as VIP and SP, are potent regulators of immunity and, as such, may modulate an inflammatory response to stress[32]. Abnormalities of neuropeptide levels have been described in both CD and UC, as well as differences in mucosal receptor expression, helping to keep a high level of interest in this line of investigation (a warm path), as well as keeping alive an interest in the complex neuroendocrine–immune interactions occurring in inflammation[33].

Finally, the last group of mediators, which is gaining more and more attention (a hot path), is reactive oxygen and nitrogen metabolites. These toxic molecules produced by neutrophils and macrophages are receiving increasing attention because they may represent a final pathway of multiple immune and non-immune cell activation, and they may directly mediate cell death and tissue injury[34]. The issue of what actually causes tissue injury is an extremely hot topic and a variety of molecules have been proposed, including all of the above as well as matrix metalloproteinases[35]. Several critical questions must be answered before a full understanding of mucosal inflammation and gut injury in IBD is reached: is tissue injury completely non-specific, or is any particular cell type targeted by the mucosal immune response? Furthermore, is any specific mediator responsible for tissue damage, or is this the result of a multiplicity of mediators all acting in an integrated deleterious fashion?

Adhesion molecules

A relatively new area of investigation in IBD is that of adhesion molecules present on the surface of essentially all cells. Adhesion molecules are indispensable, not only for cell-to-cell contact, but also for cell localization, activation and function[36]. In IBD, the cell adhesion molecules that have attracted most attention are those expressed by immune cells, T cells and monocytes in particular, since it is through the selective and timed expression of molecules that inflammatory cells travel and localize to the inflamed intestine[37]. The concentration of soluble adhesion molecules is high in the circulation of IBD patients but this represents a non-specific secondary event; more relevant is the enhanced expression of adhesion in the gut mucosa itself, where their selective expression may not only provide clues to the mechanism of inflammation but perhaps also differentiate between CD and UC[38]. Of special interest are adhesion molecules that are directly responsible for leukocyte influx during inflammation, such as MAdCAM-1, whose expression is markedly upregulated in actively inflamed IBD mucosa[39]. The expression of adhesion molecules in IBD deserves attention because it is directly linked to the process of homing of inflammatory cells into the mucosa. However, important questions that still wait for an answer are: how selective the process of recruitment during periods of activity is, how long immune cells survive after recruitment is completed, and how the survival of the newly localized immune cells is controlled in the normal and IBD intestine.

Non-immune cells and the extracellular matrix

The most recent area of investigation in IBD is that of immune–non-immune cell interactions. It is now established that inflammatory responses, regardless of the origin or organ affected, involve an extremely complex interplay between immune and non-immune cells. The latter comprise epithelial, endothelial, nerve and mesenchymal cells, as well as the acellular extracellular matrix[40]. Information is rapidly accumulating that suggests a considerably more prominent and functionally important role of diverse cell types in the pathogenesis of IBD. In both CD and UC, epithelial cells may contribute to inflammation through the inappropriate activation of helper rather than suppressor cells[41], whereas endothelial and mesenchymal cells display an enhanced capacity to bind various types of leukocytes[42,43]. Even the acellular extracellular matrix produced by intestinal fibroblasts is excessively adhesive for T cells in IBD[44]. While these multiple activities make the interpretation of the mechanisms of attraction and retention of inflammatory cells in IBD increasingly complicated, at the same time, they open up new possibilities for therapeutic intervention through the specific blockade of these multiple immune–non-immune interactions.

THE ULTIMATE QUESTION IN IBD PATHOGENESIS

Thirty years is not a long time in terms of disease evolution but it may be enough time to unravel previously unsolved problems related to the pathogenesis of a disease. The last 30 years have witnessed successively faster progress in IBD, and the description of the cold, warm and hot paths leading to the understanding of CD and UC has clearly shown the numerous difficulties encountered along the way. The most important progress has certainly occurred, not so much in discovering a specific agent causing IBD, but in unveiling some of the mechanisms of the relentless inflammatory reaction that destroys the intestines of affected individuals. Knowledge of these mechanisms of IBD is incomplete; nevertheless, it is fair to ask the ultimate question of IBD pathogenesis: has pathophysiology-based knowledge improved therapy of IBD? In other words, are we now better at treating patients after acquiring so much information about all the factors and agents discussed above? The answer is yes. The implementation of novel treatments based on cytokine blockade, and the increasing use of antibiotics in managing CD, represent examples of this success. In the next decade, we will explore several new 'biotech' paths where highly specific blockers, neutralizing antibodies or recombinant cytokines will be given to patients with very selective but different goals, but all of which aim at stopping inflammation in the gut. Our current therapeutic approaches are imperfect but benefit most patients, although at a price. Hence, will highly specific mediator-targeted therapy be more effective, in the long run, than non-specific broad immunosuppression? The answer is just around the corner, right at the beginning of the new millennium.

References

1. Fiocchi C. Inflammatory bowel disease: etiology and pathogenesis. Gastroenterology. 1998;115:185–205.
2. Fiocchi C. Immunity and inflammation: separate or unified? In: MacDermott RP, ed. Clinical Immunology in Gastroenterology and Hepatology: From Bench to Bedside. American Gastroenterological Association; 1994:182–8.
3. Sartor RB. Enteric microflora in IBD: pathogens or commensals? Inflam Bowel Dis. 1997;3:230–5.
4. Kugathasan S, Binioin DG, Itoh J, Boyle JT, Levine AD, Fiocchi C. Clonal T-cell cytokine secretion is modulated in mucosa of children with recent onset but not chronic inflammatory bowel disease. Gastroenterology. 1997;112:A1021.
5. Rhodes J, Thomas GAO. Smoking: good or bad for inflammatory bowel disease? Gastroenterology. 1994;106:807–10.
6. Hollander D. Permeability in Crohn's disease: altered barrier function in healthy relatives? Gastroenterology. 1993;104:1848–51.
7. Farmer RG, Michener WM. Association of inflammatory bowel disease in families. Front Gastrointest Res. 1986;11:17–26.
8. Duerr RH. Genetics of inflammatory bowel disease. Inflam Bowel Dis. 1996;2:48–60.
9. Polito JM, Rees RC, Childs B, Mendeloff AI, Harris ML, Bayless TM. Preliminary evidence for genetic anticipation in Crohn's disease. Lancet. 1996;347:798–800.
10. Asakura H, Tsuchiya M, Aiso S et al. Association of the human lymphocyte-DR2 antigen with Japanese ulcerative colitis. Gastroenterology. 1982;82:413–18.
11. Satsangi J, Parkes M, Louis E et al. Two stage genome-wide search in inflammatory bowel disease provides evidence for susceptibility loci on chromosones 3, 7 and 12. Nature Genet. 1996;14:199–202.
12. Hugot JP, Laurent-Puig P, Gower-Rousseau C et al. for GETAID. Linkage analysis of chromosome 6 loci, including HLA, in familial aggregations of Crohn disease. Am J Med Genet. 1994;52:207–13.
13. Vermiere S, Peeters M, Vlietinck R et al. No evidence for linkage on chromosome 16-12-7 and 3 in the Belgian population may reflect genetic heterogeneity of inflammatory bowel disease. Gastroenterology. 1998;114:A1109.

14. Brant SR, Nicolae D, LaBuda MC *et al.* A genome wide screen of Crohn's disease in a large pedigree shows evidence for linkages to chromosomes 11, 16, 8 and 15. Gastroenterology. 1998;114:A941.

15. Chiodini RJ. Crohn's disease and the mycobacterioses: a review and comparison of two disease entities. Clin Microbiol Rev. 1989;2:90–117.

16. Wakefield AJ, Ekbom A, Dhillon AP, Pittilo RM, Pounder RE. Crohn's disease: pathogenesis and persistent measles virus infection. Gastroenterology. 1995;108:911–16.

17. Elson CO, Sartor RB, Tennyson GS, Riddell RH. Experimental models of inflammatory bowel disease. Gastroenterology. 1995;109:1344–67.

18. Ruseler-van-Embden JGH, Schouten WR, vanLieshout LMC. Pouchitis: result of microbial imbalance? Gut. 1994;35:658–64.

19. D'Haens G, Geboes K, Peeters M, Baert F, Penninckx F, Rutgeerts P. Early lesions caused by infusion of intestinal contents in excluded ileum of Crohn's disease. Gastroenterology. 1998;114:262–7.

20. Elson CO, McCabe RP. The immunology of inflammatory bowel disease. In: Kirsner JB, Shorter RG, eds. Inflammatory Bowel Disease. Baltimore: Williams & Wilkins; 1995:203–51.

21. Fiocchi C. Intestinal inflammation: a complex interplay of immune–non-immune cell interactions. Am J Physiol. 1997;273:G769–75.

22. Broberger O, Perlmann P. Autoantibodies in human ulcerative colitis. J Exp Med. 1959;110:657–74.

23. Saxon A, Shanahan F, Landers C, Ganz T, Targan S. A distinct subset of anti-neutrophil cytoplasmic antibodies is associated with inflammatory bowel disease. J Allergy Clin Immunol. 1990;86:202–10.

24. Das KM, Dasgupta A, Mandal A, Geng X. Autoimmunity to cytoskeletal protein tropomyosin. A clue to the pathogenetic mechanisms for ulcerative colitis. J Immunol. 1993;150:2487–93.

25. Thompson CB. Apoptosis in the pathogenesis and treatment of disease. Science. 1995;267:1456–62.

26. Fiocchi C. Cytokines in Inflammatory Bowel Disease. Austin: RG Landes Company; 1996.

27. Romagnani S. The Th1/Th2 paradigm. Immunol Today. 1997;18:263–6.

28. Casini-Raggi V, Kam L, Chong YJT, Fiocchi C, Pizarro TT, Cominelli F. Mucosal imbalance of interleukin-1 and interleukin-1 receptor antagonist in inflammatory bowel disease: a novel mechanisms of chronic inflammation. J Immunol. 1995;154:2434–40.

29. Dignass AU, Podolsky DK. Peptide growth factors in inflammatory bowel disease. In: Fiocchi C, ed. Cytokines in Inflammatory Bowel Disease. Austin: R.G. Landes; 1996:137–55.

30. Babyatsky MW, Rossiter G, Podolsky DK. Expression of transforming growth factor α and β in colonic mucosa in inflammatory bowel disease. Gastroenterology. 1996;110:975–84.

31. Stenson WF. Arachidonic acid metabolites in inflammatory bowel disease. In: Fiocchi C, ed. Cytokines in Inflammatory Bowel Disease. Austin: R.G. Landes; 1996:157–76.

32. Reinshagen M, Egger B, Procaccino F, Eysselein VE. Neuropeptides in inflammatory bowel disease. Inflam Bowel Dis. 1997;3:303–13.

33. Reichlin S. Neuroendocrine–immune interactions. N Engl J Med. 1993;329:1245–53.

34. Grisham MB, Yamada T. Neutrophils, nitrogen oxides, and inflammatory bowel disease. Ann NY Acad Sci. 1992;664:103–15.

35. MacDonald TT, Pender SLF. Proteolytic enzymes in inflammatory bowel disease. Inflam Bowel Dis. 1998;4:157–64.

36. Frenette PS, Wagner DD. Adhesion molecules – part I. N Engl J Med. 1996;334:1526–9.

37. Panes J, Granger DN. Leukocyte–endothelial interactions: molecular mechanisms and implications in gastrointestinal disease. Gastroenterology. 1998;114:1066–90.

38. Rosenberg WMC, Prince C, Kaklamanis L *et al.* Increased expression of CD44v6 and CD44v3 in ulcerative colitis but not colonic Crohn's disease. Lancet. 1995;345:1205–9.

39. Briskin M, Winsor-Hines D, Shyjan A *et al.* Human mucosal addresin cell adhesion molecule-1 is preferentially expressed in intestinal tract and associated lymphoid tissue. Am J Pathol. 1997;151:97–110.

40. Fiocchi C, Collins SM, James SP, Mayer L, Podolsky DK, Stenson WF. Immune–non-immune cell interactions in intestinal inflammation. Inflam Bowel Dis. 1997;3:133–41.

41. Mayer L, Eisenhardt D. Lack of induction of suppressor T cells by intestinal epithelial cells from patients with inflammatory bowel disease. J Clin Invest. 1990;86:1255–60.

42. Binion DG, West GA, Ina K, Ziats NP, Emancipator SN, Fiocchi C. Enhanced leukocyte binding by intestinal microvascular endothelial cells in inflammatory bowel disease. Gastroenterology. 1997;112:1895–907.
43. Ina K, Kusugami K, Fiocchi C. Enhanced interaction of intestinal fibroblasts with T-cells in inflammatory bowel disease (IBD). Gastroenterology. 1996;110:A930.
44. Musso A, Ina K, Fiocchi C. Extracellular matrix (ECM) from inflammatory bowel disease (IBD) displays enhanced adhesiveness for T-cells. Gastroenterology. 1996;110:A977.

Section V
Standard therapies in IBD

19
Aminosalicylates in the treatment of ulcerative colitis and Crohn's disease

L. R. SUTHERLAND

INTRODUCTION

Since the discovery of the first aminosalicylate, sulphasalazine, by Svartz almost 60 years ago[1], the aminosalicylates have become one of the mainstays of therapy in inflammatory bowel disease. Following the demonstration that 5-aminosalicylic acid was the therapeutically active portion of sulphasalazine[2,3], a variety of delivery systems were developed.

Today the concepts of targeted delivery have been accepted. Physicians need to be informed as to how each aminosalicylate is formulated so that patients may gain the maximum benefit from their therapy. The aminosalicylate preparations can be conveniently divided into three categories based upon their mechanism of release: an azo bond, pH dependent or microspheres (Table 1). Topical therapy with aminosalicylate is also possible.

This paper will focus on the results of randomized controlled trials which have assessed the efficacy of the aminosalicylates in the treatment of ulcerative colitis (induction and maintenance of remission) and Crohn's disease (induction and maintenance of remission). Whenever possible, the results of meta-analyses will be used to summarize data.

Table 1 The aminosalicylates and their mechanism of release

Azo bond
  Sulphasalazine
  Olsalazine (Dipentum)
  Balsalazide (Colazide)

pH dependent
  Asacol
  Claversal, Mesasal, Salofalk

Microspheres
  Pentasa

MECHANISM OF ACTION

The mechanism of action of 5-ASA is unknown. Postulated mechanisms include: alteration in eicosanoid metabolism (leukotriene or prostaglandin), scavenging free radicals, immunological effects and colonocyte fatty acid oxidation[4]. The recent report that suppression of leukotriene production was not associated with clinical improvement suggests that interference with leukotrienes is not important clinically[5].

ULCERATIVE COLITIS

The aminosalicylates are the first line of therapy for mild to moderately active ulcerative colitis and for the maintenance of remission.

Induction of remission

Baron and associates were the first to evaluate the efficacy of sulphasalazine as first-line therapy for induction of remission[6]. Subsequent studies by Lennard-Jones and colleagues confirmed their observations[7]. It soon became apparent that the adverse events associated with the sulphapyridine component would limit the dose of sulphasalazine that could be tolerated.

The most recent meta-analysis of the newer 5-aminosalicylates[8] identified 19 randomized controlled trials that compared 5-ASA with placebo (nine trials) or sulphasalazine (10 trials). To be included in the analysis, trials had to be double-blind, controlled and of a minimum of four weeks duration. Therapeutic goals varied between trials and comparisons are limited by differences in indices used to assess outcome.

Patients who received 5-ASA did significantly better than those who received placebo. There is evidence for a dose–response curve. When compared with sulphasalazine, the newer 5-ASA preparations almost reach a statistically significant difference but the confidence intervals still include a range of results that would be clinically insignificant.

Topical therapy with mesalazine is also possible and has much to recommend it for patients with disease localized to the distal bowel. Topical therapy with either enemas or suppositories delivers drug to the area that needs it the most with minimal absorption. A recent meta-analysis by Marshall and Irvine[9] identified 19 trials which met their criteria (randomized, controlled, double blind, 4 weeks minimum duration). The odds of entering remission for patients randomized to mesalazine compared with those randomized to placebo were 7.4 (CI 4.8–11.5). In a subsequent paper, the same authors demonstrated that topical therapy with mesalazine was superior to topical corticosteroid therapy (odds ratio 2.4, CI 1.7–3.4)[10].

Combination therapy using both oral and topical forms of mesalazine has been assessed. The combination of 2.4 g mesalazine and 4 g 5-ASA enemas has been shown to be more effective than either therapy by itself[11]. Patients randomized to enemas showed improvement more rapidly than those randomized to oral medication.

4-Aminosalicylic acid (4-ASA), better known as PAS (para-aminosalicylic acid), has been used in the treatment of tuberculosis for many decades. Randomized controlled double-blind studies have demonstrated efficacy for both oral[12] and topical[13] formulations. 4-ASA is also a useful compound to assist in determining the mechanism of action of mesalazine. If a potential mechanism of action for 5-ASA cannot be confirmed using 4-ASA, then it is unlikely that it is relevant to our understanding of how 5-ASA exerts its effect.

Outstanding issues

Although much is known about the efficacy of mesalazine in the induction of remission, several issues remain to be answered. The mechanism of action of mesalazine remains a mystery. It is not clear whether we have reached the top of the dose–response curve in terms of efficacy. Whether there is a 'best' formulation of mesalazine is unknown. The usefulness of combination therapy with corticosteroid therapy for patients with more active ulcerative colitis has not been addressed.

Maintenance of remission

Although mesalazine can be demonstrated to have efficacy in the induction of remission, other medications, particularly corticosteroids, are also effective. The most significant contribution that mesalazine offers in the therapy of IBD is as the sole agent shown to be effective in the maintenance of remission. Studies of the natural history of ulcerative colitis have demonstrated that approximately 80% of untreated patients will relapse within one year following induction of remission[14]. This finding was confirmed by the analysis of placebo-treated patients[15].

Misiewicz and colleagues were the first to assess the efficacy of sulphasalazine for the maintenance of remission[16]. Subsequent studies by the Oxford group demonstrated that 2 g/day sulphasalazine offered the best trade-off between therapeutic efficacy and adverse events[17]. They also demonstrated that patients continued to gain benefit from sulphasalazine therapy regardless of the duration of ongoing therapy[18].

The meta-analysis of mesalazine for maintenance of remission demonstrated that mesalazine was superior to placebo for maintenance therapy. Included studies were randomized, controlled and of at least 6 months duration. Insufficient numbers of patients had been recruited to demonstrate a dose–response curve. An unexpected finding was the observation that sulphasalazine therapy was statistically superior to mesalazine for maintenance therapy of six months duration (OR 1.3, CI 1.1–1.6)[8]. This effect was not demonstrable at 12 months (OR 1.2, CI 0.9–1.5). There are several possible explanations for this phenomenon. First of all it could be correct and the azo bond mechanism may be a more effective mesalazine release preparation than the other formulations. Second, there is a bias in favour of sulphasalazine therapy in that an entry criterion for most sulphasalazine studies was tolerance to sulphasalazine, excluding patients who are intolerant. Third, many of the studies in the meta-analysis compared olsalazine with sulphasalazine. The early studies of olsalazine were marked by a high drop-out rate because of diarrhoea. This would benefit sulphasalazine in any comparison.

For many gastroenterologists, the concept of maintenance therapy is influenced by the maintenance therapy to prevent duodenal ulcer recurrence in the pre-*Helicobacter pylori* era when half the dose of H_2-receptor antagonist therapy was prescribed to prevent ulcer recurrence. For patients with ulcerative colitis who have a rapid relapse, consideration should be given to ongoing therapy with the dose of mesalazine used to induce remission.

Maintenance therapy with topical mesalazine is also possible. Biddle and associates demonstrated that one year of therapy with nightly mesalazine enemas was effective[19]. Various investigators have assessed the minimal frequency of enemas associated with prevention of relapse. Miner and associates reported that twice-weekly enemas were effective in maintaining remission when a placebo control was utilized[20]. Combination therapy with both enemas and tablets is a more effective maintenance therapy, in the rapid-relapse population, than either therapy alone[21].

Outstanding issues

A small proportion of patients are intolerant to mesalazine. Alternatives to mesalazine for such patients should be developed. Azathioprine therapy may be effective[22] and studies should be performed. Metronidazole may be an alternative to sulphasalazine for maintenance of remission[23]. Dickinson and associates reported that PRN sulphasalazine (3 g/day) was as effective as daily sulphasalazine (2 g/day)[24]. The study had a small sample size and the possibility of a Type II error cannot be dismissed but this may actually reflect patient behaviour.

CROHN'S DISEASE

The utility of aminosalicylates in the therapy of mild to moderately active Crohn's disease is controversial. After an initial bout of enthusiasm for the use of aminosalicylates for maintenance of remission, more recent studies have suggested that any benefit is at best modest.

Induction of remission

Despite their frequent use for the induction of remission in patients with Crohn's disease, there are few randomized controlled studies on which to base such a practice.

Because sulphasalazine requires bacterial action in order to release the mesalazine, it is not surprising that the early trials of sulphasalazine failed to demonstrate efficacy. The National Cooperative Crohn's Disease Study (NCCDS) was one of the first to report that sulphasalazine was superior to placebo in the subgroup of patients with colonic Crohn's disease[25]. The European Cooperative Crohn's Disease Study (ECCDS) also demonstrated a modest benefit for sulphasalazine-treated patients[26].

There are only six published trials of mesalazine for induction of remission of Crohn's disease[27]. Danish investigators reported that Pentasa (1.5 g/day) was no better than placebo but suggested that trials using larger doses should be performed[28]. Mahida and colleagues reported that Pentasa was no better than placebo but the trial was for only 6 weeks duration and utilized a low dose of medication (Mahida and Jewell, 1990). Singleton and associates reported that 43% of patients with mild to moderate active Crohn's disease, randomized to 4 g/day of Pentasa, entered remission compared with 18% of placebo-treated patients[29]. A second study, reported in a letter to the Editor, noted a similar response for Pentasa-treated patients but a much higher response rate for the placebo-treated patients (p = NS)[30]. The results of a third trial performed in North America are not known.

Tremaine and colleagues at the Mayo Clinic assessed Asacol in 38 patients with Crohn's disease[31]. Sixty per cent of mesalazine-treated patients achieved either partial or complete remission compared with 22% of placebo-treated patients. Wright and associates reported that olsalazine was ineffective in the treatment of patients with Crohn's disease[32].

Martin and other Canadian investigators compared Salofalk (3 g/day) with prednisone (48 mg/day tapering over 12 weeks) in 44 patients with Crohn's disease. Although prednisone-treated patients had a prompter decline in CDAI, by the end of the study both groups had an equivalent response. The possibility of a Type II error cannot, however, be ruled out[33].

Recently Thomsen and colleagues reported the results of a comparison of Pentasa (4 g/day) with budesonide (9 g/day). At the conclusion of 16 weeks of therapy, more patients treated with budesonide (62%) had entered remission than Pentasa-treated patients (36%) (p = 0.01)[34].

Outstanding issues

One of the outstanding issues is whether or not combination therapy (mesalazine with corticosteroids) is more effective than either therapy by itself. There have only been a few trials which have addressed this issue. Singleton *et al.* found that the combination of prednisone and sulphasalazine was less effective than prednisone alone[35]. The European Cooperative Crohn's Disease Study failed to show a benefit for the combination of prednisolone and sulphasalazine compared with prednisolone alone. Rijk and associates found that the addition of corticosteroids to sulphasalazine only resulted in a modest difference in van Hees index at four weeks which disappeared by the completion of therapy (16 weeks)[36].

Modigliani reported that patients who received Pentasa concurrently with prednisolone were more able to taper off steroids than those who received prednisolone alone, but this did not quite reach statistical significance[37]. Subgroup analysis of reasons for weaning failure differed significantly between the two groups.

Maintenance of remission

The initial studies of sulphasalazine for maintenance of remission were characterized by small sample size and the inclusion of a heterogeneous group of patients[38]. The only study to demonstrate efficacy was reported by Ewe and associates. This study was characterized by a large sample size (more than 200 participants) and a homogeneous patient population (post-resection)[39].

Several large studies for maintenance of medically induced remission have been equivocal. Results of subgroup analysis remain confusing with each study identifying different subgroups who respond. Three meta-analyses have been performed.

Steinhart *et al.*[40] and Messori *et al.*[41] reported similar results in 1993. In summary, they demonstrated a benefit for mesalazine-treated patients with the risk of relapse being reduced by 50%. A recent study by Camma and associates had the benefit of incorporating three large trials which had been published in the past 3 years[42]. Overall, they reported that, when all 15 studies which met their inclusion criteria were included, the reduction in risk was approximately 6% (CI 10–2). The number needed to treat (NNT) to prevent one relapse was 16. When the studies were separated by means of induction of remission (medical or surgical), different results were obtained. For the 10 studies which assessed efficacy in medically induced remission, the reduction in relative risk was 5% which did not achieve statistical significance (CI 10 to –2). The NNT was 20. For studies which reported data for the post-resection population, a statistically significant result was achieved: reduction in risk 13% (CI 22–5, NNT 8).

In my opinion, this benefit may still be exaggerated as the benefit is mainly from one study[43] which did not use a placebo but randomized patients to either mesalazine or no treatment. Such studies tend to overestimate the actual effect[44]. Also, Camma and associates failed to include the results of the largest postsurgical assessment of mesalazine which, to date, has only been published in abstract form[45]. This study, which failed to reach conventional statistical significance, might have further reduced the benefit to a statistically insignificant result.

Outstanding issues

Despite studies involving over 2000 patients, there continues to be ambiguity in terms of the dose of aminosalicylate required to maintain remission or prevent recurrence. In the future, the case for the use of maintenance therapy with aminosalicylates will depend first of all on the identification of patient subgroups at highest risk of relapse. Within that patient population, additional trials will be required to provide definitive proof that a meaningful reduction of the risk of relapse or recurrence can be achieved.

ADVERSE EFFECTS

Adverse effects are common, particularly with the first aminosalicylate, sulphasalazine. Table 2 provides a list of relatively common adverse effects. Some of the gastrointestinal side-effects reported with sulphasalazine can be reduced by using the enteric-coated formulation. Although, initially, it was thought that the newer aminosalicylates would be free of adverse events, this has not been so, but, for the most part, the frequency of adverse events is reduced[8]. The diarrhoea associated with olsalazine use results from altered chloride ion secretion in the distal terminal ileum[46]. This can be reduced by taking the olsalazine with food.

Table 2   Side-effects of the aminosalicylates

Unique to sulphasalazine
Gastrointestinal
  Nausea, vomiting
  Anorexia
  Dyspepsia
  Folate malabsorption

Haematological
  Haemolysis
  Neutropenia
  Agranulocytosis

Male infertility

Neuropathy

Common to all aminosalicylates
General
  Headaches
  Fever, rash

Gastrointestinal
  Exacerbation of colitis
  Pancreatitis
  Inflammatory liver disease
  Watery diarrhoea (olsalazine)

Other
  Pericarditis
  Pneumonitis
  Nephritis

CONCLUSIONS

The discovery that 5-ASA was the active component of sulphasalazine stimulated a decade of development resulting in numerous formulations of mesalazine. For the sulphasalazine-intolerant patient, this has been a major advance. In general, however, the introduction of mesalazine in its various forms has not produced significant benefits for patients with ulcerative colitis. The discovery that 5-ASA was the active compound led the way for the introduction of topical therapy. For Crohn's disease, however, the clinical usefulness of mesalazine remains an open question. Additional trials are required.

References

1. Svartz N. Salazyopyrin, a new sulfanilamide preparation: A. Therapeutic results in rheumatic polyarthritis. B. Therapeutic results in ulcerative colitis. C. Toxic manifestations in treatment with sulfanilamide preparation. Acta Med Scand. 1942;110:557–90.
2. Azad Khan AK, Piris J, Truelove SC. An experiment to determine the active therapeutic moiety of sulphasalazine. Lancet. 1977;2:892–5.
3. Van Hees PAM, Bakker JH, Van Tongeren JHM. Effect of sulphapyridine, 5-aminosalicylic acid, and placebo in patients with idiopathic proctitis: A study to determine the active therapeutic moiety of sulphasalazine. Gut. 1980;21:632–5.
4. Greenfield SM, Punchard NA, Teare JP, Thompson RPH. Review article: The mode of action of the aminosalicylates in inflammatory bowel disease. Aliment Pharmacol Ther. 1993;7:369–83.

5. Roberts WG, Simon TJ, Berlin RG *et al*. Leukotrienes in ulcerative colitis: Results of a multi-center trial of a leukotriene biosynthesis inhibitor, MK-591. Gastroenterology. 1997;112:725–32.

6. Baron JH, Connell AM, Lennard-Jones JE, Jones FA. Sulphasalazine and salicylazosulphadimi-dine in ulcerative colitis. Lancet. 1962;1:1094–6.

7. Lennard-Jones JE, Longmore AJ, Newell AC, Wilson CWE, Avery Jones F. An assessment of prednisone, salazyopyrin, and topical hydrocortisone hemisuccinate used as out-patient treatment for ulcerative colitis. Gut. 1960;1:217–22.

8. Sutherland LR, Roth DE, Beck PL. Alternatives to sulfasalazine: A meta-analysis of 5-ASA in the treatment of ulcerative colitis. Inflamm Bowel Dis. 1997;3:65–78.

9. Marshall JK, Irvine EJ. Rectal aminosalicylate therapy for distal ulcerative colitis: a meta-analysis. Aliment Pharmacol Ther. 1995;9:293–300.

10. Marshall JK, Irvine EJ. Rectal corticosteroids versus alternative treatments in ulcerative colitis: a meta-analysis. Gut. 1997;40:775–81.

11. Safdi M, DeMicco M, Sninsky CA *et al*. A double-blind comparison of oral versus rectal mesalamine versus combination therapy in the treatment of distal ulcerative colitis. Am J Gastroenterol. 1997;92:1867–71.

12. Ginsberg AL, Davis ND, Nochomovitz LE. Placebo-controlled trial of ulcerative colitis with oral 4-aminosalicylic acid. Gastroenterology. 1992;102:448–52.

13. Ginsberg AL, Beck LS, McIntosh TM, Nochomovitz LE. Treatment of left-sided ulcerative colitis with 4-aminosalicylic acid enemas. Ann Intern Med. 1988;108:195–9.

14. Edwards F, Truelove SC. The course and prognosis of ulcerative colitis. 1. Short-term prognosis. Gut. 1963;4:299–308.

15. Meyers S, Janowitz HD. The 'natural history' of ulcerative colitis: an analysis of the placebo response. J Clin Gastroenterol. 1989;11(1):33–7.

16. Misiewicz JJ, Lennard-Jones JE, Connell AM, Baron JH, Jones FA. Controlled trial of sul-phasalazine in maintenance therapy for ulcerative colitis. Lancet. 1965;1:185–8.

17. Azad Khan AK, Piris J, Truelove SC, Howes DT. An optimum dose of sulphasalazine for maintenance treatment in ulcerative colitis. Gut. 1980;21:232–40.

18. Dissanayake AS, Truelove SC. A controlled therapeutic trial of long-term maintenance treatment of ulcerative colitis with sulphasalazine (Salazopyrin). Gut. 1973;14:923–6.

19. Biddle WL, Miner PB Jr. Long-term use of mesalamine enemas to induce remission in ulcerative colitis. Gastroenterology. 1990;99:113–18.

20. Miner PB Jr, Daly R, Nester T *et al*. The effect of varying dose intervals of mesalamine enemas on the prevention of relapse in distal ulcerative colitis. [Abstract]. Gastroenterology. 1994;106:A736.

21. D'Albasio G, Pacini F, Camarri E *et al*. Combined therapy with 5-aminosalicylic acid tablets and enemas for maintaining remission in ulcerative colitis: A randomized, double-blind study. Am J Gastroenterol. 1997;92:1143–7.

22. Hawthorne AB, Logan RFA, Hawkey CJ *et al*. Randomised controlled trial of azathioprine withdrawal in ulcerative colitis. Br Med J. 1992;305:20–2.

23. Gilat T, Leichtman G, Delpre G, Eshchar J, Bar Meir S, Fireman Z. A comparison of metronidazole and sulfasalazine in the maintenance of remission in patients with ulcerative colitis. J Clin Gastroenterol. 1989;11:392–5.

24. Dickinson RJ, King A, Wight DGD, Hunter JO, Neale G. Is continuous sulfasalazine necessary in the management of patients with ulcerative colitis? Results of a preliminary study. Dis Colon Rectum. 1985;28:929–30.

25. Summers RW, Switz DM, Sessions JT Jr *et al*. National Cooperative Crohn's Disease Study: Results of drug treatment. Gastroenterology. 1979;77:847–69.

26. Malchow H, Ewe K, Brandes JW *et al*. European Cooperative Crohn's Disease Study (ECCDS): Results of drug treatment. Gastroenterology. 1984;86:249–66.

27. Mahida YR, Jewell DP. Slow-release 5-amino-salicylic acid (Pentasa) for the treatment of active Crohn's disease. Digestion. 1990;45:88–92.

28. Rasmussen SN, Lauritsen K, Tage-Jensen U *et al*. 5-Aminosalicylic acid in the treatment of Crohn's disease. A 16 week double-blind, placebo-controlled, multicenter study with Pentasa. Scand J Gastroenterol. 1987;22:877–83.

29. Singleton JW, Hanauer SB, Gitnick GL *et al*., Pentasa Crohn's Disease Study Group. Mesalamine capsules for the treatment of active Crohn's disease: Results of a 16-week trial. Gastroenterology. 1993;104:1293–301.

30. Singleton J. Second trial of mesalamine therapy in the treatment of active Crohn's disease. Gastroenterology. 1994;107:632–3.
31. Tremaine WJ, Schroeder KW, Harrison JM, Zinsmeister AR. A randomized, double-blind, placebo-controlled trial of the oral mesalamine (5-ASA) preparation, Asacol, in the treatment of symptomatic Crohn's colitis and ileocolitis. J Clin Gastroenterol. 1994;19:278–82.
32. Wright JP, Jewell DP, Modigliani R, Malchow H, International Organization for the Study of Inflammatory Bowel Disease (IOIBD). A randomized, double-blind, placebo-controlled trial of olsalazine for active Crohn's disease. Inflamm Bowel Dis. 1995;1:241–6.
33. Martin F, Sutherland LR, Beck IT et al. Oral 5-ASA versus prednisone in short term treatment of Crohn's disease: A multicentre controlled trial. Can J Gastroenterol. 1990:4:452–7.
34. Thomsen OO, Cortot A, Jewell D et al. Budesonide CTR is more effective than mesalazine in active Crohn's disease. A 16 week, international randomized controlled trial. [Abstract]. Gastroenterology. 1997;112:A1104.
35. Singleton JW, Summers RW, Kern F et al. A trial of sulfasalazine as adjunctive therapy in Crohn's disease. Gastroenterology. 1979;77:887–97.
36. Rijk MC, Van Hogezand RA, Van Lier HJJ, Van Tongeren JHM. Sulphasalazine and prednisone compared with sulphasalazine for treating active Crohn's disease. Ann Intern Med. 1991;114:445–50.
37. Modigliani R, Colombel JF, Dupas JL et al. Mesalamine in Crohn's disease with steroid-induced remission: Effect on steroid withdrawal and remission maintenance. Gastroenterology. 1996;110:688–93.
38. Sutherland LR. Editorial: 5-aminosalicylates for prevention of recurrence in patients with Crohn's disease: Time for a reappraisal? J Clin Gastroenterol. 1991;13:5–7.
39. Ewe K, Herfarth C, Malchow H, Jesdinsky JH. Postoperative recurrence of Crohn's disease in relation to radicality of operation and sulfasalazine prophylaxis: A multicentre trial. Digestion. 1989;42:224–32.
40. Steinhart AH, Hemphill DJ, Greenberg GR. Sulfasalazine and mesalazine for the maintenance therapy of Crohn's disease: A meta-analysis. Am J Gastroenterol. 1994;89:2116–24.
41. Messori A, Rampazzo R. Meta-analysis on the maintenance of remission in Crohn's disease. J Clin Gastroenterol. 1993;17:178–9.
42. Camma C, Giunta M, Roselli M, Cottone M. Mesalamine in the maintenance treatment of Crohn's disease: A meta-analysis adjusted for confounding. Gastroenterology. 1997;113:1465–73.
43. Caprilli R, Andreoli A, Capurso L et al. Oral mesalazine (5-aminosalicylic acid: Asacol) for the prevention of post-operative recurrence of Crohn's disease. Aliment Pharmacol Ther. 1994;8:35–43.
44. Schulz KF, Chalmers I, Hayes RJ, Altman DG. Empirical evidence of bias. Dimensions of methodological quality associated with estimates of treatment effects in controlled trials. JAMA. 1995;273:408–12.
45. Lochs H, Mayer M, Fleig WE et al. Prophylaxis of postoperative relapse in Crohn's disease with mesalazine (Pentasa) in comparison to placebo. [Abstract]. Gastroenterology. 1997;112:A1027.
46. Goerg KJ, Wanitschke R, Gabbert H, Breiling J, Franke M, Meyer zum Buschenfelde KH. Azodisalicylate (azodisal sodium) causes intestinal secretion. Digestion. 1987;37:79–87.

20
How to use steroids in inflammatory bowel disease

R. LÖFBERG

SUMMARY

Glucocorticosteroids (GCS) are the mainstay of primary medical treatment in moderate and severe attacks of Crohn's disease (CD) and ulcerative colitis (UC). Overall remission/response rate varies between 60 and 90% depending on type, site and extent of disease. However, flare-up of symptoms may occur when GCS are tapered, or after treatment cessation. A substantial proportion of patients may eventually become GCS dependent. Moreover, 10–40% of IBD patients respond poorly or not at all to GCS.

The beneficial therapeutic effects of conventional GCS may be offset by troublesome dose-related systemic side-effects. Long-term treatment should be avoided due to the risk of hazardous and irreversible complications, such as osteoporosis.

A daily dose of 40–60 mg of oral prednisolone (or equivalent) in a tapered regimen over 2–3 months induces symptomatic remission in 60–80% of patients with active Crohn's disease. The simultaneous introduction of azathioprine may increase the remission rate and facilitate steroid weaning. Antibiotic cover should be considered in certain situations (e.g. abdominal mass). Intravenous GCS therapy is often used in severe attacks of colorectal CD.

Budesonide, a GCS with high topical potency, extensive hepatic inactivation and hence low systemic availability when administered to the bowel, has become an alternative to conventional steroids in ileocaecal CD. Oral slow-release formulations of budesonide (Entocort and Budenofalk) have recently been approved in several European countries for active disease. An 8-week course with 9 mg daily is as efficacious and as rapid for induction of symptomatic remission as a standard 40 mg prednisolone regimen. However, budesonide induces less suppression of endogenous cortisol and reduces frequency and intensity of GCS-related side-effects. Oral budesonide is superior to treatment with 4 g/day of oral 5-ASA (Pentasa) in active ileal/ileocaecal CD.

If disease extent in active ulcerative colitis goes proximally beyond the splenic flexure, early introduction of systemic/oral GCS should be considered, even in mild attacks. Optimal daily dose of oral GCS for treatment of active UC ranges from 30–60 mg prednisolone (or equivalent) depending on severity and extent of disease. Intravenous GCS are used in severe/fulminant attacks of UC, shifting to the oral route when the patient starts to recover. Systemic GCS therapy in severe attacks is usually complemented with rectal GCS (or 5-ASA) enemas and the introduction also of oral 5-ASA. Prolonged high-dose GCS treatment in severe attacks should be avoided (consider colectomy if there is poor response/deterioration after 5–7 days). When a response is evident, the dose of GCS is gradually tapered (e.g. prednisolone: 5–10 mg reduction every 7–14 days).

GCS are generally not thought to have relapse-prevention properties in IBD, although certain subgroups may benefit from prolonged treatment. GCS-attained symptomatic remission in ileocolonic CD may be extended by using oral prednisolone or budesonide.

WHY SHOULD GLUCOCORTICOSTEROIDS BE USED IN IBD?

GCS remain one of the mainstays of medical treatment in active inflammatory bowel disease (IBD). The efficacy of orally given cortisone in moderate and severe attacks of ulcerative colitis (UC) was established in 1955[1] and was followed by studies using i.v. preparations[2]. GCS induce 60–90% remission in active UC, depending on extent and severity of an acute attack[1-3]. Treatment with GCS in enema form was subsequently introduced for distal UC and proctitis[4,5]. GCS was later also established in the management of Crohn's disease (CD)[6,7], inducing symptomatic improvement in the great majority of cases.

The anti-inflammatory effects of GCS in active IBD are unsurpassed by any other type of drug, and a rapid and substantial clinical response is usually seen within a few days following treatment initiation. GCS exert their actions by binding to the intracellular GCS receptor which is uniformly distributed in all types of human cells. Activation of the receptor will evoke a number of responses and effects, including inhibition of the production and action of certain key inflammatory cytokines[8-10]. Besides having very potent and broad anti-inflammatory actions, conventional GCS carry the advantages of being inexpensive and displaying well-known, and generally rather mild, toxicity problems in the short-term perspective[11]. However, long-term treatment, using e.g. oral prednisolone in doses higher than 7.5–10 mg daily for more than six months, is precluded by the risk of hazardous and sometimes irreversible complications, such as osteoporosis, osteonecrosis, cataract and diabetes mellitus[9-11]. Impact on the hypothalamic– pituitary–adrenal (HPA) function is another issue of concern. The positive effects notwithstanding, 20–30% of patients with UC or CD still respond poorly, or not at all, to GCS treatment[1-3,6-8,12]. The reasons for GCS refractority are incompletely understood, but different regulatory mechanisms involving GCS receptor expression and function are probably of fundamental importance.

WHEN IS GCS THE FIRST-LINE OPTION IN THE TREATMENT OF IBD?

Steroids should always be used as the first-line treatment for moderate and severe attacks of UC[1–3,9,10] and should also be considered as a treatment option in mild attacks if the extent of disease goes beyond the splenic flexure. GCS are also drugs of choice for moderately severe or severe attacks of ileocolonic CD[6,7,10], particularly if systemic symptoms, including fever, general malaise, anorexia and weight loss, are present. However, care should be taken when concomitant complications, such as an abdominal mass, fistula or abscess, are present. GCS should then only be given with great caution and preferably under antibiotic cover, as the risk of a septic or even fatal complication is substantial[7].

WHAT DOSE AND TYPE OF GCS SHOULD BE USED?

One of the first randomized controlled trials (RCT) in clinical medicine was carried out to establish cortisone as an efficacious treatment for moderate and severe attacks of UC in comparison with placebo[1]. Several studies have since confirmed the original results and shown that a standard regimen of 40 mg of prednisolone (or equivalent) given orally is the optimal compromise between efficacy and side-effects[13,14]. Intravenous GCS are used in severe/fulminant attacks of UC, shifting to the oral route when the patient starts to recover. Systemic GCS therapy in severe attacks is usually complemented with rectal GCS (or 5-ASA) enemas and also the subsequent introduction of oral 5-ASA or sulphasalazine. Prolonged high-dose GCS treatment in severe attacks should be avoided (consider colectomy if there is poor response/deterioration after 5–7 days of treatment). Following a clinical response and endoscopic healing/improvement, the daily GCS dose is gradually tapered by 5–10 mg per 7–14 days depending on severity of the attack in order to avoid the potential side-effects of GCS which occur during longer-term usage. A GCS course will normally last for two to three months. Overall remission rates in UC range from 50–90% depending on the extent and severity of disease[1–3].

The use of GCS in active CD has been addressed in two advanced RCTs in the USA and in Europe[6,7], demonstrating that prednisone at an initial dose of around 0.5 mg per kg body weight (or 6-methylprednisolone in an equipotent dose) is effective in inducing symptomatic remission in 60–80% of treated patients over a four-month period. Even higher remission rates, approaching 90%, have been reported from uncontrolled studies[15]. However, complete endoscopic healing is only achieved in around one third of patients, underlining that the effects of GCS in CD are mainly symptomatic[15].

TOPICALLY ACTIVE GCS FOR IBD

Recent development of GCS has resulted in compounds with 100–200 times higher affinity for the GCS receptor than hydrocortisone, coupled with a high rate of hepatic biotransformation. These new compounds have primarily been developed for asthma therapy. However, efforts to develop enhanced GCS for IBD therapy have also been made, using a topical mode of delivery to the gut, thereby causing no, or only limited, systemic side-effects[9,16]. The new highly potent non-halogenated 17-α substituted GCS budesonide has a very high receptor affinity and thus exerts potent GCS actions when given locally. The drug has less impact on the HPA-axis than beclomethasone dipropionate when used as inhalation treatment in the airways[17], and significantly less impairment on bone turn-over compared with conventional GCS treatment[18]. Due to its relatively high water solubility, budesonide is readily dissolved, and thus transport to the bowel wall is facilitated. Lipophilic properties ensure a high tissue uptake resulting in high concentrations and high activity in the target tissues when the drug is applied topically. Furthermore, budesonide remains within the mucosa for a longer period of time compared with prednisolone[19]. The rapid biotransformation in the liver via the cytochrome P450 CYP3A4 enzymes, causing very limited systemic impact, makes budesonide ideally suited for IBD treatment. Its topical selectivity for the bowel mucosa has been demonstrated in animal studies[20] and, given as an enema, in several clinical trials in active distal ulcerative colitis and proctitis[21–26].

A refined time- and pH-dependent release system for oral delivery of budesonide to more proximally affected IBD segments of the bowel has been devised by Astra Draco AB (Sweden), using mm-sized enteric-coated (Eudragit L) pellets with a rate-limiting polymer containing the active drug[27]. This preparation (Entocort) delivers around 70% of the given drug to the distal ileum and the caecum and is intended primarily for ileocaecal CD. A similar resin (Eudragit L) dissolving at pH values >6.0 has been used for another oral budesonide formulation (Budenofalk) from Falk Gmbh (Germany)[28].

A daily dose of 9 mg budesonide in any of the two oral formulations has been found to be optimal for the treatment of active ilocaecal CD in several large RCT[29–34], and has compared favourably with a standard regimen of 40 mg prednisolone/prednisone given in a tapered fashion over 8–10 weeks[30–33]. Remission rates for budesonide, assessed as a Crohn's disease activity index (CDAI) score <150, have varied between 52 and 69% (Table 1).

A 9-mg daily dose of budesonide creates significantly less suppression of endogenous plasma cortisol production[30–33] compared with prednisolone and, moreover, a 30–50% reduction in GCS-related side-effects. In a Canadian dose-ranging study, a 9-mg dose of budesonide caused GCS-related side-effects to the same extent as placebo[29]. Within the frame of that study, it was also demonstrated that patients treated with 9 mg budesonide experienced the greatest improvement in quality of life (IBD-Q) score. This finding was recently reproduced in a large European comparative study demonstrating the superiority of 9 mg budesonide vs. 4 g 5-aminosalicylic acid (Pentasa) in a 16-week trial, showing also a maximal remission rate for budesonide approaching 70%[34].

A German multicentre double-blind RCT evaluating budesonide in the Budenofalk formulation found the drug to be of benefit for the purpose of replacing prednisolone in GCS-dependent patients[35].

In an oral formulation with a retarded release profile, 10 mg budesonide was found to have similar effects on endoscopic healing in active extensive and left-sided UC to those of standard 40 mg prednisolone therapy during a 9-week

Table 1 Results from six independent randomized controlled clinical trials assessing the efficacy of the topical glucocorticosteroid budesonide given in oral formulations vs. placebo or active control therapy (prednisolone/prednisone or 5-ASA) for the treatment of active ileal or ileocaecal/ileocolonic Crohn's disease. Remission rates expressed as maximal percentage of patients achieving symptomatic remission (defined as Crohn's disease activity index score <150) after eight weeks of treatment are shown

Study (reference)	No. of patients	Treatment/dosage	8-week remission rate	p value	Remarks
Greenberg et al. 1994[29]	67	Budesonide 1.5 mg bid	33%	0.12	Entocort
	61	Budesonide 4.5 mg bid	51%	<0.001	
	64	Budesonide 7.5 mg bid	43%	0.009	
	66	Placebo	20%		
Rutgeerts et al. 1994[30]	88	Budesonide 9 mg om	52%	0.12	Entocort
	88	Prednisolone 40 mg om	65%		
Gross et al. 1996[31]	34	Budesonide 3 mg tid	56%	0.24	Budenofalk
	33	m-Prednisolone 48 mg om	73%		
Campieri et al. 1997[32]	58	Budesonide 9 mg om	60%		Entocort
	61	Budesonide 4.5 mg bid	42%	0.062	
	58	Prednisolone 40 mg om	60%		
Thomsen et al. 1998[34]	93	Budesonide 9 mg om	69%	<0.01	Entocort
	89	Mesalamine 2 g bid	45%		Pentasa
Bar-Meir et al. 1998[33]	100	Budesonide 9 mg/d	56%	NS	Budenofalk
	101	Prednisone 40 mg om	55%		

course, but without causing appreciable suppression of endogenous cortisol levels[36].

GCS IN COMBINATION WITH OTHER DRUGS FOR IBD

In the European Cooperative CD Study[7], the combined therapy of prednisolone and sulphasalazine was found to be of benefit for previously untreated patients and for those with colonic disease. 5-ASA in the form of Pentasa may be useful in the weaning of steroid treatment in certain subgroups with CD[37]. A synergistic effect has also been demonstrated for the combination of beclomethasone and 5-ASA enemas in active distal UC, as compared with treatment with either drug alone[38]. The addition of azathioprine to standard prednisolone therapy in active CD has improved time-to-remission and overall remission rates[39], and a recent controlled study indicated that azathioprine in combination with oral budesonide may be of value in delaying the time to development of significant restenosis after dilatation therapy in colorectal CD[40].

IS THERE A ROLE FOR GCS IN MAINTENANCE?

Conventional GCS have previously been evaluated at lower doses for long-term treatment to prevent exacerbations of Crohn's disease. The US

National Cooperative Crohn's Disease Study[6] reported no superiority of prednisone compared with placebo in this respect, and various other attempts to prolong the steroid-tapering phase have failed to demonstrate any significant long-term benefit in CD[41,42]. However, in the European Cooperative CD Study[7], a subgroup of patients who responded favourably to initial 6-methylprednisolone treatment, displayed a lower relapse rate during continued treatment with a decreased dose (8 mg/day). In children, alternate-day GCS dosing may prevent deleterious effects on growth, but such regimens have not been adequately investigated in adults. In clinical practice, concerns about long-term toxicity have precluded the use of conventional GCS, even at low doses, for the purpose of maintaining remission in CD as well as in UC.

As proper maintenance treatment in CD is lacking (except for the use of azathioprine or 6-mercaptopurine), the ability to prolong the time in remission using a GCS, while causing neither GCS side-effects nor HPA-axis impairment, is an important clinical goal.

A pooled analysis of three similarly designed, placebo-controlled studies, evaluating 6 or 3 mg budesonide daily (Entocort preparation) as maintenance therapy for up to one year in patients with ileocaecal CD and GCS-attained remission, was recently presented[43]. The analysis combined the results from two separate maintenance studies, previously described in detail[44,45], with the results from a study which was a continuation of the trial performed by Campieri *et al.*[32], and included a total of 270 patients. Patients treated with 6 mg of budesonide had a significantly longer median time to relapse (CDAI score >150) or discontinuation of treatment compared with the 3-mg and placebo groups (263 vs. 170 vs. 154 days, respectively, $p = 0.03$), although there were no remaining differences after one year. GCS-related side-effects were mild and did not differ between the budesonide and placebo groups.

Another RCT comprising 179 CD patients with GCS-induced remission failed to show superiority in relapse prevention properties of 3 mg daily budesonide (Budenofalk) over placebo over a one year period.[46]

Abundant data from several large studies with oral budesonide indicate a benign toxicity profile when it comes to the systemic impact of the drug[47], but further long-term experience is needed before the role of topical GCS in general and of budesonide in particular for the treatment of IBD can be fully settled. More studies addressing combination therapy (e.g. antibiotics and immunosuppressives) are in progress. Enhanced GCS with even higher potency and improved delivery systems, to the proximal colon in particular, are likely developments for the future.

References

1. Truelove SC, Witts LJ. Cortisone in ulcerative colitis. Final report on a therapeutic trial. BMJ. 1955;2:1041–8.
2. Truelove SC, Jewell DP. Intensive intravenous regimen for severe attacks of ulcerative colitis. Lancet. 1974;1:1067–70.
3. Järnerot G, Rolny P, Sandberg-Getzen H. Intensive intravenous treatment of ulcerative colitis. Gastroenterology. 1985;9:1005–13.
4. Truelove SC. Treatment of ulcerative colitis with local hydrocortisone. BMJ. 1956;2:1267–72.

5. Matts SGF. Intrarectal treatment of 100 cases of ulcerative colitis with prednisolone 21-phosphate retention enemata. BMJ. 1961;1:165–8.
6. Summers RW, Switz DM, Sessions JT Jr *et al.* National Cooperative Crohn's Disease Study. Gastroenterology. 1979;77:847–69.
7. Malchow H, Ewe K, Brandes JW *et al.* European Cooperative Crohn's Disease Study (ECCDS): results of drug treatment. Gastroenterology. 1984;86:249–66.
8. Routes J, Claman HN. Corticosteroids in inflammatory bowel disease. J Clin Gastroenterol. 1987;9:529–35.
9. Löfberg R. New steroids for inflammatory bowel disease. Inflam Bowel Dis. 1995;1:135–41.
10. Hanauer SB. Inflammatory bowel disease. Drug therapy. N Engl J Med. 1996;334:841–8.
11. Hanauer SB, Stathopoulos G. Risk–benefit assessment of drugs used in the treatment of inflammatory bowel diseases. Drug Safety. 1991;6:192–219.
12. Munkholm P, Langholz E, Davidsen M, Binder V. Frequency of glucocorticoid resistance and dependency in Crohn's disease. Gut. 1994;35:360–2.
13. Baron JH, Connel AM, Kanaghinis TG *et al.* Outpatient treatment of ulcerative colitis. BMJ. 1967;2:441–3.
14. Powell-Tuck J, Brown RL, Lennard-Jones JE. A comparison of oral prednisolone given as single or multiple doses for active proctocolitis. Scand J Gastroenterol. 1978;13:833–7.
15. Modigliani R, Mary Y, Simon JF *et al.* Clinical, biological and endoscopic picture of attacks of Crohn's disease: evolution on prednisolone. Gastroenterology. 1990;98:811–18.
16. Brattsand R. Overview of the newer glucocorticoid preparations for IBD. Can J Gastroenterol. 1990;4:407–14.
17. Brattsand R. Concepts of topical steroid therapy. Res Clin For. 1996;18:57–65.
18. Brogden RN, McTavish D. Budesonide. An updated review of its pharmacological properties and therapeutic efficacy in asthma and rhinitis. Drugs. 1992;44:375–407.
19. Hodsman AB, Toogood JH, Jennings BH, Fraker LJ, Baskerville JC. Differential effects of inhaled budesonide and oral prednisolone and serum osteocalcin. J Clin Endocrinol Metab. 1991;72:530–40.
20. Fabia R, Ar'Rajab A, Willén R, Brattsand R, Erlansson M, Svensjö E. Topical anticolitic efficacy and selectivity of the glucocorticoid budesonide in a new model of acetic acid induced acute colitis in the rat. Aliment Pharmacol Ther. 1994;8:433–46.
21. Danielsson Å, Hellers G, Lyrenäs E *et al.* A controlled randomized trial of budesonide versus prednisolone retention enemas in active ulcerative colitis. Scand J Gastroenterol. 1987;22:987–92.
22. Danielsson Å, Löfberg R, Persson T *et al.* A steroid enema, budesonide, lacking systemic effects for the treatment of distal ulcerative colitis or proctitis. Scand J Gastroenterol. 1992;27:9–12.
23. Löfberg R, Østergaard-Thomsen O, Langholz E *et al.* A comparative study of budesonide versus prednisolone retention enema in active distal ulcerative colitis. A Scandinavian multicenter study. Aliment Pharmacol Ther. 1994;8:623–9.
24. Bianchi Porro G, Prantera C, Campieri M *et al.* Comparative trial of methylprednisolone and budesonide enema in active distal ulcerative colitis. Eur J Gastroenterol Hepatol. 1994;6:125–30.
25. Hanauer S, Robinson M. A dose ranging study. Budesonide enema for the treatment of active distal ulcerative colitis and pruritus. Gastroenterology. 1998;115:525–32.
26. Lemann M, Rutgeerts P, van Heuverzwijn R *et al.* Comparison of budesonide enema and 5-ASA enema in the treatment of active distal ulcerative colitis. Aliment Pharmacol Ther. 1995;9:557–62.
27. Löfberg R. Oral formulation of budesonide for IBD. Res Clin For. 1993;15:91–6.
28. Moellmann HW, Hochhaus G, Tromm A *et al.* Pharmacokinetics and evaluation of systemic side effects of budesonide after oral administration of modified release capsules in healthy volunteers and patients with Crohn's disease. Gastroenterology. 1996;110:A972.
29. Greenberg G, Feagan B, Martin F *et al.* Oral budesonide for the treatment of active Crohn's disease. N Engl J Med. 1994;331:836–41.
30. Rutgeerts P, Löfberg R, Malchow H *et al.* A comparison of budesonide with prednisolone for active Crohn's disease. N Engl J Med. 1994;331:842–5.
31. Gross V, Andus T, Caesar I *et al.* and the German/Austrian Budesonide Study Group. Oral pH-modified release budesonide versus 6-methylprednisolone in active Crohn's disease. Eur J Gastroenterol Hepatol. 1996;8:905–9.
32. Campieri M, Ferguson A, Doe W *et al.* Oral budesonide is as effective as prednisolone in active Crohn's disease. Gut. 1997;41:209–14.

33. Bar-Meir S, Chowers Y, Lavy A *et al.* Budesonide versus prednisone in the treatment of active Crohn's disease. Gastroenterology. 1998;115:835–40.
34. Thomsen OO, Cortot A, Jewell DP *et al.* A comparison of budesonide and mesalamine for active Crohn's disease. A 16 week, international, randomized, double blind, multicentre trial. N Engl J Med. 1998;339:370–4.
35. Gross V, Caesar I, Andus T *et al.* and the German/Austrian Budesonide Study Group. Replacement of systemic steroids by oral budesonide in patients with post-active or chronic Crohn's ileocolitis – a dose-finding study. Gastroenterology. 1997;112:A987.
36. Löfberg R, Danielsson Å, Suhr O *et al.* Oral versus prednisolone in patients with active extensive and left-sided ulcerative colitis. Gastroenterology. 1996;110:1713–18.
37. Modigliani R, Colombel JF, Dupas JL. Mesalamine in Crohn's disease with steroid-induced remission: Effect on steroid withdrawal and remission maintenance. Gastroenterology. 1996;110:688–93.
38. Mulder CJJ, Fockens P, Meijer JWR, van der Heide H, Wiltink EHH, Tytgat GNJ. Beclomethasone dipropionate (3 mg) versus 5-aminosalicylic acid (2 g) versus the combination of both (3 mg/2 g) as retention enemas in active ulcerative proctitis. Eur J Gastroenterol Hepatol. 1996;8:549–53.
39. Ewe K, Press AG, Singe CC *et al.* Azathioprine combined with prednisolone or monotherapy with prednisolone in active Crohn's disease. Gastroenterology. 1993;105:367–72.
40. Raedler A, Peters I, Schreiber S. Treatment with azathioprin and budesonide prevents reoccurrence of ileocolonic stenoses after endoscopic dilatation in Crohn's disease. Gastroenterology. 1997;112:A1067.
41. Landi B, N'guyen Anh T, Cortot A *et al.* Endoscopic monitoring of Crohn's disease treatment. A prospective, randomized clinical trial. Gastroenterology. 1992;102:1647–53.
42. Brignola C, De Simone G, Belloli C *et al.* Steroid treatment in active Crohn's disease. A comparison between two regimens of different duration. Aliment Pharmacol Ther. 1994;8:465–8.
43. Feagan B, Greenberg G, Löfberg R, Ferguson A, Persson T. Budesonide controlled ileal release prolongs remission in Crohn's disease. A pooled analysis. Gastroenterology. 1997;112:A970.
44. Löfberg R, Rutgeerts P, Malchow H *et al.* Budesonide prolongs time to relapse in ileal and ileocaecal Crohn's disease. A placebo controlled one year study. Gut. 1996;39:82–6.
45. Greenberg G, Feagan B, Martin F *et al.* and the Canadian Inflammatory Bowel Disease Study Group. Oral budesonide as maintenance treatment for Crohn's disease: A placebo-controlled dose-ranging study. Gastroenterology. 1996;110:45–51.
46. Gross V, Andus T, Ecker KW *et al.* Low dose oral pH modified release budesonide for maintenance of steroid induced remission in Crohn's disease. Gut. 1998;42:493–6.
47. Østergaard-Thomsen O. Safety overview of budesonide in inflammatory bowel disease. Res Clin For. 1996;18:91–100.

21
Immunosuppression therapy in ulcerative colitis and Crohn's disease

D. H. PRESENT

I am quite pleased to see that immunosuppression therapy is now listed as a standard therapy in inflammatory bowel disease. It was not so many years ago that physicians waited for long periods of time before initiating immunomodulatory drugs in the treatment of both Crohn's disease and ulcerative colitis.

Both of these disorders are clearly genetic in basis. They are triggered by a variety of environmental factors and the bowel initially suffers a direct autoimmune injury with subsequent enhancement and amplification mediated by cytokines in the immune system. In the instance of Crohn's disease, we have highly activated Th-1 cells, which induce excess γ-interferon, TNF-α, interleukin-2, etc., which perpetuate the intestinal mucosal inflammation. Common intestinal bacteria also play a role in inducing this unregulated T-cell response.

These agents should be called immunomodulatory, not immunosuppressive, since the latter phrase tends to frighten patients who believe that you will suppress their immune system, which will then put them at greater risk for infections. In fact, you should convince patients that these agents will bring their overactive immune system back toward normality and thereby decrease the overall inflammatory process.

6-MERCAPTOPURINE AND AZATHIOPRINE

The most frequently used immunomodulatory agents in the management of inflammatory bowel disease are 6-mercaptopurine (6-MP) and azathioprine. Azathioprine is a pro-drug in which approximately 85% converts to 6-mercaptopurine. This is facilitated by sulphydryl-containing compounds such as glutathione. 6-MP is then metabolized via three enzyme systems[1]. The first, thiopurine methyltransferase (TPMT) converts 6-MP to 6-methylmercaptopurine, which may or may not have some immunomodulatory activity. Xanthine oxidase converts 6-MP to its inactive metabolite, 6-thiouric acid. Finally, hypoxanthine phosphoribosyl transferase followed by thioinosinic acid converts 6-MP to its active metabolites. Of great interest is that TPMT has significant genetic variation in the population. A deficiency may result in higher levels of active thioguanine nucleotides whereas theoretically an excess level might result in inadequate levels, thereby diminishing clinical response.

Crohn's Disease

The initial uncontrolled data in the literature up until 1972 showed a 72% response in Crohn's disease[2]. This was followed by the National Cooperative Crohn's Disease Study[3], and, retrospectively, this study was a great drawback in that it discouraged physicians from using azathioprine. In this trial, patients were randomized to a single drug and all other therapies were withdrawn. As the disease worsened, they were considered failures and removed from the trial, which subsequently showed no statistical benefit for azathioprine compared with placebo. In fact, for the azathioprine arm, the mean final CDAI was approximately 152, whereas 150 by definition was needed to attain remission. The main reason for the lack of response is that the mean time it takes to respond to azathioprine is 3.1 months and the National Cooperative Crohn's Disease Study ended at 4 months. At 4 months, almost 20% of ultimate responders would have failed to show significant improvement. Subsequently, there have been many controlled trials performed, with the majority showing efficacy[4]. The trials that were unsuccessful used small numbers of patients and usually for a duration of 4 months or less. In contradistinction, the trials that showed efficacy ranged from 6 months to one year and included larger numbers of patients. The largest and longest controlled trial was the Mount Sinai 6-mercaptopurine Crohn's study[5] in which a response rate of 67% was obtained with 6-MP compared with 8% with placebo ($p = 0.0001$). Significant steroid sparing was noted in 70% of patients, compared with 35% who were taking placebo. Fistulae were shown to heal; however, the numbers were not large enough to give any statistical significance. The drug appeared to be most effective in colonic disease. A meta-analysis by Pearson *et al.*[4] concluded that azathioprine and 6-MP were both effective in treating active Crohn's disease and maintaining remission. Steroid sparing and fistula healing were also noted and the cumulative dose appeared to be important in predicting response.

As regards fistulae, 6-MP and azathioprine have been shown to be effective in closing gastrocolic fistulae and enterovesical fistulae[6].

In an important trial by Ewe and colleagues[7], azathioprine and prednisolone were compared with prednisolone alone in active Crohn's disease. The combination of drugs demonstrated a 76% response at one year compared with only 38% response at one year using steroids alone. A recent paediatric controlled trial has shown similar results[8] and this strongly suggests that 6-MP or azathioprine should be used early in the course of Crohn's disease.

Also, in uncontrolled data from Dr Korelitz and myself, we have shown that, if a patient stays on 6-MP after remission is induced, the relapse rate in the first year is only 5%. If the patient discontinues the drug, the relapse rate is approximately 70%. This has been confirmed in a controlled trial by O'Donoghue *et al.*[9] showing again only 5% relapse in the first year after having responded to azathioprine. If a patient does not respond to azathioprine or 6-MP in 4–6 months, it is strongly suggested that the dose should be raised and the patient made leukopenic. A recent abstract by Barbe *et al.*[10] has confirmed this experience in uncontrolled data.

It is frequently asked how long the drug should be maintained and, at present, there is no definitive answer. However, a retrospective study[11] has suggested that the maintenance effect lasts for only four years and the drug may be discontinued after that time. We await results of a controlled trial which is currently underway. In an attempt to speed up the time to response, a recent controlled trial has been completed in which azathioprine was administered intravenously over 36 h for active Crohn's disease. Uncontrolled data[12] had suggested a response within four weeks and the code has thus far not been broken on the controlled trial.

Ulcerative colitis

Although there are fewer controlled trials in ulcerative colitis, the early uncontrolled literature using 6-MP and azathioprine showed a response rate of close to 80%[2]. Three of four subsequent smaller controlled trials showed a positive response; however, there has been a large accumulation of uncontrolled data clearly indicating that these drugs are as effective in ulcerative colitis as in Crohn's disease. In a large uncontrolled series[13] of 105 patients who had failed to improve with both oral and rectal steroids as well as oral and rectal 5-ASA agents, complete clinical remission was observed in 65% with partial remission in another 24%. The longer patients were maintained on the drug, the more likely they were to enter a clinical remission. Relapse was subsequently noted in 34% of patients; however, in over half of these, the relapse was mild and could be restored without initiating oral steroids. In fact, 87% of the relapsing patients went into complete remission again by either raising the dose of 6-MP, raising the dose of 5-ASA or adding topical therapy. As with Crohn's disease, if the 6-MP was discontinued a relapse rate of over 80% was observed. A controlled trial by Hawthorne *et al.*[14] has confirmed the preventive effect of azathioprine. Our own personal experience indicates that 6-MP or azathioprine will prevent colectomy in 85–90% of chronically ill ulcerative colitis patients.

Toxicity has been recorded in many large series. Acute short-term toxicity is seen in about 8% of patients[15]. This includes pancreatitis in 3–4%; allergic reactions, including rash, fever and joint pain, in 2%; and marrow depression in 2%. The latter may be related to TPMT deficiency. Starting with lower doses, 50 mg daily, may help to avoid this complication. All these abnormalities reverse with discontinuation of the 6-MP or azathioprine. A large comprehensive study in the United Kingdom which looked at bone marrow depression noted two deaths in almost 750 patients[16]. However, the significant leukopenia was not predictable and I therefore do not see the need for frequent testing of white blood cell counts after the patient has been stable on the drug for one year.

In our initial trials, we saw one cerebral lymphoma in 400 patients[15], however, there have only been scattered reports since then and there is an extensive literature documenting an increase in lymphoma in both Crohn's disease and ulcerative colitis independent of 6-MP or azathioprine. Dr Greenstein at Mount Sinai noted nine lymphomas in over 2600 patients, none of whom had been treated with azathioprine or 6-MP[17]. Similar findings have been reported by Connell *et al.*[18], in which 755 patients receiving 6-MP or azathioprine showed no significant increase in colon cancer as well as no increased incidence of non-Hodgkin's lymphomas.

Recent studies presented in abstract form looking at pregnancy associated with 6-MP have shown that, when it is used before conception and during pregnancy, 6-MP is *not* associated with increased prematurity, spontaneous abortion, congenital abnormalities, neonatal or childhood infections or neoplasia[19].

Summary

In summary, 6-MP and azathioprine are the most effective and safest immunomodulatory therapies in both ulcerative colitis and Crohn's disease. They should be used earlier in the course, especially if a patient cannot be weaned from steroids within 3 months. If there is no response within 4–6 months, leukopenia should be induced. The drug is safe in pregnancy and there appears to be no long-term neoplastic risk.

Very recently, a placebo-controlled study has demonstrated that 6-MP is superior to both 5-ASA and placebo in preventing postoperative clinical, endoscopic and radiographic recurrence[20]. A single 50-mg 6-MP pill has shown efficacy, and, since compliance should be easily obtained, strong consideration must be given in the future to the use of this drug in postoperative Crohn's disease patients.

METHOTREXATE

The exact mechanism of action of methotrexate is unknown but it appears to have both anti-inflammatory and immunosuppressive activity.

Kozarek *et al.*'s initial study and long-term follow-up[21] is quite informative with regard to the use of methotrexate in both Crohn's disease and ulcerative colitis. In their initial open-label trial, patients who were entered had failed to improve with steroids and 5-ASA drugs and approximately one third had failed to respond to 6-MP/azathioprine. Methotrexate was administered intramuscularly at a dose of 25 mg weekly for a 3-month period and good clinical response was noted in 83% of Crohn's patients. Endoscopic remission was observed in 30% although steroids could be discontinued in only 50% of patients. In ulcerative colitis, there was a 70% clinical response, but only 30% could stop taking prednisone. Maintenance of remission was less impressive. Only 44% of Crohn's patients remained well after 69 weeks of observation and only 30% of ulcerative colitis patients remained well (which is not a significant improvement compared with the placebo response in controlled trials).

A subsequent double-blind placebo-controlled trial[22] showed that methotrexate was statistically more effective than placebo (39% vs. 19%). Patients in the study were stratified for high- and low-dose steroids and improvement was noted in the Crohn's Disease Activity Index, quality of life and serum orosomucoid concentrations. Drug-related toxicity was minor. Several other uncontrolled studies[23,24] have confirmed the short-term response, which ranges from 65% to

85%. However, the long-term response, once again, was 40% or less and steroid discontinuation was seen in only 50% of patients.

Although toxicities have been minor in the reported series, they are potentially significant, including liver fibrosis and cirrhosis, an allergic interstitial pneumonitis, pancytopenia and moderate GI upset, especially when the drug is administered orally. Methotrexate is contraindicated in pregnancy, where teratogenicity is noted. In my own personal series, 3% of patients have developed cirrhosis after two years of receiving methotrexate.

In summary, methotrexate is effective in two thirds to three quarters of patients when administered at a dose of 20–25 mg intramuscularly or subcutaneously. Complete steroid sparing is possible in less than 50% of patients and fistula response is noted in approximately one third of patients. The time-to-respond is 4–12 weeks and the long-term maintenance is poor, with relapse in the majority of cases within two years. One must conclude that methotrexate is effective in refractory Crohn's disease but is likely to be used as interim therapy and not as a first-line agent.

CYCLOSPORINE

Crohn's disease

Brynskov et al.[25] reported, in the *New England Journal of Medicine*, a statistically significant 59% response to oral cyclosporine compared with 34% in placebo patients. The dose used was 5–7.5 mg daily, the response was rapid, occurring within two weeks, and appeared to be greater if the patient was receiving concurrent steroids. Malabsorption of the drug was noted in over 25% of patients.

Since that time, there have been several placebo-controlled trials showing a lack of efficacy, although the dosage in these trials was lower than that used in the Brynskov study. In a large European multicentre trial[26], 182 patients received 5 mg/kg daily. Complete and partial remission were the same in both the placebo and cyclosporine groups at four months and twelve months. In a Canadian trial[27], maintenance of remission was also ineffective using the low dose of 5 mg/kg daily.

However, it must be noted that there is erratic absorption of cyclosporine, and inadequate blood levels of cyclosporine may be obtained in the presence of active enteritis, short bowel syndrome or malabsorption, as well as when diarrhoea and anaemia are present. For this reason, studies at Mount Sinai have suggested that the use of *intravenous* cyclosporine might be more effective in the therapy of active Crohn's disease. In an initial trial looking at fistulization[28], a dose of 4 mg/kg daily was administered intravenously to 16 patients. The response rate was 88%, of which half (44%) showed complete closure of fistula. The mean duration to response was 7.4 days and steroids could be discontinued in three quarters of the patients. The toxicity was minor. Another study by Hanauer and Smith[29] has confirmed this finding.

Finally, Lemann et al.[30] reported recently that they treated 34 patients with intravenous cyclosporine, and that it was effective in active Crohn's disease in approximately two thirds of patients. Long-term remission was maintained in only 48% of responders.

In summary, recent reports on the management of Crohn's disease with cyclosporine indicate that this drug is effective when administered intravenously, the response rate being somewhere between two thirds and three quarters of patients. However, it is not effective orally at low doses either for induction or maintenance of remission, and 6-MP/azathioprine must be substituted for maintenance. Cyclosporine should be continued at a high dose until the latter drugs have had time to become effective.

Ulcerative colitis

About 15% of all patients with ulcerative colitis will experience a severe attack, requiring hospitalization and intravenous steroids. During this course of steroids, approximately one third will require a colectomy and, if the patient fails to show significant improvement, another one third will undergo colectomy within the next year[31]. It has been recommended that a colectomy be performed sometime between 5 and 10 days if the patient fails to respond to intravenous steroids. In a protocol designed at Mount Sinai Medical Center, 4 mg kg^{-1} day^{-1} intravenous cyclosporine was administered to those patients who had not improved after 10 days of intravenous steroids. The uncontrolled study showed a response rate of 81% and the controlled trial[32] data confirmed this with a response rate of 82%. The mean time to respond was approximately six days. Long-term follow-up[33] has shown that 59% of patients have been able to discontinue both steroids and cyclosporine, and have clinical and endoscopic healing. It would have been expected that, with standard therapy, almost all of these patients would have required a colectomy. Furthermore, it has been shown that the administration of 6-MP to responders maintains remission in 77% of responding patients[34]. Cyclosporine has a significant toxicity profile, which includes renal dysfunction, hepatotoxicity, neurotoxicity and seizures, electrolyte abnormalities, including magnesium deficiency, and hypertension[35]. Multiple minor side-effects, such as gingival hyperplasia, hirsutism and paraesthesias have also been noted. Renal insufficiency is the major problem and the creatinine levels as well as the cyclosporine levels should be closely monitored. If the serum creatinine increases by 33%, the cyclosporine dosage should be decreased by 25–50%. Seizures can be avoided if the serum cholesterol is checked and the cyclosporine dose halved if the cholesterol level is markedly below normal prior to administration of cyclosporine.

Lymphomas have been shown to be increased in transplantations, but we do not advocate the long-term use of cyclosporine for ulcerative colitis, and it is unlikely that this complication will be observed if the drug is used for less than one year. There should be careful observation for superinfections, especially when cyclosporine is used in combination with steroids and/or 6-MP or azathioprine. It is our preference to use prophylaxis against pneumocystis for patients who are taking three immunomodulatory drugs.

There are many unanswered questions regarding the use of cyclosporine in active ulcerative colitis. Studies have suggested a dose as low as 2 mg kg^{-1} day^{-1} may be equally effective. A recent study of 20 patients[36] showed that the response rate to intravenous cyclosporine alone was as effective, in fact slightly better than, when steroids were given alone. This raises the question of whether, for an acute severe attack, the drug of choice should be cyclosporine rather than steroids. The possibility of renal toxicity has been noted and there is still uncertainty as to whether long-term renal toxicity will surface because of the higher doses of cyclosporine that are currently being advocated.

Summary

In summary, intravenous cyclosporine is effective with and without concurrent steroid therapy in ulcerative colitis. Intravenous cyclosporine is also effective in active Crohn's disease and refractory perianal disease. 6-MP/azathioprine must be added soon after or before initiation of cyclosporine in order to maintain response in these IBD patients.

OTHER TREATMENTS

As was noted earlier, there are significant immunopathogenic alterations in inflammatory bowel disease and this gives us several treatment options. The pro-inflammatory cytokines can be down-regulated with therapy or we can increase the inhibitory cytokines. Several newer agents have been tried in the management of inflammatory bowel disease. An ICAM-1 inhibitor called ISIS-2302[37] has shown efficacy in an early small placebo-controlled trial and multicentre trials are currently being conducted. Human interleukin 10[38] has been tried in chronic active Crohn's disease as well as mild to moderate ulcerative colitis. The results have shown some success but they are certainly not dramatic. It has been suggested that mycophenolate Mofetil[39] might be effective in chronic active Crohn's disease. A single study has shown that steroid-dependent patients respond as well as those receiving azathioprine. Longer term trials are required to look at maintenance of remission as well as toxicity with this agent.

The most effective new agent is the chimeric monoclonal antibody against TNF-α. Initial controlled trials[40] showed a statistically significant response in 65% of patients compared with 17% with placebo. Remission was obtained in 33% compared with 4% receiving placebo. A subsequent retreatment phase was carried out, in which responders were randomized at 12 weeks to receive infusions at 2-month intervals of either the active antibody against TNF-α or placebo. In those patients who received the active agent, the response continued, whereas, in the placebo patients, relapse gradually occurred. It should be noted, however, that many patients stayed well for 6–8 months after a single infusion of antibody against TNF-α.

A fistula study[41] has recently been completed in which infusions of antibody against TNF-α were given at weeks 0, 2 and 6. The primary endpoint was at least 50% closure of fistulae for at least two consecutive visits (which was a minimum of 4 weeks). Secondary endpoints included the closure of all fistulae and improvement of Crohn's Disease Activity Index. The results showed a 61.9% response to the primary endpoint compared with 29.9% with placebo. Complete closure of all fistulae was seen in 46% compared with 12.9% with placebo. It would appear that the monoclonal antibody against TNF is the first agent to demonstrate a statistically significant effect on the closure of Crohn's fistulae.

CONCLUSIONS

We are still in the earliest stages of using immunomodulatory agents in the management of both ulcerative colitis and Crohn's disease. I predict that, in the next five years, newer immunomodulatory agents will become available, allowing us to use less and less steroids, and that steroids will become a third-line agent in the management of Crohn's disease.

References

1. Sandborn WJ. A review of immune modifier therapy for inflammatory bowel disease: azathioprine, 6-mercaptopurine, cyclosporine and methotrexate. Am J Gastroenterol. 1996;91:423–33.
2. Present DH. 6-Mercaptopurine and other immunosuppresive agents in the treatment of Crohn's disease and ulcerative colitis. Gastroenterol Clin N Am. 1989;18:57–71.
3. Summers RW, Switz DM, Sessions JT et al. National Cooperative Crohn's Disease Study. Results of drug treatment. Gastroenterology. 1979;77:847–69.
4. Pearson DC, May GR, Fick GH et al. Azathioprine and 6-mercaptopurine in Crohn's disease. A meta-analysis. Ann Intern Med. 1995;122:132–42.
5. Present DH, Korelitz BI, Wisch N et al. Treatment of Crohn's disease with 6-mercaptopurine in a long term, randomized, double blind study. N Engl J Med. 1980;302:981–7.
6. Korelitz BI, Present DH. The favorable effects of 6-mercaptopurine in the fistula of Crohn's disease. Dig Dis Sci. 1985;30:58–64.
7. Ewe K, Presse AG, Singe CC et al. Azathioprine combined with prednisolone or monotherapy with prednisolone in active Crohn's disease. Gastroenterology. 1993;105:367–72.
8. Markowitz J, Grancher K, Manel F et al. 6-Mercaptopurine and prednisone therapy for newly diagnosed pediatric Crohn's disease: a prospective multicenter placebo controlled clinical trial. Gastroenterology. 1998;114:A1032.
9. O'Donoghue VP, Dawson AM, Powell-Tuck J et al. Double blind withdrawal trial of azathioprine as maintenance treatment for Crohn's disease. Lancet. 1978;2:955–7.
10. Barbe L, Marteau P, Lemann M et al. Dose raising of azathioprine beyond 2.5 mg/kg/day in Crohn's disease patients who fail to improve with a standard dose. Gastroenterology. 1998;114:A925.
11. Bouhnik Y, Lemann M, Mary JY et al. Long term follow-up of patients with Crohn's disease treated with azathioprine and 6-mercaptopurine. Lancet. 1996;347:215–19.
12. Sandborn WJ, Vanose C, Zins BJ et al. An intravenous loading dose of azathioprine decreases the time to response in subjects with Crohn's disease. Gastroenterology. 1995;109:1808–17.
13. George J, Present DH, Pou R et al. The long term outcome of ulcerative colitis treated with 6-mercaptopurine. Am J Gastroenterol. 1996;91:1711–14.
14. Hawthorne AB, Logan RFA, Hawkey CJ et al. Randomized controlled trial of azathioprine withdrawal in ulcerative colitis. Br Med J. 1992;305:20–2.
15. Present DH, Meltzer SJ, Krumholz MD et al. 6-Mercaptopurine in the management of inflammatory bowel disease: short and long term toxicity. Ann Intern Med. 1989;111:641–9.
16. Connell WR, Kamm MA, Ritchie JK et al. Bone marrow toxicity caused by azathioprine in inflammatory bowel disease: twenty-seven years of experience. Gut. 1993;34:1081–5.
17. Greenstein AJ, Mullin GE, Heimann T et al. Lymphoma in inflammatory bowel disease. Cancer. 1992;69:1119–23.
18. Connell WR, Kamm MA, Dickson M et al. Long term neoplasia risk after azathioprine treatment in inflammatory bowel disease. Lancet. 1994;343:1249–52.
19. Francella A, Dayan A, Rubin P et al. 6-Mercaptopurine is safe therapy for childbearing patients with inflammatory bowel disease: a case controlled study. Gastroenterology. 1996;110:A909.
20. Korelitz D, Hanauer S, Rutgeerts T et al. Postoperative prophylaxis of 6-MP/5-ASA or placebo in Crohn's disease: a two year multicenter trial. Gastroenterology. 1998;114:A1011.

21. Kozarek PA, Patterson DJ, Gelfand MD *et al.* Methotrexate induces clinical and histologic remission in patients with refractory inflammatory bowel disease. Ann Intern Med. 1989;110:353–6.
22. Feagan BG, Rochon J, Fedorak RN *et al.* Methotrexate for the treatment of Crohn's disease. N Engl J Med. 1995;332:292–7.
23. Lemann M, Chamiot-Prieur C, Mesnard B *et al.* Methotrexate for the treatment of refractory Crohn's disease. Aliment Pharmacol Ther. 1996;10:309–14.
24. Mahadevan U, Marion J, Present DH. The place for methotrexate in the treatment of refractory Crohn's disease. Gastroenterology. 1997;112:A1031.
25. Brynskov V, Freund L, Rasmussen SN *et al.* Placebo controlled double blind randomized trial of cyclosporine therapy in active Crohn's disease. N Engl J Med. 1989;321:845–50.
26. Stange EF, Modigliani R, Pena AF *et al.* European trial of cyclosporine in chronic active Crohn's disease: a 12-month study. Gastroenterology. 1995;109:774–82.
27. Feagan BG, McDonald JW, Rochon J *et al.* Low dose cyclosporine for the treatment of Crohn's disease. N Engl J Med. 1994;330:1846–51.
28. Present DH, Lichtiger S. Efficacy of cyclosporine in treatment of fistula of Crohn's disease. Dig Dis Sci. 1994;39:374–80.
29. Hanauer SB, Smith MB. Rapid closure of Crohn's disease fistula with continuous intravenous cyclosporine A. Am J Gastroenterol. 1993;88:646–9.
30. Lemann M, de la Valussiere F, Vouhnik Y *et al.* Intravenous cyclosporine for refractory attacks of Crohn's disease: long term follow-up of patients. Gastroenterology. 1998;114:A1020.
31. Kornbluth AA, Marion JF, Salomon P *et al.* How effective is current medical therapy for severe ulcerative colitis? An analytic review of selected trials. J Clin Gastroenterol. 1995;20:280–4.
32. Lichtiger S, Present DH, Kornbluth AA *et al.* Cyclosporine in severe ulcerative colitis refractory to steroid therapy. N. Engl J Med. 1994;330:1841–5.
33. Kornbluth AA, Lichtiger S, Present DH *et al.* Long term results of oral cyclosporine in patients with severe ulcerative colitis: a double blind randomized multicenter trial. Gastroenterology. 1994;106:A714.
34. Marion JF, Present DH. 6-MP maintains cyclosporine induced response in patients with severe ulcerative colitis. Am J Gastroenterol. 1996;91:A1975.
35. Sternthal M, Present DH, Kornbluth AA *et al.* Toxicity associated with the use of cyclosporine in patients with inflammatory bowel disease. Gastroenterology. 1996;110:A1019.
36. D'Haens G, Lemmens L, Hiele M *et al.* Intravenous cyclosporine monotherapy versus methyl-prednisolone therapy in severe ulcerative colitis: a randomized double blind placebo controlled trial. Gastroenterology. 1998;114:A963.
37. Yacyshyn B, Woloschuk MB, Yacyshyn D *et al.* Efficacy and safety of ISIS 2302 in treatment of steroid-dependent Crohn's disease. Gastroenterology. 1997;112:A1123.
38. van Deventer SJH, Elson CO, Fedorak RN. For the Crohn's Disease Group. Multiple doses of interleukin-10 in steroid refractory Crohn's disease. Gastroenterology. 1997;113:383–9.
39. Neurath MF, Wanitschke R, Peters M *et al.* Randomized trial of mycophenolate mofetil versus azathioprine for treatment of chronic active Crohn's disease. Gastroenterology. 1998;114:A1050.
40. Targan SR, Hanauer SD, van Deventer SJH *et al.* A short term study of chimeric monoclonal antibody cA2 to tumor necrosis factor alpha for Crohn's disease. N Engl J Med. 1997;337:1029–35.
41. Present DH, Mayer L, Van Deventer SJH *et al.* Anti-TNF-alpha chimeric antibody (cA2) is effective in the treatment of the fistula of Crohn's disease: a multicenter randomized double blind placebo controlled study. Am J Gastroenterol. 1997;92:A1746.

22
Sequential therapy for inflammatory bowel disease

S. B. HANAUER

Until recently, the concept of step-wise, or sequential therapy has been an empiric element of therapy for ulcerative colitis and Crohn's disease. In ulcerative colitis, we have recognized sequential acute and maintenance therapies for ulcerative colitis for several decades[1]. However, in Crohn's disease, the negative results from the maintenance phases of the National Cooperative Crohn's Disease Study [2] and the European Cooperative Crohn's Disease Trial[3] led to an era of therapeutic nihilism pertaining to the maintenance therapy[4]. Two factors have led to an evolution of the concept of sequential therapy for both disorders. From the scientific side, we now have evidence-based data relating to the potential for preventing or delaying relapse in Crohn's disease (maintenance therapy)[5]. Secondly, the regulatory processes and authorities in North America and Europe have begun to recognize differing indications for approval and marketing of therapeutic agents for IBD based upon the status of disease activity[6].

The early trials by Truelove and colleagues were the first to examine the acute benefits of medical therapy (corticosteroids) in the treatment of ulcerative colitis[7]. In their trials, they defined patients according to the degree of response. Subsequent trials failed to demonstrate maintenance benefits for steroids in ulcerative colitis. However, trials with sulphasalazine did demonstrate a dose-dependent effect on prevention of relapse[5]. Unfortunately, these trials were not performed in sequence and the definitions of response and relapse were not uniform. In fact, to date, no criteria have been reproduced or validated to define either remission or relapse in ulcerative colitis[8]. Nevertheless, logic assumes that if we do have effective maintenance therapies (e.g. aminosalicylates as have been demonstrated in numerous trials), there should be a 'standardized' means of defining remission. An attempt at a regulatory definition was made in a draft guideline for drug development in the US by defining remission in ulcerative colitis as 'regeneration of the mucosa without evidence of *significant* ulceration, granularity or friability'. Relapse would, conversely, require evidence of mucosal inflammation. These 'guidelines' take into account: the lack of correlation between symptoms and mucosal inflammation (e.g. the frequency of IBS symptoms coexisting with IBD and alternative causes of rectal bleeding); the ability to directly examine the colonic mucosa; the potential failure of mucosa to completely normalize (e.g. vascular distortion or pseudopolyps in the absence of acute histological inflammation); and the uncommon clinical practice of monitoring histological activity[6].

The concept of sequential therapy for ulcerative colitis and Crohn's disease is further substantiated by differences in response to individualized treatments for acute disease or maintenance therapy. The same agents are not effective in all phases of disease. In addition, steroid-sparing therapy in ulcerative colitis and Crohn's disease and prevention of postoperative relapse in Crohn's disease are unique categories of maintenance treatment[4,9].

ACTIVE DISEASE

In ulcerative colitis, the aminosalicylates are effective at inducing remission in mild–moderate disease[1,4,9,10]. These agents are not, however, adequate for moderate or severe disease. Corticosteroids are also effective at inducing remission for all levels of severity[1,4] and cyclosporine has been demonstrated to be effective in severe colitis[11]. Subsequent to acute therapy with any of these agents, there is a predictable relapse if a maintenance therapy is not administered[12].

In Crohn's disease, the aminosalicylates are less efficacious than in ulcerative colitis but have been demonstrated to induce clinical remission in patients with mild disease. Metronidazole and ciprofloxacin have had benefits comparable to those of either sulphasalazine[13] or mesalamine. In moderate to severe disease, corticosteroids are the standard inductive agent[9], whereas cyclosporine has also been effective, either in combination with steroids or alone, for fistulizing Crohn's disease[11]. Most recently, the chimeric anti-TNF monoclonal antibody, infliximab, has also been demonstrated to be effective in the treatment of refractory Crohn's disease[14]. As with ulcerative colitis, withdrawal of therapy after acute treatment predictably leads to relapse[5,9].

MAINTENANCE THERAPY

Numerous clinical trials have proven the aminosalicylates effective at preventing relapse of ulcerative colitis[10]. The sequential treatment of patients with corticosteroids transitioning to aminosalicylates is the most common clinical scenario in IBD. Still, in some patients, it is not possible to maintain remission after steroid-induction therapy despite optimal aminosalicylate dosing. In this setting of steroid-dependent ulcerative colitis, azathioprine or 6-mercaptopurine have allowed steroid tapering while preventing relapse in a large proportion of patients[15]. Conversely, despite their benefits in active disease, neither corticosteroids nor cyclosporine have been efficacious at preventing relapse in ulcerative colitis[1,4].

Maintenance therapy in Crohn's disease is more complex due to the heterogeneity of the disease and therapies. Termination of acute therapy leads to relapse, and continuation of corticosteroids does not prevent relapse although a large proportion of patients becomes steroid dependent[9,16]. Aminosalicylates have not been effective in the prevention of relapse of steroid-treated patients[17] but do delay relapse after surgical resection[18]. Metronidazole has also been able to delay recurrence after resection[19] as does 6-mercaptopurine.

In steroid-dependent Crohn's disease, azathioprine, 6-mercaptopurine[20] and methotrexate[21] have allowed steroid withdrawal while preventing recurrence of disease activity.

PATHOPHYSIOLOGICAL CORRELATES

The drugs that are most consistently effective at inducing remission in both ulcerative colitis and Crohn's disease, corticosteroids, cyclosporine and, most recently, infliximab all impact upon proximal mediators of the immuno-inflammatory pathways[22]. These mediators include $NF\kappa\beta$ and the pro-inflammatory cytokines, IL-1, IL-2 and TNF. In contrast, the more effective maintenance therapies (i.e. aminosalicylates) impact upon distal non-specific mediators, such as prostaglandins, leukotrienes, platelet activating factor, reactive oxygen species[23]. The mechanisms of action for methotrexate and azathioprine are less understood but may be related to anti-inflammatory effects in the case of methotrexate[24] and reduction in long-lived circulating lymphocytes (NK cells) by azathioprine[25].

These observations should afford models for future drug development and positioning of agents for clinical trials. Targets for inductive agents are the proximal arms of immune activation, including nuclear factors, cytokines and lymphocytoxicity[22]. Maintenance agents are most likely to be agents that will prevent amplification of the early sequences of inflammation. As the immunoinflammatory sequences in ulcerative colitis and Crohn's disease become elucidated, therapy may be directed at initiating events. Identification of the environmental triggers will afford another direct means of inhibition or prevention of activation. In the meantime, the ability to subgroup patients with specific disease genotypes and phenotypes is proceeding rapidly[26]. Genetic markers with the potential to delineate phenotypic immune or inflammatory responses are becoming available. We can easily anticipate that sequential therapy will be defined in a preclinical state or at diagnosis rather than by the empiric basis by which our current approaches were derived and then tested in clinical trials.

References

1. Kornbluth, A, Sachar DB. Ulcerative colitis practice guidelines in adults. American College of Gastroenterology, Practice Parameters Committee. Am J Gastroenterol. 1997;92(2):204–11.
2. Summers RW *et al.* National Cooperative Crohn's Disease Study: results of drug treatment. Gastroenterology. 1979;77(4 Pt 2):847–69.
3. Malchow H *et al.* European Cooperative Crohn's Disease Study (ECCDS): results of drug treatment. Gastroenterology. 1984;86(2):249–66.
4. Hanauer SB. Review articles: Drug therapy: Inflammatory bowel disease. N Engl J Med. 1996;334(13):841–8.
5. Sachar DB. Maintenance therapy in ulcerative colitis and Crohn's disease. J Clin Gastroenterol. 1995;20:117–22.

6. Fredd S. Standards for approval of new drugs for IBD. Inflamm Bowel Dis. 1995;1(4):284–94.

7. Truelove, SC, Witts IJ. Cortisone in ulcerative colitis. Final report on a therapeutic trial. Br Med J. 1995;2:1041–7.

8. Hanauer SB. Measurement of disease activity: In Inflammatory Bowel Disease: From Bench to Bedside, Targan SR, Shanahan F, editors. Baltimore: Williams and Wilkins; 1994:429–44.

9. Hanauer SB, Meyers S. Management of Crohn's disease in adults. Am J Gastroenterol. 1997;92(4):559–66.

10. Sutherland LR, May GR, Shaffer EA. Sulfasalazine revisited: a meta-analysis of 5-aminosalicylic acid in the treatment of ulcerative colitis. Ann Intern Med. 1993;118(7):540–9.

11. Sandborn W. A critical review of cyclosporine therapy in inflammatory bowel disease. Inflamm Bowel Dis. 1995;1(1):48–63.

12. Miner PB Jr. Factors influencing the relapse of patients with inflammatory bowel disease. Am J Gastroenterol. 1997;92(12 Suppl):1S–4S.

13. Ursing B *et al.* A comparative study of metronidazole and sulphasalazine for active Crohn's disease: the Cooperative Crohn's Disease Study in Sweden II. Result. Gastroenterology. 1982;83(3):550–62.

14. Targan SR *et al.* A short-term study of chimeric monoclonal antibody cA2 to tumor necrosis factor alpha for Crohn's disease. Crohn's Disease cA2 Study Group. N Engl J Med. 1997;337(15):1029–35.

15. George J *et al.* The long-term outcome of ulcerative colitis treated with 6-mercaptopurine. Am J Gastroenterol. 1996;91:1711–14.

16. Munkholm P *et al.* Frequency of glucocorticoid resistance and dependency in Crohn's disease. Gut. 1994;35(3):360–2.

17. Modigliani R *et al.* Mesalamine in Crohn's disease with steroid-induced remission: effect on steroid withdrawal and remission maintenance, Groupe d'Etudes Therapeutiques des Affections Inflammatoires Digestives. Gastroenterology. 1996;110(3):688–93.

18. Camma C *et al.* Mesalamine in the maintenance treatment of Crohn's disease: a meta-analysis adjusted for confounding variables. Gastroenterology. 1997;113(5):1465–73.

19. Rutgeerts P *et al.* A placebo controlled trial of metronidazole for recurrence prevention of Crohn's disease after resection of the terminal ileum. Gastroenterology. 1992;102:A688.

20. Pearson D *et al.* Review: Azathioprine Maintains Remission in Crohn's Disease, but Withdrawal Rates are Higher. The Cochrane Library: The Cochrane Database of Systematic Reviews; 1998(3): 33.

21. Feagan BG *et al.* Methotrexate for the treatment of Crohn's disease. N Engl J Med. 1995;332:292–7.

22. Elson CO. The basis of current and future therapy for inflammatory bowel disease. Am J Med. 1996;100(6):656–62.

23. Greenfield SM *et al.* Review article: the mode of action of the aminosalicylates in inflammatory bowel disease. Aliment Pharmacol Ther. 1993;7(4):369–83.

24. Egan LJ, Sandborn WJ. Methotrexate for inflammatory bowel disease: pharmacology and preliminary results [see comments]. Mayo Clin Proc. 1996;71(1):69–80.

25. Sandborn WJ. Azathioprine: state of the art in inflammatory bowel disease. Scand J Gastroenterol Suppl. 1998;225:92–9.

26. Cronin CC, Shanahan F. Immunological tests to monitor inflammatory bowel disease – have they delivered yet? [editorial; comment]. Am J Gastroenterol. 1998;93(3):295–7.

Section VI
Surgery for IBD

23
Surgery for Crohn's disease: when to operate, how to operate

V. W. FAZIO

Crohn's disease is a chronic inflammatory condition of the intestinal tract that may affect any part of the intestine. The cause of the disease remains unknown. Most commonly, the condition affects the terminal ileum with or without colonic involvement or is manifested in the large bowel alone. The major clinical anatomical types seen are those of ileitis, ileocolitis and colitis (including the rectum). This type of classification is useful because of different rates with which clinical manifestations of various types occur.

The natural history of Crohn's disease has been well described over the last few decades with many reports appearing in the literature. The manifestations of the disease are protean and so there is no typical phenotype that lends itself to one type of treatment or, indeed, one type of surgery. Because of the frequency with which recurrence occurs, circumspection is required about the indications for operation in the elective case. It is also fair to say that the enigmatic nature of the disease, its capacity to undergo remission at times, and its response to both medical and surgical treatment can lead equally experienced physicians or surgeons to use different modalities of treatment and even different types of surgery. However, few contest the fact that most patients with Crohn's disease will require surgery at some point in their lives.

The frequency with which surgery is carried out has been reported by Mekhijan and others as part of the National Cooperative Crohn's Disease Study Group[1]. This study showed a 20-year reoperation rate of 78% and 30-year re-operation rate of 90%. In a separate study, Whelan *et al.* from the Cleveland Clinic reported on 5- and 10-year recurrence rates for Crohn's disease[2]. These were, respectively, for ileitis, 50% and 70%; for colitis, 50% and 70%; and for ileocolitis, 75% and 90%.

Some patients who have only recently been diagnosed with Crohn's disease, may ask, 'Why not just remove the diseased segment?' It is important that the patient and family are informed about the natural history of the disease and the limitations of treatment modalities, especially given the propensity for recurrence. Thus, patients are well advised to become educated through the gastroenterologist, surgeon, other patients and organizations, such as the Crohn's and

Colitis Foundation of America. In general, decisions regarding surgical treatment are taken jointly by the surgeon and the gastroenterologist, but obviously in concert with the patients themselves.

STRATEGIC PLAN

This will be discussed under the following headings:

    Indications
    When not to operate
    Timing
    Tactics
    Choice of operation
    Error avoidance

The clinician, realizing that there is no current cure for Crohn's disease, will be mindful of the natural history of the disease; that therapy both medical and surgical can cause harm as well as help or palliate; and, since the disease is chronic, will maintain a strategic view of the whole patient over future decades.

Indications for surgery

Indications for surgery can be relative or absolute as well as being elective or urgent. In Table 1, the commoner indications for surgery are listed along with their propensity for recurrence in the small bowel, small bowel and colon, and colon patterns of disease. Essentially, patients with small bowel and combined small bowel and colonic Crohn's disease, have bowel obstruction and intra-abdominal sepsis or fistula as the primary indications for surgery. It is relatively uncommon for these complications to occur in colonic disease, although, certainly, colonic and rectal strictures can and do occur. However, failure to thrive occurs more frequently as an indication for surgery, in the colitis pattern of disease than in the small bowel or small bowel and colon patterns. Failure to thrive includes side-effects of medication, poor response to steroids, growth retardation, extraintestinal manifestations of disease, anaemia, incontinence of stool and disabling diarrhoea. Also, toxic colitis or even megacolon are far more likely to occur in the colonic pattern of disease, as are the perianal manifestations. It is rare for either perianal disease or extraintestinal manifestations of the disease to be the major indication for surgery, but these are commonly accessory indications. Other indications for surgery include: free perforation, carcinoma, obstructive uropathy and intestinal bleeding. The large variety of fistulas that can occur will also be discussed briefly below.

When not to operate

Opinion is divided as to the role of surgery in untreated cases of Crohn's disease. The majority prevailing opinion at the present time is that untreated non-urgent cases would benefit from a trial of medical therapy. Thus, early operative intervention is rarely performed in patients who have not been through a course of

Table 1 Indications for surgery

	Small bowel	Small bowel and colon	Colon
Obstruction	+++	+++	+
Abdominal sepsis (fistula-abscess)	+++	+++	+
Failure to thrive	+	+	+++
Toxicity (+/– megacolon)	+	+	++
Perianal disease	+	++	+++
Obstructive uropathy	+	++	+
Cancer	(+)	(+)	(+)
Haemorrhage	(+)	(+)	+

Indication of frequency: (+) rare; +, uncommon; ++ indeterminant; +++ common

medical treatment or who have been on inadequate medical treatment. A contrary view has been expressed by Hulten[3] who found that operations on advanced Crohn's disease, usually associated with abscess or fistula, carry a 49% complication rate. In uncomplicated Crohn's disease, the complication rate postoperatively was 12%. Thus, the policy of operating on patients before placing them on steroids has been adopted in certain parts of Scandinavia but this is not common in North America or the rest of Europe.

Additionally, we believe that Crohn's disease alone does not constitute an indication for surgery unless there are complications. Moreover, during an operation, if one identifies areas of Crohn's disease that do not appear to be causing obstruction or are not producing symptoms, then it is inappropriate to resect these areas as well.

Similarly, there are certain complications of Crohn's disease which might be deemed minor, i.e. not producing major disability. These include, for example, small rectovaginal fistulas. If such a patient is passing only small amounts of gas through the fistula or has only minor drainage, no surgery is advised. Successful closure of such fistulas in Crohn's disease is always somewhat questionable and, while reports of cures up to 75–80% have been achieved, nonetheless, the caveat of 'first do no harm' still holds. Specifically, it is possible for the fistula to be increased in size with worsening symptomatology as a result of a failed attempt to repair. Likewise, enterocutaneous fistulas that are producing minimal amounts of drainage are possibly best left alone, especially if these have recurred on several occasions.

The patient should not undergo surgery until correction of restorable deficiencies has been carried out. These include anaemia, certain cases of malnutrition and coagulopathies. There are certain patients whose co-morbidity is so severe that the risk of the operation is excessive and, in such cases, surgery should be deferred or avoided.

Timing of surgery

An operation is advised when continued non-operative therapy would be ineffective or harmful. The goals and benefits of such surgery are stated to the patient and, when it is deemed that the risk is lower than that of alternative therapy, surgery is performed. Early surgical intervention is used selectively for patients with certain complications. These include toxic colitis or megacolon, intra-abdominal abscess, peritonitis and major colonic haemorrhage. Even with acute small bowel obstruction, however, nasogastric tube suction and intravenous fluids are usually initiated and may be successful in avoiding the need for early operation.

There are still some timing issues with respect to toxic colitis and megacolon in that the initial trial of medical therapy should be given time to produce a beneficial effect. While no hard and fast numbers can be given, usually 24–72 h passes before therapy is deemed to have failed or to have produced no improvement. In toxic colitis without megacolon, delays in surgery beyond 5–7 days are associated with increased mortality rates[4]. In our experience with toxic colitis, mortality rates were not related to whether or not colonic dilatation was present[5].

Restoration of physiological deficits

For urgent operations, those deficits that can be restored quickly are made good, e.g. electrolyte abnormalities, anaemia, coagulopathy, and hypoalbuminaemia. Malnutrition is a more vexing problem because of the continued protein-losing enteropathy that occurs despite intravenous hyperalimentation. It is difficult to answer the question of what degree of malnutrition justifies the use of preoperative parenteral nutrition (TPN). Alfonso and Rombeau[6], in a comprehensive review of the literature, concluded that, although nearly all reports of preoperative TPN and Crohn's disease showed some positive change in nutritional parameters, there were no real reductions in postoperative complications. However, hypoalbuminaemia has been associated with increased morbidity and mortality of surgery. If the operation is urgent, despite the fact that the half-life of albumin is extremely short, perioperative albumin should be used in selected cases.

With respect to identification of preoperative sepsis, such as an intra-abdominal abscess, the surgeon should have this area drained, either percutaneously or through a minilaparotomy prior to any definitive surgery. This will reduce the chances of intraoperative spillage of abscess contents as well as dissemination of sepsis. Also, any patient on immunosuppression, e.g. with azathioprine, prior to elective surgery should be advised to stop the medication. There are no hard data attesting to the need for or safety of such a practice, but most surgeons believe that immunosuppression has an adverse effect on tissue and anastomotic healing. Thus, if a patient can avoid such drugs for 2–3 weeks prior to surgery, then these should be withdrawn.

Reoperative surgery does influence the timing of operation considerably. As mentioned above, we favour preliminary abscess drainage. In certain cases, a Hartmann operation must be performed, i.e. colectomy with ileostomy and the rectal stump oversewn for toxic colitis or megacolon. In such patients, an interval of six months is advised before further surgery because of the obliterative peritonitis that tends to occur from adhesions after such an operation. There is an interval of 7–10 days after laparotomy when reoperation is technically feasible. The most common indications for such intervention are suspected bowel obstruction and enterocutaneous fistula. Despite this, early reoperation may still be impossible to perform safely. In such cases, if the adhesive barrier is so severe that the bowel loops cannot be separated, it is best for the patient to have a tube gastrostomy made, the abdomen closed and home TPN given. In such cases, the chronic obstruction will usually resolve spontaneously.

At delayed fistula after definitive bowel surgery also falls under this category and such patients are best treated by TPN and sepsis control.

Rectal stump preservation after subtotal colectomy for Crohn's colitis poses some problems for the surgeon. Should elective proctectomy be performed in the asymptomatic patient and when? The concern is the cancer risk in the out-of-circuit rectal segment. However, the counterfoil to this is the risk of impotence in young males as well as pelvic sepsis. My own practice has been to defer such surgery until or unless stomal recurrent Crohn's disease appears or some other indication for laparotomy occurs, e.g. hernia repair, cholecystectomy, etc. However, this is still an open question since, as long as continued monitoring of the rectal segment can be carried out by endoscopy and biopsy regularly, then there is no absolute indication for proctectomy.

Tactics (how to operate)

Patient counselling is of great importance when it comes to discussion of which operation is advised and how this will occur. Informed consent then, especially relating to the condition which may lead to a permanent stoma, is something which will of necessity take time for discussion with the patient. Parenthetically, the surgeon has to identify those patients for whom delaying surgery is potentially disastrous. It has been stated by Alexander Williams that one should not operate until a complication of the disease occurs. However, once this has occurred, one should not wait in case it becomes further complicated. There are exceptions to this rule: bowel obstruction is a frequent accompaniment of small bowel Crohn's disease and, although this appears as a complication, a good response to conservative measures and anti-inflammatory drugs is commonly seen. Patients with recurring obstruction while taking adequate medical therapy, especially if there is right lower quadrant fullness or mass, should usually be referred for surgery. Similarly, patients with toxic colitis while on medical therapy should undergo surgery if the toxicity persists beyond seven days.

Mechanical preparation

Mechanical bowel preparation is used in most elective cases with preference given to polyethylene glycol. Many patients have partial bowel obstruction from Crohn's disease. In these, bowel preparation may be difficult or impossible. Such patients are treated for several days with a high-protein liquid diet and given a milder aperient than PEG, such as magnesium citrate. Even so, some patients will not tolerate this. At surgery, after the patient has been placed in the Lloyd-Davies stirrups, irrigation of the rectum is carried out on table to check and improve on the bowel preparation.

Intravenous antibiotics covering Gram-negative anaerobes and aerobes are given perioperatively, mostly as an immediate preoperative and immediate post-operative dose for clean contaminated cases. With any contamination during surgery, however, the course is increased to 2–3 days. Perioperative intravenous steroids are used in 'stress' doses if the patient has been taking steroids within three months of previously taking steroids.

One other important item is to 'get a road map' where possible. What this means is that patients who are about to embark on resective surgery should have their disease location and extent identified as well as possible preoperatively. This involves recent (i.e. within 12–24 months) small bowel series as well as a recent barium enema or colonoscopy. In certain cases, if this has not been done and the patient has had a bad experience with barium or, indeed, has bowel obstruction precluding its use, then intraoperative assessment has to be made. This may include intraoperative colonoscopy as well. It is important to avoid leaving behind thickened ulcerated intestine, especially colon, as this can be difficult to identify by external viewing of the large bowel at operation.

Stoma site marking

Rehabilitation of the patient requires successful siting and construction of the stoma at the time of its construction. The 'rules' covering optimum stoma siting have been well published in the past. Basically, they include assurance of visibility on the summit of the infra-umbilical fat mound, within the surface marking of the rectus muscle, and avoidance of creases and bony prominence when the patient is in a sitting position.

Treat (only) the primary problem

The patient with obstructing or perforating ileal Crohn's disease is managed by resection of that segment. However, in the patient with diffuse non-obstructing disease, such areas are best left alone, attending to those strictured or perforative areas distally which probably cause the symptoms. In certain cases, asymptomatic gall stones may be identified and, if the procedure up to that moment has been trouble free, elective cholecystectomy can be carried out with benefit to the patient. Routine incidental appendectomy is not recommended.

The practice of bowel conservation

Controversy exists regarding the optimal extent of resection for Crohn's disease. Most surgeons favour conservative resection margins, i.e. 2–5 cm. Earlier studies by Bergman and Krause[7] favoured extensive resection. We conducted a randomized controlled trial of patients ($n = 152$)[8] with resection margins that were clear of macroscopic Crohn's disease for either 2 cm (limited group; $n = 82$) or 12 cm (extended group; $n = 70$); 131 patients received anastomoses. After 56 months (median follow-up), disease recurrence had occurred in 29 patients classified as reoperation for recurrence. These included 25% of patients in the limited group and 18% in the extended group. When the 21 cases that had been excluded because of temporary or permanent stoma were included, the surgical recurrence rates were 23% and 20% for the limited and extended groups respectively.

Microscopic changes of the macroscopically normal line of resection were also examined. Using a carefully defined set of histological criteria, margins were characterized as normal (category 1), non-specific changes (category 2), suggestive but not diagnostic of Crohn's disease (category 3), and diagnostic recurrent disease (category 4). Recurrence rates were 36% in category 2, 39% in category 3 and 21% in category 4. We concluded that extended resection margins conferred no advantage to patients in reducing cumulative recurrence rates. As with other studies which found that frozen section was of no value in helping the surgeon to reduce recurrence rates, we found that the presence of residual microscopic Crohn's disease at the resection margin did not appear to increase recurrence rates significantly compared with normal margins.

Thus, the evidence to date indicates that wide margins of resection are unnecessary. This is of some importance in that small aphthous ulcers, commonly seen at surgery, can be left *in situ* without removing more bowel.

Choice of operation

A number of different operations are used in the treatment of Crohn's disease. Incisions are generally midline to allow easy access to the abdomen and also preserve both left and right lower quadrants for possible stoma construction.

The choice of operation includes:

Stoma
Resection, anastomosis vs. stoma
Bypass
Strictureplasty
Stricture dilatation
Open vs. laparoscopic resection
Perianal surgery

Stoma surgery alone is rarely used these days. It is sometimes used in concert with definitive perianal reconstructive work, such as repair of anovaginal fistula, repair of anal sphincters, or diversion to decrease perianal sepsis prior to definitive proctocolectomy.

Resection with anastomosis is the treatment of choice for the small bowel and ileocolitis patterns of disease and, indeed, for colonic disease with rectal sparing. However, this requires an optimum physical and medical state for the patient with few comorbidities and with no intra-abdominal undrained sepsis at the end of the operation. Anastomosis is avoided in favour of a stoma in patients with toxic colitis, indeterminant colitis or colitis with major comorbidity.

The bypass procedure is also a rarely used operation. It still has a place, however, for ileocaecal Crohn's disease, especially where there has been fixity to pelvic structures or to the great vessels of the pelvis.

In addition, enteroenteric bypass surgery is sometimes used in patients with multiple skip lesions of Crohn's disease and where the inflamed segment that is causing the stricture is deemed to be unsafe for strictureplasty.

The commonest form of treatment for duodenal Crohn's disease is bypass, namely gastrojejunostomy with or without vagotomy. However, recent alternatives have included strictureplasty of the duodenum and this is discussed below.

Indications for strictureplasty include:

1. Extensive small bowel Crohn's disease as manifested by multiple strictures.
2. Rapid recurrence of Crohn's disease manifested as obstruction.
3. Stricture in the patient with short-bowel syndrome.
4. Non-phlegmonous fibrotic strictures.

The contraindications of strictureplasty are:

1. Free or contained perforation of the small bowel.
2. Phlegmonous inflammation, internal fistula or external fistula involving the affected site.
3. Multiple strictures within a short segment that lends itself to resection.
4. Stricture in close proximity to a site chosen for resection.
5. Colonic strictures.
6. Hypoalbuminaemia (less than 2.0 g/dl).

Long strictures may be approached by either the Finney strictureplasty or by the side-to-side isoperistaltic technique.

The operation is proven to be quite safe with no mortality reported from all major series. At the Cleveland Clinic, 162 patients underwent 191 operations with 698 strictureplasties and were followed for a mean of 42 months. Ninety-eight per cent were relieved of obstructive symptoms and two thirds had ceased to take steroids[9]. Reoperative recurrence affected only 28% of the patients, and most (78%) of those requiring reoperation had new strictures or perforative disease. There are still many issues attendant on the strictureplasty operation, but it seems to have found its place in the armamentarium of surgeons for patients who are vulnerable to short bowel syndrome and who have strictures or strictured segments amenable to this procedure.

Stricture dilatation

While dilatation of anorectal strictures has been common for many years, intraperitoneal dilatations have been relatively uncommon. Current reports attest to the effectiveness of such treatment with strictures remaining patent for upwards of 30 months. However, approximately 11% of patients have some form of occult or overt free perforation, serving notice to the clinician that extra care is needed in choosing the correct patient for this procedure.

Laparoscopic bowel surgery

Laparoscopic approaches for treatment of Crohn's disease of the small bowel have been increasingly reported. The majority of these report on the laparoscopic-assisted technique. A 7–8-cm incision is used to extract the mobilized ileocaecal segment. This leads to safer transection of the thickened mesentery commonly present and also allows for an extracorporeal anastomosis. Claims of the protagonists of this approach include: shorter length of stay in hospital, less pain, earlier return to work and no apparent increase in morbidity compared with the open technique. Milsom, at the Cleveland Clinic, has reported on a randomized controlled trial which shows laparoscopic surgery to be effective in the surgical treatment of Crohn's disease of the small bowel.

It is still debated whether laparoscopic surgery is appropriate for recurrent Crohn's disease, especially in patients with sepsis or fistulas.

Perianal surgery

In this brief overview, it is impossible to do justice to this subject. The conventional approach to the management of perianal fistulas has been that of conservatism with intermittent incision and drainage of abscesses when they occur. However, there have been advances in perianal disease management in the long-term treatment of high fistulas with setons, allowing avoidance of ostomies and freedom from pain without requiring surgery that may lead to incontinence or an unhealed wound.

On the other hand, many centres are now adopting selective use of fistulotomy for low lying, i.e. intersphincteric, fistulas with good effect, provided there is no active rectal Crohn's disease. Such perianal fistulas in Crohn's disease may also be treated by more advanced techniques, such as the advancement rectal flap or advancement rectal sleeve operation and, in certain cases, proctectomy with colo-anal anastomosis can be carried out.

Separate issues relate to internal pouches in Crohn's disease. While the current thinking is that such pouches are not recommended (Kock pouch or J pouch), the fact is that these operations are sometimes performed inadvertently for Crohn's disease. In these patients, complications are common and they may require pouch excision. In selected cases, however, restorative repeat procedures can be carried out with success rates of up to 60% (in the Cleveland Clinic series: Ann Surg, Nov. 98, in press).

Special situations

1. Internal fistula. In many cases, the fistula arises from the diseased small bowel and involves an otherwise normal, adjacent structure or organ (ileum, sigmoid colon, urinary bladder) by direct extension. The principles of surgery in all such fistulas are similar. The primary site, e.g. ileal Crohn's disease, is resected, the fistula is detached from the adjacent structure and, if this is a hollow viscus or organ, the defect is closed. Sepsis is drained and, in complex cases, a temporary ostomy is made.

2. Obstructive uropathy. Rarely is ureterolysis necessary. Hydroureter usually recovers with simple resection of the diseased intestine which is producing the compressive effect.

3. Intra-abdominal abscess. Drainage is provided externally. In certain cases of retroperitoneal abscess, psoas fascia is unroofed and the cavity drained.

4. Massive hemorrhage from the small bowel. Often, the source cannot be detected easily and it is useful to consider intraoperative angiopathy to assist in identifying the affected segment.

5. Rectovaginal fistula. In patients with absent or quiescent rectal Crohn's disease, an advancement rectal flap operation, or advancement sleeve achieves successful closure in 75% of patients. Initial treatment failures may still be salvageable with a repeat repair. Fistulas with associated sphincter injury (cloaca) are best repaired by the transperineal approach.

Error avoidance

While the title of this presentation is the 'when and how' of surgery for Crohn's disease, it is perhaps instructive to review commonly observed errors. One might even call these avoidable errors. Certain of these have been alluded to above.

1. Early (too early) repeat laparotomy. The window of time in which surgery should ideally be avoided is between day 10 and day 90 after surgery. The only acceptable indications for the operation within that time frame are ischaemic bowel, undrained sepsis, and massive haemorrhage. Otherwise, sequelae such as traumatic enterocutaneous fistula or massive bowel resection may result from a surgeon's well-intentioned but erroneous decision to operate on patients with persistent ileus or obstruction.

2. No road map. In the elective case, it really bears restating that contrast and/or endoscopic studies to outline the extent of the intestinal disease are important in helping the surgeon make the appropriate decisions regarding surgical treatment.

3. Right colectomy vs. ileocaecal resection. It is common practice for patients to have their right colon removed for ileal or ileocaecal Crohn's disease. Removing the hepatic flexure and ascending colon is largely unnecessary and ileo-ascending-colon anastomosis is preferred. Moreover, the ileo-transverse anastomosis comes to lie almost directly over the head of the pancreas and duodenum. A subsequent later ileocoloduodenal fistula might arise if or when recurrence occurs, producing a very complex problem for the surgeon to deal with.

4. Leaving a short rectal stump. In performing abdominal colectomy, especially for toxicity, some surgeons believe that taking more of the rectum is better than leaving a rectosigmoid stump behind. Thus, the shortened rectal stump comes to lie in the low pelvis where the apex of the stump is fused to the presacral area. This makes for an extremely difficult subsequent rectal removal and risks injury to the nervi erigentes as well as the ureters. What is more, such a short rectal stump confers no advantage to the patient in terms of reduced toxicity. Our recommendation is that the rectosigmoid be buried subcutaneously so it can be identified easily at re-operation.

5. Inadequate drainage of sepsis. Some patients with occult sepsis, e.g. a psoas abscess, or even a large pelvic abscess may not have this adequately drained and so continued smouldering occurs without defervescence of the patient's septic state.

6. Placement of mesh in contaminated cases. This is self-evident. Such mesh is likely to become infected and require a complicated operation to remove it later on. It is best to leave large hernias in contaminated cases, such as this, and repair the hernia with mesh at a later date, when all sepsis has resolved.

7. Anastomosis to strictured or ulcerated bowel. This is asking for trouble since complications of the anastomosis are considerable when such strictures are used in the anastomotic line.

8. Radical resection. This was mentioned above only to be condemned as it is totally unnecessary for patients.

9. Strictureplasty on a septic or phlegmonous segment. This was mentioned above.

10. Non-diverted anastomosis in the septic or debilitated patient.

11. Bad siting of the ostomy.

12. Leaving disease that cannot be monitored, e.g. the right colon after an ileal transverse colon bypass operation.

13. Excising indurated tags around the anus or haemorrhoid excision. While this may occasionally be safe, it is so difficult to predict who will and who will not do well that these tags and haemorrhoids are best left alone and treated conservatively.

14. Trans-sphincteric fistulotomy. This should be avoided in Crohn's disease; treatment should be by either seton or advancement rectal flap.

15. Sphincterotomy for anal fissure. This is rarely performed because of the risk of incontinence. However, certain acute fissures that are small can be treated successfully with sphincterotomy.

16. Radical proctectomy (Miles procedure). This operation renders a patient vulnerable to having an unhealed perineal wound, one of the major complications of this operation. The preferred technique is to unroof the fistulas anally, perform an intersphincteric proctectomy, close the levator plate from above and below and then leave the openings of the sinus to heal by second intention.

In summary, there are numerous problems and pitfalls that might be encountered in surgery for Crohn's disease. The clinician is well advised to keep a strategic view of the patient's entire life span and, only after obtaining the fully informed consent of the patient, and including the patient in the decision making when it comes to choices between operative and medical management, should the therapeutic plan be developed.

References

1. Mekhijan HS, Sweitz DM, Watts HD *et al*. National Cooperative Crohn's Disease Study: Factors determining recurrence of Crohn's disease after surgery. Gastroenterology. 1979;77:907–13.
2. Whelan G, Farmer RG, Fazio VW *et al*. Recurrence after surgery in Crohn's disease: Relationship to location of disease (clinical pattern) and surgical indication. Gastroenterology. 1985;88:1826–33.
3. Hulten L. Surgical treatment of Crohn's disease of the small bowel or ileocecum. World J Surg. 1988;12:180–5.
4. Goligher JC, Hoffman DC, de Domabal FT. Surgical treatment of severe attacks of ulcerative colitis, with special reference to the advantages of early operation. Br J Surg. 1970;4:703–6.
5. Fazio VW. Toxic megacolon in ulcerative colitis and Crohn's colitis. Clin Gastroenterol. 1980;9:389–407.
6. Alfonso JJ, Rombeau JL. Parenteral nutrition for patients with inflammatory bowel disease. In Rombeau JL, Caldwell M, eds. Parenteral Nutrition, 2nd edn. Philadelphia, PA: Saunders; 1993:427–41.
7. Bergman L, Krause U. Crohn's disease: A long-term study of the clinical course. Scand J Gastroenterol. 1977;12:937–44.
8. Fazio VW, Marchetti F, Church J, Goldblum J *et al*. Effective resection margins and the recurrence of Crohn's disease in the small bowel. A randomized controlled trial. Ann Surg. 1996;224:563–73.
9. Ozuner G, Fazio VW, Lavery I, Milsom J, Strong S. Reoperative rates for Crohn's disease following strictureplasty. Dis Colon Rectum. 1996;39:1199–203.

24
Natural history of Crohn's recurrence at the ileocolonic anastomosis

G. D'HAENS

INTRODUCTION

The incidence of Crohn's disease recurrence following 'curative resection' is high. Almost invariably inflammation recurs at the ileal side of the ileocolonic anastomosis. Since the neoterminal ileum can be reached by the ileocolonoscopy rather easily, postoperative recurrence in this location provides a suitable 'human model' for the study of the pathophysiological events in the earliest phases of Crohn's disease. We will review a number of important studies which have been carried out in order to unravel the mechanisms involved.

The clinical picture of recurrent disease resembles that of the preoperative disease, with regard to both length and type of inflammation. Certain risk factors for recurrence of Crohn's disease, such as smoking, parity and age, as well as disease- and surgery-related factors will be discussed.

THE INCIDENCE OF CROHN'S RECURRENCE IN THE NEOTERMINAL ILEUM

The incidence of clinical recurrence of Crohn's disease averages about 10% of all operated patients per year postoperatively[1,2]. The use of clinical parameters to diagnose recurrence, however, has serious shortcomings, for certain symptoms can be a consequence of the surgical resection itself, and the variability in individual perception and interpretation of symptoms can be significant. Fortunately, the need for repeated surgery is much lower. Reoperation rates at 10 years have varied between 16 and 65%[3,4]. A few studies have used radiological criteria to document recurrence and reported cumulative recurrence rates of 41–60% at 10 years[5,6].

The incidence of recurrence has been examined systematically by means of ileocolonoscopy, which proved to be the most sensitive method to study this phenomenon. Signs of early recurrent Crohn's disease have been observed in 73% of all patients one year and in 85% of all patients 3 years postoperatively.

The clinical disease course correlated well with the endoscopic status of the neoterminal ileum one year after surgery[7].

WHAT HAPPENS IN THE NEOTERMINAL ILEUM AFTER 'CURATIVE RESECTION'?

The role of the faecal stream: reinfusion studies

Endoscopic lesions in Crohn's disease recurrence have been observed as early as three months postoperatively. The inflammatory events, however, appear to develop within the first few days after resection. We demonstrated in a recently published study that the mucosa in the neoterminal ileum remains intact as long as the faecal stream is diverted (via loop-ileostomy). After eight days of perfusion of ileal effluent into the efferent loop of the ileostomy, massive influx of inflammatory cells was observed. The lesions showed a focal distribution and included villous architectural changes, limited patchy surface epithelial cell damage and necrosis and accumulation of eosinophils and mononuclear cells in the lamina propria in the top of the villi. Further characterization of mononuclear cells using monoclonal antibodies showed increased macrophage activation (KP1-CD 68), antigen presentation (B7-1, HLA DR), epithelioid transformation (RFD9) and active transendothelial lymphocyte recruitment (ICAM-1, LFA-1) into the mucosal compartment. Electron microscopic examination revealed damage of the epithelial cells with dilation of the rough endoplasmic reticulum and Golgi apparatus and the presence of basally located transport vesicles. This study provides further evidence for the involvement of faecal contents in the induction of early lesions in recurrent Crohn's disease[8].

In a larger study, we confirmed the finding that recurrent Crohn's lesions in the neoterminal ileum do not appear as long as the faecal stream is diverted, whereas the majority of patients (71%) develop mucosal lesions 6 months after intestinal continuity has been restored[9].

Earlier studies from Oxford observed the same phenomenon when ileal fluid was infused into defunctioned colon, previously affected by Crohn's disease. Additional infusion studies with ultrafiltration and sterilization of this effluent led to the conclusion that faecal particles >0.22 μm were responsible for the exacerbation of Crohn's disease inflammation[10,11]. Nonetheless, it remains unclear which component of the faecal stream is responsible for this phenomenon.

Cytokine studies

In the first cytokine studies in the human recurrence model, elevated levels of IL-5 mRNA accompanied by an increased number of mucosal eosinophils and overexpression of IgE mRNA and protein were observed[12,13]. This pattern was different from the findings in more chronic intestinal inflammation, which led to the conclusion that an allergic immune reaction may initiate Crohn's inflammation. The same investigators also demonstrated an enhanced expression of IL-4 in early Crohn's lesions, a cytokine classically considered to represent a typical Th-2 pattern[14]. IL-4 has been shown to attenuate epithelial barrier function[15], to cause mucosal ulcerations when used in recombinant form for cancer[16], and it is involved in the recruitment and degranulation of eosinophils[17]. Intriguingly, the receptor gene for IL-4 is located on chromosome 16. The Th-1 cytokines, IFN-γ and IL-2, on the other hand, were not increased in early lesions but clearly upregulated in chronic Crohn's inflammation[14]. Our own data showed an increased TNF-α secretion in terminal ileum biopsies affected by recurrent Crohn's disease 6 and 12 months postoperatively. The levels correlated with the severity of endoscopic and histological recurrence[18]. In conclusion, these cytokine studies suggest that there may be a shift from Th-2 to Th-1 cytokines in Crohn's recurrence and point towards an important role for IL-5, IL-4 and eosinophils as inflammatory triggers.

Permeability alterations

Increased small bowel permeability has been demonstrated repeatedly in Crohn's disease patients and healthy family members[19]. It remains a matter of discussion, however, whether these abnormalities are 'primary' and possibly involved in the pathogenesis of the disease, or rather acquired and merely a consequence of (subclinical) inflammation. The absence of a typical family pattern and the high prevalence of increased permeability in spouses of patients suggest a common environmental factor[20].

Pharmacological interventions

Numerous studies have examined the effect of drugs on the incidence and the severity of recurrent Crohn's. From a pathophysiological point of view, the metronidazole study by Rutgeerts and colleagues may be the most appealing. Patients treated with metronidazole, 10 or 20 mg per kilogram body weight per day for three months following their resection, had a significantly less-severe endoscopic stage of recurrence[21]. These results may indicate that anaerobic bacteria are involved in the initiation of Crohn's disease although metronidazole has been shown to have some immunomodulatory effect as well[22]. It is also not known whether a less-severe recurrence at 3 months predicts a milder clinical course in the years ahead. Unfortunately, the widespread use of metronidazole has been hampered by the high rate of adverse effects[21].

The role of the enteric nervous system

The question remains why Crohn's disease invariably recurs at the ileal side of the anastomosis. A possible explanation may be found in the enteric neural network. It is well known that neural inflammation is a common phenomenon in Crohn's disease[23,24]. We recently observed that the presence and the severity of 'neuritis' (both lymphocytic and eosinophilic) in the ileal section margin (*not* in the colonic margin) were predictive of severe recurrent Crohn's disease 3 months postoperatively[25]. This supports the hypothesis that the enteric nervous system may provide a network that guides intestinal inflammation. The triggering antigen could have a certain tropism for neural tissue along which inflammation could spread through the entire intestinal wall.

We conclude that the culprit in recurrent Crohn's disease is to be found in the faeces, probably linked to bacterial agents. Enhanced intestinal permeability, defective immunological downregulation with abundant cytokine production and spreading of inflammation along the neural tissue may all play an important part in the mechanisms leading to postoperative recurrence of Crohn's disease.

DISEASE PATTERNS IN POSTOPERATIVE RECURRENT CROHN'S DISEASE

The clinical presentation of recurrent Crohn's ileitis is often strikingly similar to the preoperative presentation. As early as 1971, de Dombal *et al.* suggested that there might be several subtypes of Crohn's disease: an 'indolent' one, which tends to recur slowly, and an 'aggressive' one, recurring soon after the surgical intervention[26]. These data were confirmed by a retrospective analysis by the Mount Sinai Hospitals in New York, in which patients could be classified into two subgroups: those with 'perforating' Crohn's disease (including fistulae and abscesses) and those with non-perforating or stenosing disease. Second operations for perforating indications were performed more often among cases whose surgical indication had been perforation initially. Reoperation for perforating disease was required about twice as soon for non-perforating Crohn's disease[27].

It is not only the disease behaviour but also the *length* of ileal recurrence which appears to be comparable before surgery and at the time of clinical recurrence. We studied the length of ileal inflammation on small bowel radiological studies in 23 patients before resection and at the time of symptom recurrence, and found a striking correlation between the two ($r = 0.70$, $p < 0.001$). Moreover, in 7 patients who had sequential small bowel studies without intervening surgery, the length of measured inflammation correlated with $r = 0.995$ ($p < 0.001$), which demonstrates that the extent of disease rarely changes once it is established[28].

RISK FACTORS FOR THE DEVELOPMENT OF SEVERE CROHN'S RECURRENCE: WHAT TO TELL THE PATIENTS?

Patient-related factors: age, smoking and parity

The age at the time of diagnosis of Crohn's disease does not affect the rate of postoperative recurrence. These rates are higher, however, in patients operated on at a younger age than in those undergoing resection when older[29].

The effect of cigarette smoking on the development of postoperative Crohn's recurrence has been examined thoroughly. Multiple well-designed studies have demonstrated that smoking is associated with higher recurrence rates, particularly in female patients. In a survey by Sutherland and coworkers, the need for repeat surgery at 5 and 10 years after the first intervention was significantly lower in non-smokers (20% and 41%) than in smokers (36% and 70%)[30]. Cottone *et al.* confirmed these data, with an odds ratio of 2.2 (9.5% CI 1.2–38) for endoscopic recurrence in smokers vs. non-smokers[31]. Hence, all operated patients (as well as the non-operated ones!) should be dissuaded from smoking.

Recent data have demonstrated that the need for second and third resections after the initial surgical intervention may also be influenced by the number of pregnancies[32]. The authors hypothesize that pregnancy may influence the natural history of Crohn's disease, either by decreasing immune responsiveness or by retarding fibrous stricture formation[32].

Disease-related factors: duration, location, inflammatory activity

Patients with a preoperative disease history of more than 10 years at the time of surgical intervention appear to do better than those with a shorter disease history[33]. This is in agreement with the observation that patients with 'early' recurrence had a shorter history of symptoms at operation than those with 'late' recurrence[34].

The impact of the location of the disease is also striking. Patients with combined ileocolonic disease suffer higher recurrence rates than those with isolated colonic disease[35]. Additional risk factors are related to the subtype and inflammatory activity of their Crohn's disease. Indeed, the virulence of the inflammatory activity is often comparable before and after surgery. Hence, resections should, if at all possible, be avoided if the disease appears to be clinically active.

Surgery-related factors

The recurrence rates of Crohn's disease are much lower after surgical resection with ileostomy than after resection with ileocolonic anastomosis[36–38]. Moreover, a recent review of 182 patients with an end ileostomy for Crohn's disease revealed that the site of initial Crohn's disease plays a part in the recurrence of disease in the neoterminal ileum proximal to the ileostomy: estimated overall cumulative probabilities of recurrence 20 years after the construction of the ileostomy were 64% in patients with ileocolitis as initial presentation vs. 15% in patients with colitis alone ($p < 0.001$)[38]. The number of interventions seems to be of little importance with regard to recurrence. In a Swedish study, the cumulative recurrence rates at 10 years were 65% after the second intervention vs. 60% after the third one. Again, this supports the hypothesis that disease behaviour remains unchanged throughout the patient's history. The same study reported that an ileorectal anastomosis may carry an increased risk for postoperative recurrence, up to 70% at 10 years. Two surgical techniques for the construction of an ileocolonic anastomosis have been compared and demonstrated that recurrence rates did not differ between an end-to-end anastomosis and an end-to-side anastomosis[39].

Neither the presence of granulomas in the resection specimen, nor the presence or absence of 'disease-free' resection margins (i.e. with or without inflammatory activity) have been shown to influence recurrence rates or severity[40,41]. On the other hand, the presence of neural inflammation may predict early severe endoscopic recurrence[25].

CONCLUSIONS

Although many 'prognostic factors' have been examined with regard to recurrence of Crohn's disease after surgery, only a few have been identified to really affect this process. The location of the disease in the GI tract and its inflammatory activity at the time of surgery are undoubtedly important. From a surgical point of view, an ileostomy carries lower recurrence rates than any other intervention. The only factor affecting the disease process which can be influenced by the patient and his physician is, besides perhaps medical therapy, cigarette smoking. In particular, female patients should be dissuaded from tobacco use after surgical resection for Crohn's disease.

References

1. Kyle J. Prognosis after ileal resection for Crohn's disease. Br J Surg. 1971;58:735–7.
2. Lennard-Jones JE, Stalder GA. Prognosis after resection of chronic regional enteritis. Gut. 1967;8:332–6.
3. Greenstein AJ, Sachar DB, Pasternack BS, Janowitz HD. Reoperation and recurrence in Crohn's colitis and ileocolitis. N Engl J Med. 1975;293:685–90.
4. Whelan G, Farmer RG, Fazio VW, Goormastic M. Recurrence after surgery in Crohn's disease. Gastroenterology. 1985;88:1826–33.
5. Ekberg O, Fork FT. Predictive value of small bowel radiography for recurrent Crohn's disease. AJR. 1980;135:1051–5.
6. Hildell J, Lindstrom C, Wenckert A. Radiographic appearances in Crohn's disease, IV. The new distal ileum after surgery. Acta Radiol Diagn. 1980;21:221–9.
7. Rutgeerts P, Geboes K, Vantrappen G, Beyls J, Kerremans R, Hiele M. Predictability of the postoperative course of Crohn's disease. Gastroenterology. 1990;99:956–63.
8. D'Haens G, Geboes K, Peeters M, Baert F, Pennickx F, Rutgeerts P. Early lesions of recurrent Crohn's disease caused by infusion of intestinal contents in excluded ileum. Gastroenterology. 1998;114:262–7.
9. Rutgeerts P, Geboes K, Peeters M et al. Effect of fecal stream diversion in recurrence of Crohn's disease in the neoterminal ileum. Lancet. 1991;338:771–4.
10. Harper PH, Lee ECG, Kettlewell MGW, Bennett MK, Jewell DP. Role of faecal stream in the maintenance of Crohn's colitis. Gut. 1985;26:279–84.
11. Fasoli R, Kettlewell MGW, Mortensen N, Jewell DP. Response to faecal challenge in defunctioned colonic Crohn's disease: prediction of long-term course. Br J Surg. 1990;77:616–17.
12. Dubucquoi S, Janin A, Klein O et al. Activated eosinophils and interleukin 5 expression in early recurence of Crohn's disease. Gut. 1995;37:242–6.
13. Desreumaux P, Brandt E, Gambiez L et al. Distinct cytokine patterns in early and chronic ileal lesions of Crohn's disease. Gastroenterology. 1997;113:118–26.
14. Desreumaux P, Geboes K, Gambiez L et al. Early ileal lesions of Crohn's disease are associated with the expression of IL-4 and not of inflammatory cytokines. Gastroenterology. 1998;114:A962.
15. Colgan SP, Resnick MB, Parkos CA et al. IL-4 directly modulates function of a model human intestinal epithelium. J Immunol. 1994;153:2122–9.
16. Puri RK, Siegal JP. Interleukin-4 and cancer therapy. Cancer Invest. 1993;11:473–86.
17. Favre C, Saeland S, Caux C, Duvert V, De Vries JE. Interleukin-4 has basophilic and eosinophilic cell growth-promoting activity on cord blood cells. Blood. 1990;75:67–73.
18. D'Haens G, Peeters M, Baert F et al. Increasing TNF-α and decreasing IFN-γ tissue concentrations in early recurrent Crohn's disease and correlation with endoscopic lesions. Gastroenterology. 1996;110:A894.
19. Hollander D, Vadheim CM, Brettholz E, Petersen GM, Delahunty T, Rotter JI. Increased intestinal permeability in patients with Crohn's disease and their relatives – a possible aetiological factor. Ann Intern Med. 1986;105:883–5.
20. Peeters M, Geypens B, Claus D et al. Clustering of increased small intestinal permeability in families with Crohn's disease. Gastroenterology. 1997;113:802–7.
21. Rutgeerts P, Peeters M, Hiele M et al. A placebo controlled trial of metronidazole for recurrence prevention of Crohn's disease after resection of the terminal ileum. Gastroenterology. 1995;108:1617–21.
22. Grove DI, Mahmoud AAF, Warren KS. Suppression of cell-mediated immunity by metronidazole. Int Arch Allergy Appl. Immunol. 1977;54:422–7.

23. Davis DR, Dockerty MB, Mayo CW. The myenteric plexus in regional enteritis: a study of the number of ganglion cells in the ileum in 24 cases. Surg Gynecol Obstet. 1955;101:208–16.
24. Geboes K, Rutgeerts P, Ectors N *et al.* Major histocompatibility class II expression on the small intestinal nervous system in Crohn's disease. Gastroenterology. 1992;103:439–47.
25. D'Haens G, Penninckx F, Rutgeerts P, Geboes K. The presence and severity of neural inflammation predict severe postoperative recurrence of Crohn's disease. Gastroenterology. 1998;114:A963.
26. de Dombal FT, Burton I, Goligher C. The early and late results of surgical treatment for Crohn's disease. Br J Burg. 1971;11:805–16.
27. Greenstein AJ, Lachman P, Sachar DB *et al.* Perforating and non-perforating indications for repeated operations in Crohn's disease: evidence for two clinical forms. Gut. 1988;29:588–92.
28. D'Haens G, Baert F, Gasparaitis A, Hanauer S. Length and type of recurrent ileitis after ileal resection correlate with presurgical features in Crohn's disease. Inflamm Bowel Dis. 1997;249–53.
29. Hellers G, Crohn's disease in Stockholm County 1955–1974. A study of epidemiology, results of surgical treatment and long-term prognosis. Acta Chir Scand. 1979;490(suppl.):5–81.
30. Sutherland LR, Ramcharan S, Bryant H, Fick G. Effect of cigarette smoking on recurrence of Crohn's disease. Gastroenterology. 1990;98:1123–8.
31. Cottone M, Rosselli M, Orlando A *et al.* Smoking habits and recurrence in Crohn's disease. Gastroenterology. 1994;106:643–8.
32. Nwokolo CU, Tan WC, Andrews HA, Allan RN. Surgical resections in parous patients with distal ileal and colonic Crohn's disease. Gut. 1994;35:220–3.
33. Baker WNW. The results of ileorectal anastomosis at St. Mark's Hospital from 1953 to 1968. Gut. 1970;11:235–9.
34. de Dombal FT, Burton I, Goligher JC. Recurrence of Crohn's disease after primary excisional surgery. Gut. 1971;12:519–27.
35. Sachar DB, Wolfson DM, Greenstein AJ, Goldberg J, Styczynski R, Janowitz HD. Risk factors for postoperative recurrence of Crohn's disease. Gastroenterology. 1983;85:917–21.
36. Goligher JC. The long-term results of excisional surgery for primary and recurrent Crohn's disease of the large intestine. Dis Colon Rectum. 1985;28:51–5.
37. Heimann TM, Greenstein AJ, Lewis B, Kaufman D, Heimann DM, Aufses AH. Prediction of early symptomatic recurrence after intestinal resection in Crohn's disease. Ann Surg. 1993;218:294–9.
38. Ho I, Greenstein AJ, Bodian CA, Janowitz HD. Recurrence of Crohn's disease in end ileostomies. Inflamm Bowel Dis. 1995;1:173–8.
39. Cameron JL, Hamilton SR, Coleman J, Sitzman JV, Bayless TM. Patterns of ileal recurrence in Crohn's disease. Ann Surg. 1992;215:546–51.
40. Wolfson DM, Sachar DB, Cohen A *et al.* Granulomas do not affect postoperative recurrence rates in Crohn's disease. Gastroenterology. 1982;83:405–9.
41. Kotanagi HH, Kramer K, Fazio VW, Petras RE. Do microscopic abnormalities at resection margins correlate with increased anastomotic recurrence in Crohn's disease? Retrospective analysis of 100 cases. Dis Colon Rectum. 1991;34:909–16.

25
Relapse prevention strategies in Crohn's disease

H. LOCHS

Surgical resection leads to rapid improvement of disease activity and quality of life in most patients with Crohn's disease. However relapse is a frequent and almost unavoidable event. Frequency of relapses has been demonstrated to be around 25% in the first postoperative year with a slight decrease during the next years[1,2]. However up to 80% of patients will experience a reoperation during their lifetime. Therefore relapse prevention is one of the most important therapeutic goals in these patients.

PATHOMECHANISM OF POSTOPERATIVE RELAPSE

For any relapse-preventing treatment it would of course be important to know the factors which make patients prone to have a relapse. Therefore many studies have investigated the influence of demographic, clinical and surgical factors on the frequency of postoperative relapse. Inconsistent results have been reached (Table 1). All authors had the clinical impression that they could differentiate between patients with high and patients with low risk of relapse. However, as can be seen from the table, the results were quite disappointing. Some studies found that the indication to the operation influenced the relapse rate, others found the age to be important and the preoperative course of the disease; however none of these risk factors is important enough to propose it as a selection criterion for postoperative relapse-preventing therapy. This leaves an unsatisfying situation with the only possibility to treat everybody instead of only the patients at risk, knowing that 75% of the patients would not experience a relapse during the first postoperative year without therapy and might therefore be being treated in vain. This high number of course reduces the likelihood to detect effects of postoperative treatment.

It was the group of Rutgeerts[10] who demonstrated that the first event in postoperative recurrence is the development of endoscopic lesions proximal to the anastomosis. These endoscopic changes were found very early and precede the clinical relapse by several months or even a year. Furthermore patients with

Table 1 Factors influencing postoperative recurrence in Crohn's disease

Factor	Effect on relapse rate	Study
Disease location	ileocolic higher	Whelan et al.[3]
		Raab et al.[4]
	colonic higher	Softley et al.[5]
	no influence	Lochs et al.[6]
Age	young patients	Softley et al.[5]
	higher relapse rate	Lochs et al.[6]
	no influence	Caprilli et al.[7]
Duration of disease	important	Sachar et al.[8]
		Lochs et al.[6]
Preoperative steroid intake	important	Lochs et al.[6]
Gender	important	Raab et al.[4]
	no influence	Caprilli et al.[7]
Number of anastomoses	important	Heimann et al.[9]
Fistulizing vs. stenotic	no difference	Caprilli et al.[7]
	different	Sachar et al.[8]

endoscopic relapses had a very high risk of later developing a clinical relapse, while patients without endoscopic relapses also remained in clinical remission. These endoscopic changes were therefore the best indicator of later clinical relapses. As a consequence of these studies one could use the endoscopic recurrence as a predictor of the clinical recurrence, and prevention of the endoscopic recurrence should also prevent the clinical recurrence. By using such predictive factors one could limit treatment to those patients who actually have a high risk of relapse. To our knowledge no study has yet tested this approach. Furthermore in 2 large studies on postoperative relapse the relation between endoscopic and clinical relapse was not as strong as in the study of Rutgeerts[11,12]. More data are obviously necessary to allow better selection of patients at risk.

DEFINITION OF RECURRENCE

Endoscopic recurrence, clinical recurrence and the need for reoperation have all been used as definitions of postoperative recurrence. Obviously different recurrence rates would result from these different definitions. In most studies however the clinical recurrence is used.

Despite this difficult situation several strategies have been used to prevent recurrence of CD after operation. Firstly, many studies have investigated the effect of different surgical techniques on the frequency of postoperative relapses. Secondly, different medical therapies have been investigated, and, thirdly, initiating mechanisms for postoperative relapses have been studied. This article will only deal with medical relapse prevention.

MEDICAL RELAPSE PREVENTION

Since the prevention of postoperative relapse is an urgent problem and its pathogenesis is not known, the same drugs have been used in relapse prevention as in active disease. Primarily anti-inflammatory treatment has been used to prevent relapse after operation. The basis for this strategy is the assumption that postoperative relapses are an exacerbation of continuous inflammation which is ongoing even after radical resection rather than *de novo* disease. The hypothesis for this treatment was to reduce the initial inflammatory reaction with a low dose of one of the standard drugs used for treatment of CD, as in patients after successful medical therapy of an acute phase. For this treatment, knowledge of the pathomechanisms of the postoperative relapse seems important since it might require different therapeutic strategies depending on whether relapse is an exacerbation of continuous disease or *de novo* development of disease. In the latter case initiating events could probably be prevented, avoiding the use of anti-inflammatory drugs. It has to be mentioned that there is no evidence to support the view that continuous inflammation exists in patients after radical operations. In contrast several studies showed that after radical operation there are no signs of inflammatory activity. On the other hand it could well be that the level of inflammation is too low to be detected by standard methods, and many investigators consider Crohn's disease a systemic disease which is still ongoing even if no local manifestation can be found.

Mesalazine

In relapse prevention with standard anti-inflammatory agents most experience has been accumulated with mesalazine. The advantage of this drug is that it has very few side-effects and could therefore be prescribed for long-term use. The disadvantage is the limited experience with the effect of mesalazine in Crohn's disease. While there is good evidence that mesalazine prevents a relapse in ulcerative colitis, this has not been shown in a comparable way in Crohn's disease. It appears that maintenance therapy with mesalazine after medical treatment of an active phase is effective only in a subgroup of Crohn's disease patients[4]. In a recent review on mesalazine as maintenance therapy after medical treatment, the reduction of the risk for a symptomatic relapse has been calculated as approximately 4%[17]. These data would reduce the expectations on the postoperative effect of mesalazine. However several studies have been performed to investigate the efficacy of mesalazine in postoperative Crohn's disease (Table 2).

There is a clear effect of mesalazine – better than after medical therapy – although it is still rather small with an advantage of approximately 13%[17]. This effect appears not to be dependent on the dose, since studies using 2 g/day showed a similar reduction of postoperative relapses to the study with 4 g/day. Some studies indicate[6,13] that the pharmaceutical preparation could make a difference with Salofalk® and Rowasa® being more effective in the distal intestine, while Pentasa® seems to be more effective in the small bowel.

The timepoint of the start of treatment postoperatively was quite different in the different studies, ranging from 10 days after surgery up to 8 weeks. But this also seems to have no influence on the efficacy. This is of special interest, since the endoscopic relapse occurs very early and one would expect that it is important to start therapy before this has taken place.

An interesting observation is that the effect of mesalazine becomes apparent only after more than a year with relapse rates similar to placebo during the first

Table 2 Mesalazine in postoperative Crohn's disease

Study	Patients	Follow-up (months)	Dose (g/day)	Relapse definition	Result
Caprilli et al.[11]	95	12	2, 4	Endoscopy CDAI > 150	effective
McLeod et al.[13]	163	24	3	Clinical + endoscopy/ radiology	effective
Lochs et al.[6]	308	18	4	CDAI > 200	no effect in total group, only small bowel effective
Sutherland et al.[14]	66	12	3	CDAI > 150	effective
Brignola et al.[15]	87	12	3	Endoscopy	effective
Florent et al.[16]	126	3	3	Endoscopy	no effect

postoperative year and that mesalazine does not appear to reduce the number of endoscopic relapses after operation. This could indicate that the initial event causing the relapse is not influenced by mesalazine. The effect of mesalazine might rather be prevention of the exacerbation if the disease has already recurred. In this case it would be of utmost importance to have an indicator for subclinical disease, since this would allow one to select the patients to treat with mesalazine. Lacking these data as a summary from the published studies, one can therefore conclude that treatment with mesalazine has some relapse-preventing effect in postoperative Crohn's disease; however its usefulness should be discussed since it has to be taken for a long time and the majority of patients is treated in vain.

Similarly salazosulphapyridine has been used as postoperative relapse-preventing therapy. Ewe et al.[18] report a significant effect in a 3-year study. This therapy has not been further investigated.

Immunosuppressive agents

Other anti-inflammatory drugs used for postoperative therapy are azathioprine and 6MP. Some case reports indicated that it might be effective[19] and Korelitz et al.[20] demonstrated in a recent study a reduction of the number of relapses with a low-dose treatment of 50 mg/day 6MP. Similar considerations have to be made as for mesalazine. It has however to be mentioned that in contrast to mesalazine the effect of azathioprine and 6MP in active and chronic active Crohn's disease has been well established.

Limited information exists about the effect of steroid treatment on postoperative relapse in Crohn's disease. Bergmann et al.[21] observed no reduction of postoperative relapses for 3 years after a 33-week therapy with prednisolone and salazosulphapyridine as compared to placebo. Budesonide has been used for postoperative maintenance therapy; however the results are not yet available.

Antibiotics

A completely different approach was chosen by Rutgeerts et al.[22]. In a study investigating postoperative relapses in patients with stoma vs. those with anastomosis they observed that (a) relapse is, in the majority of patients, located at the anastomosis and (b) patients with a stoma did not relapse during the observation period. They concluded therefore that the intestinal content might play an important role for the development of the postoperative relapse. In a first study they showed that patients with a stoma developed a relapse as soon as they got an anastomosis[23]. In a very elegant study they also showed that even reinfusion of the bowel contents of the proximal intestine via a catheter into the distal part of the intestine led to reappearance of Crohn's disease-specific lesions in this part[24]. They further tested whether heating, filtering or changing the pH of the reinfusate would affect the appearance of these lesions. Although the number of patients investigated was too small to draw definite conclusions these data strongly support the view that bacterial contents in the gut lumen are instrumental for the development of the postoperative relapse. An open question is, of course, why these relapses do not occur in the intestine proximal of the anastomosis, since it is constantly confronted with the same intestinal contents, which seem to lead to relapses in the distal part of the intestine. However one has to acknowledge that our understanding of the development of Crohn's disease is very limited.

A very interesting result was obtained with metronidazole. With a treatment for 3 months after an operation, the number of relapses was reduced for the following 3 years[23]. Even if that was only demonstrated in a small group of patients, this study supports the hypothesis that in the first weeks after the operation changes might happen which determine the later course of the patient. It also seems to support the importance of bacteria for the development of relapses, although metronidazole has an antibacterial as well as an immunosuppressive effect. This is certainly a concept which should be further tested.

CONCLUSION

From the data which are available by now, it has to be concluded that there is neither a convincing concept for postoperative relapse prevention in Crohn's disease nor a highly effective treatment. Obviously more studies are needed on the pathomechanism of the postoperative relapse. For the moment 5ASA and azathioprine are treatments with proven although limited efficacy.

References

1. Andrews HA, Lewis P, Allan RN. Prognosis after surgery for colonic Crohn's disease. Br J Surg. 1989;76:184–190.
2. Dirks E, Goebell H, Scharschmidt K, Förster S, Quebe-Fehling E, Eigler FW. Clinical relapse of Crohn's disease under standardized conservative treatment and after excisional surgery. Dig Dis Sci. 1989;34:1832–1840.
3 Whelan G, Fanner RG, Fazio VW, Goormastic M: Recurrence after surgery in Crohn's disease. Relationship to location of disease (clinical pattern) and surgical indication. Gastroenterology. 1985;88:1826–1833.
4. Raab Y, Bergstrom R, Ejerblad S, Graf W, Pahlman L: Factors influencing recurrence in Crohn's disease. An analysis of a consecutive series of 353 patients treated with primary surgery. Dis Colon Rectum. 1996;39:918–925.
5. Softley A, Myren J, Clamps SE, Boucier IAD, Watkinson D, de Dombal FT: Factors affecting recurrence after surgery for Crohn's disease. Scand J Gastroenterol. 1988;23:31–34.
6. Lochs H, Mayer M, Fleig, Mortensen PB, Bauer P and ECCDS VI Study Group: Prophylaxis of postoperative relapse in Crohn's disease with mesalazine (Pentasa®) in comparison to placebo. Gastroenterology. 1997;112, A1027.

7. Caprilli R, Corrao G, Taddei G, Tonelli F, Torchio P, Viscido A, Gruppo Italiano per lo Studio del Colon e del Retto: Prognostic factors for postoperative recurrence of Crohn's disease. Dis Colon Rectum. 1996;39:335–341.

8. Sachar DB, Subramani K, Mauer K, Rivera-MacMurray S, Turtel P, Bodian CA, Greenstein AJ: Patterns of postoperative recurrence in fistulizing and stenotic Crohn's disease. A retrospective cohort study of 71 patients. J Clin Gastroenterol. 1996;22:114–116.

9. Heimann TM, Greenstein AJ, Lewis B, Kaufman D, Heimann DM, Aufses AH jr: Prediction of early symptomatic recurrence after intestinal resection in Crohn's disease. Ann Surg. 1993;218:294–298.

10. Rutgeerts P, Geboes K, Vantrappen G, Beyls J, Kerremans A, Hiele M: Predictability of the postoperative course of Crohn's disease. Gastroenterology. 1990;99:956–963.

11. Caprilli R, Andreoli A, Capurso L, *et al.* Oral mesalazine (5-aminosalicylic acid; Asacol) for the prevention of post-operative recurrence of Crohn's disease. Aliment Pharmacol Ther. 1994;8:35–43.

12. McLeod RS, Wolff BG, Steinhart AH, *et al.* Risk and significance of endoscopic/radiological evidence of recurrent Crohn's disease. Gastroenterology. 1997;113:1823–1827.

13. McLeod RS, Wolff BG, Steinhart AH, *et al.* Prophylactic Mesalamine treatment decreases post-operative recurrence of Crohn's disease. Gastroenterology. 1995;109:404–413.

14. Sutherland LR, Martin F, Bailey RJ, *et al.* A randomized, placebo-controlled, double-blind trial of Mesalamine in the maintenance of remission of Crohn's disease. Gastroenterology. 1977;112:1069–1077.

15. Brignola C, Cottone M, Pera A, *et al.* Mesalamine in the prevention of endoscopic recurrence after intestinal resection of Crohn's disease. Gastroenterology. 1995;108:345–349.

16. Florent C, Cortot A, Quandale P, *et al.* Placebo-controlled clinical trial of Mesalazine in the prevention of early endoscopic recurrences after resection for Crohn's disease. Eur J Gastroenterol Hepatol. 1996;8:229–233.

17. Cammà C, Giunta M, Rosselli M, Cottone M: Mesalamine in the maintenance treatment of Crohn's disease: A meta-analysis adjusted for confounding variables. Gastroenterology. 1997;113:1465–1473.

18. Ewe K, Herfarth C, Malchow H, Jesdinsky HJ: Postoperative recurrence of Crohn's disease in relation to radicality of operation and sulfasalazine prophylaxis: A multicenter trial. Digestion. 1989;42:224–232.

19. Berrebi W, Chaussade S, Bruhl AL, Pariente A, *et al.* Treatment of Crohn's disease recurrence after ileoanal anastomosis by azathioprine. Dig Dis Sci. 1993;38:1558–1560.

20. Korelitz B, Hanauer S, Rutgeerts P, Present D, Peppercorn M: Post-operative prophylaxis with 6-MP, 5-ASA or placebo in Crohn's disease: A 2 year multicenter trial. Gastroenterology. 1988;114:4141.

21. Bergman L, Krause U: Postoperative treatment with corticosteroids and salazosulphapyridine (Salazopyrin) after radical resection for Crohn's disease. Scand J Gastroenterol. 1976;11:651–656.

22. Rutgeerts P, Hiele M, Geboes K, Peeters M, Penninckx F, Aerts R, Kerremans R: Controlled trial of Metronidazole treatment for prevention of Crohn's recurrence after ileal resection. Gastroenterology. 1995;108:1617–1621.

23. Rutgeerts P, Geboes K, Peeters M, *et al.* Effect of faecal stream diversion on recurrence of Crohn's disease in the neoterminal ileum. Lancet. 1991;338:771–774.

24. Gendre JP, Mary JY, Florent C, *et al.* Oral Mesalamine (Pentasa) as maintenance treatment in Crohn's disease: A multicenter placebo-controlled study. Gastroenterology. 1993;104:435–439.

26
Changes in prognosis for patients with inflammatory bowel disease

R. G. FARMER

Over the past fifty years, what we now refer to as inflammatory bowel diseases (IBD), ulcerative colitis and Crohn's disease, have become important chronic digestive diseases. As a result, there has been a continuous interest in the prognosis for patients with these diseases. While this is an obvious concern for physicians and patients dealing with chronic illness, the evolution of the concept of prognosis is an important factor in the assessment of the disease, its understanding, and its relationship to both the natural history of the diseases and management of them. It is the purpose of this article to review the changing prognosis for patients with IBD over the past several decades and to relate this phenomenon to our current understanding of these diseases.

Prognosis is defined by the Oxford English Dictionary[1] as being 'a recognizing beforehand, foreknowledge'. It is further defined as 'a forecast of the course and the termination of a case of disease; also the action of art of making such a forecast'[1]. Prognosis implies that the physician has an assessment of the 'natural history' of that disease and can relate this to the individual patient, and perhaps to the responses to various forms of therapy, medical and surgical.

HISTORICAL COMPARISON

Because ulcerative colitis was studied much earlier than Crohn's disease, the 'early' literature is more concerned with prognosis for patients with ulcerative colitis than with Crohn's disease. One of the first important long-term studies was published from the Mayo Clinic in 1950 by Sloan, Bargen, and Gage[2]. They reviewed 2000 patients for whom a diagnosis of ulcerative colitis had been made at the Mayo Clinic between 1918 and 1937. They observed that the mortality rate was 9% in the first year after diagnosis, that the survival rates of this entire group of patients were 71% 10 years after diagnosis and 56% 20 years after diagnosis. In other words, almost half of patients with ulcerative colitis died if they were followed for 20 years. The primary causes of death, reflecting the times, were pneumonia, emaciation and peritonitis, as well as venous thrombosis and pulmonary embolism. They were able to document that only 8 patients had died of cancer. This was a very influential paper because of: the duration of its follow up, the many other publications by Dr Bargen, and the large number and statistical analysis of these patients.

In 1963, Edwards and Truelove[3] published a series of papers on the course of prognosis in ulcerative colitis for patients seen in Oxford (UK) during the period 1938–1962 (thus giving a sequential comparison with the Bargen paper). There were 624 patients followed, and they noted that a 'severe' first attack of ulcerative colitis carried a mortality rate of 38%. A severe relapse had a mortality rate of 25%. They defined 'severity' as being the degree of diarrhoea, bleeding, fever, tachycardia, anaemia, and elevated sedimentation rate. Factors which indicated an adverse prognosis were: pancolitis, perforation of the colon, and a patient who was 'older'. In general, they observed that the overall one-year mortality rate was 16%, the ten-year mortality rate was 22%, and the twenty-year mortality rate was 40%. Thus, the mortality rate for the Oxford series was almost identical to that of the Mayo series, covering a period from 1918 to 1962.

An additional influential paper from the Mayo Clinic was by McInerney *et al.* and appeared in *Gastroenterology* in 1962[4]. This paper explored the significance of 'fulminating ulcerative colitis with marked colonic dilation' and represented an understanding of the short-term causes of death in patients with ulcerative colitis, excluding emaciation, pneumonia and pulmonary embolism. They observed 1230 patients seen at the Mayo Clinic from 1954 to 1959. There were 36 patients with dilated colon associated with ulcerative colitis (what came to be known as 'toxic megacolon'); 16 of these were observed during the first episode of colitis. It is interesting to note that the average hospital stay for these 36 patients was 49 days. Twenty-eight patients were treated medically and 5 died; 8 patients were treated surgically and 5 died. They concluded that, for patients who survived, there was 'a long and tedious post-operative convalescence'. This paper was influential since it was the largest series of toxic megacolon at the time, and also painted a very bleak picture for acute surgical intervention for such patients[4]. At the time (1960s), there was a reluctance to recommend operation, but medical therapy was only just evolving into what one could call 'modern'.

Moving ahead 30 years, a study from Stockholm on survival of patients with IBD by Persson *et al.*[5] showed that the mortality rate at 15 years was in the 6–7% range. They observed 1251 patients with Crohn's disease and 1547 patients with ulcerative colitis for whom the diagnosis had been made between 1955 and 1984 in Stockholm. The observed vs. expected survival rate at 15 years was 93.7% for Crohn's disease and 94.2% for ulcerative colitis. The causes of (related) death were colorectal cancer, respiratory diseases and alcohol-related liver disease. A similar study from Rochester, New York by Nordenholtz *et al.*[6] showed that there was a decrease in the number of deaths from Crohn's disease by 44% from the 1973–1980 period to 6% in the 1980s. In addition, colorectal cancer was a leading cause of death for patients with ulcerative colitis, 3 times as frequent as in Crohn's disease. In fact, excluding cancer, there were only 2 deaths directly due to ulcerative colitis, both in the first 2 years after diagnosis. In perhaps the most optimistic of the recent large analyses of patients with ulcerative colitis, a study from Copenhagen by Langholz, Binder, and colleagues of 1161 patients followed over 25 years (from 1962) demonstrated little or no mortality, and their concern was primarily related to the frequency and predictability of relapses[7]. They concluded that, 'although ulcerative colitis is troublesome, most patients' lives are relatively little influenced by it'.

Thus, in a period of 30 to 40 years, the mortality rate has decreased from about 40% over a 20-year period to something in the range of 5% overall; in addition, initial 'attack' mortality has decreased from 20% or so to considerably less than 5%. Obviously, much of this is related to improved therapy, both medical and surgical, but particularly in supportive therapy using antibiotics, nutritional therapy, and an understanding of the natural history of these diseases. From the perspective of the patient, the evolution of prognosis in patients with IBD has gone from mortality to quality of life.

EVOLUTION OF PROGNOSIS

Crohn's disease

Beginning in the 1960s, at the Cleveland Clinic, we began a systematic study of patients with Crohn's disease. This included an initial classification of the anatomic location of disease, which we called the 'clinical pattern'. The thesis was that location of disease was related directly to the clinical course and prognosis. The clinical patterns recognized were those of ileocolic disease (terminal ileum and proximal colon), pure small intestine involvement (predominantly ileal), and entirely confined to the colon. (This understanding did not occur until the 1960s and was a relatively new concept in the location and course of patients with Crohn's disease at the time.) In a paper published in *Gastroenterology* in 1975[8], we studied 615 patients originally diagnosed between 1966 and 1969. It was observed that the anatomic location of disease correlated with complications, indication for surgery, and prognosis. A follow-up paper the next year[9] reviewed the indications for surgery for 500 patients during approximately the same time. In Crohn's disease, it was established that complications and the need for surgery were directly correlated, and could be associated with the anatomic location. For example, patients with ileocolic disease frequently had evidence of internal fistula, generally beginning in the ileum, with development of abscess as an indication for operation (this has subsequently been referred to as 'inflammatory' or 'perforating' Crohn's disease). In contrast, patients with pure ileal disease typically had obstructive symptoms relating to inflammation and stenosis of the ileum, and these complications usually occurred later than the pure 'inflammatory' effects. Patients with colonic disease characteristically had 'systemic' manifestations, with fever, weight loss and extraintestinal manifestations[8,9].

The next step in the evolution of the understanding of prognosis was assessment of recurrence after surgery for patients with Crohn's disease, which was found to be as high as 50% if the patients were followed for 10 or 15 years[10-12]. In our subsequent follow-up of the previously described group of patients[11], we found that over 90% of patients with an ileocolic pattern of disease had required an operation during this period of time, in contrast to 58% of patients with colonic disease. About one third of patients had perianal fistulae, most characteristically associated with colonic or ileocolic disease. There was no statistical correlation between the type and duration of medical treatment and the prognosis. In the original group of 615 patients, 75 had died (12.8%); 36 of these deaths were related to the effects of Crohn's disease[11]. This led Sachar to comment in an accompanying editorial[13] that 'Crohn's disease in Cleveland was a matter of life and death'. In a subsequent follow-up study from the Cleveland Clinic[14] published in 1987, we found that 88% of patients followed for 15–25 years had undergone operation. Thus, for patients with Crohn's disease, the primary prognostic concern had evolved from mortality to recurrence requiring multiple operations.

In addition to the work at the Cleveland Clinic, others were studying the same phenomenon, including the National Cooperative Crohn's Disease Study Group[15] and those at Mt. Sinai Hospital in New York[16]. This led to a proposed classification of patient subgroups in Crohn's disease during a workshop chaired by Sachar[17] at a conference in Rome in the early 1990s, which continued the 'clinical patterns' concept[17]. More recent studies have confirmed the clinical pattern concept, from Italy[18] and Johns Hopkins in Baltimore[19], the latter emphasizing the significance of age of the patient in the long-term prognosis. Despite the significant evolution of medical and surgical therapy, there continues to be an emphasis for patients with Crohn's disease on the location of disease and the 'natural history' resulting from it. That Crohn's disease is not a homogeneous entity has been emphasized strongly by these experiences[14–19].

Ulcerative colitis

Despite the similarity with Crohn's disease, studies of ulcerative colitis have taken different forms in the past three decades. This has been partly the result of improved therapy (as also found in Crohn's disease), with significant improvement in surgical therapy (with fewer recurrences), but also the result of an increasing recognition of the significance of colorectal cancer as a complication in patients with ulcerative colitis. However, it has also been observed that the clinical pattern of patients with ulcerative colitis has changed during this time, with far more patients having distal colon ulcerative colitis (proctosigmoiditis) than was previously recognized[20]. In a study of 1116 patients from the Cleveland Clinic published in 1993[20], we observed that the primary problem in this era is that of quality of life, together with progression of disease. There was complete follow-up of these patients and it was determined that almost half had proctosigmoiditis while fewer than 40% had pancolitis. The primary thesis of this study was (as with Crohn's disease) that the clinical pattern was directly associated with the long-term prognosis; in the case of distal colon ulcerative colitis, the primary concern was that of progression of disease and the factors which might be associated with it. These were found to be: the severity of the initial clinical attack; associated extraintestinal manifestations, particularly arthritis; and younger age at the time of onset. This work followed an earlier study of patients with ulcerative proctosigmoiditis in which 359 patients were followed with 97% follow-up[21]. In that study, published in 1979, we found that progression of disease was relatively unusual, and that cancer of the colon was a rare finding for patients with proctosigmoiditis. Further, the incidence of need for operation for patients with ulcerative colitis was about half that for patients with Crohn's disease[20] and the overall prognosis was generally better than that for patients with Crohn's disease. However, a major factor in the long-term prognosis for patients with ulcerative colitis was that of the development of colorectal cancer, and we reported our retrospective experience in 1986[22]. During the ten-year period before that, and subsequent to the development of colonoscopy, endoscopic techniques to assess the potential for dysplasia and subsequent cancer were of great concern[23]. The relative frequency of cancer of the colon occurring in patients with ulcerative colitis was emphasized, and this was in contrast to its relative infrequency in Crohn's disease[24]. With the dramatic improvement in short-term mortality for patients with ulcerative colitis, the concern for long-term mortality is related primarily to the subsequent development of cancer[5,6]. An irony for patients with ulcerative colitis is that a patient whose symptoms are minimal or non-existent might be at greater risk of death than a patient who has symptoms of chronic illness. This is, of course, in contrast to patients with Crohn's disease, in which the severity of clinical illness correlates much more directly with the overall prognosis[11]. The development of surveillance programmes which are accurate in their determination of dysplasia, and the value of surgical procedures to remove the large intestine and avoid a stoma, have dominated the long-term follow-up study of patients with ulcerative colitis in recent years[5,6,20]. These studies generally relate to the observation by Binder and her colleagues[7] that ulcerative colitis can be considered primarily to be 'troublesome' at the present time.

IBD in childhood and adolescence

For patients with IBD, a significant factor is the age of onset of the disease[19]. Another Cleveland Clinic study by Michener *et al.*[25] reviewed experience with IBD in children over a 30-year period. This included 858 patients diagnosed between 1955 and 1974 and 450 between 1974 and 1984 (all under the age of 21 years). The death rate for patients in the earlier group was approximately 5% for patients with ulcerative colitis and 3% for those with Crohn's disease. For patients in the latter period, the death rate was 2.4% for those with ulcerative colitis and less than 1% for patients with Crohn's disease. However, 75% of patients with Crohn's disease and 50% of patients with ulcerative colitis had required surgery. The most significant differences in complications between the patients with ulcerative colitis and those with Crohn's disease were perianal fistulae and intestinal obstruction: frequent in Crohn's disease and rare in patients with ulcerative colitis. The most important non-gastrointestinal complication for patients with either disease was monarticular large joint arthritis. The relative severity of disease for patients with onset early in life (and particularly in the prepubertal time frame) was again emphasized[25], and is comparable with the experience at Hopkins[19]. An additional aspect of increasing concern is that of the presence of IBD among family members, with particular emphasis on children with IBD[19,26]. This work is ongoing, leading to genetic and other studies which might give clues to aetiological factors in IBD.

QUALITY OF LIFE FOR PATIENTS WITH IBD

Subsequent to the evolution of prognosis from death, operation, recurrence, clinical severity and cancer, there have been recent attempts to try to define quality of life in a systematic manner. During the National Cooperative Crohn's Disease Study (NCCDS), Best *et al.*[27] developed the Crohn's Disease Activity Index (CDAI) which attempts to define the disease activity and was primarily developed for the prediction of an adverse short-term prognosis. Despite its imperfections, the CDAI has continued to be the most widely used measure of disease activity in Crohn's disease. The CDAI is measured by the physician and is primarily concerned with the ability to predict an adverse event, or short-term clinical improvement or deterioration. Measures of quality of life by the patient are a relatively recent development, particularly in the work of Drossman *et al.*[28] and the group in Hamilton, Ontario[29]. In each of these instances, the primary focus has been on the effects of IBD and its symptoms as described by the patient, as well as the ability of the patient to give information which can be quantified. In 1992[30], we published a quality-of-life measure which attempted to assess symptoms of IBD specifically, but to correlate this with other aspects of the life of the patient, so that a more global assessment could be made. We developed a 47-question instrument which could be given by non-physicians and could be in a written or verbal form, and would require only about 20 minutes for the patient to complete.

The four categories which we assessed were:

1. The functional status of the patient and the ability to be productive economically;
2. The 'social' and recreational aspects of the life of a patient, including personal and family relationships;
3. The general effect and the attitude regarding life by the patient; and
4. The medical symptoms.

These studies were carried out with a group of 164 ambulatory patients; other instruments were used for comparison and validation studies were carried out. Subsequently, an additional 1-year follow-up for the same patients was completed. There were 18 questions which had the greatest statistical validity. These included such items as: the attitude of the patient with regard to comparison with others; the short-term daily symptoms; and the long-term outlook of the patient, indicated as optimism or pessimism for the future[30]. In a recent review article[31], we reiterated that, 'health-related quality of life encompasses the areas of physical function, somatic sensation, psychological state and social interactions that are affected by one's health status'. It is anticipated that further studies attempting to reference and quantify quality of life will continue and should be helpful in assessing both the results of medical and surgical therapy and the attitude of the patient on a short- and long-term basis.

HOW TO ASSESS THE PROGNOSIS

In order to assess the prognosis for patients with IBD, it is necessary to recognize the historical evolution of the concept of prognosis in IBD, and to try to equate the current status of the patient with what has happened previously as well as what might happen in the future based on knowledge of natural history studies. Rather than using survival rates or treating IBD as if it were cancer or a more frequently potentially fatal disease, it is important to recognize that quality of life has become the most important prognostic feature for patients with IBD[31]. Any assessment of quality must take into account global aspects of health and life, rather than simply assessing the specific medical complications[30]. Input from the patient is an essential feature despite the subjectivity of this information.

Tables 1 and 2 illustrate which aspects of prognosis have changed and why they have changed over the past several decades. Understanding of these phenomena can be useful in interpreting articles from the medical literature, as attempts to study the natural history for patients with IBD often require decades-long studies, which can usually be accomplished only in centres in which large numbers of IBD patients are followed. Because of this, there has been a tendency to emphasize adverse complications and those which might require medical or surgical intervention. Recognition of the evolution of the concept of prognosis has been evident in studies of responses to specific medications, and particularly controlled clinical trials. Despite the imperfections of the instruments available, there continues to be considerable reliance on such information and it stands to reason that improved instruments will be forthcoming as more experience from multiple centres is acquired.

On a practical clinical basis, however, there is invariably an attempt by the physician to assess the prognosis for each patient observed (usually in an ambulatory status) and this is usually considered to be 'clinical judgement'. However, quantification of the subjective opinions by the physician and

Table 1 What aspects of prognosis have changed?

Death
  Toxic megacolon

Prolonged morbidity
  Sepsis and malnutrition

Cancer surveillance/colonoscopy
  More accurate diagnosis
  Pathology
  Endoscopy
  Scanning/imaging

Table 2 Why prognosis has changed over time

Antibiotics

Nutritional support

Surgical techniques

Medical therapy
  5-ASA agents
  Immunosuppressives
  Steroids

Table 3 Factors in the prognosis for patients with IBD

1. Time from symptoms to diagnosis
2. Age at onset: childhood, prepubertal, adolescence, adult
3. Severity of onset: acute, insidious
4. Location of disease: proctitis, pancolitis, ileitis, ileocolitis, colitis
5. Symptoms: diarrhoea, bleeding, pain, weight loss, fever, arthritis
6. Duration of disease and complications: chronicity, fistulae, obstruction, etc.
7. Dysplasia/cancer
8. Medical therapy and response: type, duration, side-effects
9. Surgery: type, frequency, amount resected, recurrence
10. Quality of life

observation by the patient can be helpful, and hopefully reliable, in assessing the prognosis for the individual patient as well as putting it in the context of prognosis for patients with similar circumstances generally. Table 3 lists ten elements which can be considered to be factors for the prognosis of patients with IBD. These can be utilized, albeit quickly, by the physician in virtually every patient encountered if these clinical factors are utilized from the perspective of the physician and coupled with the subjective symptoms and observations of the patients. Using these factors, it is possible to obtain a clearer view of the prognosis for patients with IBD. One of the paradoxes of prognostic assessment is the contrast between short-term prognosis and long-term prognosis. In diseases characterized by unpredictable exacerbations, a patient may be quite concerned about the short-term prognosis (i.e. a recurrence of symptoms) and needs to be reassured that the long-term prognosis is favourable (if such is the case). Likewise, response to therapy and the assessment by both patient and physician of its efficacy, may also suffer from this same paradox and is complicated by the need to quantify qualitative information for both short- and long-term prognosis.

In summary, it has been learned over the past three decades that IBD does not represent a homogeneous condition, and, as a result, the assessment of prognosis is not homogeneous or universal either. The evolution from a life-and-death concern to a quality-of-life concern has been the most important single evolution of the concept of prognosis over the last few decades for patients with IBD. However, the ability to assess the effects of various ramifications of the diseases on the patient, and to assess the results of medical and surgical therapy continue to be major and evolving concerns. Continued development of the processes for assessment of prognosis can be helpful both to physicians in their understanding and measurement of the activity of these diseases and to patients in helping to objectify the symptoms and other subjective findings. While there is a tendency to believe that medical progress in the treatment of patients with IBD has been largely the result of diagnostic and medical and surgical therapeutic improvements, there has also been a considerable improvement in our understanding of the prognosis for patients with IBD over recent decades. Since these diseases are relatively frequent and chronic, accurate and scientific assessment of all facets of care of patients with IBD will enable better understanding of the prognosis as well as an improved response and better outcome for patients.

References

1. The compact edition of the Oxford English Dictionary. Oxford: Oxford University Press; 1971.
2. Sloan WP, Bargen, JA, Gage RP. Life histories of patients with chronic ulcerative colitis. A review of 2000 cases. Gastroenterology. 1950;16:25–38.
3. Edwards FC, Truelove SC. The course and prognosis of ulcerative colitis. Gut. 1963;4:299–315.
4. McInerney GT, Sauer WG, Baggenstoss AH *et al.* Fulminating ulcerative colitis with marked colonic dilation; A clinical pathologic study. Gastroenterology. 1962;42:244–58.
5. Persson PG, Bernell O, Leijonmarck CE *et al.* Survival and cause specific mortality and inflammatory bowel disease; A population-based cohort study. Gastroenterology. 1966;110:1339–45.
6. Nordenholtz KE, Stowe SP, Stormont JM *et al.* The cause of death in inflammatory bowel disease; A comparison of death certificates and hospital charts in Rochester, NY. Am J Gastroenterol. 1995;90:927–32.
7. Langholz E, Munkholm T, Davidsen M, Binder V. Course of ulcerative colitis; Analysis of changes and disease activity over years. Gastroenterology. 1994;107:3–11.
8. Farmer RG, Hawk WA, Turnbull RB. Clinical patterns of Crohn's disease: a statistical study of 615 cases. Gastroenterology. 1975;68:627–35.
9. Farmer RG, Hawk WA, Turnbull RB. Indications for surgery in Crohn's disease; an analysis of 500 cases. Gastroenterology. 1976;71:245–50.
10. Lock MR, Farmer RG, Fazio VW *et al.* Recurrence and reoperation for Crohn's disease: The role of disease location in prognosis. N Engl J Med. 1981;304:1585–8.
11. Farmer RG, Whelan G, Fazio VW. Long-term follow-up of patients with Crohn's disease. Gastroenterology. 1985;88:1825–33.
12. Whelan G, Farmer RG, Fazio VW, Goormastic M. Recurrence after surgery in Crohn's disease. Gastroenterology. 1985;88:1818–25.
13. Sachar DB. Crohn's disease in Cleveland: A matter of life and death. Gastroenterology. 1985;88:1996–8.
14. Harper PH, Fazio VW, Lavery IC *et al.* The long-term outcome of Crohn's disease. Dis Col Rectum. 1987;30:174–9.
15. Mekhjian HS, Switz DM, Melnyk CS *et al.* Clinical features and natural history of Crohn's disease (National Cooperative Crohn's Disease Study). Gastroenterology. 1979;77:898–906.
16. Greenstein AJ, Lachman P, Sachar DB *et al.* Perforating and non-perforating indications for repeated operations in Crohn's disease; Evidence for two clinical forms. Gut. 1988;29:588–92.
17. Sachar DB, Andrews HA, Farmer RG *et al.* Proposed classification of patient subgroups in Crohn's disease. Gastroenterol Int. 1992;5:141–54.
18. Perri F, Annese V, Napolitano G *et al.* Subgroups of patients with Crohn's disease have different clinical outcomes. Inflam Bowel Dis. 1996;2:1–5.
19. Polito JM, Childs B, Mellits ED *et al.* Crohn's disease: Influence of age at diagnosis on site and clinical type of disease. Gastroenterology. 1996;111:580–6.
20. Farmer RG, Easley KA, Rankin GB. Clinical patterns, natural history, and progression of ulcerative colitis: A long-term follow-up of 1116 patients. Dig Dis Sci. 1993;38:1117–46.
21. Farmer RG. Long-term prognosis for patients with ulcerative proctosigmoiditis (ulcerative colitis confined to the rectum and sigmoid colon). J Clin Gastroenterol. 1979;5:47–50.
22. Mir-Madjlessi H, Farmer RG, Easely KA, Beck GJ. Colorectal and extracolonic malignancy in ulcerative colitis. Cancer. 1986;58:1569–74.
23. Rosenstock E, Farmer RG, Petras R *et al.* Surveillance for colonic carcinoma in ulcerative colitis. Gastroenterology. 1985;89:1342–6.
24. Petras RE, Mir-Madjlessi SH, Farmer RG. Crohn's disease and intestinal carcinoma: a report of 11 cases with emphasis on associated epithelial dysplasia. Gastroenterology. 1987;93:1307–14.
25. Michener WM, Caulfield M, Wyllie R, Farmer RG. Management of inflammatory bowel disease: 30 years of experience. Cleveland Clin J Med. 1990;57:685–91.
26. Farmer RG, Michener WM. Association of inflammatory bowel disease in families. Front Gastroenterol. Res. 1986;11:17–26.
27. Best WR, Becktel MR, Singleton JW. Rederived values of the Crohn's Disease Activity Index (CDAI). Gastroenterology. 1979;77:843–6.
28. Drossman DA, Patrick DL, Mitchell CM *et al.* Health-related quality of life in inflammatory bowel disease: Functional status and patient worries and concern. Dig Dis Sci. 1989;34:1379–86.

29. Guyatt G, Mitchell A, Irvine EJ *et al.* A new measure of health status for clinical trials in inflammatory bowel disease. Gastroenterology. 1989;96:804–10.
30. Farmer RG, Easley KA, Farmer JM. Quality of life assessment by patients with inflammatory bowel disease. Cleveland Clin J Med. 1992;59:35–42.
31. Eisen GM, Farmer RG. Health-related quality of life in inflammatory bowel disease. Pharmacol. Econ. 1996;10:327–35.

Section VII
IBD: A systemic disease

27
Trefoil peptides and inflammatory bowel disease

D. K. PODOLSKY

The integrity of the mucosal barrier is critical to sustaining normal intestinal tract function. A continuous layer of epithelial cells is the central constituent forming this barrier. Over the past few years, substantial progress has been made in defining the structural features present in epithelial cells themselves which contribute to this barrier. These encompass a complex of proteins that form the tight junctions that demarcate apical and basolateral surfaces. These proteins include ZO-1, ZO-2 and occludin. Tight junctions and the other related components that collectively form the junctional complex are dynamic and subject to a variety of regulatory influences. As a result, permeability from the lumen to the paracellular space is modulated through signalling pathways that regulate the actinmyosin ring present in the apical pole of the cell.

Whether there are alterations in the structural features of this cellular apparatus forming the epithelial barrier or its regulation in inflammatory bowel disease remains to be determined. Thus a rigorous study of the expression of ZO-1, ZO-2 and occludin as well as other proteins that participate in the formation of junctional complexes in association with inflammatory bowel diseases would be appropriate. It will also be of interest to determine whether expression or function of these proteins are modulated by therapeutic agents.

Recent studies have provided evidence that the integrity of the intestinal mucosa is also dependent on secreted proteins present on the lumenal surface which comprise the true interface between the lumen and mucosa. Mucin glycoproteins are secreted by goblet cells (and perhaps to a lesser extent other epithelial cells). The functional roles of these large heterogeneous glycoproteins remain uncertain, though they may contribute to barrier function as well as lubrication through their ability to form a viscoelastic gel. Previous work has demonstrated alterations in the content and composition of mucin glycoproteins in patients with ulcerative colitis, though the functional importance of these changes has not been clarified.

In the last few years, new insights into the composition of this pre-epithelial compartment have emerged. In addition to the mucin glycoproteins that have long been known to be present in a continuous gel, members of a family of small proteins, designated trefoil peptides, have more recently been recognized to be present in high concentrations throughout the gastrointestinal tract[1–7]. These peptides, designated pS2, SP and ITF, have been highly conserved through mammalian evolution and they are expressed throughout the gastrointestinal tract in a regional selective manner. These peptides are characterized by the presence of a distinctive motif of six cysteine residues. Intrachain disulphide bonding results in three loops that assume a highly compact structure that may form a ligand-binding pocket. These structural features presumably also confer the protease resistance that enables them to persist structurally and functionally intact after secretion onto the mucosal surface despite exposure to the large variety of lumenal digestive and bacterial proteases that they encounter. It appears that the trefoil peptides interact directly with mucin glycoproteins, the other major product of the goblet cell population (or their counterparts)[7,8]. Although its nature remains to be determined, this interaction may contribute to enhanced viscosity and gel formation. In the stomach, the trefoil peptides substantially enhance the barrier, preventing lumenal acid from penetrating to the epithelial surface[9].

In-vitro studies provide evidence that the trefoil peptides serve to significantly enhance mucosal resistance to injury[8]. Thus, addition of trefoil peptides to the apical surface enables monolayers of model intestinal epithelial cell lines to withstand exposure from a variety of otherwise lethal insults. The latter include bacterial toxins and chemical agents (e.g. *Clostridium difficile* toxin A and ethanol, respectively). In conjunction with the epithelial contributions to the mucosal barrier, trefoil peptides in the pre-epithelial compartment ensure an effective mucosal barrier that prevents penetration of toxic and injurious agents which are present in the lumen. While the presence of a complex mucosal immune system within the lamina propria to which the epithelium is functionally linked is an essential backstop to the mucosal barrier, the barrier is the fundamental basis of mucosal protection.

A variety of data demonstrates that intrinsic alterations in the epithelial barrier can underlie chronic inflammation, perhaps a reflection, in some instances, of recurring injury due to impaired repair (see below). Thus chronic colitis has been observed in mutant murine lines with defects in intestinal epithelial function and presumably barrier integrity, e.g. chimeric mice expressing dominant-negative N-cadherin and trefoil-deficient mice[10]. In man, administration of non-metabolizable markers has suggested that patients with Crohn's disease may harbour an intrinsic defect in barrier function as reflected by increased permeability of these markers[11–13]. The report of comparable increases in some seemingly unaffected first-degree relatives suggests that this altered permeability may reflect genetically determined components of barrier function. Although the validity of these methodological approaches and interpretation of their results may be challenged, they suggest that inflammatory activity in this major form of IBD may be driven by inappropriate penetration of antigenic and pro-inflammatory factors through the mucosal barrier. However, as noted, comprehensive, rigorous assessment of expression and function of the several proteins that compose the structures that form the barrier has not yet been performed. Thus assessment of key components, including ZO-1, ZO-2 and cingulin, and their collective interaction with other cellular structural proteins as well as cadherins and relevant integrins in association with IBD are important goals for further studies.

Delineation of the factors and mechanisms that provide an effective mucosal barrier provides a basis to consider the processes which re-establish the continuity and functional integrity of the mucosa after damage in the context of inflammatory bowel disease as well as many other disorders of the gastrointestinal tract. As an understanding of the mediators which eventuate in tissue injury and the resulting clinical manifestations is increasingly refined, the central importance of repair processes which enable reconstitution of mucosal architecture in achieving clinical remission is evident. Most important is the restoration of surface epithelial continuity and re-establishment of the integrity of the mucosal barrier after ulceration. This is fundamentally achieved initially through restitution, the rapid spreading and migration of cells from the ulceration margin to cover the denuded mucosal surface[14]. This process allows resurfacing of very large areas of mucosal ulceration within several hours to a few days independent of cell proliferation. It is clear that this process is modulated by a variety of influences, including the composition of the underlying extracellular matrix and available metabolic substrate[15]. Importantly, this process is also significantly regulated through the aggregate effects of a variety of cytokines and peptide growth factors which bind receptors present on the basolateral surface of the epithelial cells[15–19]. These include interleukins 1, 2, and 15, interferon, FGFs, EGF family members HGF and TGF-β. TGF-β may be especially pivotal given that the pro-restitution effects of other cytokines and growth factors appear to act through a TGF-β-dependent mechanism in *in-vitro* model systems.

Recently, a variety of experimental approaches has underscored the complementary role of the family of trefoil peptides in promoting healing after mucosal injury. As noted, the highly protease-resistant peptides are secreted onto the mucosal surface by goblet cells or their equivalents. Functional effects may depend upon biophysical interaction with mucin glycoproteins though recent studies have demonstrated a characteristic sequence of intracellular signalling events after exposure to trefoil peptides including activation of the MAP kinase pathway which implies the potential presence of trefoil peptide specific cell surface receptors[20,21]. However, it should be noted that definitive proof of the presence of signal-transducing trefoil receptors has not yet been obtained.

Most importantly, these factors both protect epithelium from injury and promote repair through restitution after injury has occurred[22–26]. Targeted deletion of the gene encoding ITF, normally expressed throughout the small intestine and colon, results in exquisite sensitivity to colonic injury by standard agents (e.g. dextran sodium sulphate) due to an inability to repair the epithelium[23]. These observations demonstrate that deficiencies of epithelial repair mechanisms can underlie the development of 'IBD' after a focal insult. Replacement of ITF in deficient animals can reconstitute normal intestinal healing and addition of exogenous trefoil peptides can promote healing in the gastrointestinal tract of normal animals after injury as demonstrated in studies utilizing the acetic acid colitis model.

It is apparent that the pro-healing effects of trefoil peptides are active in patients with IBD. Previous work has demonstrated intense upregulation of all three peptides in immediate proximity to sites of focal ulceration in patients with

Crohn's disease[26,27]. The mechanism of this induction is uncertain given the inability to demonstrate significant regulation by cytokines or other inflammatory mediators (exclusive of neuropeptides) in model cell lines. It is possible that the peptides are the inherent distinguishing products of the reparative epithelium which emerges at sites of injury and approximating stem cells. Recent evidence suggests that trefoil peptides may be produced by committed stem cells with suppression in all lineages, other than goblet cells, during terminal differentiation. The coordinate induction at sites of ulceration of all trefoil peptide genes which are contiguous in the genome may reflect the ability of trefoil peptides to crossregulate their expression, as recently demonstrated in this laboratory[28]. Thus, addition of one trefoil peptide to model cell lines results in increased expression of the other members of the family, as well as autocrine induction of the trefoil peptide used to stimulate the cell. These observations are also compatible with observed modest reduction in expression of the other trefoil peptides (especially SP) in ITF-deficient mice, further suggesting that the ability of trefoil peptides to cross-regulate coordinate expression of all family members observed *in-vitro* reflects functional integration *in-vivo*. These findings are also consistent with histopathological observations in man, especially in association with inflammatory bowel disease. Thus, regardless of the molecular mechanism responsible for 'ectopic' induction of trefoil peptide expression, it is clear that these factors are dominant products of the phenotypically distinct epithelial cells that emerge at the edges of sites of ulceration in patients with Crohn's disease as well as other disorders which involve gastrointestinal tract ulceration. Immunohistochemical analysis has demonstrated the presence of all three trefoil peptides in reparative epithelium adjacent to mucosal ulcers associated with Crohn's disease distally, and peptic ulcer disease proximally[26,27.29,30]. It is notable that these same cells also apparently contain substantial concentrations of growth factors of the EGF family. These cells are functionally constituted to promote repair after mucosal injury.

Mucosa of patients with active ulcerative colitis, in contrast to Crohn's disease, is significantly depleted of trefoil peptide without corresponding induction of expression. This may represent a key functional deficit associated with goblet-cell depletion, a histological feature which has been long recognized as a hallmark of UC. In contrast to the observed changes in patients with Crohn's disease, it is of interest that there does not appear to be associated induction of the other trefoil peptides not normally expressed in the colon. In this sense, the ulcerative colitis may be analogous to the phenotype observed in the ITF-deficient mouse. Thus, there is an apparent dichotomy between Crohn's disease and ulcerative colitis with induction of trefoil peptides in the former and depletion of trefoil peptides in the latter. These observations suggest that reparative potential may represent a plane of mechanistic divergence between the two major forms of inflammatory bowel disease. Of note, significant IITF content is present in the mucosa of patients during periods of quiescent disease. Detailed study of ITF expression in UC patients is needed to determine whether there are intrinsic defects in ITF expression in these patients. Extrapolation from *in-vitro* and *in-vivo* models suggests that trefoil peptides could promote the restoration of mucosal integrity, enabling ultimate control of self-perpetuating inflammation.

Acknowledgements

Studies described in this chapter were supported by grants from the National Institutes of Health (P30-DK43551 and R01-DK46906).

References

1. Thim L. A new family of growth factor-like peptides. FEBS Lett. 1989;250(1):85–90.
2. Sands BE, Podolsky DK. The trefoil peptide family. Annu Rev Physiol. 1996;58:253–73.
3. Suemori S, Lynch-Devaney K, Podolsky DK. Identification and characterization of rat intestinal trefoil factor: Tissue- and cell-specific member of the trefoil protein family. Proc Natl Acad Sci USA 1991;88:11017–21.
4. Podolsky DK, Lynch-Devaney K, Stow J et al. Identification of human intestinal trefoil factor: Goblet cell specific expression of a peptide targeted for apical secretion. J Biol Chem. 1993;268(16):6694–702.
5. Poulsom R, Wright NA. Trefoil peptides: A newly recognized family of epithelial mucin-associated molecules. Am J Physiol. 1993;28:G205–13.
6. Lefebvre O, Wolf C, Kédinger M et al. The mouse one P-domain (pS2) and two P-domain (mSP) genes exhibit distinct patterns of expression. J Cell Biol. 1993;122(1):191–8.
7. Tomasetto C, Rio MC, Gautier C et al. hSP, the domain-duplicated homolog of pS2 protein is co-expressed with pS2 in stomach but not in breast carcinoma. EMBO J. 1990;9(2):407–14.
8. Kindon H, Pothoulakis H, Thim L, Lynch-Devaney K, Podolsky DK. Trefoil peptide protection of intestinal epithelial barrier function: cooperative interaction with mucin glycoprotein. Gastroenterology. 1995;109(2):516–23.
9. Tanaka S, Podolsky DK, Engel E, Guth PH, Kaunitz JD. Human spasmolytic polypeptide decreases proton permeation through gastric mucus in vivo and in vitro. Am J Physiol. 1997;35(6):G1473–80.
10. Hermiston ML, Gordon JI. Inflammatory bowel disease and adenomas in mice expressing a dominant negative n-cadherin. Science. 1995;270:1203–7.
11. Bjarnason I, MacPherson A, Hollander D. Intestinal permeability: An overview. Gastroenterology. 1995;108:1566–81.
12. Hollander D. Permeability in Crohn's disease: Altered barrier functions in healthy relatives? Gastroenterology. 1993;104:1848–73.
13. Katz KD, Hollander D, Vadheim CM et al. Intestinal permeability in patients with Crohn's disease and their healthy relatives. Gastroenterology. 1989;97:927–31.
14. Dieckgraefe BK, Stenson WF, Alpers DH. Gastrointestinal epithelial response to injury. Curr Opin Gastroenterol. 1996;12:109–14.
15. Göke MN, Zuk A, Podolsky DK. Regulation and function of extracellular matrix in intestinal epithelial restitution in vitro. Am J Physiol. 1997;271:G279–G740.
16. Dignass A, Podolsky DK. Cytokine modulation of intestinal epithelial cell restitution: Central role of transforming growth factor ϑ. Gastroenterology. 1993;105:1323–32.
17. Dignass A, Lynch-Devaney K, Podolsky DK. Hepatocyte growth factor/scatter factor modulates intestinal epithelial cell proliferation and migration. Biochem Biophys Res Commun. 1994;202(2):701–9.
18. Dignass A, Tsunekawa S, Podolsky DK. Fibroblast growth factors modulate intestinal epithelial cell growth and migration. Gastroenterology. 1994;106(5):1254–62.
19. Ciacci C, Lind SE, Podolsky DK. Transforming growth factor α regulation of migration in wounded rat intestinal epithelial monolayers. Gastroenterology. 1993;105(1):93–101.
20. Kanai M, Mullen C, Podolsky DK. Intestinal trefoil factor induces inactivation of extracellular signal-regulated protein kinase in intestinal epithelial cells. Proc Natl Acad Sci USA. 1998;95:178–82.
21. Taupin et al. MS submitted.
22. Dignass A, Lynch-Devaney K, Kindon H, Thim L, Podolsky DK. Trefoil peptides promote epithelial migration through a TGFβ-independent pathway. J Clin Invest. 1994;94:376–83.
23. Mashimo H, Wu DC, Podolsky DK, Fishman MC. Impaired defense of intestinal mucosa in mice lacking intestinal trefoil factor. Science. 1996;274:262–5.
24. Plaut AG. Trefoil peptides in the defense of the gastrointestinal tract. N Engl J Med. 1997;336(7):506–7.

25. Babyatsky MW, deBeaumont M, Thim L, Podolsky DK. Oral trefoil peptides protect against ethanol- and indomethacin-induced gastric injury in rats. Gastroenterology. 1996;110(2):489–97.
26. Playford RJ, Marchbank T, Chinery R *et al*. Human spasmolytic polypeptide is a cytoprotective agent that stimulates cell migration. Gastroenterology. 1995;108:108–16.
27. Rio MC, Chenard MP, Wolf C *et al*. Induction of pS2 and hSP genes as markers of mucosal ulceration of the digestive tract. Gastroenterology. 1991;100:375–9.
28. Taupin, Podolsky. MS submitted.
29. Wright NA, Poulsom R, Stamp G *et al*. Trefoil peptide gene expression in gastrointestinal epithelial cells in inflammatory bowel disease. Gastroenterology. 1993;104:12–20.
30. Alison MR, Chinery R, Poulsom R, Ashwood P, Longcroft JM, Wright NA. Experimental ulceration leads to sequential expression of spasmolytic polypeptide, intestinal trefoil factor, epidermal growth factor and transforming growth factor alpha mRNAs in rat stomach. J Pathol. 1995;175:405–14.

28
Functional neuroimmune interactions in IBD and their therapeutic implications

S. M. COLLINS, B. QIU and F. GALEAZZI

INTRODUCTION AND BACKGROUND

Ulcerative colitis was once considered a primary example of a psychosomatic disorder and much emphasis was placed on the role of stress in its clinical expression. Nerves were thus considered important in its pathogenesis, resulting even in the development of surgical denervation approaches to the management of refractory cases! Since the advent of anti-inflammatory therapy, the role of nerves in the pathogenesis of UC has received much less attention, with the current focus being on immune-driven inflammation, genetic susceptibility at loci responsible for immune regulation, and growing interest in the role of bacteria as triggers for the clinical expression of the disease. This stems from clear evidence in animal models that animals genetically susceptible to colitis do not express it if maintained in germ-free environments.

Recent work in the field of irritable bowel syndrome (IBS) has provided a basis for reconsidering linkages between behaviour and inflammation. About 30% of patients develop IBS following an enteric infection. A recent study suggested that patients who were stressed during the 6 months prior to the enteric infection were more likely to develop IBS[1]. This is supported by an animal study in which prior stress in rats enhanced the colitis induced by trinitrobenzene sulphonic acid[2].

The field of neuroimmunology has blossomed over recent years, based on increasingly common demonstrations of functionally active receptors for neuropeptides on immune and inflammatory cells[3] and the juxtapositioning of nerves and immune or inflammatory cells[4]. Thus, there is a clearly defined infrastructure that permits neuroimmune interactions. While it is well known that immune cell products alter neural function[5-7], it is becoming increasingly recognized that neurotransmitters alter immune cell function so that a bidirectional communication can be invoked.

OBSERVATIONS SUGGESTING NEUROMODULATION OF INFLAMMATION IN HUMAN IBD

The observation that cigarette smoking is beneficial in ulcerative colitis, yet deleterious in Crohn's disease, is suggestive of the notion that nicotinic nerves have both positive and negative effects on inflammatory processes in the gut. Quitting smoking is a risk factor for the development or exacerbation of UC and this beneficial effect is also associated with the use of nicotine in UC. Taken at face value, these observations suggest that the beneficial effect of smoking in UC is mediated via nicotine receptors and can thus be construed as an example of neuromodulation of colitis. In contrast, smoking is an acknowledged risk factor in Crohn's disease where it is associated with more aggressive and recurrent disease.

Certain therapeutic agents, such as the α-adrenergic agonist clonidine, have been shown to be of benefit in some patients with ulcerative colitis and this suggests that the sympathetic component of the autonomic nervous system also modulates inflammation in the gut. It is also known that there is an imbalance of the autonomic nervous system in IBD, in both Crohn's disease and ulcerative colitis[8,9]. Could it be that this imbalance might predict those who will respond, positively or negatively, to agents that modulate the autonomic nervous system, including nicotine, smoking and sympathomimetic drugs?

The apparent benefit obtained by intrarectal administration of lidocaine may also be construed as evidence of neuromodulation of the inflammatory process in ulcerative colitis[10]. Taken at face value, these data suggest that afferent nerves play a role in UC. As the patients used in that study had distal diseases and some had painful proctitis, it is possible that symptom relief altered autonomic, particularly sympathetic, outflow and this could have had a bearing on the underlying mechanism. The alternative is that afferent nerves have a proinflammatory effect and certainly this is the case with one sensory transmitter, substance P. By dampening afferent nerves, it is possible that the release of substance P is attenuated with resulting improvement in colitis. Studies by Mantyh *et al.* have shown an increase in substance P binding sites on lymphoid and vascular tissue in the gut. If these observations reflect increased substance-P-mediated activity, it would suggest actions on immune cells, blood flow and might perhaps implicate neurogenic inflammation. This process involves the antidromic release of substance P from sensory nerves, acting on postcapillary venules to cause plasma extravasation and the onset of tissue inflammation.

What about stress and colitis? In this author's experience, stressful life events do seem to be temporally corelated with clinical relapses of IBD yet the literature is ambivalent on this point. There are as many studies that suggest a positive relationship as there are that do not. Theoretically, stress has a number of effects on gut function including motor activity, mucus production and blood flow, not to mention the growing evidence that stress alters immune cell function. Thus, it is perhaps surprising that the clinical literature on the relationship between stress and IBD is so weak.

Finally, there is some very exciting recent evidence suggesting that the involvement of nerves in the inflammatory process may be a predictor of relapse of Crohn's disease. Studies by D'Haens *et al.* have shown that the presence of neuritis or ganglionitis in the myenteric plexus of the resected margin of surgical specimens of Crohn's disease is positively correlated with the development of endoscopically evident relapse at 3 months postoperatively[11]. It is important to emphasize that the mucosal compartment of these specimens was free from inflammation. If confirmed, these exciting preliminary data support the notion that nerves may play a more active role in the inflammatory process of IBD than was previously suspected.

ANIMAL STUDIES

Involvement of the autonomic nervous system

Studies of the effect of chemical sympathectomy in rats with colitis induced by trinitrobenzene sulphonic acid (TNBS) reveal an exacerbation of colitis, indicating a protective effect of sympathetic neurotransmission[12]. This would be consistent with the clinical observation that the α-adrenergic agonist clonidine may confer benefit in UC[13]. Studies in our laboratory have looked at colitis induced by DNBS in rats exposed to first-hand cigarette smoke using a specialized chamber[14]. In these studies, exposure to cigarette smoke was accompanied by a worsening of the colitis. This was not seen in rats exposed to the sham smoking protocol. The effect of cigarette smoke could be blocked by hexamethonium, suggesting the involvement of nicotinic receptors and autonomic neural transmission. In a separate study in our laboratory, we gave nicotine dissolved in the drinking water to rats with TNBS-induced colitis. Nicotine was present prior to and during the colitis[15]. At low concentrations (<50 μg/ml) nicotine reduced the severity of the colitis and the effect could be blocked by hexamethonium. Interestingly, at higher concentrations of nicotine, the colitis was exacerbated. This probably reflects the fact that, at high doses, nicotine inhibits its own receptor. It may be that the deleterious effect of smoking in our study reflects autoinhibition of the nicotine receptor, although we did not use particularly high levels of cigarette smoke.

Sensory nerves and their neurotransmitters

Evidence that sensory nerves may be protective in intestinal inflammation is based on demonstrations that ablation of primary afferents using capsaicin results in marked worsening of experimental colitis[12,16]. This implies either that the circuitry, of which afferent nerves are a part, is in itself protective (e.g. via changes in mucosal blood flow) and contains neurotransmitters that exert anti-inflammatory properties, such as CGRP, or that it is the removal of substance P which is critical. There is evidence that CGRP is anti-inflammatory in the DNBS colitis model and that using a CGRP antagonist worsens colitis[17]. In contrast, using substance P antagonists improves colitis. Thus, substance P is pro-inflammatory in every system tested including the gut. Neutral endopeptidase degrades substance P and bradykinin, two important mediators of neurogenic inflammation. Transgenic mice lacking the NEP-encoding gene have recently been shown to be more susceptible to DNBS-induced colitis and develop a greater degree of inflammation which lasts longer than in NEP-expressing mice[18].

The relationship between stress and experimental colitis

It has been shown that when animals are exposed to restraint stress *prior* to the induction of colitis by TNB, there is an increased inflammatory response. In contrast, when stress was applied simultaneously with the induction of colitis, no change in the colitis was seen[2]. These findings indicate that the timing of stress in relation to the induction of colitis is important in determining the severity of colitis. Clinically, this may be reflected in the observation made by some patients that their IBD was first diagnosed at a time of stress. It could be that such patients have a predisposition to IBD, and have been exposed to a number of noxious insults that have the potential to trigger the disease. Thus, if stress 'primes' the gut beforehand, subsequent exposure to one of these insults could precipitate the clinical expression of the disease. This does not mean that the stress caused the disease but simply that it enhanced the inflammatory response to a level at which it became clinically manifest.

A more common clinical scenario is that stress is associated with exacerbations of quiescent disease. We have tried to develop a model of this in the rat. We allowed rats to recover from acute colitis induced by TNB and subjected them to mild restraint stress for 3 days 6 weeks later. Although we were successful in increasing the activity of myeloperoxidase activity with stress, we were unable to produce sufficient tissue damage to warrant a claim of reactivated 'colitis'[19]. In preliminary work in the mouse[20], we have modified the protocol to enable us to reactivate a clinically relevant level of colitis. In this study, acute colitis was induced by dinitrobenzene sulphonic acid and then the mice were allowed to recover for 8 weeks. Mice then received a subthreshold dose of DNBS intrarectally followed by three days of restraint plus acoustic stress. This resulted in ulceration and inflammation of the distal colon. The reactivation could not be achieved in athymic mice or mice with severe combined immune deficiency (SCID), suggesting that there was an immunological prerequisite. To investigate this, we first studied the phenomenon in transgenic mice lacking certain T-cell subpopulations. Reactivation was evident in CD-8 knockout mice but not in CD-4 knockout mice. This suggests a critical role for CD-4-positive cells. We next isolated an enriched CD-4 population of T cells from the spleen and mesenteric lymph nodes of mice recovering from acute colitis. Transfer of these cells to naive SCID mice produced no evidence of inflammation for at least 12 weeks after receipt of the cells. However, when the recipient mice were stressed after receiving a subthreshold challenge of DNB, colitis was induced. These findings indicate that stress can reactivate colitis and that there is an immunological prerequisite in which T cells play a critical role.

What are the clinical implications of this? First, proof of the concept of a relationship has now been provided – it was lacking in previous observations and experimentation. Second, the results imply that aggressive treatment of acute attacks directed against the immune system is likely to generate resistance to reactivation by stress as the immunological prerequisite has been suppressed.

References

1. Gwee KA, Graham JC, McKendrick MW, Collins SM, Marshall JS, Read NW. Psychological scores and persistence of irritable bowel after infectious diarrhea. Lancet. 1996;347:150–3.
2. Gue M, Bonbonne C, Fioramonti J *et al.* Stress-induced enhancement of colitis in rats: CRF and arginine vasopressin are not involved. Am J Physiol. 1997;272:G84–91.
3. Payan DG. Neuropeptides and inflammation: the role of substance P. Annu Rev Med. 1989;40:341–52.
4. Stead RH. Innervation of mucosal immune cells in the gastrointestinal tract. Reg Immunol. 1992;4:91–9.
5. Hurst SM, Collins SM. Mechanism underlying tumor necrosis factor-alpha suppression of norepinephrine release from rat myenteric plexus. Am J Physiol. 1994;266:G1123–9.
6. Hurst SM, Stanisz AM, Sharkey KA, Collins SM. Interleukin 1 beta-induced increase in substance P in rat myenteric plexus. Gastroenterology. 1993;105:1754–60.
7. Main C, Blennerhassett P, Collins SM. Human recombinant interleukin 1 beta suppresses acetylcholine release from rat myenteric plexus. Gastroenterology. 1993;104:1648–54.
8. Lindgren S, Stewenius J, Sjölund K, Lilja B, Sundkvist G. Autonomic vagal nerve dysfunction in patients with ulcerative colitis. Scand J Gastroenterol. 1993;28:638–42.
9. Lindgren S, Lilja B, Rosén I, Sundkvist G. Disturbed autonomic nerve function in patients with Crohn's disease. Scand J Gastroenterol. 1991;26:361–6.
10. Bjorck S, Dahlstrom A, Johansson L, Ahlman H. Treatment of the mucosa with local anaesthetics in ulcerative colitis. Agents Actions. 1992;10:C61–72.
11. D'Haens G, Colpaert FC, Peeters F *et al.* The presence and severity of neural inflammation predict severe post-operative recurrence of Crohn's disease [Abstract]. Gastroenterology. 1998;114:A963.
12. McCafferty DM, Wallace JL, Sharkey KA. Effects of chemical sympathectomy and sensory nerve ablation on experimental colitis in the rat. Am J Physiol. 1997;272:G272–80.
13. Lechin F, van der Dijs B, Insausti CLE. Treatment of ulcerative colitis with clonidine. J Clin Pharmacol. 1985;25:255–62.
14. Galleazzi F, Collins SM. Smoking aggravates colitis in rats [Abstract]. Gastroenterology. 1997;
15. Qiu B, Collins SM. Nicotine improves experimental colitis in rats [Abstract]. Gastroenterology. 1997;112:A1065.
16. Swain MG, Agro A, Blennerhassett P, Stanisz A, Collins SM. Increased levels of substance P in the myenteric plexus of Trichinella-infected rats. Gastroenterology. 1992;102:1913–19.
17. Black IB, Kessler JA, Adler JE, Bohn MC. Regulation of substance P expression and metabolism in vivo and in vitro. Ciba Found Symp. 1982:107–22.
18. Sturiale S, Barbara G, Qiu B *et al.* The onset and chronicity of experimental colitis is modulated by pro-inflammatory peptides [Abstract]. Gastroenterology. 1998;114:A1092.
19. Collins SM, McHugh K, Jacobson K *et al.* Previous inflammation alters the response of the rat colon to stress. Gastroenterology. 1996;111:1509–15.
20. Qiu B, Vallance B, Blennerhassett P *et al.* The susceptibility to stress-induced reactivation of colitis requires CD4+ve but not CD8+ve T lymphocytes [Abstract]. Gastroenterology. 1998;114:A1065.
21. Manlyh CR, Gates TS, Zimmerman RP *et al.* Receptor binding sites for substance P but not substance K or neuromedin K are expressed in high concentrations by arterioles, venules and lymph nodules in surgical specimens obtained from patients with ulcerative colitis and Crohn's disease. Proc Natl Acad Sci USA. 1998; 85:3235–9.

29
Inflammatory arthropathy and inflammatory bowel disease

M. DE VOS, H. MIELANTS, F. DE KEYSER, C. CUVELIER and
E. M. VEYS

The important link between gut and joint is supported by the articular findings in
IBD and by the intestinal abnormalities in articular diseases like spondyloarthropathy (SpA).

ARTHROPATHY IN IBD

Arthropathy is the most frequent extraintestinal manifestation in IBD. It includes
peripheral arthritis and axial syndromes.

Peripheral arthropathy

Recently, a large retrospective study from Orchard et al.[1] recognized two types
of peripheral arthropathy in IBD:

- Type 1 with an oligoarticular, mostly asymmetrical, involvement, a self-
  limited evolution in 80% of the cases and a clear temporal association with
  relapse of the gut symptoms. Furthermore, this type of arthropathy was
  strongly associated with other extraintestinal manifestations, such as erythema nodosum and uveitis.

- Type 2 arthropathy, in contrast, had a different natural history, with persistent symptoms for months to years, involvement of many joints, mostly on a
  symmetrical basis and a course independent of IBD.

According to these data and previous definitions[2], peripheral arthropathy in IBD
involves large and small joints of the lower limbs in a pauciarticular asymmetrical way. Frequently, an enthesiopathy or inflammation of the insertion of the
tendon to the bone accompanies the clinical picture. Usually, the arthritis is transient, migratory and non-deforming. Generally, it subsides over 6–8 weeks but
evolves into chronic arthritis in 10% of cases. In the majority of cases,

radiographs of the affected joints are normal although erosive lesions have been described. Synovial fluid analysis reveals inflammation, with leukocyte counts ranging from 1000 to 50 000 cells, consisting predominantly of neutrophils. Histopathology of the synovium reveals a mild chronic inflammation. In contrast to other enterogenic arthritides, there is no increased incidence in the HLA B27 phenotype.

Because data about the prevalence of arthropathy in IBD are disparate in the literature, we performed a prospective clinical study on 75 consecutive patients presenting at our GI unit irrespective of the presence or not of articular symptoms[3]. Peripheral synovitis was detected in 9% of patients. As we consider enthesiopathy to be a specific feature of SpA, we evaluated this clinical sign separately and found it in 11% of patients, mostly as the only clinical sign (Figure 1).

No differences were observed between CD and UC. No relationship was found with the duration of gut disease.

These prevalences correspond very well with those observed in the retrospective study of Orchard *et al.*[1] who described a peripheral arthropathy type 1 in 5% of patients. However, no data were available about enthesiopathy. So, in general, we can state that the prevalence of peripheral arthropathy varies between 5 and 10%.

Axial involvement

Axial involvement includes spondylitis and sacroiliitis[2].

The clinical picture of *symptomatic spondylitis* is similar to that of idiopathic ankylosing spondylitis (AS) and includes: inflammatory spinal pain occurring at night and at rest, morning stiffness and a decreased mobility of spine and/or chest expansion. Radiographic lesions compatible with spondylitis are present. In contrast to the very high incidence of HLA B27 in idiopathic AS, the reported incidence in IBD is much lower and varies between 50 and 75%.

Sacroiliitis (SI) is a mostly asymptomatic radiological diagnosis.

In contrast to peripheral arthropathy, the onset and evolution of axial involvement is independent of the severity, extent, location and duration of bowel disease. Estimates of the prevalence of axial involvement are probably underestimated because they are clinically less impressive and need to be detected actively. In our prospective study, we found inflammatory back pain in 23%, clinical diagnosis of AS in 8% and radiological diagnosis of SI in 13% of patients (Figure 1)[3]. These prevalences are higher than those in the retrospective study of Orchard *et al.* with the presence of low back pain in 5% of patients and AS in 1%. No data are available about sacroiliitis[1].

In general, our prospective study illustrates that arthropathy is a very frequent extraintestinal manifestation of IBD, affecting about half of the patients. In 28% of patients, this manifestation is symptomatic and corresponds to the criteria of spondyloarthropathy (SpA), in 8% it consists of an enthesiopathy, and in 13% it remains an asymptomatic SI.

Treatment of SpA is difficult to evaluate because of the natural history of flares and remission of the arthropathy.

Most patients respond rapidly to a treatment with NSAIDs. However, caution is necessary since these drugs may activate quiescent IBD[4].

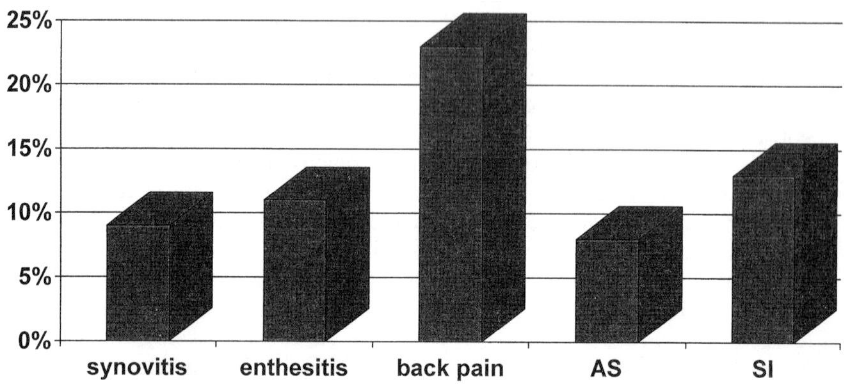

Figure 1 Prevalence of different types of inflammatory arthropathy in IBD. AS = ankylosing spondylitis; SI = sacroiliitis

Since peripheral arthropathy follows intestinal activity, maximal treatment of the gut is mandatory and will resolve articular disease in the majority of patients. As SASP has proved to be efficacious in the treatment of reactive arthritis[5] and peripheral arthritis associated with AS[6,7], its use can be recommended for maintenance therapy. Data about other 5-ASA preparations are extremely scarce, and no clear benefit has been demonstrated[8].

GUT INFLAMMATION IN SPONDYLOARTHROPATHY

Since the arthritis of IBD is a type of SpA, a possible role of gut inflammation in the aetiopathogenesis of other forms of SpA deserved interest and has led to exploration of the gut in these patients.

The concept of SpA includes several chronic diseases with common clinical, biological, genetic and therapeutic characteristics. The target organs are not only the joints and the axial skeleton, but also the eyes, the gut and the urogenital tract. Its prevalence in the general population can be estimated as 1%.

The criteria of SpA elaborated by the European study group[9] include: an inflammatory spinal pain and/or an asymmetric synovitis of the lower limbs associated with one of the following criteria:

– Positive personal history of SpA, IBD or psoriasis,
– A recent history of urethritis, cervicitis or diarrhoea,
– Presence of alternating buttock pain, enthesiopathy or sacroiliitis.

Several authors have confirmed the presence of asymptomatic gut inflammation on ileocolonoscopy and histology in the different forms of SpA[10-16].

We found, as expected, the highest prevalences of gut inflammation in enterogenic forms of ReA, but also observed inflammation in 57% of AS patients (principally those with associated peripheral arthritis) and 72% of patients with undifferentiated SpA, a group of patients with the clinical criteria of SpA but without clear aetiology[12,13].

The prevalence in psoriatic arthritis was much lower (25%)[17] and inflammation was seldom found in urogenital forms of reactive arthritis. A study of 27 patients with acute anterior uveitis, with or without axial joint inflammation, revealed gut inflammation in 66% of patients[18].

On histology, we distinguished two types of inflammation: an acute inflammation resembling infectious colitis and a chronic form of inflammation suggestive of Crohn's disease[19]. Gut inflammation, predominantly chronic inflammation, was more frequently present in patients with pauciarticular involvement (55%) than polyarticular involvement ($30\% - p < 0.0001$), supporting the link between gut and joint inflammation in this particular form of peripheral arthropathy.

The relationship between this gut inflammation and arthritis in SpA was further supported by the evolution of gut and articular inflammation[20].

- Evolution to overt IBD was observed in 7% of patients. In all except one patient, subclinical gut lesions were already present at the initial endoscopy, mostly as chronic inflammation[20].

- In patients who underwent a second ileocolonoscopy, disappearance of the lesions was observed in all patients who went into clinical articular remission whereas gut inflammation persisted in most patients with persistent articular symptoms[20].

- Evolution to CD was more frequently observed in patients with pauciarticular (6.5%) than polyarticular arthritis (2.5%).

The challenging link between gut inflammation and arthropathy has also been documented in some animal models. The most convincing model is the HLA B27/β2 microglobulin transgenic rat model, developing a spontaneous, multisystem inflammatory disorder with skin, nails, gut and joint inflammation[21].

The essential role of bacterial flora in the induction of inflammation became apparent as transgenic rats bred in germ-free conditions developed no gut or joint lesions, although skin lesions persisted[22]. Later exposure of these germ-free animals to conventional flora induced both gut and joint inflammation.

RELATIONSHIP BETWEEN GUT AND JOINT

Several potential mechanisms may explain the relationship between gut and joint inflammation.

A first hypothesis includes the transport of exogenous antigens by macrophages from the gut to the joint.

Arguments for this hypothesis are:

- The *in-vitro* studies demonstrating the binding of mucosal macrophages to the inflamed synovial high endothelial venules (HEV)[23].

- The detection of components of bacterial lipopolysaccharides in synovial fluid and membrane of patients with reactive arthritis following an enteric infection[24–27].

– The demonstration of a synovial immune response against specific *Yersinia* antigens[28,29].

– The finding of HLA B27 restricted cytotoxic CD8+ T cells with specificity for arthritogenic bacteria in synovial fluid of patients with *Yersinia*- or *Salmonella*-triggered reactive arthritis, suggesting that the presentation of bacterial peptides by HLA B27 may be disturbed[30].

The second hypothesis takes into account the homing properties of activated gut-derived lymphocytes to the joints.

Lymphocytes continuously circulate between lymphoid tissues. This trafficking is regulated by adhesion molecules expressed on leukocytes and endothelial cells, allowing specific immune reactions throughout the body and facilitating the cell–cell interactions. Lymphocytes leave blood by recognizing and binding to vascular endothelial cells and migrate between the endothelial cells into the surrounding tissues.

The differentiation of lymphocytes into memory and effector lymphocytes in the secondary lymphoid tissue in response to antigen, is accompanied by the development of tissue-selective homing properties. This selective circulation or homing is determined by the type of adhesion molecule: for example, the combination of MadCAM-1 (mucosal addressin cell adhesion molecule) on mucosal endothelial cells (venules in lamina propria and HEVs in organized GALT) and $\alpha4\beta7$ on lymphocytes regulates the very important lymphocyte homing to GI mucosa and gut-associated lymphoid tissue. MadCAM-1 appears to be also responsible for the attraction of macrophages and eosinophils to normal gut because they also express $\alpha4\beta7$[31,32].

Vascular adhesion protein (VAP-1) seems to be involved mainly in the trafficking of lymphocytes and immunoblasts to synovium. This adhesion molecule is expressed on HEV-like venules in synovial membranes[33]. It is also expressed on the majority of HEV at non-mucosal sites.

Binding of macrophages isolated from lamina propria of the gut to synovial endothelium seems to be almost entirely P-selectin dependent[34].

In the case of inflammation, activation of endothelial cells induces changes in adhesion molecule status. These changes determine the magnitude and type of leukocyte influx into the affected tissue.

The role of $\alpha4\beta7$–MadCAM in the recruitment of immune cells into the chronically inflamed gut is supported by several observations:

– An upregulation of MadCAM and P-selectin has been observed at inflammatory loci[35].

– An attenuation of spontaneous colitis in the cotton-top tamarin by parenteral administration of monoclonal antibodies against the $\alpha4$ integrin subunit and against $\alpha4\beta7$ has been described[36,37].

– Experiments with knock-out mice deficient in this subfamily of adhesion molecule have shown the dominant role of $\beta7$ integrins in lymphocyte extravasation[38].

– Efficient blocking of lymphocyte extravasation and reduced disease severity in colitis of SCID mice reconstituted with CD4+ T cells after systemic administration of monoclonal antibodies to $\beta7$ as well as to MadCAM-1 also supports the role of these molecules[39].

— A downregulation of $\alpha4\beta7$ and an upregulation of the epithelial adhesion molecule $\alpha E\beta7$ has been observed in IL-2-expanded cell lines from the gut of CD patients[40]. The epithelial affinity appears to be explained by a downregulation of $\alpha4\beta7$ and an increased expression and migration of $\alpha E\beta7$ to the epithelium where they are retained as IEL by the binding to E-cadherin present on epithelial cells and upregulated in IBD[31,41].

Adhesion molecules playing a role at the synovial site are less known. We observed an increased expression of $\alpha4\beta7$ and $\alpha E\beta7$ in activated T cells in synovium of SpA patients as compared with RA patients. An inverse correlation between $\alpha4\beta7$ and $\alpha E\beta7$ was seen in SpA and contrasted with the linear correlation in rheumatoid arthritis, suggesting a mucosal origin of $\beta7$ cells in SpA and a systemic origin from peripheral circulation in rheumatoid arthritis[42].

A strong upregulation of VAP-1 has been observed in joint, skin and gut in inflammatory conditions[43].

In conclusion, gut-derived lymphoblasts adhere equally well to mucosal and inflamed synovial venules. The mucosal affinity is mainly mediated by lymphocyte homing receptor $\alpha4\beta7$ integrin and CD 44 glycoproteins. Synovial affinity of mucosal immunoblasts and small lymphocytes seems to be mediated by VAP-1, adherence of mucosal macrophages by binding to P-selectin[34]. A working model explaining gut–joint interaction proposed by Salmi starts with the uptake and processing of antigen by mucosal macrophages, followed by systemic circulation to synovium and adherence to endothelial P-selectin which is upregulated by the systemic effects of inflammation, cytokines and lipopolysaccharides.

This allows the entry of macrophages carrying exogenous antigens into the synovium. Introduced antigen induces local inflammation which results in a further cytokine-mediated endothelial activation.

Synovial adhesion molecules, such as VAP-1, become upregulated and bind preactivated mucosal lymphoblasts and lymphocytes and *circulus vitiosus* becomes established. Sustained activation of the endothelial cells and/or inappropriate elimination of the target antigen may lead to the development of arthritis.

This model may have direct therapeutic implications as several antiadhesive therapies would interfere with the synovial homing of various subclasses of mononuclear cells originating from the gut at different stages in the cascade.

References

1. Orchard TR, Wordsworth BP, Jewell DP. Peripheral arthropathies in inflammatory bowel disease: their articular distribution and natural history. Gut. 1998;42:309–11.
2. De Vos M, Mielants H, Cuvelier C. Ileitis in the spondylarthropathies. In: Allan RN, Rhodes JM, Hanauer SB, eds. Inflammatory bowel diseases. Edinburgh: Churchill Livingstone; 1997:451–60.
3. De Vos M, De Vlam K, Mielants H *et al.* Prevalence of clinical and subclinical spondyloarthropathy in patients with inflammatory bowel disease. Gastroenterology. 1998;114:4,G3947.
4. Davies NM. Toxicity of nonsteroidal anti-inflammatory drugs in the large intestine. Dis Colon Rectum. 1995;38:1311–21.
5. Clegg DO, Reda DJ, Weisman MH *et al.* Comparison of sulfasalazine and placebo in the treatment of reactive arthritis (Reiter's syndrome). Arthritis Rheum. 1996;39:2021–7.

6. Clegg DO, Reda DJ, Weisman MH *et al.* Comparison of sulfasalazine and placebo in the treatment of ankylosing spondylitis. Arthritis Rheum. 1996;39:2004–12.

7. Dougados M, van der Linder S, Leirisalo-Repo M *et al.* Sulfasalazine in the treatment of spondylarthropathy. A randomized, multicenter, double-blind, placebo-controlled study. Arthritis Rheum. 1995;38:618–27.

8. Taggart AJ, Gardiner P, McEvoy FM *et al.* Which is the active moiety of sulphasalazine in ankylosing spondylitis? Arthritis Rheum. 1996;39:1400–5.

9. Dougados M, van der Linden J, Juhlin R *et al.* The European Spondylarthropathy Study Group preliminary criteria for the classification of spondylarthropathy. Arthritis Rheum. 1991;34:1218–26.

10. Dougados M, Allemanni M, Tulliez M *et al.* Iléocolonoscopie systématique au cours de spondylarthropathies séronégatives. Rev Rheum. 1987;54:279–83.

11. Grillet B, De Clerck L, Dequeker J *et al.* Systematic ileocolonoscopy and bowel biopsy in spondylarthropathy. Br J Rheumatol. 1987;26:338–40.

12. Mielants H, Veys EM, Cuvelier C, De Vos M. Ileocolonscopic findings in seronegative spondylarthropathies. Br J Rheumatol. 1988;27(suppl II): 95–105.

13. De Vos M, Cuvelier C, Mielants H *et al.* Ileocolonoscopy in seronegative spondylarthropathy. Gastroenterology. 1989;96:339–44.

14. Simenon G, Van Gossum A, Adler M *et al.* Macroscopic and microscopic gut lesions in seronegative spondylarthropathies. J Rheumatol. 1990;17:491–4.

15. Altomente L, Zoli A, Veneziana A *et al.* Clinical silent inflammatory gut lesions in undifferentiated spondyloarthropathies. Clin Rheumatol. 1994;13:565–70.

16. Leirisalo-Repo M, Turunen U, Stenman S *et al.* High frequency of silent inflammatory bowel disease in spondylarthropathy. Arthritis Rheum. 1994;37:23–31.

17. Schatteman L, Mielants H, Veys EM *et al.* Gut inflammation in psoriatic arthritis: a prospective ileocolonoscopic study. J Rheumatol. 1995;22:680–3.

18. Banares AA, Jover JA, Fernandez-Gutierrez B *et al.* Bowel inflammation in anterior uveitis and spondylarthropathy. J Rheumatol. 1995;22:1112–17.

19. Cuvelier C, Barbatis C, Mielants H *et al.* Histopathology of intestinal inflammation related to reactive arthritis. Gut. 1987;28:394–401.

20. De Vos M, Mielants H, Cuvelier C, Elewaut A, Veys E. Long-term evolution of gut inflammation in patients with spondylarthropathy. Gastroenterology. 1996;110:1696–703.

21. Hammer RE, Maika SD, Richardson JA *et al.* Spontaneous inflammatory disease in transgenic rats expressing HLA-B27 and human b2m: an animal model of HLA-B27 associated human disorders. Cell. 1990;63:1099–112.

22. Taurog JD, Richardson JA, Croft JAT *et al.* The germfree state prevents development of gut and joint inflammatory disease in HLA-B27 transgenic rats. J Exp Med. 1994;180:2359–64.

23. Salmi M, Andrew DP, Butchers EC, Jalkanen S. Dual binding capacity of mucosal immunoblasts to mucosal and synovial endothelium in humans: dissection of the molecular mechanisms. J Exp Med. 1995;181:137–49.

24. Granfors K, Jalkanen S, von Essen R *et al.* Yersinia antigens in synovial fluid cells from patients with reactive arthritis. N Engl J Med. 1989;320:216–21.

25. Granfors K, Jalkanen S, Lindberg AA *et al.* Salmonella lipopolysaccharide in synovial cells from patients with reactive arthritis. Lancet. 1990;335:685–8.

26. Granfors K, Jalkanen S, Toivanen P *et al.* Bacterial lipopolysaccharide in synovial fluid cells in Shigella-triggered reactive arthritis. J Rheumatol. 1992;19:500.

27. Merilahti-Palo R, Pelliniemi LJ, Granfors K *et al.* Electron microscopy and immunolabeling of Yersinia antigens in human synovial fluid cells. Clin Exp Rheumatol. 1994;12:255–60.

28. Sieper J, Braun J, Wu P, Kingsley G. T cells are responsible for the enhanced synovial cellular immune response to triggering antigen in reactive arthritis. Clin Exp Immunol. 1993;91:96–103.

29. Viner NJ, Bailey LC, Life PF *et al.* Isolation of Yersinia-specific T cells clones from the synovial membrane and synovial fluid of a patient with reactive arthritis. Arthritis Rheum. 1991;34:1151–7.

30. Hermann E, Yu DTY, Meyer zum Büschenfelde KH, Fleischer B. HLA-B27-restricted CD8 T cells derived from synovial fluid of patients with reactive arthritis and ankylosing spondylitis. Lancet. 1993;342:646–50.

31. Brandtzaeg P. Review article: Homing of mucosal immune cells – a possible connection between intestinal and articular inflammation. Aliment Pharmacol Ther. 1997;11(suppl 3):24–39.

32. Erle DJ, Briskin MJ, Butcher EC *et al.* Expression and function of the MAdCAM-1 receptor, integrin a4b7, on human leukocytes. J Immunol. 1994;153:517–28.
33. Salmi M, Jalkanen S. A 90-kilodalton endothelial cell molecule mediating lymphocyte binding in humans. Science. 1992;257:1407–9.
34. Salmi M, Rajala P, Jalkanen S. Homing of mucosal leukocytes to joints. Distinct endothelial ligands in synovium mediate leukocyte-subtype specific adhesion. J Clin Invest. 1997;99:2165–72.
35. Briskin M, Winsor-Hines D, Shyjan A *et al.* Human mucosal addressin cell adhesion molecule-1 is preferentially expressed in intestinal tract and associated lymphoid tissue. Am J Pathol. 1997;151:97–110.
36. Podolsky DK, Lobb R, King N *et al.* Attenuation of colitis in the cotton-top tamarin by anti-α4 integrin monoclonal antibody. J Clin Invest. 1993;92:372–80.
37. Hesterberg PE, Winsor-Hines D, Briskin MJ *et al.* Rapid resolution of chronic colitis in the cotton-top tamarin with an antibody to a gut-homing integrin α4β7. Gastroenterology. 1996;111:1373–80.
38. Wagner N, Löhler J, Kunkel EJ *et al.* Critical role for β7 integrins in formation of the gut-associated lymphoid tissue. Nature. 1996;382:366–70.
39. Picarella D, Hurlbut P, Rottman J *et al.* Monoclonal antibodies specific for β7 integrin and mucosal addressin cell adhesion molecule-1 (MAdCAM-1) reduce inflammation in the colon of scid mice reconstituted with CD4 45Rbhigh CD4+ T cells. J Immunol. 1997;158:2099–106.
40. Elewaut D, De Keyser F, Cuvelier C *et al.* Distinctive activated cellular subsets in colon from patients with Crohn's disease and ulcerative colitis. Scand J Gastroenterol. 1998;33:743–8.
41. Demetter P, Cesmeli E, De Vos M *et al.* Upregulation of E-cadherin and associated molecules (α-, β-, and γ-catenins) in inflamed bowel mucosa. Gastroenterology. 1998;114:4,G3943.
42. Elewaut D, De Keyser F, Van Den Bosch F *et al.* Enrichment of T cells carrying β7 integrins in inflamed synovial tissue from patients with early spondyloarthropathy, compared to rheumatoid arthritis. J Rheumatol. 1998;25:1932–7.
43. Salmi M, Kalimo K, Jalkanen S. Induction and function of vascular adhesion protein-1 at sites of inflammation. J Exp Med. 1993;178:2255–60.

30
Refractory anaemia and iron deficiency in IBD

C. GASCHE

Anaemia in IBD is a frequent and relevant problem. Most studies demonstrate that 30% of the IBD population suffer from anaemia. The patients are usually young and seem to tolerate severe anaemic disease states for long periods. However, also in this population, anaemia goes with impairments of quality of life, cognitive functions and ability to work[1]. Thus, effective treatment for anaemia in IBD is needed.

IBD-assciated anaemia is a multifactorial event with two major proponents: iron deficiency and chronic inflammatory disease. Beside these two important factors, anaemia may occasionally result from deficiencies in cobalamin (sometimes after ileal resection) or folic acid[2]. Glucose-6-phosphate dehydrogenase deficiency[3], autoimmune haemolysis[4] or myelodysplastic syndromes[5] are anecdotal contributors to the occurrence of anaemia in IBD.

IRON METABOLISM IN HUMANS

Iron uptake

Iron absorption takes place in the duodenum and upper jejunum. The iron balance is maintained by regulation of iron absorption. Usually, 1–2 mg/day are absorbed and the same quantity is lost through epithelial turnover in the skin and gut (Figure 1).

Internalized iron binds to transferrin and is transported in the plasma. This plasma iron pool, however, represents a very small percentage of the total iron which is between 4 and 5 g in adult humans and mainly bound to haemoglobin (Figure 2). The bilobal nature of transferrin contains two iron binding sites. Under physiological conditions, about 30–40% of these binding sites are occupied. Transferrin bound iron is taken up by the transferrin receptor into target cells, mainly erythroid progenitor cells but also immune or liver cells. Indeed, iron is an important cofactor of many intracellular proteins or enzymes, such as mitochondrial cytochromes or ribonucleotide reductase. Actually, iron is needed in every cell of the body.

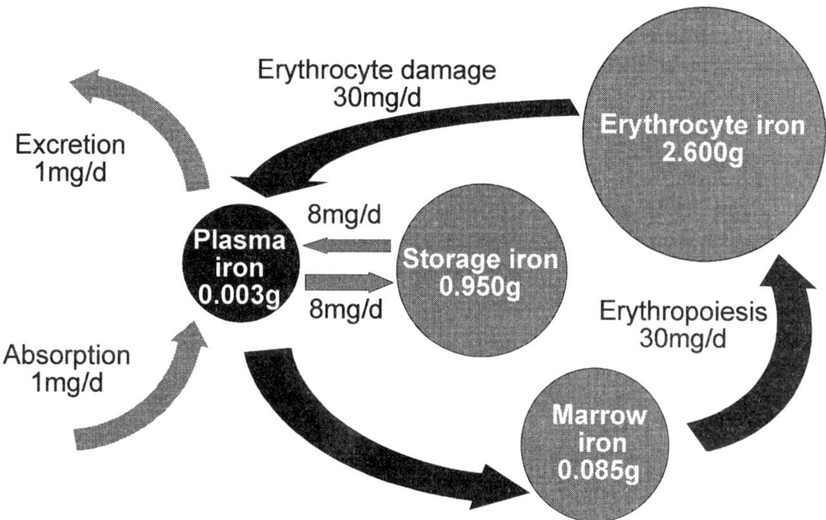

Figure 1 Iron metabolism in healthy adults. Every day, about 1–2 mg elemental iron are absorbed in the proximal small bowel and bound to transferrin. Transferrin-bound plasma iron may be transported to the bone marrow and used for erythropoiesis (30 mg/day). The same amount of iron is released after erythrocyte damage. In addition, there is continuous exchange of iron between the storage pool (RES) and the plasma pool. The daily excreted amount of iron balances iron absorption (1–2 mg)

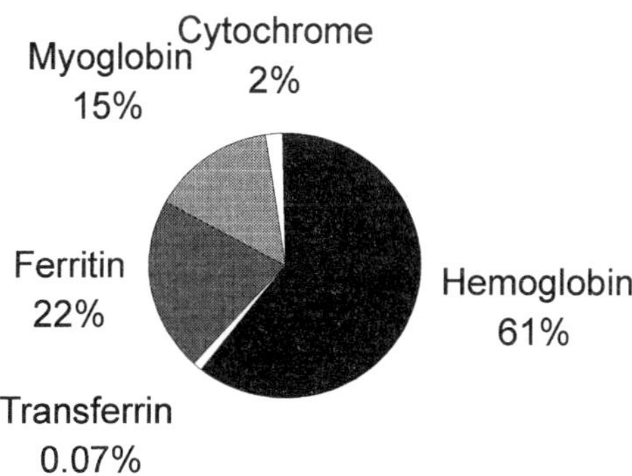

Figure 2 Distribution of total body iron (4–5 g) in adults

After the binding of the iron–transferrin complex to the receptor, the complex enters the cell by formation of a coated pit and then a vesical, which sheds its clathrin and is called an endosome. The pH within the endosome is lowered to approximately 5 by an energy-dependent proton pump, and iron is released into the cytoplasm. The apotransferrin receptor is then returned to the plasma membrane where apotransferrin (which has a lower affinity than transferrin for the receptor) is released. A truncated form of the transferrin receptor molecule (lacking the cytoplasmic and the transmembrane domains) can be detected in human serum[6]. This soluble molecule is a sensitive measure of erythropoiesis and iron deficiency[7,8].

The transferrin receptor expression is regulated posttranscriptionally by interaction between the iron regulatory protein (IRP) and the iron responsive elements (IRE) present on the 3'-untranslated region of the transferrin receptor mRNA. Low intracellular iron levels activate the iron-regulatory protein-binding activity, which then may bind to these iron-responsive elements on the untranslated mRNA regions of the transferrin receptor, leading to stabilization of the transferrin receptor mRNA and to increase in translation and consecutive up-regulation of receptor expression.

In contrast to transferrin, ferritin serves as soluble store of iron within body cells. It consists of an apoprotein shell (24 subunits) enclosing a core of iron which may contain up to 4500 iron atoms. Regulation of ferritin synthesis is also related to binding of the iron-regulatory protein to iron responsive elements of the ferritin in RNA. High intracellular iron levels inactivate the iron-regulatory protein-binding activity to iron-responsive elements of the 5' untranslated region of the ferritin mRNA and induce translation of ferritin. The main function of ferritin is to provide an intracellular store of iron which may be used for synthesis of iron-containing proteins when required.

Role of iron for haemoglobin synthesis

Most importantly, haemoglobin synthesis depends on the availability of intracellular iron in erythroid precursor cells. In parallel to ferritin mRNA, ε-aminolaevulinic acid synthesis (the key enzyme of haemoglobin biosynthesis) is also regulated by the iron-regulatory protein interaction with iron-responsive elements of its mRNA. High intracellular iron concentrations thereby lead to increased mRNA translation and as a consequence to increased haemoglobin biosynthesis. Haemoglobin itself binds about 60% of total body iron (Figure 2). As iron itself regulates the synthesis of related proteins, iron metabolism can be observed by measurement of such proteins.

Immunological properties of iron

Iron is not only essential for erythropoiesis, growing micro-organisms and tumour cells, but also crucial for proliferation of immune cells. Iron plays a critical role in macrophage-mediated cytotoxicity by contributing to the production of several reactive oxygen species. Th1-type cytokines like interferon-γ or IL-2 may strongly enhance the expression of the transferrin receptor. In contrast, iron itself is able to influence cytokine activity. Low-molecular-weight iron as well as transferrin-bound or haem iron reduced the effects of interferon-γ on the monocytic cell line THP-1 by approximately 70%. In contrast, iron starvation caused a considerable increase interferon-γ activity. Similar interactions exist between iron and TNF-α or its receptor (for review, see Weiss et al.[9]).

IRON METABOLISM IN IBD

Iron deficiency in IBD results mostly from chronic intestinal blood loss[10]. Occasionally, iron absorption may be impaired in CD patients in the duodenum or upper jejunum[11]. In general, however, no data support an impaired iron absorption capacity in Crohn's disease or ulcerative colitis. It is obvious that, in a proportion of IBD patients, the increase in iron loss is not compensated by an increase in iron absorption, leading to a negative iron balance. Dietary restrictions may also contribute to a general reduction in total body iron. During the late 1970s, the ability of ferritin to reflect body iron stores was explored and also studied in patients with anaemia of chronic diseases[12]. For patients with IBD, only ferritin levels above 55 μg/L were able to rule out iron-depleted bone marrows as the basis of anaemia[13]. Beside deficiencies in total body iron, chronic intestinal inflammation mediates mechanisms of iron withholding from the plasma pool. Upregulation of ferritin and downregulation of transferrin synthesis are part of the acute-phase response. This leads to a shortening of available transferrin bound plasma iron, the so-called 'functional iron deficiency'.

ANAEMIA OF CHRONIC DISEASES

For a review, see Reference 14. The production of inflammatory cytokines within inflamed bowel segments not only perpetuates the inflammatory reaction within the bowel, but also has systemic effects. The term anaemia of chronic diseases (ACD) was first invented by Cartwright[15]. Our understanding of the interaction between inflammatory cytokines and erythropoieses has grown in recent decades. Interferon-γ, IL-1 and TNF-α as well as IL-6 are actors in this field. These mechanisms are comparable in different disease states, such as rheumatoid arthritis, IBD, chronic infection and malignancy. Both ineffective erythropoiesis and reduced red blood cell life span contribute to ACD.

Three important mechanisms have been identified (Figure 3):

1. Direct inhibition of erythropoieses on BFU-E and CFU-E level (IFN-γ);
2. Inhibition of erythropoietin production[16] (IL-1, TNF-α, IL-6);
3. Iron withholding from the plasma (IL-1, TNF-α).

Indeed, a number of studies have shown reduced serum erythropoietin levels in anaemic patients with inflammatory bowel disease[17]. *In-vitro* studies have shown that IFN-γ-induced inhibition of erythropoiesis may be overcome by

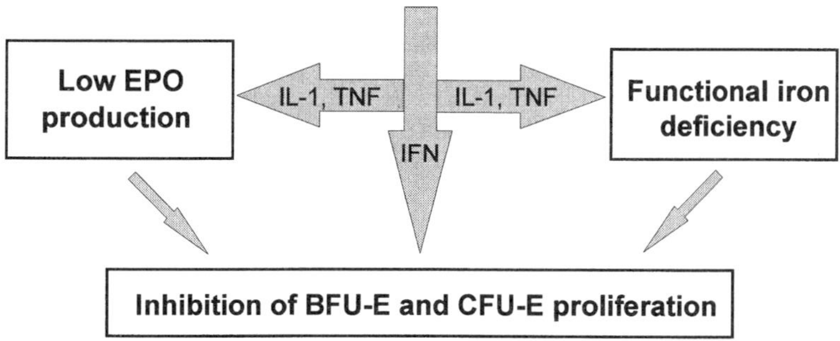

Figure 3 Important mechanisms of pro-inflammatory cytokine inducing anaemia of chronic diseases

erythropoietin supplementation[18]. In fact, in IBD patients, the pathogenesis of anaemia is a combination of iron deficiency and ACD.

TREATMENT OF IBD-ASSOCIATED ANAEMIA

As shown above, the mechanisms of IBD-associated anaemia are well understood. Treatment strategies should be directed to correct both iron deficiency and ACD.

Oral iron preparations

Most oral iron supplements contain iron in the form of ferrous salts or iron polysaccharide (Table 1). Although there are different formulations available, no clear evidence supports the superiority of any specific agent. In general, enteric-coated formulations should be avoided because they may release their iron content beyond the intestinal sites of maximal iron absorption. The efficacy of oral iron preparations in patients with IBD may be hindered by two important factors:

1. Patient compliance in taking oral iron preparations decreases with gastrointestinal side-effects. Nausea, bloating and increase in diarrhoea, as well as upper gastrointestinal pain, are frequently observed symptoms in this population. The causes of these symptoms are not well understood but they may be due to the production of free oxygen radicals[19].
2. High level of iron deficiency. The iron needed to correct anaemia in IBD can be estimated as approximately: an increase of 1 g/dl serum haemoglobin corresponds to 150 mg iron. In a case with a haemoglobin of 8.0 g/dl and a therapeutic goal of 13.0 g/dl, the difference would be 750 mg (5 × 150). Anaemic disease states in IBD are associated with exhausted iron storage pools. Therefore, additional iron is needed to fill the storage pool; this can also be estimated[14]. The protected iron requirement for a patient with a haemoglobin of 8.0 g/dl and a ferritin level of 15 μg/L would be aproximately 1000 mg. Presuming there is normal iron absorption, a high patient compliance and no continuous blood loss, oral iron therapy would be needed for more than 3 months (150 mg Fe^{2+}/day) to replace such an iron deficit. Many patients, however, are continuously losing blood. Controlled trials have shown that oral iron substitution is not sufficient to compensate for ongoing iron loss[21].

Intravenous parenteral iron supplements

For effective iron substitution, parenteral iron preparations are needed. The direct administration of iron into the circulation requires a formulation that avoids the

Table 1 Oral iron preparations

Ferrous sulphate
Ferrous gluconate
Ferrous fumarate
Ferric polysaccharide
Recomendations for use:
Daily dose: at least 150 mg, away from meals
Combined with vitamin C (prevents oxidation)
No concomitant therapy with antacids, H2-blockers or proton pump inhibitors
Avoid slow-release preparations

Table 2 Intravenous iron preparations

- *Iron dextran*
  100–500 kDa, robust type (low degradation), uptake by RES, half-life 3–4 days, anaphylactoid potency

- *Iron saccharate*
  30–100 kDa, half robust type (medium degradation), uptake by transferrin/apoferritin and RES, half-life about 90 min

- *Iron gluconate*
  <50 kDa, labile type (fast degradation), uptake to transferrin/apoferritin/other proteins, very short half-life, risk of transferrin oversaturation

cellular toxicity of iron salts (Table 2; for pharmacological overview, see Reference 22). Three different products are available. Iron dextran is a robust and strong type of parenteral iron product. Its molecular weight is between 100 and 500 kDa. This iron complex shows high structural homogeneity and thus a slow and competitive delivery of complexed iron to endogenous iron-binding proteins. They are taken up from the plasma by the RES (half-life about 3–4 days). After intracellular degradation, the iron re-enters the plasma and becomes available for haemoglobin synthesis. Since this preparation is stable, even high doses are clinically safe. The dextran molecule may cause well-known dextran-induced anaphylactic reactions.

Since the molecular weight of iron saccharate is much lower (30–100 kDa), almost no allergic reactions are observed. Iron saccharate is a half robust type of intravenous iron with medium degradation and partial uptake of released iron by apotransferrin or apoferritin but also by the RES. Its half-life is therefore relatively short (about 90 min).

Iron gluconate is a labile type with fast degradation and only direct uptake to plasma proteins (apotransferrin, apoferritin, etc.). Potential toxicity of iron gluconate is attributed to oversaturation of transferrin-binding capacity[23]. Free iron induces cell damage with clinical symptoms of a capillary leak syndrome (dyspnoea, hypotension, oedema).

For all of our IBD studies, we decided to use iron saccharate. Iron saccharate is tolerated well, particularly when it is used as a dilute solution[24–26]. In the past, over 1000 intravenous iron saccharate infusions have been administered at our centre as part of controlled trials with no serious adverse events[27,28]. One infusion is prepared from 10 ml iron saccharate, corresponding to 200 mg Fe^{3+} (Venofer, previously called Ferrum Hausmann, Vifor AG, St. Gallen, Switzerland), diluted in 250 ml of a 0.9% sodium chloride solution and given intravenously over 60 min. During the first two weeks infusions are given twice a week and afterwards once a week. Over 8 weeks, 75% of patients respond to iron saccharate (Figure 4).

Erythropoietin

Specific treatment of ACD is not available at the moment. Anti-inflammatory drugs may have the potency to inhibit cytokine production but may also inhibit erythropoiesis themselves (e.g. azathioprine). Because erythropoietin serum levels in ACD are inadequate recombinant human erythropoietin (r-HuEPO) has been studied in a variety of different types of ACD[29–31]. r-HuEPO can also correct the direct inhibitory effect of IFN-γ on erythropoietic progenitor cells (see above). Early reports in selected IBD cases were positive[32]. Controlled data

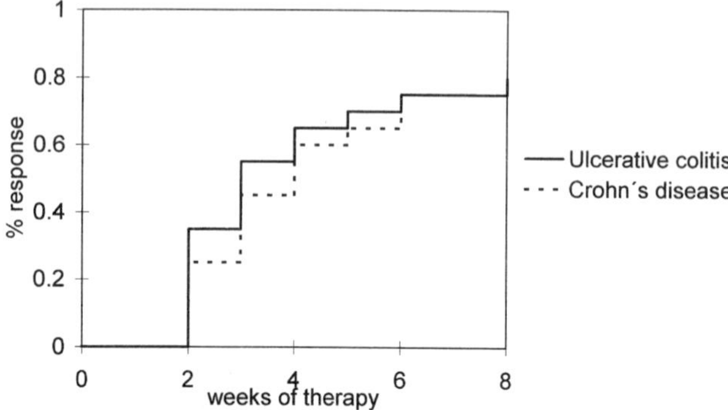

Figure 4   Response of patients with IBD-associated anaemia (haemoglobin <10.5 g/dl) to repeated intravenous iron saccharate infusions (total 2000 mg). Response was defined as an increase in haemoglobin >2.0 g/dl. There is no difference in response rate between Crohn's disease and ulcerative colitis[27,28]. There is a significant rise in the haemoglobin of most patients within 4 weeks

were able to confirm the efficacy of r-HuEPO in the treatment of IBD-associated anaemia[21]. However, concomitant iron deficiency limited the potency of r-HuEPO to a haemoglobin increase of 1.7 g/dl after 12 weeks (Figure 5). Because of the importance of iron deficiency in this population, another controlled trial was performed using iron saccharate[27]. Again, the rise in haemoglobin concentration was superior (4.9 g/dl within 8 weeks) in the r-HuEPO group compared with iron saccharate alone (Figure 5). A high proportion of patients (75%), however, responded to intravenous iron alone, highlighting the high cost efficacy of intravenous iron preparations in IBD.

Prediction of response to intravenous iron therapy

Since it was clear that intravenous iron saccharate is the most cost-effective therapy for IBD-associated anaemia, we tried to improve the treatment protocol

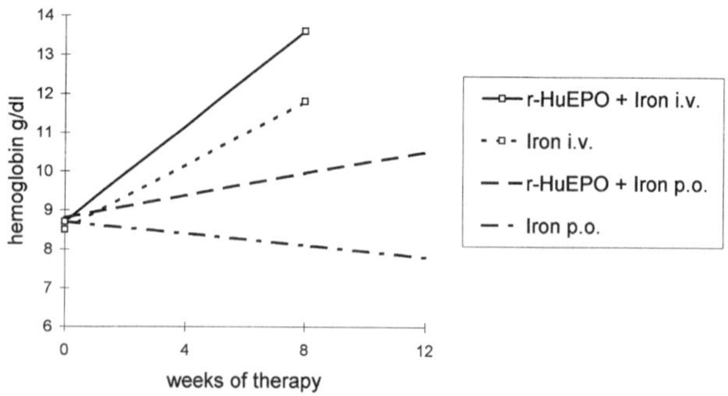

Figure 5   Results of two randomized controlled trials using r-HuEPO combined with oral or intravenous iron therapy. The mean increase in the r-HuEPO groups was superior in both trials. A comparison of intravenous iron treatment alone (Ann Intern Med. 1997) with r-HuEPO plus oral iron (N Engl J Med. 1996) demonstrates the high cost efficacy of iron saccharate infusions (US$ 215 vs US$ 3420). Oral iron alone is cheap (US$ 25) but ineffective

and to test the efficacy of this product, in a multicentre design[33]. The number of iron saccharate infusions was reduced to 6 within 4 weeks and predictors of a response to iron saccharate were evaluated.

A number of parameters (CRP, orosomucoid, serum erythropoietin, transferrin, transferrin saturation, ferritin, soluble transferrin-receptor, clinical activity) were measured at baseline and analysed for their ability to predict the response to iron therapy. In this trial, 65% of IBD patients responded within 4 weeks. Both high transferrin levels (>300 mg/dl) and low C-reactive protein levels (<2.0 mg/dl) were good predictors of response to iron saccharate. Again, in this multicentre trial, no serious side-effects were observed when 65 patients were treated. Iron non-responders improved significantly on subsequent erythropoietin therapy.

CONCLUSIONS

With regard to limited medical resources and the high costs of r-HuEPO, we consider that therapy with r-HuEPO should be restricted to those patients who do not respond to intravenous iron therapy. The ability to predict which patients will not respond to intravenous iron therapy by measurement of baseline transferrin and C-reactive protein levels is the basis for early stratification of patients with IBD-associated anaemia. Those with low transferrin levels and high C-reactive protein will benefit from concomitant r-HuEPO therapy. The backbone of therapy for IBD-associated anaemia is, in any case, intravenous iron supplementation. It is clear that supportive treatment does not change the chronic illness of our patients. However, successful treatment of IBD-associated anaemia results in better quality of life and increases the productive power of these patients. Thus, gastroenterologists in charge of IBD patients should care, not only for bowel movements, but also for the haemoglobin levels of their patients.

Acknowledgement

The author is grateful to Alexandra Weisgram for all her efforts in preparing this manuscript.

References

1. Schreiber S, Wedel S. Diagnosis and treatment of anemia in inflammatory bowel diseases. Inflamm. Bowel Dis. 1997;3:204–16
2. Plum P, Warburg E. Hematological changes, especially megalocytic anemia, in regional ileitis. Acta Med Scand. 1939;102:449–75.
3. Sheehan RG, Necheles TF, Lindeman RJ, Meyer HJ, Patterson JF. Regional enteritis and granulomatous colitis associated with erythrocyte glucose-6-phosphate dehydrogenase deficiency. N Engl J Med. 1967;23:1124–6.
4. Yates P, Macht LM, Williams NA, Elson CJ. Red cell autoantibody production by colonic mononuclear cells from a patient with ulcerative colitis and autoimmune haemolytic anemia. Br J Haematol. 1992;82:753–6.
5. Eng C, Farraye FA, Shulman LN *et al.* The association between myelodysplastic syndromes and Crohn's disease. Ann Intern Med. 1992;117:661–2.
6. Shih YJ, Baynes RD, Hudson BG, Flowers CH, Sikikne BS, Cook JD. Serum transferrin receptor is a truncated form of tissue receptor. J Biol Chem. 1990;265:19077–81.

7. Beguin Y, Clemons GK, Pootrakul P, Fillet G. Quantitative assessment of erythropoietin and functional classification of anemia based on measurements of serum transferrin receptor and erythropoietin. Blood. 1993;81:1067–76.

8. Skikne BS, Flowers CH, Cook JD. Serum transferrin receptor: a quantitative measure of tissue iron deficiency. Blood. 1990;75:1870–6.

9. Weiss G, Wachter H, Fuchs D. Linkage of cell-mediated immunity to iron metabolism. Immunol Today. 1995;16:495–500.

10. Child JA, Brozovic B, Dyer NH, Mollin DL, Dawson AM. The diagnosis of iron deficiency in patients with Crohn's disease. Gut. 1973;14:642–8.

11. Bartels U, Strandberg Pedersen N, Jarnum S. Iron absorption and serum ferritin in chronic inflammatory bowel disease. Scand J Gastroenterol. 1978;13:649–56.

12. Hansen TM, Hansen NE, Birgens HS, Holund B, Lorenz I. Serum ferritin and the assessment of iron deficiency in rheumatoid arthritis. Scand J Rheumatol. 1983;12:353–9.

13. Thomson ABR, Brust R, Ali MAN, Mant MJ, Valberg LS. Iron deficiency in inflammatory bowel disease. Diagnostic efficacy of serum ferritin. Dig Dis. 1978;23:705–9.

14. Means RT, Krantz SB. Progress in understanding the pathogenesis of the anemia of chronic disease. Blood. 1992;80:1639–47.

15. Cartwright GE. The anemia of chronic disorders. Semin Hematol. 1966;3351–75.

16. Jelkmann W, Pagel H, Wolff M, Fandrey J. Monokines inhibiting erythropoietin production in human hepatoma cultures and in isolated perfused rat kidneys. Life Sci. 1992;50:301–8.

17. Gasche C, Reinisch W, Lochs H et al. Anemia in Crohn's disease: Importance of inadequate erythropoietin production and iron deficiency. Dig Dis Sci. 1994;39:1930–4.

18. Means RT, Krantz SB. Inhibition of human erythroid colony-forming units by γ interferon can be corrected by recombinant human erythropoietin. Blood. 1991;78:2564–7

19. Babbs C. Oxygen radicals in ulcerative colitis. Free Rad Biol Med. 1992;13:169–81.

20. Van Wyck DB, Stivelman JC, Ruiz J, Kirlin LF, Katz MA, Ogden DA. Iron status in patients receiving erythropoietin for dialysis-associated anemia. Kidney Int. 1989;35:712–16.

21. Schreiber S, Howaldt S, Schnoor M et al. Recombinant erythropoietin for the treatment of anemia in inflammatory bowel disease. N Engl J Med. 1996;334:619–23.

22. Geisser P, Baer M, Schaub E. Structure/histotoxicity relationship of parenteral iron preparations. Drug Res. 1992;42:1439–52.

23. Zanen AL, Adriaansen HJ, van Bommel EFH, Posthuma R, de Jong GM. Oversaturation of transferrin after intravenous ferric gluconate (Ferrlecit®) in haemodialysis patients. Nephrol Dial Transplant. 1996;11:820–4.

24. Nyvad O, Danielsen H, Madsen S. Intravenous iron–sucrose complex to reduce epoietin demand in dialysis patients. Lancet. 1994;344:1305–6.

25. Mercuriali F, Gualtieri G, Sinigaglia L et al. Use of recombinant human erythropoietin to assist autologous blood donation by anemic rheumatoid arthritis patients undergoing major orthopedic surgery. Transfusion. 1994;34:501–6.

26. Sunder-Plassmann G, Hörl W. Importance of iron supply for erythropoietin therapy. Nephrol Dial Transplant. 1995;10:2070–6.

27. Gasche C, Dejaco C, Waldhoer T et al. Intravenous iron and erythropoietin for anemia associated with Crohn disease. A randomized, controlled trial. Ann Intern Med. 1997;126:782–7.

28. Gasche C, Dejaco C, Reinisch W et al. Sequential treatment of anemia in ulcerative colitis with intravenous iron and erythropoietin. Digestion. 1998; (in press).

29. Ludwig H, Fritz E, Kotzmann H, Höcker P, Gisslinger H, Barnas U. Erythropoietin treatment of anemia associated with multiple myeloma. N Engl J Med. 1990;322:1693–9.

30. Miller CB, Platanias LC, Mills SR et al. Phase I-II trial of erythropoietin in the treatment of cisplatin-associated anemia. J Natl Cancer Inst. 1992;84:98.

31. Pincus T, Olsen NJ, Russell J et al. Multicenter study of recombinant human erythropoietin in correction of anemia in rheumatoid arthritis. Am J Med. 1990;89:161–8.

32. Horina JH, Petritsch W, Schmid CR et al. Treatment of anemia in inflammatory bowel disease with recombinant human erythropoietin: results in three patients. Gastroenterology. 1993;104:1828–31.

33. Gasche C, Mittermaier C, Waldhoer T, Petritsch W and The Austrian IBD Study Group. Transferrin and C-reactive protein predict iron resistance in IBD-associated anemia. Gastroenterology. 1997;112:A980.

31
Manipulation of intestinal microflora

M. CAMPIERI and P. GIONCHETTI

THE INTESTINAL FLORA AND INTESTINAL DEFENCE MECHANISMS

The human body meets the environment mainly through two large mucosal surfaces, the respiratory system with an approximate surface area similar to that of a soccer field, and the gastrointestinal tract with an approximate surface area similar to that of a tennis court (200–250 m^2). Although the gastrointestinal mucosal surface is much smaller than that of the lung, its functions are much more complex. In fact the gastrointestinal tract can be regarded as a reservoir with an internal surface separating 10^{13} eucaryotic cells of the human host from 10^{14} bacterial cells[1]. There is a marked variation in bacterial pattern and concentration between different levels of the gastrointestinal tract. The number of ingested bacteria is reduced dramatically by contact with gastric acid; the microflora of the stomach is predominantly Gram-positive and aerobic, and the bacterial concentration is usually $<10^3$ colony-forming units/ml (CFU/ml). The small intestine represents a transitional zone between the sparse population of aerobic flora found in the stomach and the very dense bacterial flora of the colon. The microflora of the proximal small bowel is similar to that of the stomach and the bacterial concentration is 10^3–10^4 CFU/ml. In the distal ileum the concentration of micro-organisms increases to levels of 10^5–10^9 CFU/ml and the Gram-concentration of micro-organisms increases to 10^5–10^9 CFU/ml; Gram-negative bacteria begin to outnumber Gram-positive organisms. Within the colon the total number of micro-organisms increases dramatically to 10^{10}–10^{12} CFU/ml; nearly one third of the faecal dry weight consists of viable bacteria, and anaerobic bacteria outnumber aerobes by a ratio of about 1000:1. The complexity of colonic flora is illustrated by the presence of more than 400 bacterial species[2].

The gut represents a complex ecosystem in which a delicate balance exists between the intestinal microflora and the host. The mechanisms by which the intestinal microflora interacts with the intestinal immune system are not well understood. The presence of the indigenous flora is crucial for maturation of the immune system, development of normal intestinal morphology, and to maintain a chronic and immunologically balanced intestinal inflammatory response ('physiological inflammation')[3]. However, to maintain this delicate balance, the host has to acquire various protective defence mechanisms which include the barrier provided by the epithelial layer, mechanical factors such as peristalsis and desquamation, and factors which interfere with bacterial attachment, such as the mucus layer and secretory IgA (sIgA), which represent the primary immune barrier against pathogens. In addition, recent studies have suggested the presence of a novel type of innate immunity in gastrointestinal tract in the form of antimicrobial peptides[4].

EVIDENCE FOR THE ROLE OF THE INTESTINAL FLORA IN IBD

A body of evidence from clinical and experimental observations indicates a role for intestinal microflora in the pathogenesis of IBD. The distal ileum and the colon are the areas with highest luminal bacterial concentration and represent the sites of inflammation in IBD. Also pouchitis, a non-specific disease of the ileal reservoir, occurs in presence of a bacterial overgrowth and dysbiosis. Enteric bacteria and their phlogistic products (chemotactic peptides, such as FMLP, and cell wall polymers, such as lipopolysaccharide and peptidoglycan–polysaccharide) cross the inflamed mucosa and can be seen deep in the mucosa in Crohn's disease (CD)[5]. Recently, two studies have shown convincing evidence of a breakdown of tolerance to the normal commensal flora in active IBD, supporting the theory that hyperreactivity to ubiquitous antigens from the intestinal microflora is implicated at least in perpetuation of IBD[6,7]. Suppression of the microflora with antibiotics, faecal stream diversion and bowel rest decrease the activity of CD but have less effect in patients with ulcerative colitis (UC)[8,9]. As in CD, antibiotic treatment attenuates or prevents experimental colitis in several models and are the treatment of choice for active pouchitis. Purified bacterial products are able to determine and perpetuate experimental inflammation; lipopolysaccharide and FMLP can induce an acute enterocolitis, while peptidoglycan–polysaccharide, injected into the gut wall of rats, produces a transmural inflammation which resembles CD. The importance of normal luminal bacterial flora is further emphasized by the absence of spontaneous intestinal inflammation in HLA-B27/β_2-microglobulin transgenic rats and IL-2 and IL-10 knock-out mice in the germ-free environment, and by the presence of attenuated colitis in HLA-B27, IL-2 and IL-10 knock-out mice in pathogen-free conditions[10].

PROBIOTICS IN IBD

Very few data have been published on probiotics and IBD.

Recently, a significant decrease in lactobacilli concentration was found in patients with active UC and in rats with acetic-acid-induced colitis[11]; the same authors have subsequently shown the efficacy of exogenous administration of lactobacilli in preventing the development of acetic-acid-induced colitis in the rat[12]. In a study evaluating the effect of oral bacteriotherapy with *Lactobacillus* GG in patients with CD, it was shown that this approach has the potential to increase gut IgA immune response, promoting the gut immunological barrier[13].

Interestingly, treatment with *Lactobacillus* spp. was able to prevent the development[14] and to attenuate established spontaneous colitis in IL-10-deficient mice[15].

We recently had the opportunity to use a new highly concentrated probiotic preparation (VSL ≠ 3) containing 5×10^{11} cells/g of viable lyophilized bacteria of 3 strains of bifidobacteria (*B. longum, B. infantis* and *B. brevis*), 4 strains of lactobacilli (*L. acidophilus, L. casei, L. delbrueckii* subsp. *bulgaricus* and *L. plantarum*) and one strain of *Streptococcus salivarius* subsp. *thermophilus*. We administered, as maintenance treatment, 6 g/day VSL ≠ 3 to 15 patients with UC, intolerant or allergic to 5-aminosalicylic acid, for 12 months. Twelve of the 15 patients remained in remission at the end of the trial, and faecal concentration of lactobacilli, bifidobacteria and *Streptococcus salivarius* subsp. *thermophilus* increased significantly in all patients after the 15th day of treatment. We also performed a double-blind randomized trial comparing VSL ≠ 3 with placebo in the maintenance treatment of patients with chronic relapsing pouchitis. Forty patients were randomized to receive 6 g/day of VSL ≠ 3 ($n = 20$) or placebo for 9 months. Relapse was defined as an increase of ≥2 points in the clinical portion of the Pouchitis Disease Activity Index (PDAI)[16]; clinical assessment and stool culture were performed every month, while endoscopic and histological assessment were performed every 2 months. At the end of the study, 17/20 patients remained in remission in the VSL ≠ 3 group compared with 0/20 in the placebo group. Faecal concentrations of lactobacilli, bifidobacteria and *S. salivarius* subsp. *thermophilus* increased significantly only in the VSL ≠ 3 group after the 15th day and remained stable during the 9-month treatment. No side-effects were registered.

CONCLUSIONS

Several observations support the hypothesis that intestinal microflora play a role at least in the perpetuation of IBD. Treatment with exogenous probiotics may enhance the concentration of protective bacteria in intestinal microflora and therefore may be of therapeutic benefit for patients with IBD and pouchitis.

References

1. Tancrede C. Role of human interflora in health and disease. Eur Clin Microbiol Infect Dis. 1992;11:1012–15.
2. Simon GL, Gorbach SL. Intestinal flora in health and disease. Gastroenterology. 1984;86:174–93.
3. Kenworthy R. Observations on the reaction of the intestinal mucosa to bacterial challenge. J Clin Pathol. 1971;24:138–42.
4. Mahida YR, Rose F, Chan WC. Antimicrobial peptides in the gastrointestinal tract. Gut. 1997;40:161–3.
5. Klasen IS, Melief MJ, Van Halteren AGS *et al.* The presence of peptidoglycan–polysaccharide complexes in the bowel wall and the cellular responses to these complexes in Crohn's disease. Clin Immunol Immunopathol. 1994;71:303–8.
6. Duchmann R, Kaiser I, Hermann E, Mayet W, Ewe K, Meyer zum Büschenfelde K-H. Tolerance exists towards resident intestinal flora but is broken in active inflammatory bowel disease (IBD). Clin Exp Immunol. 1995;102:448–55.
7. Macpherson A, Khoo UY, Forgacs I, Philpott-Howard J, Bjarnason I. Mucosal antibodies in inflammatory bowel disease are directed against intestinal bacteria. Gut. 1996;38:365–75.

8. Rutgeerts P, Hiele M, Geboes K *et al.* Controlled trial of metronidazole treatment for prevention of Crohn's recurrence after ileal resection. Gastroenterology. 1995;108:1617–21.

9. Rutgeerts P, Goboes K, Peeters M *et al.* Effect of faecal stream diversion on recurrence of Crohn's disease in the neoterminal ileum. Lancet. 1991;338:771–4.

10. Sartor RB. Role of the intestinal microflora in pathogenesis and complications. In: Schölmerich J, Kruis W, Goebbell H, Hohenberger W, Gross V, eds. Inflammatory Bowel Disease: Pathophysiology as Basis of Treatment. Falk symposium No. 67. Lancaster: Kluwer Academic Publishers; 1993:175–87.

11. Fabia R, Ar'Rajab A, Johansson M-L *et al.* Impairment of bacterial flora in human ulcerative colitis and experimental colitis in the rat. Digestion. 1993;54:248–55.

12. Fabia R, Ar'Rajab A, Johansson M-L *et al.* The effect of exogenous administration of *Lactobacillus reuteri* R2LC and oat fiber on acetic acid-induced colitis in the rat. Scand J Gastroenterol. 1993;28:155–62.

13. Malin M, Suomalainen H, Saxelin M, Isolauri E. Promotion of IgA immune response in patients with Crohn's disease by oral Bacteriotherapy with *Lactobacillus* GG. Ann Nutr Metab. 1996;40:137–45.

14. Madsen KL, Tavernini MM, Doyle JSG, Fedorak RN. *Lactobacillus* sp. prevents development of enterocolitis in interleukin-10 gene-deficient mice. Gastroenterology. 1997;112:A1030.

15. Schultz M, Veltkamp C, Dieleman LA, Wyrick, PB, Tonkonogy SL, Sartor RB. Continuous feeding of *Lactobacillus plantarum* attenuates established colitis in interleukin-10 deficient mice. Gastroenterology. 1998; (in press).

16. Sandborn WJ, Tremaine WJ, Batts KP, Pemberton JH, Phillips SF. Pouchitis following ileal pouch–anal anastomosis: a pouchitis disease activity index. Mayo Clin Proc. 1994;69:409–15.

32
Pathogenesis and treatment of pouchitis

D. P. JEWELL

Restorative proctocolectomy, i.e. colectomy with an ileal pouch–anal anastomosis, has been a major advance in the surgical management of patients with ulcerative colitis since the pioneering operations of Sir Allan Parkes and Dr Utsunomiya. Avoidance of a life-long ileostomy appeals to both patients and their doctors but pouch surgery has been inevitably associated with unique complications which have provided major challenges in management and considerable academic stimulation in terms of pathogenesis. Nevertheless, when the operation has been performed for severe colitis or for chronic continuous disease, there is no doubt about its value in providing excellent quality of life and a favourable clinical course. For asymptomatic patients, e.g. those colitics being operated on for dysplasia or patients with familial adenomatous polyposis, there is inevitably a deterioration in quality of life even though the cancer risk may have been considerably reduced, or possibly abolished.

POUCHITIS – EPIDEMIOLOGY AND CLINICAL FEATURES

A high proportion of patients who have had a pouch procedure for ulcerative colitis will have at least one attack of acute pouchitis. However, the precise frequency of pouchitis is difficult to assess from published series, not only because definitions vary from centre to centre but also because the nature (telephone or personal interview) and length of follow-up varies[1–4]. Most patients who develop acute pouchitis do so within the first year but some may suffer their first attack some years following surgery. About two thirds of patients will have more than one attack. There is a tendency for the frequency of attacks to diminish with time although this has not been seen in all series. Certainly, in many major centres for pouch surgery, there is an impression that pouchitis is seen less commonly than hitherto but this is poorly documented. If the impression is true, it is suggestive that surgical technique has improved although there is no evidence to support this. On the other hand, patients may have learnt to self-medicate with antibiotics and thus avoid coming back to the clinic. Nevertheless, the cumulative rate of acute attacks of pouchitis is probably 30–50%[1–4] but only in patients who previously had ulcerative colitis. Well-documented attacks of 'idiopathic' pouchitis are extremely rare in patients who have had a colectomy for familial adenomatous polyposis.

The symptomatology of acute pouchitis is similar to a relapse of ulcerative colitis. Pouch contents become more liquid, often containing blood, and there is an accompanying increase in the frequency of defaecation with urgency, often with incontinence. Pelvic or lower abdominal discomfort is common, patients may have fever, and they readily become dehydrated. An acute arthropathy, uveitis or erythema nodosum can develop during an episode of acute pouchitis[5,6]. Pyoderma gangrenosum has also been seen. Although there may be few abnormal physical signs, some patients look ill, with fever and tachycardia, are anaemic, and have lower abdominal tenderness. Introducing an endoscope into the pouch can be painful (lignocaine gel often helps) and reveals an acutely inflamed mucosa. Inflammation is usually diffuse but, in milder cases, is frequently more severe on the posterior wall[7]. Biopsy specimens should be obtained from both anterior and posterior walls of the pouch, preferably in the upper as well as the lower part of the pouch. The prepouch ileum should also be examined and biopsied, as should the columnar cuff immediately above the anal–transitional zone (ATZ). The pouch–anal anastomosis should be assessed for stricturing. Pouch contents should be cultured for pathogens, including *Clostridium difficile*; the presence of Clostridial toxin should also be excluded.

A small proportion of patients (perhaps 5–10%) with an IPAA develop a chronic or refractory pouchitis. This group is clearly different from those who just have an occasional acute attack and represents the major challenge in management. This is discussed later in the chapter.

PATHOGENESIS OF POUCHITIS

Some risk factors have been clearly identified which may predict the occurrence of pouchitis. These are:

1. Ulcerative colitis as the original diagnosis
2. HLA-DRB1*0103
3. Presence of serum antibody to pANCA
4. Extraintestinal manifestations prior to surgery
5. Non-smoking

Ulcerative colitis

As already mentioned, the problem of pouchitis is confined to patients who had an IPAA for ulcerative colitis. Pouchitis is extremely rare in patients who had their pouch for familial adenomatous polyposis. Despite this, all pouches undergo varying degrees of colonic metaplasia, regardless of the indication for the surgery. Thus, the villous height usually shortens with increasing crypt depth; total mucosal thickness does not usually change[18]. In some pouches, the mucosa becomes entirely flat, and therefore colonic, even in the absence of inflammation. There is an increased rate of crypt cell proliferation[9,10] and this has been reported to be greater in pouches of patients with previous colitis than those with FAP[11]. Epithelial and goblet cells also resemble colonocytes in so far as the epithelial cells express colonic antigens[8,12] and the goblet cells express much more sulphomucin than sialomucin[8]. The factors that drive the colonic metaplasia are unknown but almost certainly relate to stasis because similar metaplastic change can be seen just proximal to small intestinal strictures[13]. Should this be the case, then it is likely that bacterial or chemical stimuli in the pouch contents are influencing crypt cell proliferation. This is known to be increased, even in the uninflamed pouch[9,10], but studies on the expression of transcripts and protein of TGF-α and TGF-β (two growth factors which exert a major influence on crypt proliferation) have not clearly elucidated a mechanism[14]. The cytokines, IL-1 and IL-8, occur more frequently in a healthy UC pouch than in normal healthy ileum[15] but no data are available for an FAP pouch. mRNA transcripts for IL-2 are increased in the healthy UC pouch compared with an FAP pouch[11] but there was no difference between them for IL-6, γ-interferon and TNF-α.

Luminal factors, such as bacterial counts, deficiencies of glutamine or short-chain fatty acids, and ischaemia, have all been proposed as potential mechanisms for metaplastic change and/or the induction of acute pouchitis. Ischaemic pouchitis can certainly occur but this happens soon after the pouch is formed and it is not a cause of intermittent acute pouchitis nor, probably, chronic refractory pouchitis. Ischaemia is certainly not the cause of the colonic metaplasia. These various hypotheses have been reviewed recently[16]. The possibility that bile acids or other chemical substances in the lumen may influence epithelial proliferation has been poorly studied although one *in-vitro* study failed to find convincing evidence for an effect of pouch dialysate on the integrity of epithelial cell monolayers[17].

Thus, whatever the mechanism of colonic metaplasia, it is probably common to all patients with a pouch. This has given rise to the concept that the factors which rendered the patient susceptible to developing ulcerative colitis initially are still operating, so that the colonic metaplastic mucosa is also susceptible to becoming inflamed. Some of these factors may well be genetic since it is now known that a number of genes confer susceptibility to developing chronic intestinal disease. For ulcerative colitis, the genes are located on chromosomes 2, 3, 6, 7 and 12 (see Chapter 2). The problem now is to narrow these areas of linkage to small enough regions to allow attempts to be made to determine the precise genes involved. The areas of linkage so far detected are known to contain genes for cytokines or their receptors, growth factors and mucins, all of which could be important candidate genes influencing both susceptibility to and pathogenesis of chronic inflammation. Thus, the genes for IL-1β and the IL-1 receptor antagonist are near the area of linkage on chromosome 2 and have been implicated in determining disease extent by at least some investigators. Similarly, some of the Class II genes on the short arm of chromosome 6 may influence extent and severity and yet other HLA genes may determine which patients develop extraintestinal manifestations. It seems very likely, therefore, that understanding the pathogenesis of pouchitis will largely depend on understanding the role of all the different genes involved in determining susceptibility to chronic colonic inflammation and the behaviour of that inflammation.

HLA antigens

A preliminary study suggested that there is a higher frequency of HLA-DRB1*0103 in patients who develop pouchitis than in those pouch patients who do not have this complication[18]. However, this was not confirmed in a larger study of 100 patients with an IPAA for ulcerative colitis[19]. Nevertheless, much larger cohorts of patients should be studied before safe conclusions can be drawn, especially as the pouchitis group will have to be stratified into patients with intermittent attacks of acute pouchitis and those with chronic refractory inflammation. Other HLA antigens which may be relevant include the HLA-DR3 DQ2 haplotype and HLA-B27 (see later).

Presence of antibody to pANCA

A circulating antibody to a neutropil antigen is frequently present in patients with ulcerative colitis[20]. It is termed a perinuclear cytoplasmic antibody because of the pattern seen by immunofluorescence or immunoperoxidase staining. However, most of the antibody is now known to be directed towards a nuclear histone protein[21,22]. Why colitics develop these antibodies, in contrast to patients with Crohn's disease, is unknown. In some populations of colitics, increased frequency of pANCA is associated with HLA-DR2[23] whereas, in other populations, it is associated with HLA-DR3, DQ2, TNF-α2[24]. Whether the antibody has any pathogenic significance is also unknown but patients with IPAA who are pANCA positive, especially with a high titre, tend to develop frequent attacks or refractory pouchitis[25–27]. On the other hand, other series have been unable to demonstrate any difference in pANCA positivity between patients with and those without pouchitis[28,29].

Extraintestinal manifestations

Patients with ulcerative colitis and primary sclerosing cholangitis (PSC) are at risk of recurrent pouchitis or refractory pouchitis following colectomy and IPAA[2]. The mechanisms are unknown but the HLA-DR3, DQ2 haplotype is frequently associated with PSC[30] and these patients also have a high prevalence and titre of pANCA[20]. Whether the Class II alleles, pANCA or an altered luminal milieu (as a result of defective secretion of bile) are responsible for the pouchitis is unclear.

Patients with an acute arthropathy, uveitis or erythema nodosum associated with attacks of ulcerative colitis also appear to be at risk of developing pouchitis following colectomy and IPAA, and these extraintestinal manifestations often develop in association with actue pouchitis[5,6]. Whether or not patients develop such manifestations also seems to be influenced by genetic factors, especially HLA Class I and II alleles (see Chapter 2), which again suggests that susceptibility to pouchitis is partly under genetic control. Two of the most refractory cases of pouchitis that we have seen in Oxford had ankylosing spondylitis and HLA-B27. Studies of idiopathic ankylosing spondylitis have demonstrated increased permeability and intestinal inflammation which may therefore be relevant in terms of developing chronic pouchitis. Few studies of pouch permeability have been performed. Merrett *et al.*[17] have shown that the permeability of the ileal mucosa falls towards colonic levels as colonic metaplasia takes place but the results were not correlated with HLA status.

Smoking

In one small study, smokers with an IPAA following colectomy for ulcerative colitis had a significantly lower incidence of pouchitis than non-smokers[31]. This is consistent with the decreased relative risk of ulcerative colitis in smokers compared with non-smokers. This is an interesting observation which requires confirmation. It is of interest that former smoking also appears to be a protective factor for pouchitis[3].

Pathogenesis – Conclusions

Inflammation of an ileo-anal pouch may be caused by a recognized pathogen (e.g. *Campylobacter*) or by stasis due to poor emptying, e.g. stenosis of the pouch–anal anastomosis. However, the majority of cases are of unknown aetiology. At present, it is probably wise to regard refractory pouchitis as a separate entity from acute intermittent pouchitis while accepting that they may be part of a similar underlying pathogenic process. From the previous discussion, it seems likely that the genes which rendered the patient susceptible to ulcerative colitis in the first place are also operating when the ileal mucosa of the pouch undergoes colonic metaplasia. This does not exclude a role for luminal or other environmental factors (e.g. smoking) but, so far, no consistent or convincing data have emerged from studies of microbiology, food substances or bile acids. Perhaps the major challenge is to determine the mechanisms by which stasis induces colonic metaplasia even in the absence of inflammation.

ASSESSMENT OF POUCHITIS

Criteria for the diagnosis, classification and measurement of activity are not yet uniformly agreed, which has led to some confusion in reporting the frequency of pouchitis and in the assessment of therapy. Most clinicians regard it as essential to confirm the clinical diagnosis by endoscopy and biopsy, and scoring systems have been devised based on these findings[32]. The histological scoring system scores acute and chronic changes separately and an aggregate score greater than 6/12 defines acute pouchitis. This system has proved robust and valuable and is widely used. However, marked inflammation giving a high score can occur in the absence of symptoms which, of course, also occurs in colitic patients prior to colectomy. To overcome this problem, a Pouchitis Disease Activity Index (PDAI) has been developed which is based on symptoms and endoscopic appearance as well as histological features of acute inflammation[33]. This should be a useful assessment but can be distorted when other causes of pouch dysfunction co-exist with mild pouchitis, thereby giving a much higher score than would be obtained using the Shepherd scoring system[32]. Therefore, until knowledge increases, it may be preferable to separate symptoms from histological scores and use the two assessments in parallel. This is similar to virtually all the scoring systems in use for ulcerative colitis.

TREATMENT

Acute pouchitis

Samples of pouch effluent should be cultured for pathogens. This should include *Clostridium difficile* and detection of its toxin since these patients frequently have antibiotics. Even if no pathogen is isolated, the majority of attacks respond well to a course of antibiotics. Metronidazole, ciprofloxacin, amoxycillin/clavulanic acid or tetracycline are used most frequently. However, only one controlled trial has been reported – a double-blind placebo-controlled crossover trial of oral metronidazole (400 mg tds) for 7 days[34]. Only 13 patients were enrolled and 11 completed both arms of the study. Metronidazole was significantly more effective in reducing stool frequency than placebo.

Refractory (chronic–active) pouchitis

There is no agreed definition of this entity but it includes patients who fail to respond to antibiotics as well as those who continually relapse once antibiotics are stopped. Treatment is often difficult and, if all else fails, defunctioning the pouch with an ileostomy may allow the inflammation to settle. If not, there is little to offer other than excision of the pouch and an end-ileostomy but this is a fairly unusual sequel and applies to less than 5% of all IPAA patients. The following approach to refractory pouchitis is logical and is the algorithm we use in Oxford.

1. Check the pouch to ensure that there is histological pouchitis. If that is confirmed, a prolonged course of an antibiotic may be helpful (e.g. ciprofloxacin 500 mg bd for 4 weeks). Delayed emptying due to stasis may be one explanation: pouch-emptying studies using isotopic scans are useful if available but stenosis of the pouch–anal anastomosis can be readily assessed by digital examination. If delayed emptying is suspected, 2-hourly emptying of the pouch with a Medena catheter can result in major improvement.

2. If these measures fail, then topical steroids or mesalazine can be used as foams or suppositories. Some patients find that foams cause acute discomfort, as they expand within the pouch, and find suppositories more acceptable. Failure to control symptoms inevitably means oral steroids and/or mesalazine and some patients even need immunosuppressants, e.g. azathioprine.

3. Several novel therapies are being tested in patients with chronic pouchitis. Bismuth–carbomer foam enemas appeared to have some benefit in open studies but failed to have an advantage over placebo in a double-blind trial[35]. Uncontrolled studies have failed to show any benefit from butyrate enemas[36]. However, a comparative trial of butyrate versus glutamate suppositories showed no difference in response rate[37] but, as no placebo group was included, it is not possible to conclude whether these treatments were equally effective or ineffective. An interesting trial has been reported using a cocktail of bacteria as probiotic therapy[38]. This study was designed as a maintenance trial and showed significantly less relapses in the probiotic

Table 1   Causes of pouch dysfunction

Pouchitis, prepouch ileitis, cuffitis
Pelvic infection, pouch–vaginal fistula
Small volume, non-compliant pouch
Partial ileal obstruction
Small-bowel motility disorder
Dietary intolerance
Crohn's disease

group than the placebo group. If confirmed, this result is fascinating and might lead to insights in terms of pathogenesis.

4.   Other causes of pouch dysfunction, as listed in Table 1, must also be excluded, especially if there is only minimal acute inflammatory activity on biopsy.

Prepouch ileitis and cuffitis

These entities have only been recognized recently and little information is available.

Prepouch ileitis is inflammation of the ileum just proximal to the pouch. It is usually confined to 10–20 cm but we have seen patients with virtually all of the small intestine involved. Radiologically, it can resemble Crohn's disease but histopathologically there are no specific features to suggest Crohn's disease (Dr Bryan Warren, personal communication). It resembles the prestomal ileitis that is occasionally seen in patients with an ileostomy and both conditions are probably due to stasis although no direct evidence exists for this. Prepouch ileitis responds well to antibiotics and corticosteroids although we have seen one patient who only recovered when given an ileostomy.

Cuffitis represents inflammation in the columnar cuff above the anal transitional zone in patients who have had a stapled anastomosis between the pouch and the top of the anal canal. The cuff should only be 1.5–2.0 cm in length but, in practice, can be much longer. The inflammation is usually mild, persists over time, is frequently asymptomatic and is not necessarily related to inflammation of the pouch[39–41]. However, cuffitis can give rise to symptoms, which include anal discomfort or pain, perianal irritation, and mucus and pouch dysfunction but there is no correlation between the histological appearance of the cuff and the degree of symptoms. Treatment includes mesalazine or steroid suppositories and exclusion of an undetected pouch–vaginal fistula. For patients with marked discomfort or tenesmus, application of 1% lignocaine gel can be beneficial.

CONCLUSIONS

Medical management of pouchitis remains largely empirical. Acute, intermittent attacks respond well to antibiotics but refractory pouchitis usually requires mesalazine and corticosteroids. If, indeed, refractory pouchitis represents a similar process to the original ulcerative colitis occurring in the metaplastic mucosa of the pouch, then this approach to treatment would seem inevitable.

References

1. McIntyre PB, Pemberton JH, Wolff BG, Beart RW, Dozois RR. Comparing functional results one year and ten years after ileal pouch–anal anastomosis for chronic ulcerative colitis. Dis Colon Rectum. 1994;37:303–7.
2. Penna C, Dozois R, Tremaine W *et al.* Pouchitis after ileal–anal anastomosis for ulcerative colitis occurs with increased frequency in patients with associated primary sclerosing cholangitis. Gut. 1996;38:234–9.
3. Stahlberg D, Gullberg K, Liljeqvist L, Hellers G, Lofberg R. Pouchitis following pelvic pouch operation for ulcerative colitis: incidence, cumulative risk, and risk factors. Dis Colon Rectum. 1996;39:1012–18.
4. Romanos J, Samarasekera DN, Stebbing JF, Jewell DP, Kettlewell MGW, Mortensen NJM. Outcome of 200 restorative proctocolectomy operations: the John Radcliffe Hospital experience. Br J Surg. 1997;84:814–18.
5. Lohmuller JL, Pemberton JH, Dozois RR, Illstrup D, van Heerden J. Pouchitis and extra-intestinal manifestations of inflammatory bowel disease after ileal pouch–anal anastomosis. Ann Surg. 1990;211:622–7.
6. de Silva HJ, de Angelis CP, Soper N, Kettlewell MGW, Mortensen NJ, Jewell DP. Clinical and functional outcome after restorative proctocolectomy. Br J Surg. 1991;78:1039–44.
7. Shepherd NA, Healey CJ, Warren BF, Thompson WHF, Wilkinson SP. The distribution of pathological changes and an assessment of colonic phenotypic change in the pelvic ileal reservoir. Gut. 1992;34:101–5.
8. de Silva HJ, Millard PR, Kettlewell M, Mortensen NJ, Prince C, Jewell DP. Mucosal characteristics of pelvic ileal pouches. Gut. 1991;32:61–5.
9. de Silva HJ, Millard PP, Soper N, Kettlewell MGW, Mortensen NJ, Jewell DP. Effects of the faecal stream and stasis on the ileal pouch mucosa. Gut. 1991;32:1166–9.
10. Apel R, Cohen Z, Andrews CW *et al.* Prospective evaluation of early morphological changes in pelvic ileal pouches. Gastroenterology. 1994;107:435–43.
11. Goldberg IA, Herbst F, Beckett CG *et al.* Leucocyte typing, cytokine expression and epithelial turnover in the ileal pouch in patients with ulcerative colitis and familial adenomatous polyposis. Gut. 1996;38:549–53.
12. Campbell AP, Merrett MN, Kettlewell MGW, Mortensen NJ, Jewell DP. Expression of colonic antigens by goblet and columnar epithelial cells in ileal pouch mucosa: their association with inflammatory change and faecal stasis. J Clin Pathol. 1994;47:834–8.
13. Merrett MN, de-Silva HJ, Rhodes JM *et al.* Colonic type mucin occurs in the ileal pouch and small intestinal Crohn's strictures, but not in coeliac disease. Gut. 1991;32:A1254–5.
14. Campbell AP, Smithson JE, Lewis C *et al.* Altered expression of TGFα and TGFβ1 in the mucosa of a functioning pelvic ileo–anal pouch. J Pathol. 1996;180(4):407–14.
15. Gionchetti P, Campieri M, Belluzzi A *et al.* Mucosal concentrations of interleukin-1, interleukin-6 and tumour necrosis factor α in pelvic ileal pouches. Dig Dis Sci. 1994;39:1525–31.
16. Merrett MN. Ileal pouches: adaptation and inflammation. Baillieres Clin Gastroenterol. 1997;11:175–93.
17. Merrett MN, Soper N, Mortensen N, Jewell DP. Intestinal permeability in the ileal pouch. Gut. 1996;39:226–30.
18. Merrett MN, Bunce M, Mortensen N, Kettlewell MGW, Jewell DP. HLA DRB1*0103 (HLA-DR-BON) may predict pouchitis in patients who have an ileal pouch–anal anastomosis (IPAA) for ulcerative colitis (UC). Gastroenterology. 1992;102(4):A935.
19. Roussomoustakaki M, Satsangi J, Welsh KI *et al.* Genetic markers may predict disease behaviour in patients with ulcerative colitis. Gastroenterology. 1997;112(6):1845–53.
20. Duerr RH, Targan SR, Landers CJ, Sutherland LR, Shanahan F. Antineutrophil cytoplasmic antibodies in ulcerative colitis: comparison with other colitides/diarrhoeal illnesses. Gastroenterology. 1992;100:1590–6.
21. Billing P, Tahir S, Calfin B *et al.* Nuclear localisation of the antigen detected by ulcerative colitis-associated perinuclear antineutrophil cytoplasmic antibodies. Am J Pathol. 1995;147(4):979–87.
22. Eggena MP, Targan SR, Vidrich A, Clemons DF, Iwancyzk L, Braun J. Histone H1: the UC-specific pANCA target antigen. FASEB J. 1996;10:463.
23. Yang H, Rotter JI, Toyoda H *et al.* Ulcerative colitis: a genetically heterogeneous disorder defined by genetic (HLA Class II) and subclinical (antineutrophil cytoplasmic antibodies) markers. J Clin Invest. 1993;92:1080–4.

24. Satsangi J, Landers CJ, Welsh KI, Koss K, Targan S, Jewell DP. The presence of anti-neutrophil antibodies reflects clinical and genetic heterogeneity within inflammatory bowel disease. Inflamm Bowel Dis. 1998;4(1):18–26.
25. Sandborn WJ, Landers CJ, Tremaine WJ, Targan SR. Antineutrophil cytoplasmic antibody correlates with chronic pouchitis after ileal pouch–anal anastomosis. Am J Gastroenterol. 1995;90(5):740–7.
26. Yang P, Oresland T, Jarnerot G, Hulton L, Danielsson D. Perinuclear antineutrophil cytoplasmic antibody in pouchitis after proctocolectomy with ileal pouch–anal anastomosis for ulcerative colitis. Scand J Gastroenterol. 1996;31:594–8.
27. Vecchi M, Gionchetti P, Bianchi MB *et al.* pANCA and development of pouchitis in ulcerative colitis patients after proctocolectomy and ileo anal pouch anastomosis. Lancet. 1994;344:886–7.
28. Brett PM, Yasuda N, Yiannakou JY *et al.* Genetic and immunological markers in pouchitis. Eur J Gastroenterol Hepatol. 1996;8:951–5.
29. Esteve M, Mallolas J, Klaassen J *et al.* Antineutrophil cytoplasmic antibodies in sera from colectomised ulcerative colitis patients and its relation to the presence of pouchitis. Gut. 1996;38(6):894–8.
30. Olerup O, Olsson R, Hulterantz R, Broome U. HLA-DR and HLA-DQ are not markers for rapid disease progression in primary sclerosing cholangitis. Gastroenterology. 1995;21:959–62.
31. Merrett M, Mortensen N, Kettlewell M, Jewell DP. Smoking may prevent pouchitis in patients with restorative proctocolectomy for ulcerative colitis. Gut. 1996;38(3):362–4.
32. Shepherd NA, Jass JR, Duval J, Moskowitz RL, Nichols RJ, Morson BC. Restorative proctocolectomy with ileal reservoir: pathological and histochemical study of mucosal biopsy specimens. J Clin Pathol. 1987;40:601–7.
33. Sandborn WJ, Tremaine WJ, Batts KP, Pemberton JH, Phillips SF. Pouchitis after ileal pouch–anal anastomosis: a Pouchitis Disease Activity Index. Mayo Clin Proc. 1994;69(5):409–15.
34. Maddon MV, McIntyre AS, Nicolls RJ. Double blind cross-over trial of metronidazole versus placebo in chronic unremitting pouchitis. Dig Dis Sci. 1994;39:1193–6.
35. Tremaine WJ, Sandborn WJ, Wolff BG, Carpenter HA, Zinweister AR, Metzger PP. Bismuth carbomer foam enemas for active chronic pouchitis: a randomized, double-blind, placebo-controlled trial. Aliment Pharmacol Ther. 1997;11:1041–6.
36. de Silva HJ, Ireland A, Kettlewell M, Mortensen N, Jewell DP. Short-chain fatty acid irrigation in severe pouchitis. N Engl J Med. 1989;321:416–17.
37. Wischmeyer P, Pemberton JH, Philips SF. Chronic pouchitis after ileal pouch–anal anastomosis: response to butyrate and glutamine suppositories in a pilot study. Mayo Clin Proc. 1993;68:978–81.
38. Gionchetti P, Rizzello F, Venturi A *et al.* Maintenance treatment of chronic pouchitis: a randomised placebo-controlled, double-blind trial with a new probiotic preparation. Gastroenterology. 1998;114:A985.
39. Lavery IC, Sirimarco MT, Ziv Y, Fazio VW. Anal canal inflammation after ileal pouch–anal anastomosis. Dis Colon Rectum. 1995;38:803–6.
40. Schmitt SL, Wexner SD, Lucas FV, James K, Nogueras JJ, Jagleman DG. Retained mucosa after doubled stapled ileal reservoir and ileo anal anastomosis. Dis Colon Rectum. 1992;35:1051–6.
41. Thompson-Fawcett MW, Mortensen NJM, Warren BF. 'Cuffitis' and inflammatory changes in the columnar cuff, anal transitional zone and ileal reservoir after a stapled pouch anal anastomosis. Dis Colon Rectum. 1998; (in press).

Index

α-haemolysin   75
activation-induced apoptosis   137
acute pouchitis   306
adhesion molecules   194
adolescents   261
adrenocorticotrophic hormone (ACTH),
    nicotine effect   45
adverse effects
    aminosalicylates   206–7
    azathioprine   220
    cyclosporine   223
    glucocorticosteroids   210, 211–12, 213
    6MP   220
    nicotine treatment   47–8, 49
aetiology   1–51
aetiopathogenesis   188–97
age   3–4, 68, 247
age at onset   4, 29–30, 34, 160, 169, 261
aminosalicylates   178, 201–9, 227, 228–9
4-aminosalicylic acid   203
5-aminosalicylic acid (5-ASA)   201–2, 207,
    211, 214, 282
anaemia   288–96
anal carcinoma   178
anastomosis   239, 242, 246, 254–5
ANCA *see* antineutrophil cytoplasmic
    antibodies
aneuploidy   162–3, 174
animal models   105–11
    bacteria   190
    IFN-γ   114–17, 120–4
    mucosal inflammation   148–50
animal studies
    candidate genes   12
    neuroimmune interactions   277–8
anti-CD3 antibody-induced syndrome   116
anti-cytokines   145–55
anti-inflammatory molecules   107–8
anti-inflammatory treatment   253–4
anti-*Saccharomyces cerevisiae* antibodies
    (ASCA)   10, 25, 30, 73, 187
anti-TNF-α antibodies   146–7, 150–1, 152–3,
    224, 228
antibiotics   69, 237, 254–5, 306
antigen presentation   117–18

antineutrophil cytoplasmic antibodies (ANCA)
    25, 28, 152
antineutrophil cytoplasmic antibody with
    perinuclear staining (pANCA)   10, 28,
    30, 187, 304
antinuclear cytoplasmic antibodies   191
aphthoid ulcers   68
apoptosis
    activation-induced   137
    T cells   192
arachidonic acid   84, 98
arginine   82–3
arthritis   124, 282, 283, 285
arthropathy   20, 280–7
arthropometry   90
ASA *see* aminosalicylic acid
Asacol   205
ASCA *see* anti-*Saccharomyces cerevisiae*
    antibodies
association studies   6–10, 12
autoimmune diabetes   120
autonomic nervous system   277
axial involvement   281–2
axonal changes   57–8
axonal damage   62
azathioprine   178–9, 204, 210, 214, 218–21,
    228, 229, 236, 254

B12 absorption   91
bacteria   190–1, 297–300
Bacteroides   73, 74
barium enemas   179–80, 238
bifidobacteria   299
bowel conservation   238–9
bowel rest   92, 98
budesonide   186, 205, 210–11, 213–14, 215
butyrate oxidation   81–2
bypass procedure   239

Caco-2 cells   74
cancer   157–97, 237
    see also colorectal cancer; hereditary non-
        polyposis colorectal cancer
    early detection   168–84
    nicotine   47–8

Candida albicans 73
candidate genes 6–10, 12–13, 19–20
CD4+ T-lymphocytes 118, 140
CD11b/CD18 expression 137
CD45RB 108, 149
CDP571 150
cell-mediated immunity 191–2
CGRP 277
chemokines 114, 192
chemoprevention, colon cancer 164
children 189, 261
cholangiocarcinoma 177
chromium-51 labelled ethylenediaminetetra-
    acetic acid ($[^{51}Cr]EDTA$) 45
chromosome 12 11, 21
chromosome 16 11, 21, 26, 27–8
chronic enterocolitis 106–7
CIA 124
cingulin 270
ciprofloxacin 228
clonidine 276, 277
Clostridium 73
  C. difficile 302, 306
colectomy 35–6, 172, 236, 237, 242
colitis 233
collagen, Crohn's disease 56, 58
collagen-induced arthritis 124
colonic haemorrhage 236
colonic metaplasia 303, 305
colonoscopy 159, 164–5, 172, 173–4, 180,
    238
colorectal cancer 261
  early detection 168–84
  risk factors 159–67
combination therapy 205, 214, 219
computed tomography (CT) 180
ConA-induced lethal hepatitis syndrome 116
contraceptives, Crohn's disease 37–9
corticosteroids 45, 203, 205, 227, 228, 229
cortisone 211, 212
counselling 237
Crohn's colitis, smoking 39–41
Crohn's disease
  aetiopathogenesis 188–97
  animal models 105–11
  cancer 157–97
  classification 185–7
  colorectal cancer 159–67, 169, 173, 181
  cytokines 135–44
  genetic heterogeneity 17–23
  genetics 24–33
  IFN-γ role 112–29
  immunomodulation therapy 145–55
  infectious track 68–79
  inflammatory arthropathy 280–7
  interleukin-12 130–4
  intestinal microflora 298–9
  myenteric plexus inflammatory lesions
      55–67

neuroimmune interactions 275–9
nutrition role 80–8
nutritional therapy 89–101
prognosis 257–66
recurrence 244–50
refractory anaemia 288–96
relapse prevention strategies 251–6
smoking 34, 37–9, 41
standard therapies 199–230
surgery 233–66
susceptibility genes 3–16
trefoil peptides 269–74
Crohn's Disease Activity Index (CDAI) 262
cuffitis 307
cyclo-oxygenase 2 (COX-2) 193
cyclosporine 179, 222–4, 228, 229
cytokines 20, 135–44, 145–55, 192–3, 271, 272
  see also interleukins; tumour necrosis
      factor-α
  anaemia 291
  animal models 106
  Crohns' disease recurrence 245–6
  iron 289
  lupus-like syndrome 122
  nicotine effect 45

delayed-release oral nicotine 48, 49
diabetes 120, 122
diet 189
dietary fat 84–5, 98–9
dietary fibre 80–1, 82
DNA mismatch repair 9, 163
DR3/DQ2 186, 187
DR103 186
DTH reactions, IFN-γ 120
dysplasia 159, 162–3, 170–1, 173, 174, 175,
    176, 180

E-cadherin 270, 271
E-selectin 136
EAE *see* experimental autoimmune
    encephalomyelysis
EAT *see* experimental autoimmune thyroiditis
EAU *see* experimental autoimmune uveitis
eicosanoids 45, 84, 98
eicosapentaenoic acid 84
EIMs *see* extraintestinal manifestations
eisinophils 63, 65
elemental diets 92, 96, 97, 98
endogenous bacteria 73–5
endoscopic relapses 252, 253–4
endothelial cells 194
endotoxin, IFN-γ 116
enemas
  barium 179–80, 238
  nicotine 48, 49
enteral nutrition 91, 92–9
enteric nervous system 55–66, 246–7
enteroenteric bypass surgery 239

environmental factors   25, 189–90
environmental importance   34–42
environmental risk factors   4–5
epidemiology   3–5
epithelial cells   194
erythropoeitin   291, 293–4
Escherichia coli   73–5
essential fatty acids   84, 85
ethnic groups   4, 10, 19, 26, 27
European variation   4
experimental autoimmune encephalomyelysis (EAE)   120, 124
experimental autoimmune thyroiditis (EAT)   124
experimental autoimmune uveitis (EAU)   120
extracellular matrix   194
extraintestinal manifestations (EIMs)   7, 20, 234, 280, 304–5

failure to thrive   234
familial factors   190
family history   34
family studies   5–6, 17–18, 25–6, 27, 28–9
fat absorption   91
fat (dietary)   84–5, 98–9
fatty acids   84–5, 98
fibroblast growth factors (FGFs)   193, 271
Finney strictureplasty   240
fish oil   84–5
fistulas   235, 236–7, 240–3
fistulizing Crohn's disease   186, 228
folate deficiency   164
folic acid   91, 177
functional iron deficiency   291

gastrojejunostomy   239
genetic anticipation   12, 30
genetic factors   190
genetic heterogeneity   17–23
genetics, telling patients   24–33
genome-wide scanning   10–13, 18–19, 20–2, 27
glucocorticoids, smoking effect   35, 36
glucocorticosteroids   210–17
glutamine   83–4
graft versus host (GVH) disease   117, 122, 124
granulomas   248
growth effects   90
growth factors   193

haematinic deficiency   91
haemoglobin synthesis   289
haemorrhage   241
Hartmann operation   236
Helicobacter hepaticus   72
hereditary non-polyposis colorectal cancer (HNPCC)   9, 29, 163
heritability coefficient   17–18, 26
heterogeneity   26, 28, 31
HGF   271

HLA *see* human leukocyte antigen
human leukocyte antigen (HLA)   19–20, 59, 304
  complex   27, 30
  genes   6–7
  phenotypes   137
humoral immunity   191–2
hypoalbuminaemia   236
hypoallergenic diets   98

iatrogenic malignancy   178–9
IBD1   11, 21, 26, 27
ICAM-1   114, 137, 140
identity by descent method   11
IFNγ *see* interferon (IFN)-γ
IL *see* interleukins
ileitis   233, 247, 307
ileocaecal resection   242
ileocolectomy   63
ileocolitis   233, 239
ileocolonic anastomosis   244–50
ileorectal anastomosis   248
ileostomy   236, 248
immune factors   191–4
immune response
  IFN-γ   117–24
  interleukin-10   140
  TNF   136–7
immunomodulation   145–55, 218–26
immunoregulation   107–8
immunostat hypothesis   146
immunosuppressants   178–9, 254
immunosuppression   107–8, 218–26, 236
in vivo modulation   120–4
inducible NO synthases (iNOS)   83
infection   68–79
  see also bacteria
inflammatory arthropathy   280–7
inflammatory Crohn's disease   186
inflammatory lesions, myenteric plexus   55–67
infliximab   228, 229
intercellular adhesion molecule-1 (ICAM-1)   9
interferon   271
interferon (IFN)-γ   112–29, 192
interleukins   8–9, 271
  IL-1   107, 192–3
  IL-1 receptor antagonist   20
  IL-1a   8–9
  IL-1b   8–9
  IL-1β   114
  IL-1ra   8–9
  IL-2   20, 124, 192, 246
  IL-4   192, 245–6
  IL-6   192
  IL-8   137, 192
  IL-10   20, 139–41, 145, 148, 149–50, 151–2, 192, 224
  IL-10 receptor   139–40
  IL-12   124, 130–4

intestinal microflora manipulation   297–300
intestinal mucin genes   20
intestinal permeability   28, 45, 190, 270
intra-abdominal abscess   236, 241
intravenous parenteral iron   292–3, 294–5
iron   84
   deficiency   91, 288–96
   metabolism   288–91
ischaemic bowel disease   185
ISIS-2302   224
ITF   270, 271, 272

janus family tyrosine kinases   131
joint inflammation   283–4

keratinocyte growth factor   193
Ki-67 antigen   175

Lactobacillus   298–9
lamina propria mononuclear cells (LPMC)
   131–2
laparoscopic bowel surgery   240
laparotomy   241–2
leukotrienes   202
lidocaine   276
linkage analyses   19
linoleic acid   84, 98
α-linolenic acid   84
lipid mediators   193
Listeria   72
   L. monocytogenes   72
lupus-like disease   120, 122
lymphocytes   284
lymphocytic neuropathy   63
lymphomas   220–1, 223

macrophages   132
MAdCAM-1   194, 284–5
magnesium citrate   237
magnesium deficiency   91
maintenance therapy   227, 228–9, 253
malnutrition   89–90, 236
MAP kinase   271
mast cells   65
matrix metalloproteinases   193
measles virus   5, 70–1, 190
mercaptopurine   178, 179
6-mercaptopurine (6MP)   218–21, 228–9,
   254
mesalazine   82, 202, 203–5, 206, 253–4
mesenchymal cells   194
methotrexate   179, 221–2, 229
6-methyl prednisolone   214
metronidazole   204, 228, 246, 255, 306
MHC Class I molecules   122
MHC Class II   120
   antigens   58–9, 190
   expression   63–4
   molecules   117

MHC molecules   55
microbial agents   190–1
Miles procedure   243
mineral deficiency   91
minimal residue diets   98
MLH1   9
model-free analysis   10–11
6MP *see* 6-mercaptopurine
MSH2 gene   163
MUC 2 and 3   20
mucin glycoproteins   30–1
mucosal macrophages   106
mucus production   45
mycobacteria   5, 68–9
Mycobacterium paratuberculosis   68–9, 190
mycophenolate mofetil   224
myenteric plexus, inflammatory lesions
   55–67
Myobacterium
   M. avium   118
   M. lepraemurium   117–18

NADPH diaphorase-positive cells   60–1
neoplasia   159, 161, 172–3, 176, 179–80
neoterminal ileum, recurrence   244–7, 248
nerve fibre hypertrophy   57, 62
neuritis   246
neuroimmune interactions   275–9
neuromatous lesions   62
neuromodulation   276–7
neuropeptides   193
neurotransmitters   277
neutral endopeptidase   277
neutrophil stimulation, TNF-   137
NGF receptor   57
nicotine   190, 277
   see also smoking
   gum   45–8
   patches   5, 34, 35, 37, 45–8
   ulcerative colitis   43–51
nitrergic innervation   59
nitric oxide   118
nitric oxide synthases (NOS)   59, 83, 114
nitrogen balance   90
nitrogen metabolites   193
non-immune cells   194
non-steroidal anti-inflammatory drugs
   (NSAIDs)   28, 176
nutrition   80–8
nutritional therapy   89–101

obstructive uropathy   241
occludin   269
oleic acid   84, 85
oligomeric diets   92, 93
olsalazine   206
oral contraceptives, Crohn's disease   37–9
oral iron preparations   292
oxygen metabolites   193

p53 tumour suppressor gene   162, 174–5
palmitoleic acid   84
pANCA *see* antineutrophil cytoplasmic
    antibody with perinuclear staining
pancolitis   160
para-aminosalicylic acid *see* 4-aminosalicylic
    acid
paramyxovirus-like structures   70
parenteral nutrition   92
pathogenesis   53–101
pauci-articular asymmetrical arthropathy   20
Pentasa   204–5, 211, 214, 253
peptide growth factors   271
peptidergic nerves   59
perianal disease   234
perianal surgery   239, 240–3
peripheral arthropathy   280–1
peritonitis   236
peroperative sepsis   236
Peyer's patches   68
Plantago ovata   82
platelet-activating factor (PFA)   137
polyethylene glycol   237
polymeric diets   92, 93, 96, 97, 98
population stratification   10
pouches   241
pouchitis   191, 298, 301–9
Pouchitis Disease Activity Index (PDAI)   305
prednisolone   47, 210, 214, 219
prednisone   205
pregnancy, Crohns' disease recurrence   248
primary sclerosing cholangitis   160–1, 175–6,
    177, 179, 304
probiotics   298–9
proctitis   160, 185
proctocolitis   185
prognosis   257–66
proinflammatory molecules   107–8
proliferating cell nuclear antigen (PCNA)   175
prostaglandins   118
protein   98
    metabolism   90
    protein-energy malnutrition   90
pS2   270
psoriasis   7

quality of life   262, 263

radiation exposure   179–80
radical proctectomy   243
RANTES   147
reactive metabolites   193
recombinant human erythropoeitin (r-HuEPO)
    293–4, 295
rectovaginal fistula   241
recurrence
    Crohn's disease   233
    definition   252
refractory anaemia   288–96

refractory pouchitis   306–7
relapse
    neuromodulation   277
    prevention
        Crohn's disease   251–6
        ulcerative colitis   253
remission
    definition   227
    induction   201–3, 204–5, 210, 228, 229
    maintenance   201, 203–4, 205–6, 211,
        214–15
resection margins   238–9, 248
restorative proctocolectomy   301
risk factors
    colorectal cancer   159–67
    Crohns' disease recurrence   247–8
Rowasa   253

Saccharomyces cerevisiae   73
sacroilitis   281–2
salazosulphapyridine   254
Salofalk   205, 253
SASP   282
SEB, IL-12   132
sensory nerves   277–8
sepsis   242
sequential therapy   227–30
short-chain fatty acids (SCFA)   80–1
Shwartzman reaction   115, 116, 117
sialosyl-Tn   163, 175
side effects *see* adverse effects
side-to-side isoperistaltic technique   240
small bowel
    cancer   177–8
    obstruction   236
    permeability   25, 246
smoking   5, 34–42, 189–90
    see also nicotine
    Crohns' disease recurrence   247
    neuromodulation   276, 277
    pouchitis   305
socioeconomics   4
SP   193, 270, 272
sphincterotomy   243
spondylitis   281–2
spondyloarthropathy (SpA)   280, 281, 282–3,
    285
STAT-4 molecule   131
steatorrhoea   91
stenotic Crohn's disease   186
step-wise therapy   227–30
steroids   210–17, 237
stoma   254–5
    site marking   238
    surgery   239
Streptococcus salivarius subsp. *thermophilus*
    299
streptozotocin-induced diabetes   120
stress   275, 276, 278

stricture dilatation 240
strictureplasty 239–40, 242
substance P 59, 276, 277
sulphasalazine 201, 202, 203, 204, 205–7, 214, 227
sulphate-containing compounds 80–1
sulphide 81–2
superantigen-induced shock syndrome 116
surgery 233–66
surveillance 164, 168–84, 261
susceptibility genes 3–16, 17, 18, 19, 21–2, 24, 26, 27
symmetrical polyarthropathy 20

T cells
    activation 130
    apoptosis 192
T lymphocytes 106, 107, 117–18, 137, 140
T-helper-1 (Th-1) 118–20
    cytokines 146, 148, 149, 150
    immune response 192
    lymphocytes 130, 133
T-helper-2 (Th-2) 118–20
    cytokines 122, 146, 148
    immune response 192
    lymphocytes 130–1
T-lamina propria lymphocytes (T-LPL) 132
TAP proteins 8
targeted delivery 201
TGF-β 271
TNF-α see tumour necrosis factor-α
tobacco 5
topical treatment
    glucocorticosteroids 213–14
    mesalazine 202, 204
    nicotine 48
total parenteral nutrition (TPN) 92, 236, 237
toxic colitis 234, 236, 237
toxic megacolon 59, 234, 236, 258
TPN see total parenteral nutrition
trans-sphincteric fistulotomy 243
transferrin 288–9
transmission disequilibrium test (TDT) 10
transmittable-agent hypothesis 72
trefoil peptides 193, 269–74
tropomyosin fraction 5 191
Trypanosoma brucei 118
tumour necrosis factor (TNF)
    receptor I (TNFRI) 136
    receptor II (TNFRII) 136
tumour necrosis factor-α (TNF-α) 7–8, 20, 135–9, 145, 146–8, 149–51, 192, 246
    IFN-γ 114

iron 290
nicotine effect 45
tumour necrosis factor-α converting enzyme (TACE) 135
tumour-associated cachexia 116
twin studies 5–6, 17–18, 26, 31

ulcerative colitis
    aetiopathogenesis 188–97
    animal models 105–11
    cancer 157–97
    classification 185–7
    colorectal cancer 159–67, 168–9, 170–3, 175, 180–1
    cytokines 135–44
    genetic heterogeneity 17–23
    genetics 24–33
    IFN-γ role 112–29
    immunomodulation therapy 145–55
    infectious track 68–79
    inflammatory arthropathy 280–7
    interleukin-12 130–4
    intestinal microflora 298–9
    neuroimmune interactions 275–9
    nicotine treatment 43–51
    nutrition role 80–8
    nutritional therapy 89–101
    pouchitis 302–3
    prognosis 257–66
    refractory anaemia 288–96
    relapse prevention 253
    smoking 34–7
    standard therapies 199–230
    susceptibility genes 3–16
    trefoil peptides 269–74

vagotomy 239
vascular adhesion protein 284, 285
vascular theory 5
vasculitis 70–1, 190
vasoactive intestinal peptide (VIP) 59, 65, 193
viruses 190
vitamin deficiency 91

weight loss 90
whole genome research 10–13

yeasts 73

zinc deficiency 91
ZO-1 269, 270
ZO-2 269, 270

Falk Symposium Series

43. Reutter W, Popper H, Arias IM, Heinrich PC, Keppler D, Landmann L, eds.: *Modulation of Liver Cell Expression*. Falk Symposium No. 43. 1987   ISBN: 0-85200-677-2*

44. Boyer JL, Bianchi L, eds.: *Liver Cirrhosis*. Falk Symposium No. 44. 1987
      ISBN: 0-85200-993-3*

45. Paumgartner G, Stiehl A, Gerok W, eds.: *Bile Acids and the Liver*. Falk Symposium No. 45. 1987   ISBN: 0-85200-675-6*

46. Goebell H, Peskar BM, Malchow H, eds.: *Inflammatory Bowel Diseases – Basic Research & Clinical Implications*. Falk Symposium No. 46. 1988   ISBN: 0-7462-0067-6*

47. Bianchi L, Holt P, James OFW, Butler RN, eds.: *Aging in Liver and Gastrointestinal Tract*. Falk Symposium No. 47. 1988   ISBN: 0-7462-0066-8*

48. Heilmann C, ed.: *Calcium-Dependent Processes in the Liver*. Falk Symposium No. 48. 1988   ISBN: 0-7462-0075-7*

50. Singer MV, Goebell H, eds.: *Nerves and the Gastrointestinal Tract*. Falk Symposium No. 50. 1989   ISBN: 0-7462-0114-1

51. Bannasch P, Keppler D, Weber G, eds.: *Liver Cell Carcinoma*. Falk Symposium No. 51. 1989   ISBN: 0-7462-0111-7

52. Paumgartner G, Stiehl A, Gerok W, eds.: *Trends in Bile Acid Research*. Falk Symposium No. 52. 1989   ISBN: 0-7462-0112-5

53. Paumgartner G, Stiehl A, Barbara L, Roda E, eds.: *Strategies for the Treatment of Hepatobiliary Diseases*. Falk Symposium No. 53. 1990   ISBN: 0-7923-8903-4

54. Bianchi L, Gerok W, Maier K-P, Deinhardt F, eds.: *Infectious Diseases of the Liver*. Falk Symposium No. 54. 1990   ISBN: 0-7923-8902-6

55. Falk Symposium No. 55 not published

55B. Hadziselimovic F, Herzog B, Bürgin-Wolff A, eds.: *Inflammatory Bowel Disease and Coeliac Disease in Children*. International Falk Symposium. 1990 ISBN 0-7462-0125-7

56. Williams CN, eds.: *Trends in Inflammatory Bowel Disease Therapy*. Falk Symposium No. 56. 1990   ISBN: 0-7923-8952-2

57. Bock KW, Gerok W, Matern S, Schmid R, eds.: *Hepatic Metabolism and Disposition of Endo- and Xenobiotics*. Falk Symposium No. 57. 1991   ISBN: 0-7923-8953-0

58. Paumgartner G, Stiehl A, Gerok W, eds.: *Bile Acids as Therapeutic Agents: From Basic Science to Clinical Practice*. Falk Symposium No. 58. 1991   ISBN: 0-7923-8954-9

59. Halter F, Garner A, Tytgat GNJ, eds.: *Mechanisms of Peptic Ulcer Healing*. Falk Symposium No. 59. 1991   ISBN: 0-7923-8955-7

60. Goebell H, Ewe K, Malchow H, Koelbel Ch, eds.: *Inflammatory Bowel Diseases – Progress in Basic Research and Clinical Implications*. Falk Symposium No. 60. 1991
      ISBN: 0-7923-8956-5

61. Falk Symposium No. 61 not published

62. Dowling RH, Folsch UR, Löser Ch, eds.: *Polyamines in the Gastrointestinal Tract*. Falk Symposium No. 62. 1992   ISBN: 0-7923-8976-X

63. Lentze MJ, Reichen J, eds.: *Paediatric Cholestasis: Novel Approaches to Treatment*. Falk Symposium No. 63. 1992   ISBN: 0-7923-8977-8

64. Demling L, Frühmorgen P, eds.: *Non-Neoplastic Diseases of the Anorectum*. Falk Symposium No. 64. 1992   ISBN: 0-7923-8979-4

64B. Gressner AM, Ramadori G, eds.: *Molecular and Cell Biology of Liver Fibrogenesis*. International Falk Symposium. 1992   ISBN: 0-7923-8980-8

*These titles were published under the MTP Press imprint.

Falk Symposium Series

65. Hadziselimovic F, Herzog B, eds.: *Inflammatory Bowel Diseases and Morbus Hirschprung*. Falk Symposium No. 65. 1992   ISBN: 0-7923-8995-6

66. Martin F, McLeod RS, Sutherland LR, Williams CN, eds.: *Trends in Inflammatory Bowel Disease Therapy*. Falk Symposium No. 66. 1993   ISBN: 0-7923-8827-5

67. Schölmerich J, Kruis W, Goebell H, Hohenberger W, Gross V, eds.: *Inflammatory Bowel Diseases – Pathophysiology as Basis of Treatment*. Falk Symposium No. 67. 1993   ISBN: 0-7923-8996-4

68. Paumgartner G, Stiehl A, Gerok W, eds.: *Bile Acids and The Hepatobiliary System: From Basic Science to Clinical Practice*. Falk Symposium No. 68. 1993   ISBN: 0-7923-8829-1

69. Schmid R, Bianchi L, Gerok W, Maier K-P, eds.: *Extrahepatic Manifestations in Liver Diseases*. Falk Symposium No. 69. 1993   ISBN: 0-7923-8821-6

70. Meyer zum Büschenfelde K-H, Hoofnagle J, Manns M, eds.: *Immunology and Liver*. Falk Symposium No. 70. 1993   ISBN: 0-7923-8830-5

71. Surrenti C, Casini A, Milani S, Pinzani M , eds.: *Fat-Storing Cells and Liver Fibrosis*. Falk Symposium No. 71. 1994   ISBN: 0-7923-8842-9

72. Rachmilewitz D, ed.: *Inflammatory Bowel Diseases – 1994*. Falk Symposium No. 72. 1994   ISBN: 0-7923-8845-3

73. Binder HJ, Cummings J, Soergel KH, eds.: *Short Chain Fatty Acids*. Falk Symposium No. 73. 1994   ISBN: 0-7923-8849-6

73B. Möllmann HW, May B, eds.: *Glucocorticoid Therapy in Chronic Inflammatory Bowel Disease: from basic principles to rational therapy*. International Falk Workshop. 1996   ISBN 0-7923-8708-2

74. Keppler D, Jungermann K, eds.: *Transport in the Liver*. Falk Symposium No. 74. 1994   ISBN: 0-7923-8858-5

74B. Stange EF, ed.: *Chronic Inflammatory Bowel Disease*. Falk Symposium. 1995   ISBN: 0-7923-8876-3

75. van Berge Henegouwen GP, van Hoek B, De Groote J, Matern S, Stockbrügger RW, eds.: *Cholestatic Liver Diseases: New Strategies for Prevention and Treatment of Hepatobiliary and Cholestatic Liver Diseases*. Falk Symposium 75. 1994.   ISBN: 0-7923-8867-4

76. Monteiro E, Tavarela Veloso F, eds.: *Inflammatory Bowel Diseases: New Insights into Mechanisms of Inflammation and Challenges in Diagnosis and Treatment*. Falk Symposium 76. 1995.   ISBN 0-7923-8884-4

77. Singer MV, Ziegler R, Rohr G, eds.: *Gastrointestinal Tract and Endocrine System*. Falk Symposium 77. 1995.   ISBN 0-7923-8877-1

78. Decker K, Gerok W, Andus T, Gross V, eds.: *Cytokines and the Liver*. Falk Symposium 78. 1995.   ISBN 0-7923-8878-X

79. Holstege A, Schölmerich J, Hahn EG, eds.: *Portal Hypertension*. Falk Symposium 79. 1995.   ISBN 0-7923-8879-8

80. Hofmann AF, Paumgartner G, Stiehl A, eds.: *Bile Acids in Gastroenterology: Basic and Clinical Aspects*. Falk Symposium 80. 1995   ISBN 0-7923-8880-1

81. Riecken EO, Stallmach A, Zeitz M, Heise W, eds.: *Malignancy and Chronic Inflammation in the Gastrointestinal Tract – New Concepts*. Falk Symposium 81. 1995   ISBN 0-7923-8889-5

82. Fleig WE, ed.: *Inflammatory Bowel Diseases: New Developments and Standards*. Falk Symposium 82. 1995   ISBN 0-7923-8890-6

Falk Symposium Series

82B. Paumgartner G, Beuers U, eds.: *Bile Acids in Liver Diseases*. International Falk Workshop. 1995   ISBN 0-7923-8891-7

83. Dobrilla G, Felder M, de Pretis G, eds.: *Advances in Hepatobiliary and Pancreatic Diseases: Special Clinical Topics*. Falk Symposium 83. 1995.   ISBN 0-7923-8892-5

84. Fromm H, Leuschner U, eds.: *Bile Acids – Cholestasis – Gallstones: Advances in Basic and Clinical Bile Acid Research*. Falk Symposium 84. 1995   ISBN 0-7923-8893-3

85. Tytgat GNJ, Bartelsman JFWM, van Deventer SJH, eds.: *Inflammatory Bowel Diseases*. Falk Symposium 85. 1995   ISBN 0-7923-8894-1

86. Berg PA, Leuschner U, eds.: *Bile Acids and Immunology*. Falk Symposium 86. 1996   ISBN 0-7923-8700-7

87. Schmid R, Bianchi L, Blum HE, Gerok W, Maier KP, Stalder GA, eds.: *Acute and Chronic Liver Diseases: Molecular Biology and Clinics*. Falk Symposium 87. 1996   ISBN 0-7923-8701-5

88. Blum HE, Wu GY, Wu CH, eds.: *Molecular Diagnosis and Gene Therapy*. Falk Symposium 88. 1996   ISBN 0-7923-8702-3

88B. Poupon RE, Reichen J, eds.: *Surrogate Markers to Assess Efficacy of TReatment in Chronic Liver Diseases*. International Falk Workshop. 1996   ISBN 0-7923-8705-8

89. Reyes HB, Leuschner U, Arias IM, eds.: *Pregnancy, Sex Hormones and the Liver*. Falk Symposium 89. 1996   ISBN 0-7923-8704-X

89B. Broelsch CE, Burdelski M, Rogiers X, eds.: *Cholestatic Liver Diseases in Children and Adults*. International Falk Workshop. 1996   ISBN 0-7923-8710-4

90. Lam S-K, Paumgartner P, Wang B, eds.: *Update on Hepatobiliary Diseases 1996*. Falk Symposium 90. 1996   ISBN 0-7923-8715-5

91. Hadziselimovic F, Herzog B, eds.: *Inflammatory Bowel Diseases and Chronic Recurrent Abdominal Pain*. Falk Symposium 91. 1996   ISBN 0-7923-8722-8

91B. Alvaro D, Benedetti A, Strazzabosco M, eds.: *Vanishing Bile Duct Syndrome – Pathophysiology and Treatment*. International Falk Workshop. 1996   ISBN 0-7923-8721-X

92. Gerok W, Loginov AS, Pokrowskij VI, eds.: *New Trends in Hepatology 1996*. Falk Symposium 92. 1997   ISBN 0-7923-8723-6

93. Paumgartner G, Stiehl A, Gerok W, eds.: *Bile Acids in Hepatobiliary Diseases – Basic Research and Clinical Application*. Falk Symposium 93. 1997   ISBN 0-7923-8725-2

94. Halter F, Winton D, Wright NA, eds.: *The Gut as a Model in Cell and Molecular Biology*. Falk Symposium 94. 1997   ISBN 0-7923-8726-0

94B. Kruse-Jarres JD, Schölmerich J, eds.: *Zinc and Diseases of the Digestive Tract*. International Falk Workshop. 1997   ISBN 0-7923-8724-4

95. Ewe K, Eckardt VF, Enck P, eds.: *Constipation and Anorectal Insufficiency*. Falk Symposium 95. 1997   ISBN 0-7923-8727-9

96. Andus T, Goebell H, Layer P, Schölmerich J, eds.: *Inflammatory Bowel Disease – from Bench to Bedside*. Falk Symposium 96. 1997   ISBN 0-7923-8728-7

97. Campieri M, Bianchi-Porro G, Fiocchi C, Schölmerich J, eds. *Clinical Challenges in Inflammatory Bowel Diseases: Diagnosis, Prognosis and Treatment*. Falk Symposium 97. 1998   ISBN 0-7923-8733-3

98. Lembcke B, Kruis W, Sartor RB, eds. *Systemic Manifestations of IBD: The Pending Challenge for Subtle Diagnosis and Treatment*. Falk Symposium 98. 1998   ISBN 0-7923-8734-1

Falk Symposium Series

99.   Goebell H, Holtmann G, Talley NJ, eds. *Functional Dyspepsia and Irritable Bowel Syndrome: Concepts and Controversies.* Falk Symposium 99. 1998
ISBN 0-7923-8735-X

100.   Blum HE, Bode Ch, Bode JCh, Sartor RB, eds. *Gut and the Liver.* Falk Symposium 100. 1998
ISBN 0-7923-8736-8

101.   Rachmilewitz D, ed. *V International Symposium on Inflammatory Bowel Diseases.* Falk Symposium 101. 1998
ISBN 0-7923-8743-0

102.   Manns MP, Boyer JL, Jansen PLM, Reichen J, eds. *Cholestatic Liver Diseases.* Falk Symposium 102. 1998
ISBN 0-7923-8746-5

102B. Manns MP, Chapman RW, Stiehl A, Wiesner R, eds. *Primary Sclerosing Cholangitis.* International Falk Workshop. 1998.
ISBN 0-7923-8745-7

103.   Häussinger D, Jungermann K, eds. *Liver and Nervous System.* Falk Symposium 102. 1998
ISBN 0-7924-8742-2

103B. Häussinger D, Heinrich PC, eds. *Signalling in the Liver.* International Falk Workshop. 1998
ISBN 0-7923-8744-9

103C. Fleig W, ed. *Normal and Malignant Liver Cell Growth.* International Falk Workshop. 1998
ISBN 0-7923-8748-1

104.   Stallmach A, Zeitz M, Strober W, MacDonald TT, Lochs H, eds. *Induction and Modulation of Gastrointestinal Inflammation.* Falk Symposium 104. 1998
ISBN 0-7923-8747-3

105.   Emmrich J, Liebe S, Stange EF, eds. *Innovative Concepts in Inflammatory Bowel Diseases.* Falk Symposium 105. 1999
ISBN 0-7923-8749-X

106.   Rutgeerts P, Colombel J-F, Hanauer SB, Schölmerich J, Tytgat GNJ, van Gossum A, eds. *Advances in Inflammatory Bowel Diseases.* Falk Symposium 106. 1999
ISBN 0-7923-8750-3

Immunosuppression in Inflammatory Bowel Diseases

Standards, New Developments, Future Trends

Immunosuppression in Inflammatory Bowel Diseases

Standards, New Developments, Future Trends

Edited by

K. Fellermann

Medizinische Klinik I
Medizinische Universität zu Lübeck
Lübeck
Germany

W. J. Sandborn

Division of Gastroenterology
Mayo Clinic
Rochester, MN 55905
USA

D. P. Jewell

Gastroenterology Unit
The Radcliffe Infirmary
Oxford
United Kingdom

J. Schölmerich

Klinik und Poliklinik für Innere
Medizin I
Klinikum der Universität
Regensburg
Regensburg
Germany

E. F. Stange

Zentrum Innere Medizin
Robert Bosch Krankenhaus
Stuttgart
Germany

Proceedings of Falk Symposium 119 held in Freiburg, Germany,
October 3–4, 2000

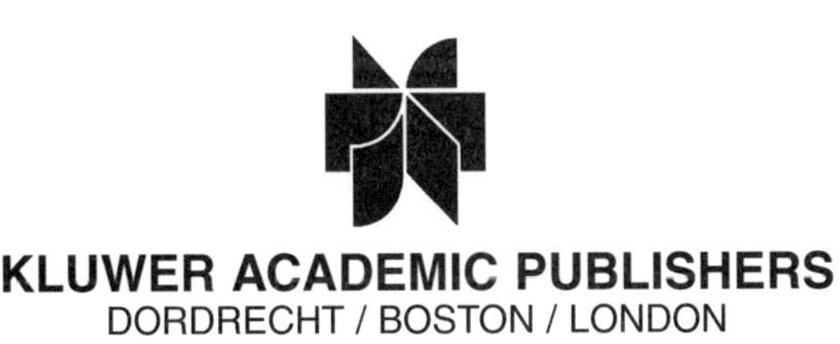

KLUWER ACADEMIC PUBLISHERS
DORDRECHT / BOSTON / LONDON

Library of Congress Cataloging-in-Publication Data is available.

ISBN 0–7923–8767–8

Published by Kluwer Academic Publishers, BV
P.O. Box 17, 3300 AA Dordrecht, The Netherlands.

Sold and distributed in North, Central and South America
by Kluwer Academic Publishers, PO Box 358,
Accord Station, Hingham, MA 02018-0358, USA.

In all other countries, sold and distributed
by Kluwer Academic Publishers, Distribution Center,
P.O. Box 322, 3300 AH Dordrecht, The Netherlands.

Printed on acid-free paper

Printed and bound in Great Britain by MPG Books, Bodmin, Cornwall.

Contents

List of Principal Contributors   ix

SECTION I: PATHOPHYSIOLOGY AND IMMUNOLOGY

1   Genetics of inflammatory bowel disease – progress, prospects and problems   3
J. Satsangi

2   Bacteria and immunological response in inflammatory bowel disease   11
J. Wehkamp

3   Mucosal immunity and gut epithelium   18
L. Mayer

4   Immunology of the lamina propria   25
R. Duchmann and M. Zeitz

5   Immunosuppression in inflammatory bowel disease: a personal view   37
D. H. Present

SECTION II: DISEASE STATES AND THERAPEUTIC PROBLEMS IN INFLAMMATORY BOWEL DISEASES

6   Chronic active and steroid-refractory inflammatory bowel disease: definition   47
C. Gasché

7   Mechanisms of refractory disease   54
G. Rogler

CONTENTS

8   Limitations of standard therapy for inflammatory
bowel disease
D. P. B. McGovern, T. Ahmad and D. P. Jewell   68

**SECTION III: STANDARDS: AZATHIOPRINE/
6-MERCAPTOPURINE**

9   Azathioprine/6-mercaptopurine: mechanisms of action,
pharmacology and toxicology
W. J. Sandborn   91

10   Azathioprine and 6-mercaptopurine in Crohn's
disease: acute and chronic active
L. R. Sutherland   101

11   Azathioprine/6-mercaptopurine for the treatment of
ulcerative colitis: evidence-based standards for therapy
J. F. Marion   106

SECTION IV: STANDARDS: METHOTREXATE

12   Methotrexate: mechanisms of action, pharmacology
and toxicology
A. Schnabel   113

13   Methotrexate therapy for Crohn's disease
B. G. Feagan   119

14   Methotrexate therapy for ulcerative colitis
T. Gilat, M. Moshkowitz and R. Oren   128

**SECTION V: NEW DEVELOPMENTS:
MYCOPHENOLATE MOFETIL**

15   Mycophenolate mofetil – an introduction to its
pharmacology
K. Fellermann   133

16   Mycophenolate mofetil in Crohn's disease
W. Petritsch   137

17   Mycophenolate mofetil in ulcerative colitis: acute
and chronic
K. Fellermann   144

CONTENTS

SECTION VI: NEW DEVELOPMENTS: CYCLOSPORIN/TACROLIMUS

18 Cyclosporin and tacrolimus in acute and chronic Crohn's disease   149
J. Brynskov

19 Cyclosporin – what have we learned in the past 15 years?   155
S. Lichtiger

SECTION VII: NEW DEVELOPMENTS: ANTI-TNF ANTIBODIES

20 Inhibition of tumour necrosis factor α as a therapeutic strategy in Crohn's disease   163
S. J. H. van Deventer

21 Anti-tumour necrosis factor antibodies in Crohn's disease and ulcerative colitis   170
B. E. Sands

SECTION VIII: FUTURE TRENDS: MOLECULAR THERAPY

22 Development of antisense to intercellular adhesion molecule-1 (ISIS 2302) for inflammatory bowel disease therapy   179
B. R. Yacyshyn

23 NF-κB: a key transcription factor in chronic intestinal inflammation   185
M. F. Neurath

24 Cellular and molecular mechanisms of anti-interleukin-12 therapy in the treatment of inflammatory bowel disease   191
I. Fuss, M. Boirivant, T. Marth, W. Strober and M. F. Neurath

25 Interleukin-2-related strategies in experimental models of inflammatory bowel disease   197
A. Stallmach

SECTION IX: FUTURE TRENDS: SPECIAL SITUATIONS

26 Immunosuppressive therapy and pregnancy   207
A. Dignass

27	Immunosuppressive therapy during childhood and adolescence *B. S. Kirschner*	213
28	Immunosuppressive therapy and extraintestinal manifestations in inflammatory bowel disease *G. D'Haens*	222
29	Classical immunosuppressive therapy and malignancy *T. Andus*	225
30	Anti-tumour necrosis factor α therapy and malignancy in Crohn's disease *S. R. Targan and E. A. Vasiliauskas*	233

SECTION X: CONSENSUS ON IMMUNOSUPPRESSIVE THERAPY

31	The use of immunosuppressors in active ulcerative colitis *M. Campieri*	243
32	Consensus on immunosuppressive therapy for ulcerative colitis: chronic active disease *D. B. Sachar*	246
	Index	249

List of Principal Contributors

T. Andus
Department of Internal Medicine
Krankenhaus Bad Cannstatt
Klinikum Stuttgart
Priessnitzweg 24
D-72374 Stuttgart
Germany

J. Brynskov
Herlev University Hospital
Department of Medical
   Gastroenterology
C 112
75 Herlev Ringvej
DK-2730 Herlev
Denmark

M. Campieri
Istituto di Clinica Medica I
Policlinico S. Orsola
Via Massarenti, 9
I-40138 Bologna
Italy

G. D'Haens
Department of Gastroenterology
University Hospital Gasthuisberg
University of Leuven
Herestraat 49
B-3000 Leuven
Belgium

A. Dignass
Medizinische Klinik mit
Schwerpunkt Gastroenterologie
Campus Virchow-Klinikum des
   Universitätsklinikums Charité
Augustenburger Platz 1

D-13353 Berlin
Germany

R. Duchmann
Medizinische Klinik I
Universitätsklinikum Benjamin Franklin
Freie Universität Berlin
Hindenburgdamm 30
D-12200 Berlin
Germany

B. G. Feagan
The University of Western Ontario
Robarts Research Institute
100 Perth Drive
London, Ontario N6A 5K8
Canada

K. Fellermann
Medizinische Klinik I
Medizinische Universität
   zu Lübeck
Ratzeburger Allee 160
D-23538 Lübeck
Germany

I. Fuss
National Institute of Health
Mucosal Immunity Section
10 Center Drive
Bldg. 10, Tm. 11N238
Bethesda, MD 20892-1890
USA

C. Gasché
Clinic of Internal Medicine IV
Department of Gastroenterology and
   Hepatology
Vienna General Hospital

Währinger Gürtel 18–20
A-1090 Vienna
Austria

T. Gilat
Department of Gastroenterology
Ichilov Hospital
Tel Aviv and Sackler
  Faculty of Medicine
Tel Aviv University
Tel Aviv
Israel

D. P. Jewell
Gastroenterology Unit
The Radcliffe Infirmary
Woodstock Road
Oxford
OX2 6HE
UK

B. S. Kirschner
The University of Chicago
  Children's Hospital
5839 S. Maryland Avenue, MC-4065
Chicago, IL 60637
USA

S. Lichtiger
Division of Immunology
The Mount Sinai School of Medicine
1185 Park Avenue
New York, NY 10128
USA

J. F. Marion
Mount Sinai School of Medicine
12 East 86th Street
New York, NY 10028
USA

L. Mayer
Mount Sinai Medical Center
Immunobiology Center
1425 Madison Avenue –
  Room 11-20
New York, NY 10029
USA

M. R. Neurath
I. Medizinische Klinik
Klinikum der Universität
Langenbeckstr. 1
D-55101 Mainz
Germany

W. Petritsch
Medizinische Klinik
Karl-Franzens-Universität Graz
Auenbruggerplatz 15
A-8036 Graz
Austria

D. H. Present
Mount Sinai Medical Center
12 East 86th Street
New York, NY 10028
USA

G. Rogler
Cellular and Molecular Medicine
University of California at San Diego
  UCSD
9500 Gilman Drive
La Jolla, CA 92093-0651
USA

D. B. Sachar
Division of Gastroenterology
The Mount Sinai Medical Center
Box 1069
One Gustave L. Levy Place
New York, NY 10029-6574
USA

W. J. Sandborn
E19B
Division of Gastroenterology
Mayo Clinic
200 First Street SW
Rochester, MN 55905
USA

B. E. Sands
Gastrointestinal Unit and Center for
  the Study of Inflammatory Bowel
  Disease
Massachusetts General Hospital and
  Harvard Medical School
55 Fruit Street, GRJ-724
Boston, MA 02114
USA

J. Satsangi
Gastroenterology Unit
The University of Edinburgh
Western General Hospital
Edinburgh
EH4 2XU
UK

A. Schnabel
Poliklinik für Rheumatologie
Rheumaklinik Bad Bramstedt
Universität zu Lübeck
Ratzeburger Allee 160
D-23538 Lübeck
Germany

J. Schölmerich
Klinik und Poliklinik für Innere
  Medizin I
Klinikum der Universität Regensburg
D-93042 Regensburg
Germany

A. Stallmach
Innere Medizin II
Medizinische Klinik und Poliklinik
Universität des Saarlandes
Kirrberger Str.
D-66421 Homburg
Germany

E. F. Stange
Zentrum Innere Medizin
Robert Bosch Krankenhaus
Auerbachstr. 110
D-70376 Stuttgart
Germany

L. R. Sutherland
Department of Community Health
  Sciences
University of Calgary
3330 Hospital Drive NW
Calgary, Alberta
Canada

S. R. Targan
Cedars-Sinai IBD Center
Davis Research Center #D-4063
8700 Beverly Blvd
Los Angeles, CA 90048-1865
USA

S. J. F. van Deventer
Department of Gastroenterology
Academic Medical Center
University of Amsterdam
Meibergdreef 9
NL-1105 AZ Amsterdam
The Netherlands

J. Wehkamp
Abt. für Gastroenterologie
Medizinische Klinik I
Medizinische Universität zu Lübeck
Ratzeburger Allee 160
D-23538 Lübeck
Germany

B. R. Yacyshyn
Department of Medicine
Division of Gastroenterology
2E3.11 Walter Mackenzie Center
University of Alberta
Edmonton, Alberta T6G 2R7
Canada

Section I
Pathophysiology and immunology

1
Genetics of inflammatory bowel disease – progress, prospects and problems

J. SATSANGI

INTRODUCTION

The epidemiological data which have accumulated in recent years provide very strong evidence that genetic factors are important in the pathogenesis of both Crohn's disease and ulcerative colitis. The study which catalysed the recent molecular genetics studies was the systematic review of the Swedish Twin Registry, carried out by Curt Tysk and colleagues[1]. Eighty twin pairs were identified from the Swedish records, in whom at least one twin was known to have inflammatory bowel disease. The investigators compared concordance for disease in the monozygotic and dizygotic twin pairs. These data were consistent with a substantial genetic contribution to the pathogenesis of Crohn's disease, and a lesser contribution in ulcerative colitis. These data were further supplemented by reports from the United Kingdom[2], and from Denmark[3]. In total 322 twin pairs have been reported in these three studies. The overall concordance rates in Crohn's disease were 37% and 7% for monozygotic and dizygotic twin pairs, respectively, and the corresponding results for ulcerative colitis are 10% and 3%. The derived coefficient of heritability from these data in Crohn's disease is consistent with a strong genetic contribution, equivalent to that in insulin-dependent diabetes or multiple sclerosis.

Further support for the importance of inherited susceptibility in disease predisposition is evident in the familial aggregation of disease[4]. Between 6% and 32% of patients with inflammatory bowel disease have affected first- or second-degree relatives. The prevalence of a positive family history varies among ethnic groups, being highest in the Ashkenazi Jewish population. Of first-degree relatives, siblings of patients with Crohn's disease and ulcerative colitis are at greatest risk of developing disease. The relative risk to a sibling of patients with Crohn's disease has been estimated as between 13 and 36, when compared with the population prevalence. For ulcerative colitis the corresponding figure varies between 7 and 17. In comparison the relative risk to siblings (λ_s) in cystic fibrosis is 500, and in type 1 diabetes is 15.

Although these data do support the importance of genetic factors, it is clear that there is no simple Mendelian mode of inheritance which is pertinent to Crohn's disease and ulcerative colitis. The genetic contribution is more complex. The presence of common susceptibility genes in both Crohn's disease and ulcerative colitis is suggested by the fact that both forms of the inflammatory bowel diseases may coexist in a family, at a frequency greater than that expected by chance alone. The model which seems most pertinent to the inflammatory bowel diseases is that Crohn's disease and ulcerative colitis are related polygenic diseases, sharing some but not all susceptibility genes (and perhaps environmental factors). However, even this model may represent an oversimplification. There is now increasing molecular evidence to suggest that the clinical variability within either Crohn's disease or ulcerative colitis may be genetically determined, and reflect extensive genetic heterogeneity. Thus any particular phenotype of inflammatory bowel disease may reflect not only the interaction of a number of different genes with one another, but also the effect of allelic variation within these genes and the further confounding issue of gene–environmental interaction.

GENOME-WIDE SCANNING IN INFLAMMATORY BOWEL DISEASE

In recent years it has been feasible to search systemically the entire human genome for the chromosomal location of genes involved in disease susceptibility, and then to identify these genes. This advance has become possible as a direct result of the development of linkage maps of the genome involving anonymous markers – 'microsatellites' – of known chromosomal location. These markers are informative in linkage analysis and highly polymorphic, and therefore may be used in linkage analysis studies of multiple-affected pedigrees with disease. Co-segregation of disease with a given marker provides evidence for the location of the susceptibility gene, without any '*a priori*' hypothesis as to gene function.

In single-gene disorders the technique is relatively straightforward – few large pedigrees are required and established methods for parametric linkage analysis may be applied. However, for complex multifactorial disease the techniques are continuing to develop and problems continue to be identified. Experience since the first genome-wide studies (in insulin-dependent diabetes and psychiatric disorders), has served to emphasize the need for access to large numbers of families, rigorous definition of disease genotype and ethnicity, and painstaking statistical design and analysis.

The latter point is of particular concern, given the fact that any single gene in a complex disorder is likely to make a relatively small contribution. Genomewide scans in complex diseases now typically involve approximately 400 microsatellite markers across the whole genome. Sub-chromosomal regions of interest may be identified by studying large numbers of affected relative pairs (typically siblings). The degree of allele sharing in affected individuals is significantly different from that expected by chance alone in a region of linkage.

Such an approach involves multiple comparisons and is at risk of engendering both type 1 and type 2 errors. Many authors have considered the statistical difficulties involved in these studies. Lander and Kruglyak suggested guidelines, which have been widely publicized[5], and are based on the number of times one would expect to see a result at random in genome-wide scanning. The threshold suggested for 'significant linkage' (maximum logarithm of odds (LOD) score >3.6 for sibling pairs, $p<2\times10^{-5}$) allows for one false-positive finding in every 20 genome scans; whereas 'suggestive' linkage (LOD >2.2, $p<7\times10^{-4}$) is likely to occur once by chance only in one genome scan.

In spite of all of the potential complexities related to disease heterogeneity and study design, genome-wide scanning in inflammatory bowel disease has been remarkably successful and fruitful, compared with other complex diseases.

Eight whole genome scans[6–13] and many replication studies have been reported since 1996. In these studies four sub-chromosomal regions – the peri-centromeric region of chromosome 16 (*IBD 1*), chromosome 12q13 (*IBD 2*), 6p23 (the major histocompatibility complex – *IBD 3*) and most recently chromosome 14 (*IBD 4*) have achieved significant linkage in initial and replication sets. A further area of 'significant linkage' on chromosome 19 awaits replication, as do nine other areas with less strong evidence for linkage – these would be defined as showing 'suggestive' linkage, according to Lander and Kruglyak guidelines.

CHROMOSOME 16 (IBD 1)

The locus which has received the most attention lies in the pericentromeric region of chromosome 16, and was first reported in a relatively small study from the European collaborative group based in Paris. In a two-stage study, involving a total of 78 families, the investigators identified the IBD 1 region and estimated the sibling risk ratio (λ_s) as 1.3. In spite of worries related to the sample size and the relatively small contribution of this region, the linkage has been widely replicated in studies from Oxford[14], United States[15], Europe[9,16], and Australia[17]. The data from Australia are most compelling, as a LOD score in this data set of 6.3 in Crohn's disease was obtained.

The international IBD genetics consortium, set up in 1997 to replicate and try to fine-map these putative regions of linkage, has recently reported data from 581 affected sibling pairs, and has demonstrated the strength of the *IBD 1* linkage[18]. A LOD score of 5.2 was obtained in the Crohn's disease data set.

The peri-centromeric region on chromosome 16 contains a number of potential candidate genes. Strongly negative data are reported for the interleukin 4 receptor[19]. Other candidates under investigation include the E-cadherin gene, encoding a transmembrane glycoprotein which mediates intercellular adhesion in the intestinal epithelium. Other positional candidates include the CD 19 and CD 43 genes, involved in B cell function and intercellular adhesion in molecule 1 (ICAM-1 interaction, respectively).

CHROMOSOME 12 (IBD 2)

The genome scan from Oxford identified significant linkage between inflammatory bowel disease overall, and a broad region on chromosome 12, spanning

41 centimorgans. In the initial paper a peak LOD score for inflammatory bowel disease was reported of 5.47, at the marker D12S83. The investigators reported a loci-specific relative risk of 2.0 from this study. Again positive replication data were provided in Europe[20], Los Angeles[12] and Pittsburgh[21]. However, the recent IBD consortium data showed that, when all 581 sibling pairs were analysed, the maximum LOD scores for inflammatory bowel disease, ulcerative colitis and Crohn's disease pertaining to this locus were 1.8, 1.2 and 1.1, respectively. The explanation for these apparent discrepancies may involve a combination of statistical and clinical factors. It is particularly noteworthy with respect to this controversy that the region has been studied more extensively in collaboration between the investigators in Oxford and Pittsburgh; these data suggest that the *IBD 2* locus may be significantly more strongly linked to ulcerative colitis than to Crohn's disease. Given the relatively small number of ulcerative colitis sibling pairs in the international consortium data set, this is perhaps the most plausible explanation for the group's findings in relation to this locus.[30]

Of positional candidate genes on chromosome 12, the gene encoding the vitamin D receptor has been investigated in view of the fact that vitamin D has multiple immune functions, including suppression of lymphocyte function and cytokine activity. Early positive data are reported from the Oxford group showing association in Crohn's disease, but not ulcerative colitis[22].

Strongly negative data are now available for the natural resistance associated macrophage protein 2 (NRAMP2) which lies within the linkage interval[23]. Several other genes have been mapped to this region recently, including the genes encoding β_7 integrin and matrix metalloproteinase 19 (MMP19), and Hamlin and his colleagues in Leeds have constructed an informative physical map[24].

CHROMOSOME 6 (HLA REGION, IBD 3)

The HLA region has been the subject of many candidate gene studies and most recently has also been implicated by the results of genome-wide scanning. In the early literature there are a number of confusing and contradictory reports. It seems likely that the confusion and apparent contradiction are attributable to a number of factors – small studies of insufficient power, the use of serological typing, ethnic admixture and disease heterogeneity appear to have contributed to the complexities. Most recently there is strong evidence that the region is important in predisposition towards inflammatory bowel disease. Association studies are most consistent with the fact that the HLA region has a stronger role to play in susceptibility in ulcerative colitis than in Crohn's disease[25]. The data are particularly compelling in the Japanese population, in which strong replicated evidence of association between susceptibility to ulcerative colitis and the DRB1*1502 allele representing HLA DR 2 is evident.

Stokkers and colleagues[26] have analysed the association data to date in the Caucasian population. This analysis and more recent data provide strong evidence that the HLA region is important in terms of susceptibility, but also behaviour. The data from the United Kingdom, now replicated elsewhere, suggest that the HLA DRB1*0103 allele is important in predicting severe disease, and the presence of extra-intestinal manifestations of inflammatory bowel disease.

Moreover, detailed clinical immunogenetic analysis of the HLA region[27] has allowed reclassification of the arthropathy associated with inflammatory bowel disease, into an asymmetrical large-joint arthropathy (seen in active disease, and associated with the DRB1*0103 allele), and a symmetrical small-joint pattern.

CHROMOSOME 14

Most recently, Ma and her collaborating investigators in Los Angeles[12] reported evidence for linkage between Crohn's disease and the region of chromosome 14. The suggested linkage reported by these investigators was most strong in non-Jewish families. Duerr *et al.*[11] subsequently confirmed this finding in 127 affected relative pairs in the United States, and some recent data from Belgium, in abstract, also replicate this locus[28]. There are a number of interesting positional candidature genes on chromosome 14, including the T cell receptor alpha and delta genes, a cluster of genes encoding proteasomes involved in antigen presentation, and the leukotriene B4 receptor.

FROM LINKAGE TO GENE

The consistent replication of the loci detailed above has excited scientists and clinicians working in the field. However, the challenge now – to narrow the region of linkage and identify the true genes – poses a number of problems. Although some reports suggest successful fine-mapping, there is no consensus that any of the regions implicated by genome-wide scanning has been narrowed to a size where physical mapping might be possible. Several strategies for fine-mapping and gene identification are being applied and it may well be that a combination of these is the most logical method to gene identification.

The international IBD consortium has allowed the accumulation of large numbers of affected sibling pairs with inflammatory bowel disease in an attempt to resolve linkage regions. However, linkage analysis alone has been unsuccessful in narrowing these regions, and it may well be that, given the relatively small contribution of any individual gene, sibling pair analysis or relative pair analysis does not have the power for detailed resolution. Association studies, either family-based (transmission disequilibrium test, TDT) or population-based (the case–control design) exploit linkage disequilibrium in populations, and therefore involve a large number of recombination events over several generations. Thus this strategy may be of considerably increased power compared with the sibling pair strategy, which involves a limited number of meioses. The technique might be further refined by studying individuals of a particular disease behaviour. For example, disease with early age of onset may well have a stronger genetic contribution than disease with late adult onset. There are certainly epidemiological data in inflammatory bowel disease to support this hypothesis, and support from the analogy with early-onset breast cancer and other common disorders.

Ethnic admixture is a particular problem in population-based association studies. It is of particular note and credit that Cho and colleagues[13] have identified a small number of families in the American Chaldean population with multiple-affected relatives. Cho and colleagues performed linkage analysis in these families, and have been able to report preliminary data narrowing the region of suggestive linkage on chromosome 1, which had been demonstrated in the same group's studies of the outbred US population. The authors have replicated the linkage with a multipoint LOD score of 3.01 and report refinement of the region of less than 1 cM, using detailed haplotype analysis in the four families studied.

To date, genome-wide scanning has relied on the use of genome maps involving microsatellite markers. However, recent interest has focused not on these polymorphic markers, but on single nucleotide polymorphisms (SNPs), which are found frequently throughout the genome, and are easier to genotype with confidence. Although genome-wide SNP mapping has not yet been successfully developed for use in complex disease, this area may prove to be most helpful in narrowing regions of linkage. The technique would be most readily applied to association study data, and Risch has calculated the number of individuals necessary to identify genes of relatively low genetic contribution, using both linkage analysis and association study designs[29].

Complementary strategies to genome-wide scanning may aid gene identification. In particular, analysis of gene expression, detected either by more conventional techniques or by expression microarray technology[31], will complement genome-wide scanning. In addition, animal models of inflammatory bowel disease induced by genetic manipulation are available to give insight into the genes implicated, and the pathogenic mechanisms responsible.

PERSPECTIVES

The molecular genetics of inflammatory bowel disease now attract enormous excitement and considerable financial investment. Progress has been made, and there are a number of avenues for further development, which may lead to gene identification. The clinician will hope to see some benefit from the investment that has been made. What might be expected? Perhaps the most realistic hope is that these studies will provide an insight into the pathogenesis of inflammatory bowel disease – the primary mechanisms involved in disease pathogenesis, and some insight into the heterogeneity of disease and the relationship between Crohn's disease and ulcerative colitis. It is hoped that these insights may allow more accurate counselling as to family risk, and also to the course of disease.

Allied to this is the hope that one might be able to select more appropriate treatment for each patient, on the basis of that patient's genotype. This might be achieved either in terms of avoiding drug side-effects, or prediction of drug efficacy. Preliminary data regarding azathioprine and the thiopurine methyl transferase polymorphism are pertinent, as are the data regarding the polymorphism of the tumour necrosis alpha (TNF-α) gene and the response to monoclonal antibodies against TNF in Crohn's disease. The great hope is that genome analysis may lead to the discovery of a new modality of therapy for Crohn's disease and ulcerative colitis, which is specific to the disease and is also free of the side-effects of present therapies. Whether this is indeed a realistic proposition will become evident within the next few years.

References

1. Tysk C, Lindberg E, Järnerot G, Flodérus-Myrhed B. Ulcerative colitis and Crohn's disease in an unselected population of monozygotic and dizygotic twins. A study of heritability and the influence of smoking. Gut. 1988;29:990–6.

2. Thompson NP, Driscoll R, Pounder RE, Wakefield AJ. Genetics versus environment in inflammatory bowel disease: results of a British twin study. Br Med J. 1996;12:95–6.

3. Orholm M, Binder V, Sorensen T, Kyvik K. Inflammatory bowel disease in a Danish twin register. Gut. 1996;39(Suppl. 3):A187.

4. Parkes M, Satsangi J, Jewell DP. Mapping susceptibility loci in inflammatory bowel disease: why and how? Mol Med Today. 1997;546–55.

5. Lander ES, Kruglyak L. Genetic dissection of complex traits: guidelines for interpreting and reporting linkage results. Nature Genet. 1995;11:241–7.

6. Hugot JP, Laurent-Puig P, Gower-Rousseau C *et al.* Mapping of a susceptibility locus for Crohn's disease on chromosome 16. Nature. 1996;379:821–2.

7. Satsangi J, Parkes M, Louis E *et al.* Two-stage genome-wide search in inflammatory bowel disease provides evidence for susceptibility loci on chromosomes 3, 7 and 12. Nat Genet. 1996;14:199–202.

8. Cho JH, Nicolae DL, Gold LH *et al.* Identification of novel susceptibility loci for inflammatory bowel disease on chromosomes 1p, 3q, and 4q: evidence for epistasis between 1p and IBD1. Proc Natl Acad Sci USA. 1998;95:7502–7.

9. Hampe J, Schreiber S, Shaw S *et al.* A genomewide analysis provides evidence for novel linkages in inflammatory bowel disease in a large European cohort. Am J Hum Genet. 1999;64:808–16.

10. Rioux J, Silverberg M, Daly M *et al.* Genomewide search in Canadian families with inflammatory bowel disease reveals two novel susceptibility loci. Am J Hum Genet. 2000;66:1863–70.

11. Duerr R, Barmada M, Zhang L, Pfutzer R, Weeks D. High-density genome scan in Crohn's disease shows confirmed linkage to chromosome 14q11–12. Am J Hum Genet. 2000;66:1857–62.

12. Ma Y, Ohmen J, Li Z *et al.* A genome wide search identifies potential new susceptibility loci for Crohn's disease. Inflam Bowel Dis. 1999;5:271–8.

13. Cho JU. Linkage and linkage disequilibrium in chromosome 1p36 in American Chaldeans with inflammatory bowel disease. Hum Mol Genet. 2000;9:1425–32.

14. Parkes M, Satsangi J, Lathrop GM, Bell JI, Jewell DP. Susceptibility loci in inflammatory bowel disease (Letter). Lancet. 1996;348:1588.

15. Brant SR, Fu Y, Fields CT *et al.* American families with Crohn's disease have strong evidence for linkage to chromosome 16 but not chromosome 12. Gastroenterology. 1998;115:1056–61.

16. Annese V, Latiano A, Bovio P *et al.* Genetic analysis in Italian families with inflammatory bowel disease supports linkage to IBD1 locus – a GISC study. Eur J Hum Genet. 1999;7:567–73.

17. Cavanaugh JA, Callen DF, Wilson SR *et al.* Analysis of Australian Crohn's disease pedigrees refines the localisation for susceptibility to inflammatory bowel disease on chromosome 16. Ann Hum Genet. 1998;2:291–8.

18. The IBD Consortium. The International IBD genetics consortium confirms linkage of Crohn's disease to a locus on chromosome 16 (IBD1). Gastroenterology. 2000;118:A3862.

19. Olavesen M, Hampe J, Mirza M *et al.* Analysis of single-nucleotide polymorphisms in the interleukin-4 receptor gene for association with inflammatory bowel disease. Immunogenetics. 2000; 51:1–7.

20. Curran ME, Lau KF, Hampe J *et al.* Genetic analysis of inflammatory bowel disease in a large European cohort supports linkage to chromosomes 12 and 16. Gastroenterology. 1998;115:1066–71.

21. Duerr RH, Barmada MM, Zhang L *et al.* Linkage and association between inflammatory bowel disease and a locus on chromosome 12. Am J Hum Genet. 1998;63:95–100.

22. Simmons JD, Mullighan C, Welsh KI, Jewell DP. Vitamin D receptor gene polymorphism: association with Crohn's disease susceptibility. Gut. 2000;47:211–14.

23. Mirza M, Rowley G, Hampe J *et al.* Analysis of single nucleotide polymorphisms in the NRAMP2 gene, for association with inflammatory bowel disease. Gut. 2000;46(Suppl. 11):A4.

24. Hamlin P, Komolmit P, Bransfield K *et al.* Identification of multiple candidate genes for IBD susceptibility using high density transcript mapping in the IBD2 locus on chromosome 12q. Gastroenterology. 1999;117:1029–31.

25. Satsangi J, Welsh KI, Bunce M *et al.* Contribution of genes of the major histocompatibility complex to susceptibility and disease phenotype in inflammatory bowel disease. Lancet. 1996;347:1212–17.
26. Stokkers PC, Reitsma PH, Tygat GN, van Deventer SJ. HLA-DR and -DQ phenotypes in inflammatory bowel disease: a meta-analysis. Gut. 1999;45:395–401.
27. Orchard T, Thiyagaraja S, Welsh K, Wordsworth B, Gaston J, Jewell D. Clinical phenotype is related to HLA genotype in the peripheral arthropathies of inflammatory bowel disease. Gastroenterology. 2000;118:274–8.
28. Vermeire S, Vlietinck R, Groenen P, Peeters M, Rutgeers P. Replication of linkage on 14q11–12 in inflammatory bowel disease. Gastroenterology. 2000;118(4 Suppl. 2):A338.
29. Risch NJ. Searching for genetic determinants in the new millennium. Nature. 2000;405:847–56.
30. Parkes M, Barmada MM, Satsangi J, Weeks DE, Jewell DP, Duerr RW. The IBD2 locus shows linkage heterogeneity between ulcerative colitis and Crohn's disease. Am J Hum Genet. 2000;67: 1605–10.
31. Lawrance IC, Fiocchi C, Chakravarti S. Ulcerative colitis and Crohn's disease: distinctive gene expression profiles and novel susceptibility candidate genes. Hum Mol Genet. 2001;105: 445–456.

2
Bacteria and immunological response in inflammatory bowel disease

J. WEHKAMP

BACKGROUND

Various findings suggest that the mucosal barrier function in the major idiopathic inflammatory bowel diseases, Crohn's disease and ulcerative colitis, may be altered. Thus, the normal bacterial flora may gain a pathogenic role under circumstances of an impaired host defence. For example, diversion of the faecal stream is effective in ameliorating Crohn's disease distally[1,2], suggesting that luminal contents trigger inflammation[3]. A recent study demonstrated T cell responses against the autologous bacterial flora in Crohn's disease but not in controls[4], implying a defective tolerance. Antibiotics appear to provide a benefit both in acute flares[5] and maintenance of remission[6]. Furthermore, a germ-free environment prevents gut inflammation in TCR-, IL-2- and IL-10 knock out animal models of inflammatory bowel disease[7–11].

Mucosal surfaces are protected by an unspecific innate antimicrobial system consisting of numerous peptides which confer epithelial barrier integrity as an adjunct to specific immunity. One important class of antimicrobial peptides is the family of defensins, small arginine-rich peptides with characteristic disulphide bonds between cysteine residues and a mass of 3–5 kDa[12–14]. Distinct members are present on virtually every surface of the human body and abundantly in neutrophils. Defensins exert antimicrobial activity against bacteria, fungi and some enveloped viruses by perforating the cell wall through formation of multimeric pores[15,16]. They appear to be functionally important since enteric β-defensin expression is induced in bovine infection with *Cryptosporidium parvum*[17] and increased defensin levels have been noted in bronchiolar epithelium upon infection[18,19].

Defensins are classified as α- and β-defensins based on the position of three intramolecular disulphide bonds. Till now, eight human defensins have been isolated. The α-defensins comprise human neutrophil peptide (HNP) 1–4 of neutrophilic origin as well as intestinal human defensin 5 (HD-5) and human defensin 6 (HD-6). Human β-defensin 1 (HBD-1) and 2 (HBD-2) belong to the β-defensins, and are formed by epithelia. All intestinal defensins have a genomic 2 exon structure in common, conserved through phylogeny. Analogous peptides have been isolated in several species, e.g. as cryptdins in mice[14], tracheal antimicrobial peptide (TAP)[20], lingual antimicrobial peptide (LAP)[21] and enteric β-defensin[17] in cattle. Unlike the multitude of cryptdins in mice[13], the diversity of human intestinal defensins appears to be much more limited. The known human defensin genes have been mapped to chromosome 8p22-p23[22–25]. Polymerase chain reaction (PCR) analysis and *in-situ* hybridization revealed HD-5 and HD-6 transcripts in Paneth cells of the small intestine[26,27] and the corresponding HD-5 peptide was immunolocalized in corresponding cellular granules[28]. HD-5 was also found in fetal but not yet in adult colon[29]. HBD-1 is considered constitutive, whereas HD-5, HD-6 and HBD-2 are inducible under certain conditions[30–32].

A recent report detected β-defensins in inflamed colonic tissue[33] by immunohistochemistry. However, to the best of our knowledge no defensin RNA has been found in adult human colonic tissue so far, and there is no information on the localization of α-defensins in the human colon. Since Crohn's disease mucosa, unlike normal epithelium, is characterized by the presence of adherent *Escherichia coli*[34] and sometimes other bacteria such as *Mycobacterium paratuberculosis*[35,36], we hypothesized that the defensin profile in these diseases may be altered. Therefore, the aim of the present study was to systematically compare defensin expression in normal colonic mucosa to that in inflammatory bowel diseases. We demonstrated that there is a differential induction of certain defensins in Crohn's disease and ulcerative colitis[37,38]. In addition, it was shown that the various defensins differ with respect to mucosal localization and inflammatory response.

METHODS

Reverse-transcription PCR (RT-PCR) was performed with primers for human defensin 5 or 6 (HD-5, HD-6) and β-defensin 1 or 2 (HBD-1, HBD-2)[39]. Paraffin-embedded tissue from colonic resections was tested for HD-5, HBD-1 and HBD-2 by immunohistochemistry.

RESULTS

HD-5 and HD-6 expression is enhanced in both inflammatory bowel diseases, whereas HBD-2 is induced preferentially in UC. These findings are based on the RT-PCR and could be confirmed by immunohistochemistry.

DISCUSSION

The discovery of antimicrobial peptides has extended the knowledge of unspecific defence mechanisms. In principle, deficiencies in this system with a breakdown of barrier function may account for increased invasion of infectious pathogens leading to inflammation or a potentially deleterious immune response. It may be hypothesized that chronic inflammatory bowel diseases originate from an alteration in mucosal defensins. We report herein differences in defensin expression in normal and inflamed colon by RT-PCR analysis and immunohistochemistry.

Transcripts of HD-5 and HD-6 were rarely seen in normals, but more often in inflammatory bowel disease, which is reminiscent of the unspecific induction of heat-shock proteins in both Crohn's disease and ulcerative colitis[40,41]. This might reflect an increased expression in diseased mucosa, as has already been reported in necrotizing enterocolitis[31]. Both defensin transcripts were absent from the native CaCo-2 cell line but both were inducible by cytokines. This is in agreement with their inducible status. Results by PCR analysis were paralleled by positive findings of HD-5 peptide in inflamed tissue and its virtual absence in control samples. Interestingly, positive cells were confined to the basal crypts. This raises the question of whether HD-5 originated from metaplastic Paneth cells[42] or rapidly dividing enterocytes due to increased cell turnover. Further histological characterization is under way. Mallow *et al.* observed a developmental expression pattern of defensins in the gastrointestinal tract paralleling the appearance of Paneth cells. HD-5 but not HD-6 were present in colonic tissue at gestational week 13.5, but disappeared during further fetal development[29]. Outside Paneth cells, HD-5 transcripts and peptide have been detected in epithelia of the female reproductive tract[43,44]. A lambda cDNA library of adult human colon has been reported to be negative for HD-5 and HD-6[26,27], whereas our positive signal was obtained in fresh snap-frozen biopsies. A false-positive spurious finding is unlikely because negative controls including PBMNC were consistently negative and the PCR products were confirmed by sequencing.

HBD-1 mRNA was present similarly in the majority of non-inflamed biopsies, in accordance with a constitutive nature of this antimicrobial peptide, but surprisingly less frequent in inflamed biopsies. The HBD-1 gene bears an IL-6 recognition site but lacks a NF-κB transcription site upstream of the gene and expression does not respond to various cytokines or proinflammatory mediators *in vitro*[30,44,45]. Using Northern blot a widespread expression on epithelial surfaces has been reported with the notable exception of the colon[30]. Our data are further substantiated by the positive finding in human cultured CaCo-2 cells derived from human colon carcinoma. It is likely that the low transcript level requires PCR for amplification rather than Northern blots. Immunohistochemistry revealed that many differentiated epithelial colonic cells were the source of HBD-1 peptide, quite complementary to HD-5.

HBD-2 protein was originally isolated from squamous psoriatic lesions and the genomic sequence was deduced from protein sequence analysis. A lack of HBD-2 in the intestine was reported initially[32], but a widespread distribution including colon has been found using customizable RNA libraries just recently[46]. Interestingly, *in-situ* hybridization revealed a broad unrestricted epithelial staining – not limited to Paneth cells – throughout the intestine. Moreover, increased HBD-2 peptide levels have been determined in pneumonia locally and systemically[18,19]. Inactivated defensins have been linked to recurrent bronchopulmonary infections in cystic fibrosis based on their salt-sensitive properties[47,48]. Homologous peptides have been isolated from several species.

The bovine LAP and TAP genes bear a NF-κB recognition site and are inducible following challenge with LPS, IL-1β or TNF-α *in vitro*[21,49]. An inducible enteric β-defensin has been isolated from cattle upon *Cryptosporidium parvum* infection[17]. Highest levels were detected in the distal ileum, coincident with the maximal density of Paneth cells.

Whereas a positive signal for HBD-2 mRNA was a rare event in controls, transcripts were significantly more frequent in ulcerative colitis than in Crohn's disease. Although immunohistochemistry is no reliable method to evaluate quantitative differences, a positive staining in ulcerative colitis was both more frequent and extensive, with many positive cells underlining this difference. Stained cells were exclusively localized in the apical region and their shape suggests prior injury.

Harder *et al.*[32] detected HBD-2 mRNA in inflamed but not in normal skin. A focally induced HBD-2 transcript and peptide pattern in skin keratinocytes of inflamed areas extends this observation[23]. This response is possibly mediated through the NF-κB activation pathway[23,32], which is activated in inflammatory bowel disease[50,51]. O'Neil *et al.*[33] have elegantly shown HBD-2 in some inflammatory bowel disease patients, and activation mediated by NF-κB-dependent transcription in CaCo-2 cells. Moreover, certain bacteria were able to induce HBD-2. Therefore an enhanced detectability in a case of ulcerative colitis may have been expected, but the apparent defect in some patients with Crohn's disease is intriguing. The mucosal Th1 cytokine pattern in Crohn's disease[52,53], greatly enhancing NF-κB, would suggest an up-regulation of this inducible defensin. Thus, other factors may counteract HBD-2 induction or the NF-κB binding to the defensin promoter is impaired in Crohn's disease. Another possible explanation for this finding is a more extensive epithelial damage by the inflammation diminishing the antimicrobial response. However, we cannot definitely rule out that the changes are due to the patients' therapy, although Crohn's disease and ulcerative colitis were treated similarly.

In conclusion, Crohn's disease and ulcerative colitis appeared to differ from each other, as well as from normal controls, with respect to their defensin profile. We detected defensin transcripts by RT-PCR and the respective peptides by immunohistochemistry in colonic mucosa. The nearly universal expression of HBD-1 in normal colonic tissue gives further evidence for its constitutive nature. HD-5 and HD-6 are induced in both inflammatory bowel diseases, whereas HBD-2 is characteristic, although not exclusive, for ulcerative colitis. Therefore it can be hypothesized that HBD-1 may provide a baseline function in preventing colonization of epithelial surfaces, while HD-5 as well as HD-6, and especially HBD-2, are related to the inflammatory process in inflammatory bowel disease. The apparent lack of HBD-2 despite frank inflammation in a significant number of Crohn's disease patients provides preliminary evidence for an impaired unspecific host defence predisposing to bacterial invasion in this group.

References

1. Harper PH, Truelove SC, Lee ECG, Kettlewell MGW, Jewell DP. Split ileostomy and ileocolostomy for Crohn's disease of the colon and ulcerative colitis: a 20-year survey. Gut. 1983;24:106–13.

2. Rutgeerts P, Geboes K, Peeters M *et al*. Effect of faecal stream diversion on recurrence of Crohn's disease in the neoterminal ileum. Lancet. 1991;338:771–4.

3. D'Haens G, Geboes K, Peeters M, Baert F, Penninckx F, Rutgeerts P. Early lesions of recurrent Crohn's disease caused by infusion of intestinal contents in excluded ileum. Gastroenterology. 1998;114:262–7.

4. Duchmann R, May E, Heike M *et al*. T cell specificity and cross reactivity towards enterobacteria, *Bacteroides*, *Bifidobacterium*, and antigens from resident intestinal flora in humans. Gut. 1999;44:812–18.

5. Prantera C, Zannoni F, Scribano ML *et al*. An antibiotic regimen for the treatment of active Crohn's disease: a randomized, controlled clinical trial of metronidazole plus ciprofloxacin. Am J Gastroenterol. 1996;91:328–32.

6. Rutgeerts P, Hiele M, Geboes K *et al*. Controlled trial of metronidazole treatment for prevention of Crohn's recurrence after ileal resection. Gastroenterology. 1995;108:1617–21.

7. Kühn R, Löhler J, Rennick D, Rajewski K, Müller W. Interleukin-10-deficient mice develop chronic enterocolitis. Cell. 1993;75:263–74.

8. Mombaerts P, Mizoguchi E, Grusby MJ, Glimcher LH, Bhan AK, Tonegawa S. Spontaneous development of inflammatory bowel disease in T cell receptor mutant mice. Cell. 1993;75:275–82.

9. Sadlack B, Merz H, Schorle H, Schimpl A, Feller AC, Horak I. Ulcerative colitis-like disease in mice with a disrupted interleukin-2 gene. Cell. 1993;75:253–61.

10. Dianda L, Hanby AM, Wright NA, Sebesteny A, Hayday AC, Owen MJ. T cell receptor-alpha beta-deficient mice fail to develop colitis in the absence of a microbial environment. Am J Pathol. 1997;150:91–7.

11. Elson CO, Sartor RB, Tennyson GS, Riddell RH. Experimental models of inflammatory bowel disease. Gastroenterology. 1995;109:1344–67.

12. Ganz T, Lehrer RI. Defensins. Curr Opin Immunol. 1994;6:584–9.

13. Ouellette AJ, Hsieh MM, Nosek MT *et al*. Mouse Paneth cell defensins: primary structures and antibacterial activities of numerous cryptdin isoforms. Infect Immun. 1994;62:5040–7.

14. Selsted ME, Miller SI, Henschen AH, Ouellette AJ. Enteric defensins: antibiotic peptide components of intestinal host defense. J Cell Biol. 1992;118:929–36.

15. Lehrer RI, Barton A, Daher KA, Harwig SS, Ganz T, Selsted ME. Interaction of human defensins with *Escherichia coli*. Mechanism of bactericidal activity. J Clin Invest. 1989;84:553–61.

16. Kagan BL, Selsted ME, Ganz T, Lehrer RI. Antimicrobial defensin peptides form voltage-dependent ion-permeable channels in planar lipid bilayer membranes. Proc Natl Acad Sci USA. 1990;87:210–14.

17. Tarver AP, Clark DP, Diamond G *et al*. Enteric beta-defensin: molecular cloning and characterization of a gene with inducible intestinal epithelial cell expression associated with *Cryptosporidium parvum* infection. Infect Immun. 1998;66:1045–56.

18. Hiratsuka T, Nakazato M, Date Y *et al*. Identification of human beta-defensin-2 in respiratory tract and plasma and its increase in bacterial pneumonia. Biochem Biophys Res Commun. 1998;249:943–7.

19. Singh PK, Jia HP, Wiles K *et al*. Production of beta-defensins by human airway epithelia. Proc Natl Acad Sci USA. 1998;95:14961–6.

20. Diamond G, Zasloff M, Eck H, Brasseur M, Maloy WL, Bevins CL. Tracheal antimicrobial peptide, a cysteine-rich peptide from mammalian tracheal mucosa: peptide isolation and cloning of a cDNA. Proc Natl Acad Sci USA. 1991;88:3952–6.

21. Schonwetter BS, Stolzenberg ED, Zasloff MA. Epithelial antibiotics induced at sites of inflammation. Science. 1995;267:1645–8.

22. Liu L, Zhao C, Heng HH, Ganz T. The human beta-defensin-1 and alpha-defensins are encoded by adjacent genes: two peptide families with differing disulfide topology share a common ancestry. Genomics. 1997;43:316–20.

23. Liu L, Wang L, Jia HP *et al*. Structure and mapping of the human beta-defensin HBD-2 gene and its expression at sites of inflammation. Gene. 1998;222:237–44.

24. Harder J, Siebert R, Zhang Y *et al*. Mapping of the gene encoding human beta-defensin-2 (DEFB2) to chromosome region 8p22-p23.1. Genomics. 1997;46:472–5.

25. Bevins CL, Jones DE, Dutra A, Schaffzin J, Muenke M. Human enteric defensin genes: chromosomal map position and a model for possible evolutionary relationships. Genomics. 1996;31:95–106.

26. Jones DE, Bevins CL. Paneth cells of the human small intestine express an antimicrobial peptide gene. J Biol Chem. 1992;267:23216–25.
27. Jones DE, Bevins CL. Defensin-6 mRNA in human Paneth cells: implications for antimicrobial peptides in host defense of the human bowel. FEBS Lett. 1993;315:187–92.
28. Porter EM, van-Dam E, Valore EV, Ganz T. Broad-spectrum antimicrobial activity of human intestinal defensin 5. Infect Immun. 1997;65:2396–401.
29. Mallow EB, Harris A, Salzman N *et al.* Human enteric defensins. Gene structure and developmental expression. J Biol Chem. 1996;271:4038–45.
30. Zhao C, Wang I, Lehrer RI. Widespread expression of beta-defensin hBD-1 in human secretory glands and epithelial cells. FEBS Lett. 1996;396:319–22.
31. Salzman NH, Polin RA, Harris MC *et al.* Enteric defensin expression in necrotizing enterocolitis. Pediatr Res. 1998;44:20–6.
32. Harder J, Bartels J, Christophers E, Schroder JM. A peptide antibiotic from human skin. Nature. 1997;387:861.
33. O'Neil DA, Porter EM, Elewaut D *et al.* Expression and regulation of the human β-defensins hBD-1 and hBD-2 in intestinal epithelium. J Immunol. 1999;163:6718–24.
34. Darfeuille-Michaud A, Neut C, Barnich N *et al.* Presence of adherent *Escherichia coli* strains in ileal mucosa of patients with Crohn's disease. Gastroenterology. 1998;115:1405–13.
35. Fidler HM, Thurrell W, Johnson NM, Rook GA, McFadden JJ. Specific detection of *Mycobacterium paratuberculosis* DNA associated with granulomatous tissue in Crohn's disease. Gut. 1994;35:506–10.
36. Lisby G, Andersen J, Engbaek K, Binder V. *Mycobacterium paratuberculosis* in intestinal tissue from patients with Crohn's disease demonstrated by a nested primer polymerase chain reaction. Scand J Gastroenterol. 1994;29:923–9.
37. Jewell DP. Ulcerative colitis. In: Feldman M, Scharschmidt BF, Sleisenger MH, editors. Sleisenger and Fordtran's Gastrointestinal and Liver Disease: Pathophysiology/Diagnosis/Management. Philadelphia: Saunders, 1998:1735–58.
38. Kornbluth A, Sachar DB, Salomon P. Crohn's disease. In: Feldman M, Scharschmidt BF, Sleisenger MH, editors. Sleisenger and Fordtran's Gastrointestinal and Liver Disease: Pathophysiology/Diagnosis/Management. Philadelphia: Saunders, 1998:1708–34.
39. Valore EV, Park CH, Quayle AJ, Wiles KR, McCray-PB J, Ganz T. Human beta-defensin-1: an antimicrobial peptide of urogenital tissues. J Clin Invest. 1998;101:1633–42.
40. Stahl M, Ludwig D, Fellermann K, Stange EF. Intestinal expression of human heat shock protein 90 in patients with Crohn's disease and ulcerative colitis. Dig Dis Sci. 1998;43:1079–87.
41. Ludwig D, Stahl M, Ibrahim MT *et al.* Enhanced intestinal expression of heat shock protein 70 in patients with inflammatory bowel disease. Dig Dis Sci. 1999;44:1440–7.
42. Symonds DA. Paneth cell metaplasia in diseases of the colon and rectum. Arch Pathol. 1974;97:343–7.
43. Svinarich DM, Wolf NA, Gomez R, Gonik B, Romero R. Detection of human defensin 5 in reproductive tissues. Am J Obstet Gynecol. 1997;176:470–5.
44. Quayle AJ, Porter EM, Nussbaum AA *et al.* Gene expression, immunolocalization, and secretion of human defensin-5 in human female reproductive tract. Am J Pathol. 1998;152:1247–58.
45. Krisanaprakornkit S, Weinberg A, Perez CN, Dale BA. Expression of the peptide antibiotic human beta-defensin 1 in cultured gingival epithelial cells and gingival tissue. Infect Immun. 1998;66:4222–8.
46. Bals R, Wang X, Wu Z *et al.* Human beta-defensin 2 is a salt-sensitive peptide antibiotic expressed in human lung. J Clin Invest. 1998;102:874–80.
47. Goldman MJ, Anderson GM, Stolzenberg ED, Kari UP, Zasloff M, Wilson JM. Human beta-defensin-1 is a salt-sensitive antibiotic in lung that is inactivated in cystic fibrosis. Cell. 1997;88:553–60.
48. Smith JJ, Travis SM, Greenberg EP, Welsh MJ. Cystic fibrosis airway epithelia fail to kill bacteria because of abnormal airway surface fluid. Cell. 1996;85:229–36.
49. Diamond G, Russell JP, Bevins CL. Inducible expression of an antibiotic peptide gene in lipopolysaccharide-challenged tracheal epithelial cells. Proc Natl Acad Sci USA. 1996;93:5156–60.
50. Rogler G, Brand K, Vogl D *et al.* Nuclear factor κB is activated in macrophages and epithelial cells of inflamed intestinal mucosa. Gastroenterology. 1998;115:357–69.
51. Schreiber S, Nikolaus S, Hampe J. Activation of nuclear factor κB in inflammatory bowel disease. Gut. 1998;42:477–84.

52. Woywodt A, Ludwig D, Neustock P *et al*. Mucosal cytokine expression, cellular markers and adhesion molecules in inflammatory bowel disease. Eur J Gastroenterol Hepatol. 1999; 11:267–76.
53. Reimund JM, Wittersheim C, Dumont S *et al*. Increased production of tumour necrosis factor-alpha interleukin-1 beta, and interleukin-6 by morphologically normal intestinal biopsies from patients with Crohn's disease. Gut. 1996;39:684–9.

3
Mucosal immunity and gut epithelium

L. MAYER

INTRODUCTION

There are three major factors which dictate immune responses: (1) the nature of the antigen (Ag) driving the response, (2) the nature of the microenvironment in which the Ag is delivered (e.g. cytokines), and (3) the nature of the cell type presenting the Ag to responsive cells. In the gastrointestinal tract several scenarios exist allowing for a myriad of responses, especially in an antigen-overloaded system. However, it is intriguing to note that the majority of immune responses in the gastrointestinal tract are either non-responses or suppressed responses[1,2]. Studies from a number of laboratories have suggested that this results from multiple processes, all of which impact on the three factors described above. Clearly the nature of Ag is unique in the gut, being affected by luminal enzymes, pH extremes and detergents. Most antigens are rendered non-antigenic by virtue of their digestion to non-immunogenic peptides of two or three amino acids in length. Bacterial products which are abundant in the colon either fail to elicit a response or at best elicit a weak response. This may relate to processes which reduce the ability of various cell types to interact with or respond to Lipo-polysaccharide (LPS). Epithelial cells and intestinal microphages do not express a classical component of the LPS receptor (CD14), reducing their ability to generate a full-blown inflammatory response. The cytokine microenvironment in the normal gut is generally proposed to be suppressive in nature (Th2/Th3). The focus of this chapter, however, will be on the nature of the antigen-presenting cell (APC) in the mucosa-associated lymphoid tissue. The lamina propria is replete with classical APCs (dendritic cells, macrophages and B cells) but a barrier of epithelial cells lies between the lumen and these APCs and the Ag-rich lumen. The concept that this is a purely physical barrier has been questioned over the past 10 years, and there is increasing evidence that the intestinal epithelium contributes in many ways to regulate mucosal immune responses.

IECs SECRETE CYTOKINES AND CHEMOKINES WHICH REGULATE IMMUNE RESPONSES

One of the first lines of evidence that intestinal epithelial cells (IECs) could modify mucosal immune responses came from observations from several laboratories that these cells produce cytokines. As shown in Fig. 1, these cytokines range from proinflammatory (e.g. IL-6, GM-CSF) to chemoattractive (e.g. IL-8, ENA-78, MCP-1) to immunoregulatory (IL-10, TGFβ). While it is well documented that invasive bacteria trigger a chemokine response, it is less clear as to what factors induce the secretion of other cytokines. An organized repertoire of cytokines/chemokines could orchestrate a directed immune/inflammatory response. The presence of cytokine receptors on IECs further speaks to the interaction of the various components of the mucosal microenvironment[3]. It is certainly conceivable that the IEC responds to environmental stimuli to promote the growth and differentiation of these cells, creation of a mucus barrier, as well as the secretion of factors which maintain intestinal homeostasis. Animal models with a focus on selective alterations in IEC function/barrier function will provide valuable clues as to the critical importance of this cell type.

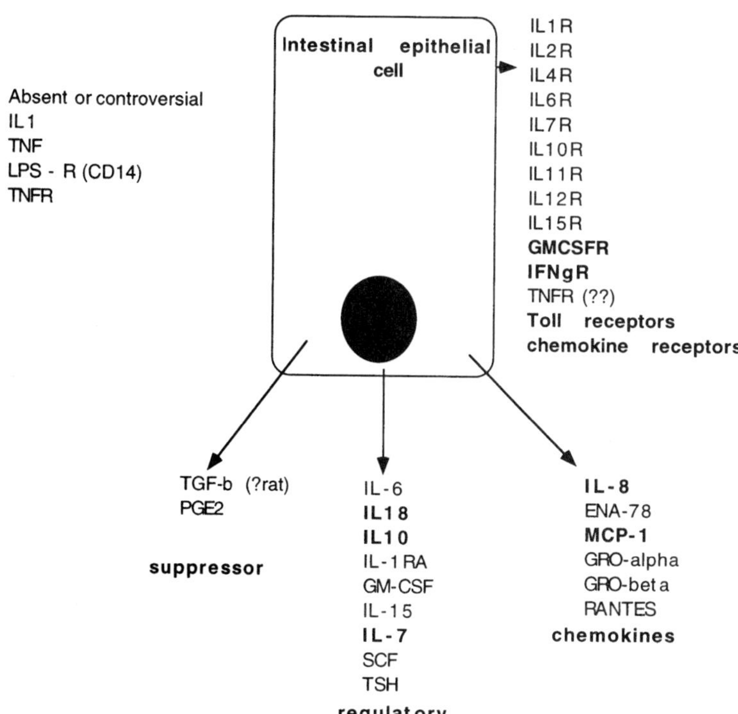

Figure 1   Intestinal epithelial cell cytokine secretion and receptor expression

IECs SAMPLE AGs AND DIRECT THEM INTO SPECIFIC PROCESSING COMPARTMENTS

In order to generate an appropriate T cell response, large antigenic moieties require processing to generate a form of antigen that can be recognized by the T cell's antigen receptor. Several lines of evidence suggest that IECs can take up Ags *in vitro* and *in vivo*. Gonnella *et al.*[4] and Brandeis *et al.*[5] localized soluble protein Ags in endolysosomal pathways within IECs when the Ag was given orally or into an isolated intestinal loop. Berin *et al.*[7–9] demonstrated facilitated uptake in an allergen model in which HRP (horseradish peroxidase) was used (primary systemic immunization with alum-Th2 biased response – followed by oral feeding). Uptake was mediated by low-affinity Fc receptors for IgE. So *et al.*[10] defined the nature of Ags taken up by IECs as soluble proteins as opposed to particulate Ags or carbohydrates. Here too Ag localization was within processing compartments (Fig. 2). When compared to uptake by conventional APCs, the IEC was more limited in the speed in which Ags were taken up and moved through the compartments. Studies by Hershberg's group[11,12] supported a polar transport process, with Ag uptake maximal on the apical surface followed by transcytosis of antigen to the basolateral surface. It is at these surfaces where processed Ag might interact with lamina propria T cells. Electron microscopic studies have noted the extension of epithelial cell foot processes through fenestrations in the basement membrane underlying the IEC. This would facilitate IEC–T cell interactions[16].

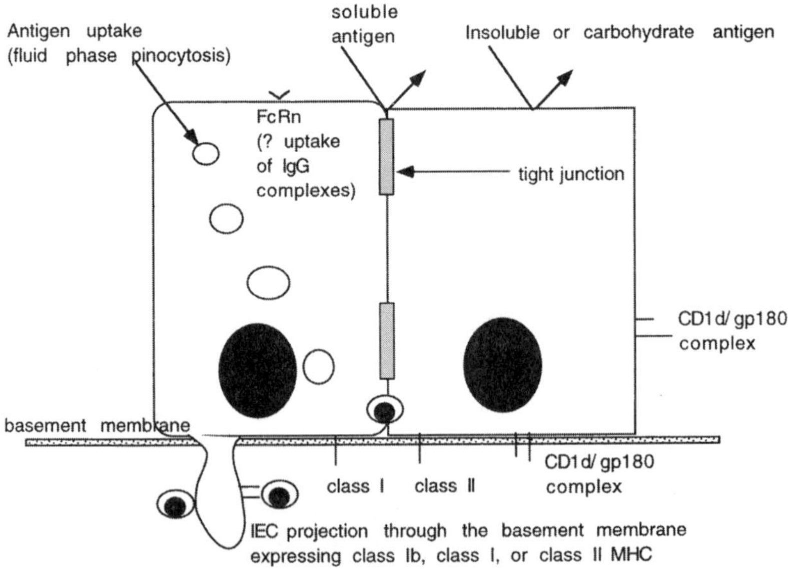

Figure 2 Antigen uptake and trafficking within intestinal epithelium

IECs EXPRESS CLASSICAL AND NON-CLASSICAL RESTRICTION ELEMENTS

It is the nature of the T cell–IEC interactions which remains to be defined. Early as well as more recent studies demonstrated not only that IECs constitutively express MHC class II molecules, but also that these restriction elements serve to activate Ag-specific CD4[+] memory T cells. Studies by Kaiserlian[13–15] and Hershberg[11,12] used T cell hybridomas to demonstrate such an interaction. However, the requirements for activation of hybridomas are less stringent than those of primary T cells. No evidence exists to date to support the possibility that CD4[+] T cells can be primed by Ags presented by IEC.

By contrast, initial studies by Bland et al.[17,18], and Shlien and Mayer[19], suggested that Ags presented to non-primed T cell populations by IEC would selectively activate CD8[+] Ag non-specific suppressor T cells. Despite the expression of the classical CD8[+] T cell restriction element, MHC class I, on normal IECs, the data from Li et al.[20] suggested that conventional class I MHC did not participate in the activation of CD8[+] T cells by IEC. Parallel studies by Bleicher et al.[21], Blumberg et al.[22–25], Spies[22–25], and Simester[24] reported the expression of non-classical class I MHC molecules (class Ib) by IECs. These included CD1d, MICA/B and the neonatal FcγR (FcR$_N$) (Fig. 3). Panja et al.[26] presented evidence that *in-vitro* co-culture of T cells and IECs required the interaction of CD1d on the IEC with the T cell receptor on a population of CD8[+] T cells. The concept which has evolved is that regulatory CD8[+] T cell populations may exist in the gut, and that different populations may be restricted by unique class Ib molecules.

It is interesting to speculate on the nature of the Ag presented by the class Ib molecules. The CD1 family of molecules have been shown to have the capacity to present lipids, glycolipids, or carbohydrate Ags. Hershberg et al.[27] suggested that TL, a murine class Ib molecule, recognizes an epithelial cell Ag expressed

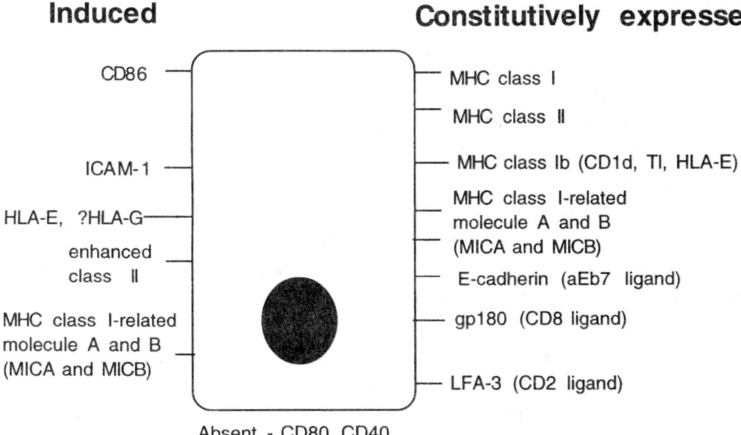

Figure 3 Surface molecule expression by IEC (related to potential T cell interactions)

by stressed IECs. If class Ib molecules have a limited repertoire of Ag binding capacity, then one can envision presentation of luminal bacteria products (non-pathogenic) or normal epithelial cell-surface Ags to regulatory T cells to dampen immune responses or eliminate dying cells in the mucosa. Such presentation may explain the normally immunosuppressed tone of the gut and the presence of similar oligoclonal T cells in diverse segments of the bowel.

IECs EXPRESS NOVEL COSTIMULATORY MOLECULES

To maximally and effectively activate T cells there is a requirement for costimulatory pathways. Conventional costimulatory molecules (B7-1, B7-2, CD40) are not normally expressed by IEC. We have identified a novel costimulatory pathway for IEC-activated CD8[+] T cells. IECs express a surface glycoprotein, gp180, on both the apical and basolateral surface[28]. mAbs generated against this glycoprotein selectively inhibit IEC-induced CD8[+] T cell activation. The mechanism of action of gp180 has recently been elucidated: gp180 forms a complex on the surface of IEC with the class Ib molecule CD1d[29]; gp180 interacts with CD8 on the T cell activating the CD8-associated tyrosine kinase p56lck. CD1d presents Ag to the TcR receptor. The gp180:CD1d complex on the IEC allows for the formation of the TcR co-receptor complex promoting optimal T cell activation. Neither gp180 nor CD1d alone is sufficient to drive CD8[+] T cell proliferation. Current studies are focusing on the nature of these interactions as well as the Ag(s) involved in this response.

ALTERATION OF gp180 EXPRESSION IS ASSOCIATED WITH DISEASE STATES

If gp180 is required for activation of regulatory suppressor T cells in the gut, it is conceivable that it plays a similar role in other tissues where this glycoprotein is expressed. Such may be the case in the placenta, where gp180 is expressed by syncytiotrophoblasts. CD1d is not expressed by this cell type, so it is possible that other class Ib molecules may be involved (?HLA-E, HLA-G). There is a syndrome of recurrent spontaneous abortion which usually occurs between 8 and 12 weeks of gestation. gp180 expression in the normal placenta is seen at 6 weeks, but expression peaks by 12 weeks and is persistent at a constant level thereafter. We have studied placentas from 12 patients with recurrent spontaneous abortion. Nine of the 12 failed to express gp180 by Western blot. Only one of 10 control age-matched (induced abortions) placentas failed to express gp180. Since suppression of maternal immune responses to paternal MHC is obviously required to maintain successful pregnancy, it is intriguing to speculate that gp180 plays a role in this process.

In the intestine similar defects may also result in disease. Studies by Toy et al.[30] demonstrated a defect in the expression of gp180 in CD epithelium and an alteration in the form expressed (apical only) in ulcerative colitis. These findings correlated well with the inability of inflammatory bowel disease IEC to activate CD8[+] T cells. The nature of this defect is currently under investigation.

SUMMARY

This chapter has cited evidence for a role for the IEC in Ag processing and presentation in the gut. What is lacking is a true *in-vivo* correlate which would solidify the concepts proposed. The ability to generate murine models of mucosal immunoregulation will be critical to these efforts.

Acknowledgements

This work was supported by PHS grants AI23504, AI24671 and AI44236.

References

1. Mestecky J. The common mucosal immune system and current strategies for induction of immune responses in external secretions. J Clin Immunol. 1987;7:265–76.
2. Mayer, L. Review article: Local and systemic regulation of mucosal immunity. Aliment Pharmacol Ther. 11 Suppl 1997;3:81–5; discussion 85–8.
3. Panja A, Goldberg S, Eckmann L, Krishen P, Mayer L. The regulation and functional consequence of proinflammatory cytokine binding on human intestinal epithelial cells. J Immunol. 1998;161:3675–84.
4. Gonnella PA, Wilmore DW. Co-localization of class II antigen and exogenous antigen in the rat enterocyte. J Cell Sci. 1993;106:937–40.
5. Brandeis JM, Sayegh MH, Gallon L, Blumberg RS, Carpenter CB. Rat intestinal epithelial cells present major histocompatibility complex allopeptides to primed T cells. Gastroenterology. 1994;107:1537–42.
6. Berg DJ, Davidson N, Kuhn R *et al.* Enterocolitis and colon cancer in interleukin-10-deficient mice are associated with aberrant cytokine production and CD4(+) TH1-like responses. J Clin Invest. 1996;98:1010–20.
7. Berin MC, Kiliaan AJ, Yang PC, Groot JA, Taminiau JA, Perdue MH. Rapid transepithelial antigen transport in rat jejunum: impact of sensitization and the hypersensitivity reaction Gastroenterology. 1997;113:856–64.
8. Berin MC, Yang PC, Ciok L, Waserman S, Perdue MH. Role for IL-4 in macromolecular transport across human intestinal epithelium. Am J Physiol. 1999;276:C1046–52.
9. Berin MC, McKay DM, Perdue MH. Immune-epithelial interactions in host defense. Am J Trop Med Hyg. 1999;60:16–25.
10. So AL, Small G, Sperber K, Becker K, Oei E, Tyorkin M, Mayer L. Factors affecting antigen uptake by human intestinal epithelial cell lines. Dig Dis Sci. 2000;45:1130–7.
11. Hershberg RM, Framson PE, Cho DH *et al.* Intestinal epithelial cells use two distinct pathways for HLA class II antigen processing. J Clin Invest. 1997;100:204–15.
12. Hershberg RM, Cho DH, Youakim A *et al.* Highly polarized HLA class II antigen processing and presentation by human intestinal epithelial cells. J Clin Invest. 1998;102:792–803.
13. Kaiserlian D, Vidal K, Revillard JP. Murine enterocytes can present soluble antigen to specific class II- restricted CD4+ T cells. Eur J Immunol. 1989;19:1513–16.
14. Kaiserlian D, Nicolas JF, Revillard JP. Constitutive expression of Ia molecules by murine epithelial cells: a comparison between keratinocytes and enterocytes. J Invest Dermatol. 1990; 94:385–6.
15. Kaiserlian D. Murine gut epithelial cells express Ia molecules antigenically distinct from those of conventional antigen-presenting cells. Immunol Res. 1991;10:360–4.
16. Hughson EJ, Cutler DF, Hopkins CR. Basolateral secretion of kappa light chain in the polarised epithelial cell line, Caco-2. J Cell Sci. 1989;94:327–32.
17. Bland PW, Warren LG. Antigen presentation by epithelial cells of the rat small intestine. I. Kinetics, antigen specificity and blocking by anti-Ia antisera. Immunology. 1986;58:1–7.
18. Bland PW, Warren LG. Antigen presentation by epithelial cells of the rat small intestine. II. Selective induction of suppressor T cells. Immunology. 1986;58:9–14.
19. Mayer L, Shlien R. Evidence for function of Ia molecules on gut epithelial cells in man. J Exp Med. 1987;166:1471–83.

20. Li Y, Yio XY, Mayer L. Human intestinal epithelial cell-induced CD8+ T cell activation is mediated through CD8 and the activation of CD8-associated p56lck. J Exp Med. 1995; 182:1079–88.
21. Bleicher PA, Balk SP, Hagen SJ, Blumberg RS, Flotte TJ, Terhorst C. Expression of murine CD1 on gastrointestinal epithelium. Science. 1990;250:679–82.
22. Blumberg RS, Terhorst C, Bleicher P *et al*. Expression of a nonpolymorphic MHC class I-like molecule, CD1D, by human intestinal epithelial cells. J Immunol. 1991;147:2518–24.
23. Blumberg RS, Gerdes D, Chott A, Porcelli SA, Balk SP. Structure and function of the CD1 family of MHC-like cell surface proteins. Immunol Rev. 1995;147:5–29.
24. Blumberg RS, Koss T, Story CM *et al*. A major histocompatibility complex class I-related Fc receptor for IgG on rat hepatocytes. J Clin Invest. 1995;95:2397–402.
25. Blumberg RS, Colgan SP, Balk SP. CD1d: outside-in antigen presentation in the intestinal epithelium? Clin Exp Immunol. 1997;109:223–5.
26. Panja A, Blumberg RS, Balk SP, Mayer L. CD1d is involved in T cell-intestinal epithelial cell interactions. J Exp Med. 1993;178:1115–19.
27. Hershberg R, Eghtesady P, Sydora B, Brorson K, Cheroutre H, Modlin R, Kronenberg M. Expression of the thymus leukemia antigen in mouse intestinal epithelium. Proc Natl Acad Sci USA. 1990;87:9727–31.
28. Yio XY, Mayer L. Characterization of a 180-kDa intestinal epithelial cell membrane glycoprotein, gp180. A candidate molecule mediating t cell-epithelial cell interactions. J Biol Chem. 1997;272:12786–92.
29. Campbell NA, Kim HS, Blumberg RS, Mayer L. The nonclassical Class I molecule CD1d associates with the novel CD8 ligand gp180 on intestinal epithelial cells. J Biol Chem. 1999; 274:26259–65.
30. Toy LS, Yio XY, Lin A, Honig S, Mayer L. Defective expression of gp180, a novel CD8 ligand on intestinal epithelial cells, in inflammatory bowel disease. J Clin Invest. 1997;100:2062–71.

4
Immunology of the lamina propria

R. DUCHMANN and M. ZEITZ

INTRODUCTION

The connective tissue of the intestinal lamina propria contains a plethora of immunologically active cells. These include T lymphocytes, macrophages and dendritic cells, B lymphocytes and plasma cells, eosinophils, mast cells and mesenchymal cells and some cells that express surface markers of NK cells (Fig. 1). The function of these different cell types and their abnormalities in chronic intestinal inflammation will be discussed, with a focus on T cells, B cells and antigen-presenting cells (APC).

After primary stimulation within classical mucosal inductive follicular tissues, lymphocytes home to the lamina propria guided by adhesion molecules present on the lymphocyte/endothelial surfaces[1]. Once arrived in the lamina propria, T cells and B cells show a high degree of differentiation and, upon restimulation, are well prepared to express their definitive effector functions, the production of helper or suppressor cytokines, mediation of cytotoxicity or antibody production[2,3]. The above scenario of a primary stimulation in classical inductive mucosal follicular tissues probably holds true for the majority of lamina propria lymphocytes, but it seems not to be exclusive. Recent experiments demonstrate that mucosal Ig responses can also be induced in the absence of organized Peyer's patches[4,5]. In addition, there is increasing evidence for a role of the intestinal epithelium as a T cell inductive site and immune regulatory compartment. Thus, although identical structures were not identified in humans[6], crypt lamina propria patches (cryptopatches, CP)[7] are sites of extrathymic T cell maturation[8,9] in mice and epithelial-derived growth factors[10] are important for the development of γδ T cells and Peyer's patches. Furthermore, there is increasing evidence that intestinal epithelial cells can function as APCs and regulate T-cell responses of intraepithelial lymphocytes. It has also been speculated that they regulate lamina propria T lymphocytes by contacting them through basolateral projections[11].

T CELLS

In humans, T cells constitute about 25–40% of lymphocytes in the lamina propria. Most intestinal lamina propria T cells express the αβ T cell receptor (95%)

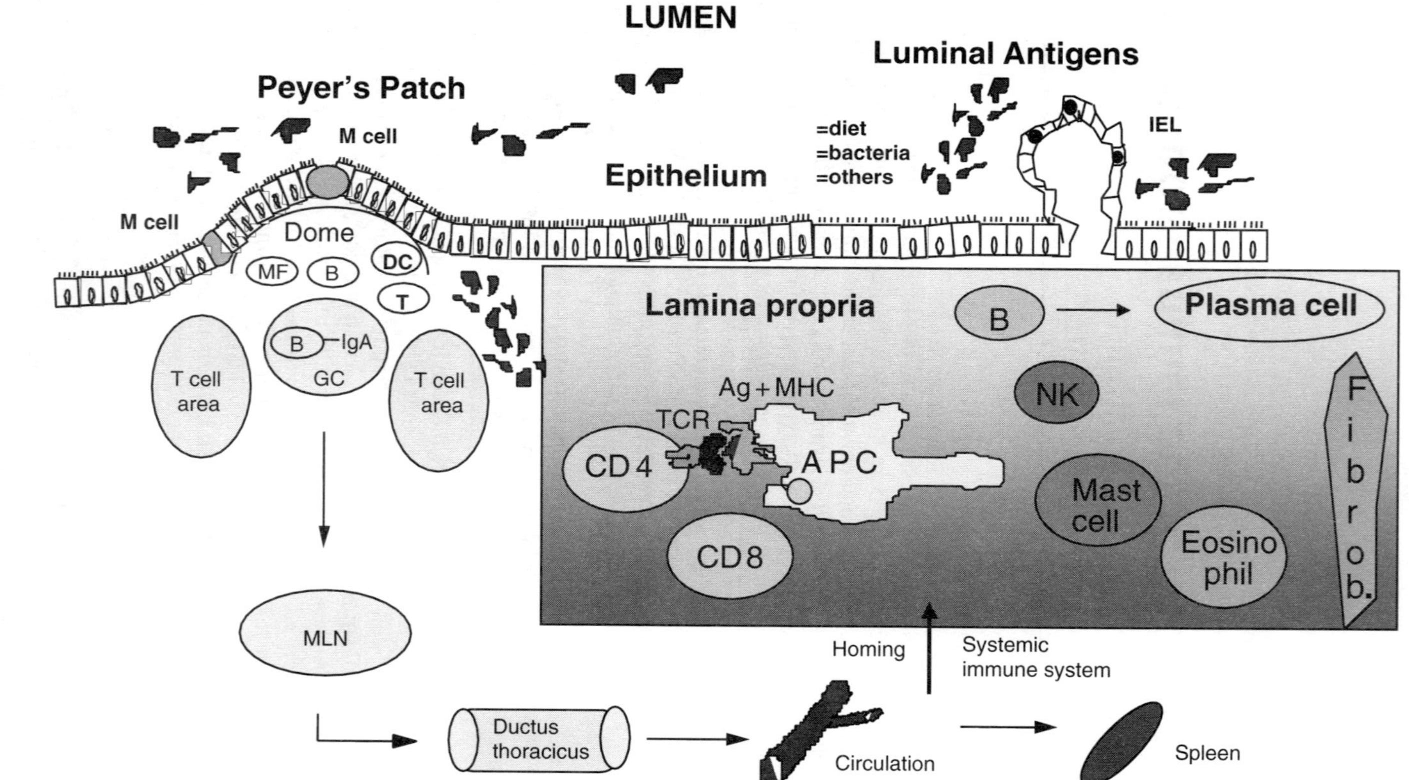

Figure 1 Immune cells within the lamina propria and their relation with the intestinal and systemic immune system

with a CD4[+]:CD8[+] ratio > 2:1, similar to the peripheral blood. Phenotype and functional analyses indicate that CD4[+] lamina propria T cells represent a highly specialized subset of memory T cells which perform important regulatory and effector functions[12,13]. Normal lamina propria T cells (LP-T) do not proliferate well to TCR/CD3 stimulation alone *in vitro* compared with peripheral blood T cells, yet demonstrate largely preserved or even enhanced proliferation and cytokine production (e.g. IL-2, IFN-γ, TNF-α, IL-4, IL-10) to CD2 and CD28 triggering, i.e. stimulation via accessory pathways[14–18]. This requirement for accessory signals may be interpreted to protect intestinal T cells from being stimulated by ubiquitous antigens presented on non-professional Ag-presenting cells (i.e. TCR/CD3 alone), while preserving their ability to respond to immuno-logically important antigens presented on professional APCs displaying appro-priate costimulatory molecules. Molecular differences in the intracellular pathways which lead to increased responsiveness and cytokine release of LP-T cells to CD2 and CD2/CD28 stimulation are being unravelled[19,20]. Such studies will also be helpful to determine the clinically important relative insensi-tivity of LP-T cells to some immunosuppressive drugs[21,22].

Determined by surface expression of CD25 (interleukin-2 receptor), CD71 (transferrin receptor) and other early activation markers, LP-T cells show signs of increased activation[12,13] and activation is further increased in IBD, in both the circulation and in the mucosa[23–25]. With regard to cytokine production it was shown, using defined T cell stimuli, that lamina propria CD4[+] T cells isolated from CD patients produce more IFN-γ but less IL-4 or IL-5 than control T cells. In contrast, LP-T cells from UC patients produced more IL-5 and did not show increased production of IFN-γ[26].

The cause of the increased activation of LP-T cells and the immunoregulatory abnormalities in IBD is still unknown. Several mechanisms, including aberrant instruction of T cells through primitive pattern-recognition receptors of the innate immune system and specific receptors of the adaptive immune system during host–microbe interactions, have been suggested[27,28].

Activation of LP-T cells can directly contribute to epithelial cell destruction since soluble factors released from activated T cells decrease the viability and proliferation of intestinal epithelial cell lines[29]. In addition, in an *in-vitro* model using fetal intestinal explant cultures, T cell activation induced mucosal trans-formation and destruction[30]. Mucosal pathology was strongly enhanced by the activating effect of IL-12 on Th1 T cell responses[31].

The importance of CD4[+] T lymphocytes in IBD pathogenesis has recently been highlighted in a variety of animal models of IBD. In one of these models, CD45RB[high] CD4[+] cells induced colitis when injected into immunodeficient (SCID or RAG) mice, whereas cotransfer of the CD45RB[low] CD4[+] subset prevented disease[32]. Similar to findings in other animal models of IBD, colitis was induced by Th1 cells[33] and down-regulated by TGF-β[34] and IL-10[35]. Pheno-typically and functionally distinct populations of T regulatory cells (Treg) which control intestinal inflammation in mice were further shown to display a CD25[+]CD45RB[low]CD4[+] phenotype and to act through signalling via CTLA-4 and secretion of TGF-β[36]. Interestingly, colitis was also dependent on compo-nents of the normal flora[37] and showed signs of antigen-driven activation and oligoclonal expansion of T cells[38].

When the immune response of intestinal CD4[+] T cells towards enterobacteria was analysed in humans using T cell clones, these studies indicated that enterobacteria express dominant discrete protein antigens and that these are recognized by a network of antigen-specific CD4[+] TCRαβ[+] T cells[39] with broad crossreactivity within and between enterobacteria and indigenous bacteria[40]. In IBD the relative frequency of enterobacteria-specific T cell clones was increased in involved intestine of both CD and UC patients, providing evidence that the increased responsiveness of intestinal IBD T cells to bacterial antigens *in vitro*[27,41] leads to expansion of bacteria-reactive T cells in the intestinal tissue. Thus, these data support the view that in the normal situation a protective immune response towards luminal bacteria is regulated by a tight network of T cell specificities and that increased numbers of T cells recognizing luminal bacteria contribute to the immune dysregulation and increased level of immune stimulation characteristic for IBD.

Human studies determining the regional variation and diversity of the T cell receptor β (TCRB) repertoire by a detailed analysis of multiple colonic biopsy specimens from non-inflammatory controls and CD patients revealed that expanded T cells in the intestine show either a focal or a continuous segmental or even ubiquitous distribution[42]. Since the regional distribution and diversity of expanded T cells was similar in the non-inflamed colon of controls, and involved and non-involved colon of CD patients, additional functional studies which determine the inflammatory profile of *in-vivo* expanded T cells will be extremely helpful to distinguish disease-related T cells from physiologically expanded T cells. Evidence that disease-related T cell expansions occur within the intestinal mucosa was suggested by the expansion of identical T cell clones in the intestine and synovia of patients with enterogenic spondyloarthropathy[43]. Nakajima *et al.* showed that the same T cell clones were expanded in different early CD lesions but not in intervening non-involved mucosa[44]. Similar investigations performed in more chronically involved intestine from colonic resections showed that identical CD4[+] T cell clones are more frequently detected in the lamina propria of inflamed sites compared to non-involved tissue[45]. In addition, a public motif, i.e. one shared by different individuals, was found among lamina propria CD8[+] T cells from UC patients undergoing colectomy[46] and shared private and public TCRB-CDR3 motifs were present among activated CD4[+] and CD8[+] T cells from involved CD mucosa, isolated after culture with recombinant IL-2[47].

In a model of IBD pathogenesis (Fig. 2) it is suggested that IBD is a consequence of an as-yet-undefined abnormality which leads to a dysregulated immune response of lamina propria T cells to luminal, most likely bacterial, antigens. Although this may be a single abnormality with different phenotypic expression, current data seem to favour the presence of more than one abnormality (e.g. indicated by the large number of different abnormalities leading to chronic intestinal inflammation in animal models). In IBD these abnormalities may eventually combine into individual or subgroup-specific patterns and overrule the normally counterinflammatory tone of the mucosal immune system, mediated by regulatory T cells, T cell anergy and apoptosis.

In Crohn's disease (Fig. 2a) it is suggested that production of the soluble mediator IL-12[48], interleukin 6 *trans* signalling[49] as well as cell–cell interactions mediated by CD44 variants[50,51] drive the differentiation of T cells into regulators of inflammation and prevent them from apoptosis[52,53]. During these processes, IL-12 increases the action of IL-18, which is also increased in CD[54], through up-regulation of its receptor on T cells[55], counterregulates tolerance to normal intestinal flora[56] and induces LP-T cells to produce IFN-γ, which in turn activates macrophages to produce proinflammatory cytokines. In UC (Fig. 2b), in contrast, low levels of IL-12 seem to favour the differentiation of T cells more prone to B cell help and the production of autoantibodies[57].

B CELLS

It has been estimated that around 80% of all Ig-producing cells of the body, i.e. 10^{10} per metre of small bowel, are present in the intestinal lamina propria[58]. Here, in contrast to the predominant production of IgG at other sites, approximately 75–90% of lamina propria B lymphocytes and plasma cells produce IgA, whereas only 15–20% produce IgM, 3% produce IgG and 2% produce IgE. Secretory IgA antibodies act as a first line of defence by performing antigen exclusion in mucus on the epithelial surface and against luminal antigens. They are generated from J-chain containing polymeric IgA (pIgA) released by plasma cells and are transported to the lumen by the polymeric Ig receptor (pIgR) together with unoccupied receptor released as free secretory component. Although most of the IgA B cells in the lamina propria derive from precursors in Peyer's patches, it was recently shown, in rodents, that a significant proportion of specific IgA induction against commensal flora antigens is through a pathway independent of T cell help and of follicular lymphoid tissue organization[4,5].

In IBD there is increased secretion of IgG. This is dominated by IgG2 in CD, whereas secretion of IgG1 dominates in UC. Furthermore, intestinal mononuclear cells (MNC) from involved CD intestine secrete less total IgA but high percentages of monomeric IgA and IgA1 compared to control intestinal MNC[59]. Changes in Ig-isotype production observed in IBD may affect mucosal defence mechanisms and contribute to inflammation. Whereas secretory IgA (SIgA) antibodies, and to a lesser extent, secretory IgM antibodies are thought to play an important role in preserving mucosal integrity by neutralizing toxins and viruses, and by preventing epithelial adherence and penetration of pathogenic microorganisms and foreign proteins, inflammatory properties of IgG antibodies may contribute to damage of the intestinal barrier. In addition, the observed shift from mucosal IgA2 to IgA1 immunocytes in IBD may compromise local defence, since IgA2 but not IgA1 is resistant to most IgA-specific bacterial proteases. Furthermore, irrespective of antibody activity, IgA2 may play a superior role in protection against Enterobacteriaceae because of its relatively strong mannose-mediated agglutination of *Escherichia coli*.

The reason for the increased state of activation of B cells in IBD is unclear, but it may result from increased exposure to luminal immunogenic substances, e.g. the commensal flora[60]. Thus, it has been shown in children that the mucosal densities of immunocytes decrease considerably after defunctioning colostomy[61]. Using hybridomas generated from activated B cells from mesenteric lymph nodes from patients with CD or UC, the majority of mucosal B cells produced antibodies against intestinal bacteria[62]. Only a relatively small percentage of

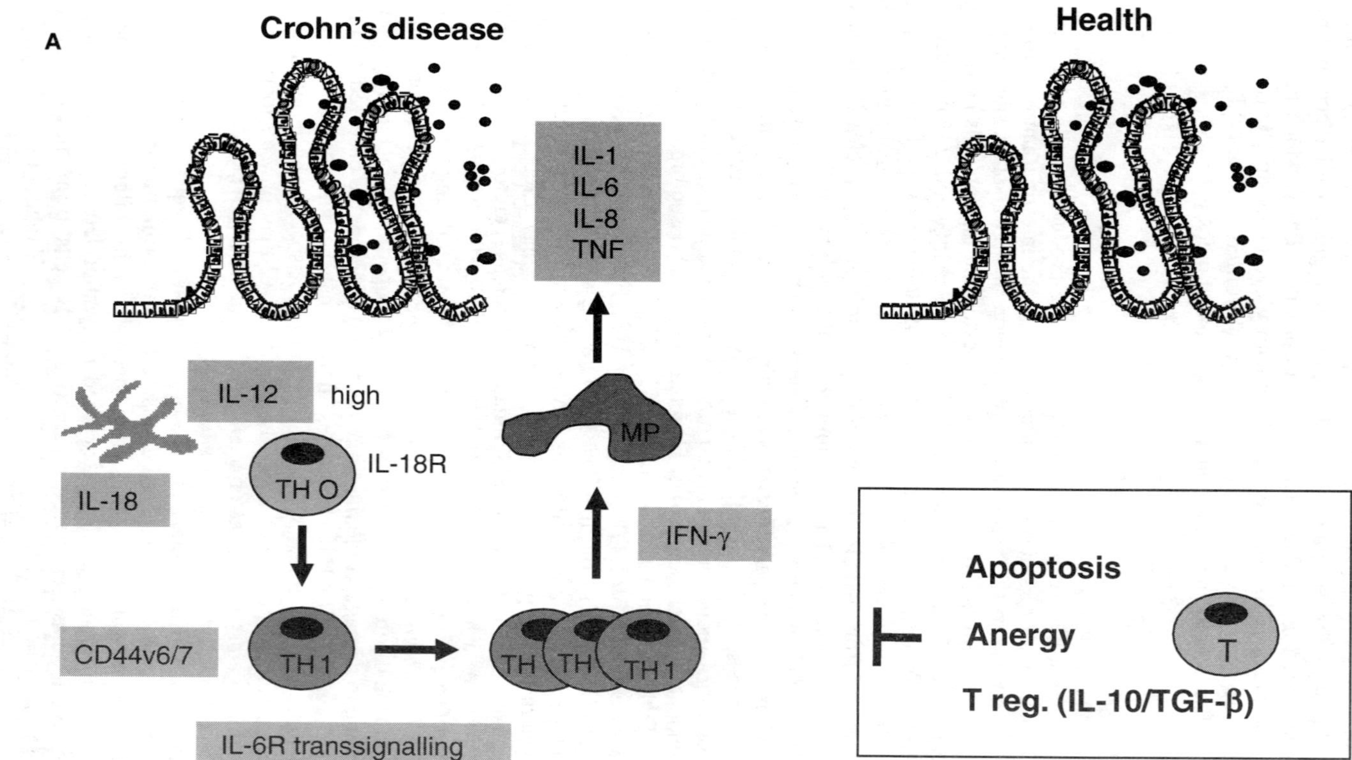

Figure 2 Model of the involvement of lamina propria lymphocytes in IBD immune pathogenesis

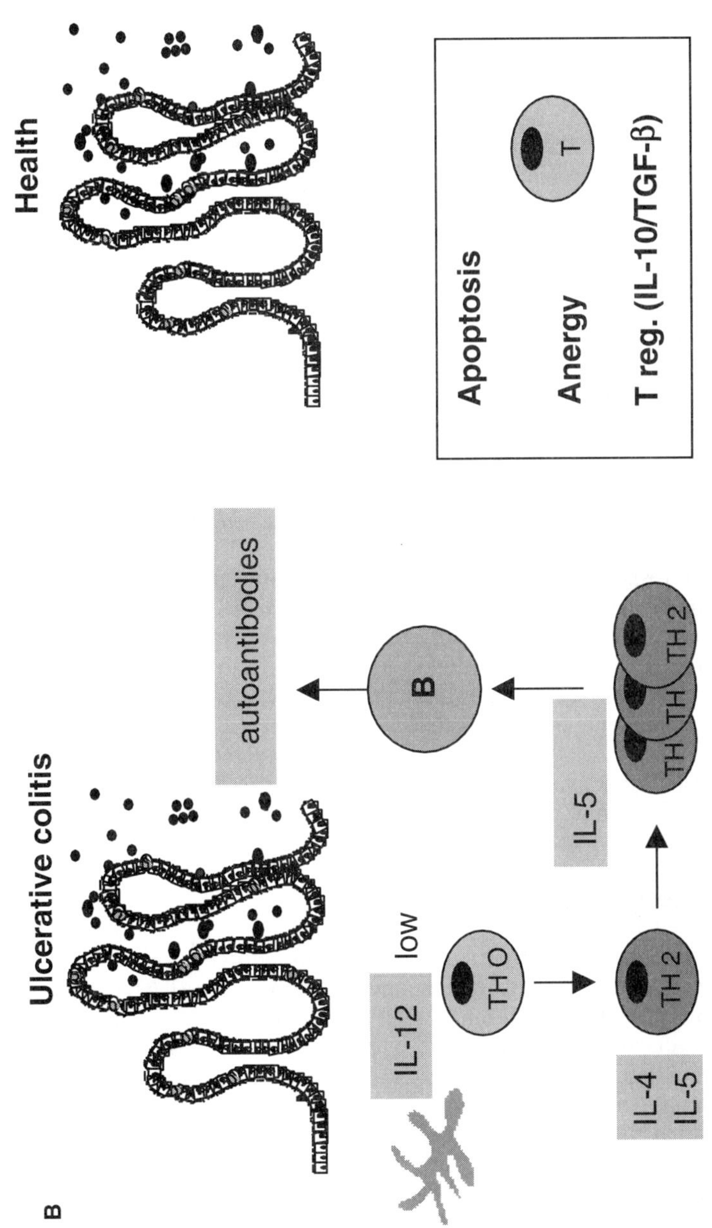

Health
Apoptosis
Anergy
T reg. (IL-10/TGF-β)
T
Ulcerative colitis
B
autoantibodies
IL-5
TH TH TH 2
IL-12
low
TH O
TH 2
IL-4
IL-5

these hybridomas secreted antibodies reactive with food antigens or intestinal autoantigens.

Differential IgG subtype secretion in CD vs UC may result from differences in the cytokine profiles of both diseases, with CD rather expressing a Th1-type cytokine pattern associated with IgG2 induction, and UC rather expressing a Th2-type cytokine pattern associated with IgG1 induction. Animal models of IBD, characteristic for CD and UC, showed development of an oligoclonal antibody response to enteric bacteria[63,64]. Furthermore, recent results indicate that mature B cells play an important role in TCRalpha($-/-$) mice by directly regulating the pathogenic T cells (CD4$^+$ TCRalpha-beta$^+$ T cells)[65].

ANTIGEN-PRESENTING CELLS

Under appropriate conditions, macrophages have the capacity to present antigens and to stimulate components of the specific immune system. In the normal gut this antigen-presenting function has been largely ascribed to dendritic cells[66]. Using monoclonal antibodies it has been shown that, in the human, colon macrophages are concentrated in a band immediately beneath the luminal epithelium. Thus, macrophages might normally serve as a first line of defence by non-specifically eliminating particles or organisms which have penetrated from the intestinal lumen. In contrast, dendritic cells are the most potent stimulators of primary T cell responses and have been demonstrated to form a reticular network throughout the lamina propria and beneath the basement membrane of the crypts. Here dendritic cells may normally act as 'immune adjuvants' by recruiting T cell responses when foreign antigens breach the macrophage barrier[67]. In CD mucosa numbers of macrophages and antigen-presenting dendritic cells are increased and include subpopulations that are rarely present in normal tissue[68] with surface markers indicating the presence of an increased activation state[69]. This increased state of activation is associated with increased functional activity and increased production of proinflammatory mediators.

OTHER IMMUNE CELLS

Lamina propria lymphocytes exhibit little spontaneous cytolytic function against classic NK targets, but cells with lymphokine-activated killer (LAK) function are easily demonstrated. In addition, CD8$^+$ LP-T cells can be activated to exhibit cytolytic or suppressor function[70,71]. NK T cells, suggested to interact with intestinal epithelial cells expressing CD1d, can act as regulatory cells and protect against colitis in mice[72].

Human intestinal mast cells can be isolated and cultured by recently established techniques[73] and, in addition to releasing a plethora of preformed mediators (histamine, proteases and others), were shown to be an important source for a variety of proinflammatory and regulatory cytokines[74–77]. Mast cell number determined in lamina propria from biopsy specimens was reduced in inflamed IBD lesions, probably due to degranulation, whereas eosinophil numbers were found increased[78]. Eosinophils and mast cells seem to be involved in IBD;

however, their role is not yet clear. Mesenchymal cells, especially intestinal subepithelial myofibroblasts (ISEMF), are known to respond to and to secrete growth factors and cytokines. They are important promoters for wound repair and may be critically involved in Crohn's fibrosis[79].

References

1. Brandtzaeg P, Farstad IN, Haraldsen G. Regional specialization in the mucosal immune system: primed cells do not always home along the same track. Immunol Today. 1999;20:267–77.
2. McIntyre T, Strober W. Gut-associated lymphoid tissue. Regulation of IgA B-cell development. In: Orgra PL, Mestecky J, Lamm ME, Strober W, Bienenstock J, McGhee J, editors. Mucosal Immunology, 2nd edn. New York: Academic Press, 1999:319–56.
3. Kelsall B, Strober W. Gut-associated lymphoid tissue. Antigen handling and T lymphocyte responses. In: Orgra PL, Mestecky J, Lamm ME, Strober W, Bienenstock J, McGhee J, editors. Mucosal Immunology, 2nd edn. Academic Press, 1999:293–318.
4. Macpherson AJ, Gatto D, Sainsbury E, Harriman GR, Hengartner H, Zinkernagel RM. A primitive T cell-independent mechanism of intestinal mucosal IgA responses to commensal bacteria. Science. 2000;288:2222–6.
5. Yamamoto M, Rennert P, McGhee JR et al. Alternate mucosal immune system: organized Peyer's patches are not required for IgA responses in the gastrointestinal tract. J Immunol. 2000; 164:5184–91.
6. Moghaddami M, Cummins A, Mayrhofer G. Lymphocyte-filled villi: comparison with other lymphoid aggregations in the mucosa of the human small intestine. Gastroenterology. 1998;115:1414–25.
7. Kanamori Y, Ishimaru K, Nanno M et al. Identification of novel lymphoid tissues in murine intestinal mucosa where clusters of c-kit+ IL-7R+ Thy1+ lympho-hemopoietic progenitors develop. J Exp Med. 1996;184:1449–59.
8. Saito H, Kanamori Y, Takemori T et al. Generation of intestinal T cells from progenitors residing in gut cryptopatches. Science. 1998;280:275–8.
9. Oida T, Suzuki K, Nanno M et al. Role of gut cryptopatches in early extrathymic maturation of intestinal intraepithelial T cells. J Immunol. 2000;164:3616–26.
10. Laky K, Lefrancois L, Lingenheld EG et al. Enterocyte expression of interleukin 7 induces development of gamma-delta T cells and Peyer's patches. J Exp Med. 2000;191:1569–80.
11. Hershberg RM, Mayer LF. Antigen processing and presentation by intestinal epithelial cells – polarity and complexity. Immunol Today. 2000;21:123–8.
12. James S, Kiyono H. Gastrointestinal lamina propria T cells. In: Orgra PL, Mestecky J, Lamm ME, Strober W, Bienenstock J, McGhee J, editors. Mucosal Immunology, 2nd edn. New York: Academic Press, 1999:381–96.
13. Zeitz M, Schieferdecker HL, Ullrich R, Jahn HU, James SP, Riecken EO. Phenotype and function of lamina propria T lymphocytes. Immunol Res. 1991;10:199–206.
14. Zeitz M, Quinn TC, Graeff AS, James SP. Mucosal T cells provide helper function but do not proliferate when stimulated by specific antigen in lymphogranuloma venereum proctitis in nonhuman primates. Gastroenterology. 1988;94:353–66.
15. Qiao L, Schurmann G, Betzler M, Meuer SC. Activation and signaling status of human lamina propria T lymphocytes. Gastroenterology. 1991;101:1529–36.
16. Pirzer UC, Schurmann G, Post S, Betzler M, Meuer SC. Differential responsiveness to CD3-Ti vs. CD2-dependent activation of human intestinal T lymphocytes. Eur J Immunol. 1990;20: 2339–42.
17. Targan SR, Deem RL, Liu M, Wang S, Nel A. Definition of a lamina propria T cell responsive state. Enhanced cytokine responsiveness of T cells stimulated through the CD2 pathway. J Immunol. 1995;154:664–75.
18. Braunstein J, Qiao L, Autschbach F, Schurmann G, Meuer S. T cells of the human intestinal lamina propria are high producers of interleukin-10. Gut. 1997;41:215–20.
19. Gonsky R, Deem RL, Bream JH, Lee DH, Young HA, Targan SR. Mucosa-specific targets for regulation of IFN-gamma expression: lamina propria T cells use different cis-elements than peripheral blood T cells to regulate transactivation of IFN-gamma expression. J Immunol. 2000;164:1399–407.

20. Gonsky R, Deem RL, Lee DH, Chen A, Targan SR. CD28 costimulation augments IL-2 secretion of activated lamina propria T cells by increasing mRNA stability without enhancing IL-2 gene transactivation. J Immunol. 1999;162:6621–9.
21. Braunstein J, Autschbach F, Sido B *et al.* Insensitivity towards inhibition by cyclosporin A, rapamycin, and tacrolimus in human intestinal lamina propria lymphocytes. In: Stallmach A, Zeitz M, Strober W, McDonald TT, Lochs H, editors. Induction and Modulation of Gastrointestinal Inflammation. Lancaster: Kluwer, 1999:199.
22. Zeitz M, Quinn TC, Graeff AS, Schwarting R, James SP. Oral administration of cyclosporin does not prevent expansion of antigen-specific, gut-associated, and spleen lymphocyte populations during *Chlamydia trachomatis* proctitis in nonhuman primates. Dig Dis Sci. 1989;34:585–95.
23. Schreiber S, MacDermott RP, Raedler A, Pinnau R, Bertovich MJ, Nash GS. Increased activation of isolated intestinal lamina propria mononuclear cells in inflammatory bowel disease. Gastroenterology. 1991;101:1020–30.
24. Pallone F, Fais S, Squarcia O, Biancone L, Pozzilli P, Boirivant M. Activation of peripheral blood and intestinal lamina propria lymphocytes in Crohn's disease. *In vivo* state of activation and *in vitro* response to stimulation as defined by the expression of early activation antigens. Gut. 1987;28:745–53.
25. Choy MY, Walker-Smith JA, Williams CB, MacDonald TT. Differential expression of CD25 (interleukin-2 receptor) on lamina propria T cells and macrophages in the intestinal lesions in Crohn's disease and ulcerative colitis. Gut. 1990;31:1365–70.
26. Fuss IJ, Neurath M, Boirivant M *et al.* Disparate CD4+ lamina propria (LP) lymphokine secretion profiles in inflammatory bowel disease. Crohn's disease LP cells manifest increased secretion of IFN-gamma, whereas ulcerative colitis LP cells manifest increased secretion of IL-5. J Immunol. 1996;157:1261–70.
27. Duchmann R, Kaiser I, Hermann E, Mayet W, Ewe K, Meyer zum Büschenfelde KH. Tolerance exists towards resident intestinal flora but is broken in active inflammatory bowel disease (IBD). Clin Exp Immunol. 1995;102:448–55.
28. French N, Pettersson S. Microbe–host interactions in the alimentary tract: the gateway to understanding inflammatory bowel disease. Gut. 2000;47:162–3.
29. Deem RL, Shanahan F, Targan SR. Triggered human mucosal T cells release tumour necrosis factor-alpha and interferon-gamma which kill human colonic epithelial cells. Clin Exp Immunol. 1991;83:79–84.
30. MacDonald TT, Bajaj-Elliott M, Pender SL. T cells orchestrate intestinal mucosal shape and integrity. Immunol Today. 1999;20:505–10.
31. Monteleone G, MacDonald TT, Wathen NC, Pallone F, Pender SL. Enhancing lamina propria Th1 cell responses with interleukin 12 produces severe tissue injury. Gastroenterology. 1999;117:1069–77.
32. Powrie F, Leach MW, Mauze S, Caddle LB, Coffman RL. Phenotypically distinct subsets of CD4+ T cells induce or protect from chronic intestinal inflammation in C. B-17 scid mice. Int Immunol. 1993;5:1461–71.
33. Powrie F, Mauze S, Coffman RL. CD4+ T-cells in the regulation of inflammatory responses in the intestine. Res Immunol. 1997;148:576–81.
34. Powrie F, Carlino J, Leach MW, Mauze S, Coffman RL. A critical role for transforming growth factor-beta but not interleukin 4 in the suppression of T helper type 1-mediated colitis by CD45RB(low) CD4+ T cells. J Exp Med. 1996;183:2669–74.
35. Asseman C, Mauze S, Leach MW, Coffman RL, Powrie F. An essential role for interleukin 10 in the function of regulatory T cells that inhibit intestinal inflammation. J Exp Med. 1999;190:995–1004.
36. Read S, Malmstrom V, Powrie F. Cytotoxic T lymphocyte-associated antigen 4 plays an essential role in the function of CD25(+)CD4(+) regulatory cells that control intestinal inflammation. J Exp Med. 2000;192:295–302.
37. Aranda R, Sydora BC, McAllister PL *et al.* Analysis of intestinal lymphocytes in mouse colitis mediated by transfer of CD4+, CD45RBhigh T cells to SCID recipients. J Immunol. 1997;158:3464–73.
38. Matsuda JL, Gapin L, Sydora BC *et al.* Systemic activation and antigen-driven oligoclonal expansion of T cells in a mouse model of colitis. J Immunol. 2000;164:2797–806.
39. Duchmann R, Marker-Hermann E, Meyer zum Büschenfelde KH. Bacteria-specific T-cell clones are selective in their reactivity towards different enterobacteria or *H. pylori* and increased in inflammatory bowel disease. Scand J Immunol. 1996;44:71–9.

40. Duchmann R, May E, Heike M, Knolle P, Neurath M, Meyer zum Büschenfelde KH. T cell specificity and cross reactivity towards enterobacteria, bacteroides, bifidobacterium, and antigens from resident intestinal flora in humans. Gut. 1999;44:812–18.

41. Pirzer U, Schonhaar A, Fleischer B, Hermann E, Meyer zum Büschenfelde KH. Reactivity of infiltrating T lymphocytes with microbial antigens in Crohn's disease. Lancet. 1991;338:1238–9.

42. May E, Lambert C, Holtmeier W, Hennemann A, Zeitz M, Duchmann R. Regional variation of the αβ T cell repertoire in the colon of healthy individuals and patients with Crohn's disease (Submitted).

43. May E, Märker-Hermann E, Wittig B, Zeitz M, Meyer zum Büschenfelde KH, Duchmann R. Identical T cell expansions in the colon mucosa and the synovium of a patient with enterogenic spondylarthropathy. Gastroenterology. 2000;119:1745–55.

44. Nakajima A, Kodama T, Yazaki Y *et al*. Specific clonal T cell accumulation in intestinal lesions of Crohn's disease. J Immunol. 1996;157:5683–8.

45. Gulwani-Akolkar B, Akolkar PN, Minassian A *et al*. Selective expansion of specific T cell receptors in the inflamed colon of Crohn's disease. J Clin Invest. 1996;98:1344–54.

46. Chott A, Probert CS, Gross GG, Blumberg RS, Balk SP. A common TCR beta-chain expressed by CD8 + intestinal mucosa T cells in ulcerative colitis. J Immunol. 1996;156:3024–35.

47. Saubermann LJ, Probert CS, Christ AD *et al*. Evidence of T cell receptor beta-chain patterns in inflammatory and noninflammatory bowel disease states. Am J Physiol. 1999;276:G613–21.

48. Monteleone G, Biancone L, Marasco R *et al*. Interleukin 12 is expressed and actively released by Crohn's disease intestinal lamina propria mononuclear cells. Gastroenterology. 1997;112:1169–78.

49. Atreya R, Mudter J, Finotto S *et al*. Blockade of interleukin 6 *trans* signaling suppresses T-cell resistance against apoptosis in chronic intestinal inflammation: evidence in Crohn disease and experimental colitis *in vivo*. Nat Med. 2000;6:583–8.

50. Wittig BM, Johansson B, Zoller M, Schwarzler C, Gunthert U. Abrogation of experimental colitis correlates with increased apoptosis in mice deficient for CD44 variant exon 7 (CD44v7). J Exp Med. 2000;191:2053–64.

51. Wittig B, Seiter S, Schmidt DS, Zuber M, Neurath M, Zoller M. CD44 variant isoforms on blood leukocytes in chronic inflammatory bowel disease and other systemic autoimmune diseases. Lab Invest. 1999;79:747–59.

52. Boirivant M, Pica R, DeMaria R, Testi R, Pallone F, Strober W. Stimulated human lamina propria T cells manifest enhanced Fas-mediated apoptosis. J Clin Invest. 1996;98:2616–22.

53. Boirivant M, Marini M, Di Felice G *et al*. Lamina propria T cells in Crohn's disease and other gastrointestinal inflammation show defective CD2 pathway-induced apoptosis. Gastroenterology. 1999;116:557–65.

54. Monteleone G, Trapasso F, Parrello T *et al*. Bioactive IL-18 expression is up-regulated in Crohn's disease. J Immunol. 1999;163:143–7.

55. Sareneva T, Julkunen I, Matikainen S. IFN-alpha and IL-12 induce IL-18 receptor gene expression in human NK and T cells. J Immunol. 2000;165:1933–8.

56. Duchmann R, Schmitt E, Knolle P, Meyer zum Büschenfelde KH, Neurath M. Tolerance towards resident intestinal flora in mice is abrogated in experimental colitis and restored by treatment with interleukin-10 or antibodies to interleukin-12. Eur J Immunol. 1996;26:934–8.

57. Seibold F, Brandwein S, Simpson S, Terhorst C, Elson CO. pANCA represents a cross-reactivity to enteric bacterial antigens. J Clin Immunol. 1998;18:153–60.

58. Brandtzaeg P, Halstensen TS, Kett K *et al*. Immunobiology and immunopathology of human gut mucosa: humoral immunity and intraepithelial lymphocytes. Gastroenterology. 1989;97:1562–84.

59. Duchmann R, Zeitz M. Crohn's disease. In: Orgra PL, Mestecky J, Lamm ME, Strober W, Bienenstock J, McGhee J, editors. Mucosal Immunology, 2nd edn. New York: Academic Press, 1999:1055–80.

60. Macpherson A, Khoo UY, Forgacs I, Philpott-Howard J, Bjarnason I. Mucosal antibodies in inflammatory bowel disease are directed against intestinal bacteria. Gut. 1996;38:365–75.

61. Wijesinha SS, Steer HW. Studies of the immunoglobulin-producing cells of the human intestine: the defunctioned bowel. Gut. 1982;23:211–14.

62. Chao LP, Steele J, Rodrigues C *et al*. Specificity of antibodies secreted by hybridomas generated from activated B cells in the mesenteric lymph nodes of patients with inflammatory bowel disease. Gut. 1988;29:35 40.

63. Mizoguchi A, Mizoguchi E, Tonegawa S, Bhan AK. Alteration of a polyclonal to an oligoclonal immune response to cecal aerobic bacterial antigens in TCR alpha mutant mice with inflammatory bowel disease. Int Immunol. 1996;8:1387–94.
64. Brandwein SL, McCabe RP, Cong Y *et al*. Spontaneously colitic C3H/HeJBir mice demonstrate selective antibody reactivity to antigens of the enteric bacterial flora. J Immunol. 1997;159:44–52.
65. Mizoguchi E, Mizoguchi A, Preffer FI, Bhan AK. Regulatory role of mature B cells in a murine model of inflammatory bowel disease. Int Immunol. 2000;12:597–605.
66. Pavli P, Hume DA, Van De Pol E, Doe WF. Dendritic cells, the major antigen-presenting cells of the human colonic lamina propria. Immunology. 1993;78:132–41.
67. Pavli P, Maxwell L, Van de Pol E, Doe F. Distribution of human colonic dendritic cells and macrophages. Clin Exp Immunol. 1996;104:124–32.
68. Rogler G, Andus T, Aschenbrenner E *et al*. Alterations of the phenotype of colonic macrophages in inflammatory bowel disease. Eur J Gastroenterol Hepatol. 1997;9:893–9.
69. Rogler G, Hausmann M, Spottl T *et al*. T-cell co-stimulatory molecules are upregulated on intestinal macrophages from inflammatory bowel disease mucosa. Eur J Gastroenterol Hepatol. 1999;11:1105–11.
70. James SP, Graeff AS. Spontaneous and lymphokine-induced cytotoxic activity of monkey intestinal mucosal lymphocytes. Cell Immunol. 1985;93:387–97.
71. Fiocchi C, Tubbs RR, Youngman KR. Human intestinal mucosal mononuclear cells exhibit lymphokine-activated killer cell activity. Gastroenterology. 1985;88:625–37.
72. Saubermann LJ, Beck P, De Jong YP *et al*. Activation of natural killer T cells by alpha-galactosylceramide in the presence of CD1d provides protection against colitis in mice. Gastroenterology. 2000;119:119–28.
73. Bischoff SC, Schwengberg S, Raab R, Manns MP. Functional properties of human intestinal mast cells cultured in a new culture system: enhancement of IgE receptor-dependent mediator release and response to stem cell factor. J Immunol. 1997;159:5560–7.
74. Lorentz A, Schwengberg S, Sellge G, Manns MP, Bischoff SC. Human intestinal mast cells are capable of producing different cytokine profiles: role of IgE receptor cross-linking and IL-4. J Immunol. 2000;164:43–8.
75. Bischoff SC, Sellge G, Lorentz A, Sebald W, Raab R, Manns MP. IL-4 enhances proliferation and mediator release in mature human mast cells. Proc Natl Acad Sci USA. 1999;96:8080–5.
76. Lorentz A, Schwengberg S, Mierke C, Manns MP, Bischoff SC. Human intestinal mast cells produce IL-5 *in vitro* upon IgE receptor cross-linking and *in vivo* in the course of intestinal inflammatory disease. Eur J Immunol. 1999;29:1496–503.
77. Bischoff SC, Lorentz A, Schwengberg S, Weier G, Raab R, Manns MP. Mast cells are an important cellular source of tumour necrosis factor alpha in human intestinal tissue. Gut. 1999;44:643–52.
78. Bischoff SC, Wedemeyer J, Herrmann A *et al*. Quantitative assessment of intestinal eosinophils and mast cells in inflammatory bowel disease. Histopathology. 1996;28:1–13.
79. Powell DW, Mifflin RC, Valentich JD, Crowe SE, Saada JI, West AB. Myofibroblasts. II. Intestinal subepithelial myofibroblasts. Am J Physiol. 1999; 277:C183–201.

5
Immunosuppression in inflammatory bowel disease: a personal view

D. H. PRESENT

The organizers of this symposium have asked me to give a personal view and a historical perspective of immunomodulatory therapy for inflammatory bowel disease (IBD). Considering the time it has taken for immunomodulatory drugs to be accepted, to now have a full symposium on this topic is very gratifying to me, since I was fortunate enough to start my clinical research career at the beginning of immunomodulatory therapy.

On the other hand, when someone is asked to give a historical perspective, does this mean that the speaker's major research time has passed and that he is 'over the hill'? I would hope that this would not be true.

I was fortunate to be in the right place at the right time when immunomodulatory therapy for IBD was starting. I had finished my fellowship in gastroenterology at Mount Sinai under the tutelage of Dr Henry D. Janowitz in 1966. Dr Janowitz invited me to help care for his busy practice while I was developing my own clinical practice. At the same time the Foundation for Ileitis and Colitis came into being, with its founders, the Rosenthals and the Modells, as well as Dr Henry Janowitz.

I received the first grant from the National Foundation for Ileitis and Colitis for $10 000 a year. The Foundation, which was renamed the Crohn's and Colitis Foundation of America (incidentally this name was chosen by my wife, Jane Present, when she was the national president) now dispenses several million dollars in research each year. I looked for a research topic, and on reviewing the literature, the first paper on immunomodulatory therapy was that of Bean[1], who published his experience with 6-mercaptopurine (6-MP) and ulcerative colitis in the *Medical Journal of Australia* in 1962. He used a high dose of 300 mg daily and later lowered it to 50–100 mg daily and demonstrated dramatic remission. Also intriguing was the early article by Dr Brian Brooke and co-workers, published in the *Lancet* in 1969[2], at which time he used azathioprine for Crohn's disease and demonstrated a dramatic response in six patients. A year later he reported on 24 patients with similar results. These studies were so dramatic that it stimulated me to become involved in a prospective placebo-controlled trial looking at 6-MP in the treatment of Crohn's disease.

From a historical perspective it was Dr Gertrude Elion and George Hitchings who studied purine metabolites while working at Burroughs Wellcome, which led to the drugs 6-MP, azathioprine and allopurinol. They were the first having come from industry to win a Nobel Prize.

I did not have the vaguest idea how to conduct a control trial, but I developed an initial protocol and a meeting was held at Mount Sinai funded by the Crohn's and Colitis Foundation to discuss my protocol. Those people attending included Drs Joseph Kirsner, Burton Korelitz, Fred Kern, and Thomas Chalmers, as well as Dr Henry Janowitz. Dr Chalmers was an expert in control trials, who subsequently became the Dean of the Mount Sinai Medical School.

Our initial plans called for a control trial in both Crohn's disease and ulcerative colitis, but I was 'incorrectly' convinced by many colleagues and friends that 6-MP was a toxic agent and could be fatal, and that since there was a cure for ulcerative colitis, namely a colectomy and ileostomy, we should not study this group of patients. This turned out to be my first major error in planning controlled trials, and Dr Tom Chalmers later said it would have been quite ethical to do such a study until the drug was definitely proved to be toxic. Dr Korelitz and I created our own index for evaluating activity, called the Goals of Therapy. We still believe that this index is the best for this chronic illness with multiple manifestations. I am often asked why we did not use the Crohn's Disease Activity Index (CDAI), and the simple answer was that 'it did not exist'. Our study preceded the National Cooperative Crohn's Disease Study[3]. The CDAI provided a computerized analysis of clinical activity but it had its faults, especially with subjectivity. For example if a patient with an irritable bowel syndrome calculated his or her CDAI it could range up to 220, which is considered moderately active disease.

In looking at the National Cooperative Study retrospectively, it was initiated in 1970 and there were no prior control trials to determine the efficacy or safety of medications used in the treatment of Crohn's disease. The organizers selected prednisone, sulphasalazine, and azathioprine as agents meriting a clinical trial, and the design attempted to model as closely as possible the process of contemporary management of Crohn's disease.

The study was well conceived for steroids and sulphasalazine, but retrospectively it was a poor design for a slow-acting drug such as azathioprine. Also as noted, the CDAI was quite subjective; nevertheless, it has become the standard through the years for control trials in Crohn's disease. The study demonstrated the efficacy of both sulphasalazine and steroids in active Crohn's disease, but did not 'emphasize' the lack of the long-term efficacy of prednisone, or its significant long-term toxicity. The study also did not detect the efficacy for azathioprine, and overestimated its toxicity, which significantly retarded physicians' use of azathioprine and 6-MP in chronically ill Crohn's disease patients.

Dr Korelitz and I completed our study on 6-MP about 1 year after the first report of the National Cooperative Study[4]. We demonstrated statistical efficacy as regards overall clinical improvement, steroid sparing and fistula healing. This was the first control trial to randomize patients with and without fistulization, and up until the recent infliximab studies no other controlled trials have randomized for fistula. This has been a never-ending source of amazement to me, since approximately one-third of Crohn's patients have fistulization, and there are clinical data showing that these patients behave differently compared with those with the inflammatory type of Crohn's disease. Papers by Greenstein *et al.*[5] and Aeberhardt *et al.*[6] have shown that the fistulizing patients have more aggressive disease, have earlier recurrence of disease and require earlier re-operation.

Although I do believe in control trials, and what is now euphemistically called evidence-based medicine, the design of a trial is the most important part of the study. For example, to demonstrate the efficacy of 6-MP and azathioprine you required a longer time to show response, and when the National Cooperative Crohn's Disease Study ended at 17 weeks, it lost approximately 20% of the responders. The medical community did not believe the study of Dr Korelitz and myself until a meta-analysis was performed by Pearson *et al.*[7]. As noted earlier, I very much regret the fact that we did not use 6-MP in studying ulcerative colitis in a control trial. Although control data are lacking, it is quite clear from the uncontrolled data that this drug is equally as effective with ulcerative colitis. I personally have used 6-MP to treat several hundred patients with ulcerative colitis, and have observed many dramatic responses[8]. After this extensive experience I do not need a control trial to convince me of efficacy, but nevertheless, under the auspices of the IOIBD and the CCFA, the Mount Sinai group will be leading a study in the near future using azathioprine to prevent relapse after a severe attack of ulcerative colitis. Although many new drugs are on the horizon, 6-MP and azathioprine appear to be the best currently available agents for both Crohn's disease and ulcerative colitis, and I personally credit Dr William Sandborn from the Mayo Clinic, who has rejuvenated the field while looking at the pharmacology and mechanisms of action of these drugs. We still are not certain how long patients should be maintained on 6-MP/azathioprine, but I would refer you to an excellent review by Professor Modigliani, who has summarized this topic and points out clearly that we must look at the risks versus benefits of this drug[9]. He emphasizes that we should look at the rate of relapse after withdrawal as compared to the risk of prolonged therapy. We must also ask whether response can be repeated after a withdrawal relapse? As is pointed out, we will have to await controlled withdrawal trials. What I am fairly certain of, as presented in our toxicity paper[10], is that there is little risk from prolonged therapy, and that these drugs are extraordinarily safe. The short-term toxicity consists of pancreatitis (3–4%), allergy, including rash and fever (2%), and leukopenia, which theoretically should occur in about 10% of patients with TPMT deficiency. We personally have not seen any long-term toxicity, including neoplasia or an increase in infections. A recent large series presented in abstract form at the American Gastroenterological Association confirms this lack of long-term toxicity[11].

I was privileged to help mentor Dr Simon Lichtiger when he came up with the concept of using intravenous cyclosporin in the treatment of Crohn's disease and ulcerative colitis. We, as well as others, had embarked on uncontrolled studies to evaluate the efficacy of this agent, but it was Dr Lichtiger's idea to use an intravenous loading dose of cyclosporin in order to try to drive the patients into rapid remission. He had noted that there was a lack of absorption with the oral agent, and that continuous intravenous infusions resulted in stable blood levels of cyclosporin. We negotiated with the pharmaceutical company, Sandoz, to do a control trial. However, they managed to procrastinate for 7 years, and when we were finally given the funds to start a control trial we completed it within 9 months, with publication in the *New England Journal of Medicine*[12]. The results of our controlled and uncontrolled data were similar and showed a response rate of over 80%. We terminated the control trial early because none of the placebo patients responded, whereas the active drug was effective once again, in over 80% of patients. This study has been criticized for being too small, but it must be pointed out that, prior to the trial, we studied 32 patients in an uncontrolled manner while awaiting funding, with similar results. Much still needs to be done in this field since other investigators have shown that the efficacy of cyclosporin when given alone is equal to that of steroids when given alone. Another study has shown that the combination of steroids with cyclosporin administered concurrently shows a higher positive response than either alone.

When we turn to cyclosporin in Crohn's disease, once again control trials have given us the 'wrong answers'. Brynskov *et al.*'s initial study administering up to 7.5 mg/kg daily showed statistical efficacy in active Crohn's disease in a publication in the *New England Journal of Medicine*[13]. I was present at the meeting conducted by Sandoz in which they were planning future controlled trials. Dr Lichtiger and I pointed out that they were using too low a dose of cyclosporin and that our dose of 4 mg/kg daily, administered intravenously, really represented 8–9 mg daily of an oral dose. Nevertheless, the company decided to conduct the studies at a low dose because of the potential nephrotoxicity of higher doses. This resulted in three studies showing a lack of efficacy of low-dose oral cyclosporin in the treatment of Crohn's disease. A meta-analysis[14] reported that oral cyclosporin was ineffective for Crohn's disease, but it is unfortunately a meta-analysis of three studies that were designed using too low a dose. Cyclosporin was safe at this dose but not effective. In fact, several uncontrolled studies have shown that cyclosporin is effective in active Crohn's disease in about two-thirds of patients, and very effective in the management of fistula. Uncontrolled studies by Hanauer and Smith[15], as well as by our Mount Sinai group[16], clearly demonstrate clinical response in 86% and complete closure in 61% within 4–7 days. Unfortunately relapse occurred on oral cyclosporin in 42%; however, we saw little toxicity. It was our feeling that prospective control trials were required using intravenous cyclosporin but adding maintenance with 6-MP/azathioprine. I feel that a placebo control trial is also advisable, administering intravenous cyclosporin for treatment of very active Crohn's disease. My personal opinion is that cyclosporin remains a very effective therapeutic agent for Crohn's disease and should not be overlooked, although the long-term renal toxicity is uncertain and remains a concern. We would recommend maintenance with either 6-MP/azathioprine or methotrexate.

In looking at the latter drug, Dr Brian Feagan designed a study that showed that methotrexate was effective in the treatment of Crohn's disease, but his design was rather unique[17]. All patients had to start at 20 mg of prednisone, so if you were taking a lower dose, it was raised to 20 mg, and if you were taking a higher dose, you were lowered to 20 mg. The data showed efficacy, but if you break it down as to steroid dose, statistical significance was reached only in those patients who started higher than 20 mg daily. Frankly, I am not sure how to translate this into private practice. Feagan and co-workers have now successfully demonstrated that methotrexate will maintain remission[18]. The long-term toxicity data are not as complete as those seen with 6-MP or azathioprine. My conclusion is that, as of the year 2000, 6-MP and methotrexate are both effective in about two-thirds of patients with active Crohn's disease and that both will maintain remission. The allergic pneumonitis, teratogenicity and potential hepatotoxicity of methotrexate make 6-MP or azathioprine the initial drug of choice. However, methotrexate remains a good alternative if the patient is allergic or non-responsive to 6-MP or azathioprine. On the other hand, methotrexate may prove to be more effective than 6-MP/azathioprine when used in combination with other newer immunomodulatory agents. An example of this would be the methotrexate–infliximab combination in treating rheumatoid arthritis.

6-MP has recently shown another valuable facet in the treatment of postoperative prevention of Crohn's disease. In a study using low-dose 6-MP (50 mg daily) compared to 3 g of mesalamine versus placebo, the 6-MP was shown to be statistically more effective than the placebo in preventing both clinical and endoscopic recurrence[19]. Mesalamine just missed significance when compared to placebo. Future work is needed in this field to find out the optimal dose. For example, should we use higher doses of 6-MP and/or should we use 6-MP in combination with 5-aminosalicylates?

As I have continued to age, I have been fortunate enough to continue to be involved with control trials, and most recently I participated in designing the studies for infliximab in the treatment of Crohn's disease. Dr Stephan Targan was the lead author on the paper showing the efficacy of this mouse–human antibody against tumour necrosis factor (TNF) alpha. About 7–8 years ago Dr Targan embarrassed me by calling me the Grandfather of Immunomodulatory Therapy, which was long before I was an actual grandfather. I forgive him, since I am now a grandfather of four. The clinical results of these trials are known to everyone[20–22]. Targan showed statistically significant remission in 48% using a 5 mg/kg dose as compared to 4% with placebo. Dr Rutgeerts showed that administering infliximab every 8 weeks maintained the response, although there were several patients who received only one infusion, and were randomized to placebo, who continued to do well for up to 1 year. Our paper in the *New England Journal of Medicine* showed complete closure of almost 55% of fistulas compared to 13% with placebo. Thus far there have been 150 000 infusions with this agent, but further studies are required to show whether it should be a first-line agent in the treatment of Crohn's disease while, of course, observing closely for any long-term toxicity, especially neoplasia.

It would appear that infliximab has been a breakthrough, because we have now seen a marked increase in the number of studies being performed using immunomodulatory drugs for both Crohn's disease and ulcerative colitis. We have recently seen two uncontrolled trials[23,24] showing efficacy of thalidomide in the treatment of active Crohn's disease with a rapid progression and steroid sparing. Toxicity, however, remains uncertain. We have also seen the recent report of the efficacy of a more humanized antibody against TNF (CDP571)[25]. Efficacy with this agent has been shown in active disease, steroid sparing and fistula healing. Tacrolimus, like cyclosporin, has shown efficacy in uncontrolled studies in the treatment of active Crohn's disease, as well as fistula[26]. This response has been rapid and tacrolimus may be used in combination with 6-MP or azathioprine.

In summing up, I believe that over the years I may have been somewhat evangelical in advocating immunomodulatory agents. However, I was impatient because early on in my career our successful 6-MP study was faced with a negative National Cooperative Crohn's Disease Study and I observed many patients going to colectomy without a prior trial of immunomodulatory agents. Immunomodulatory drugs will significantly improve quality of life in both Crohn's disease and ulcerative colitis patients.

Recently, the use of laparoscopic techniques has altered my approach to limited Crohn's disease, and I do advise surgery earlier in localized disease, especially when scarring has taken place and obstruction has developed. However, when there is extensive disease in Crohn's and/or ulcerative colitis then immunomodulatory therapy, early in the course, is indicated.

I have been fortunate in being exposed to some of the most brilliant gastroenterologists during my career, and I appreciate and acknowledge their help, but most especially Drs Burton Korelitz, David Sachar, and Henry Janowitz. My collaborations with Drs Stephan Targan and Steven Hanauer have stimulated me to continue to be active and productive in the research field.

What have I learned about control trials? Monotherapy studies are out of date and combination therapies will be required for the treatment of IBD in the future. I believe that the design of the control trial should be a reflection of, and have relevance to, clinical practice. I have learned that one large, well-designed control trial is probably better than a meta-analysis of several smaller trials.

What will the future bring? I am not a basic scientist, nor am I an immunologist; however, I believe that our colleagues who are experts in this field will come up with agents to either enhance those cytokines which quiet the immune system, or to lower or eliminate those cytokines which cause excessive immunological activity. However, when they do, and no matter what the theoretical rationale, and no matter whatever they demonstrate in the test tube or laboratory animals, they will have to test the agents in human control trials. My motto, after listening to immunological lectures about mechanism, especially by my close colleague, Dr Lloyd Mayer, is 'let's try it in patients'. I believe that through immunological therapy and genetic alterations we will be able to cure both Crohn's disease and ulcerative colitis in the near future.

Finally, I would like to thank my wife, Jane Present, for her continued support, and thank my children, children-in-law, and grandchildren for the great pleasure they have given me in the past, and for allowing me to take my 'work' seriously but not take 'myself' seriously.

References

1. Bean RHD. The treatment of chronic ulcerative colitis with 6 mercaptopurine. Med J Aust. 1962;2:592–3.
2. Brooke BN, Hoffmann DC *et al*. Azathioprine for Crohn's disease. Lancet. 1969;2:612–14.
3. Summers RW, Switz DM *et al*. National Cooperative Crohn's Disease Study: Results of drug treatment. Gastroenterology. 1979;77:847–69.
4. Present DH, Korelitz BI *et al*. Treatment of Crohn's disease with 6 mercaptopurine: a long term randomized, double-blind study. N Engl J Med. 1980;302:981–7.

5. Greenstein AJ, Lachman P *et al*. Perforating and non-perforating: indications for surgery in Crohn's disease. Evidence for two clinical forms. Gut. 1986;29:588–92.

6. Aberhardt P. Berchtold W *et al*. Surgical recurrence of perforating and non-perforating Crohn's disease. Dis Colon Rectum. 1996;39:80–7.

7. Pearson DC, May GR *et al*. Azathioprine and 6 mercaptopurine in Crohn's disease. A meta-analysis. Ann Intern Med. 1995;122:132–42.

8. George J, Present DH *et al*. The long term outcome of ulcerative colitis treated with 6 mercaptopurine. Am J Gastroenterol. 1996;91:1711–14.

9. Modigliani R. Immunosuppressors for inflammatory bowel disease: how long is long enough? Inflam Bowel Dis. 2000;6:251–7.

10. Present DH, Meltzer SJ *et al*. 6-Mercaptopurine in the management of inflammatory bowel disease: short and long term toxicity. Ann Intern Med. 1989;111:641–9.

11. Fraser AG, Jewell DP. Side effects of azathioprine treatment given for inflammatory bowel disease – a 30 year audit. Gastroenterology. 2000;118:A787.

12. Lichtiger S, Present DH *et al*. Cyclosporine in severe ulcerative colitis refractory to steroid therapy. N Engl J Med. 1994;330:1841–5.

13. Brynskov V, Freund L, Rasmussen SN *et al*. Placebo controlled double blind randomized trial of cyclosporine therapy in active Crohn's disease. N Engl J Med. 1984;321:845–50.

14. Present DH. Cyclosporine: indications in inflammatory bowel disease. In: Yocum DE, editor. Clinical Application in Autoimmune Disease. Philadelphia, PA: Mosby Wolfe, 2000:125–38.

15. Hanauer SB, Smith MB. Rapid closure of Crohn's disease fistula with continuous intravenous cyclosporine. Am J Gastroenterol. 1993;88:646–9.

16. Present DH, Lichtiger S. Efficacy of cyclosporine in treatment of fistula of Crohn's disease. Dig Dis Sci. 1994;39:374–80.

17. Feagan BG, Rochon J *et al*. Methotrexate for the treatment of Crohn's disease. N Engl J Med. 1995;332:292–7.

18. Feagan BG, Fedorak RN *et al*. A comparison of methotrexate with placebo for the maintenance of remission in Crohn's disease. N Engl J Med. 2000;342:1627–32.

19. Korelitz D, Hanauer S *et al*. Postoperative prophylaxis of 6 MP/5 ASA or placebo in Crohn's disease: a two year multicenter trial. Gastroenterology. 1998;114A:1011.

20. Targan SR, Hanauer SB *et al*. A short term study of chimeric monoclonal antibody cA2 to tumor necrosis factor alpha for Crohn's disease. N Engl J Med. 1997;337:1029–35.

21. Rutgeerts P, D'Haens G *et al*. Efficacy and safety of retreatment with anti-tumor necrosis factor antibody to maintain remission in Crohn's disease. Gastroenterology. 1999;117:761–9.

22. Present DH, Rutgeerts P *et al*. Infliximab treatment of fistulas in patients with Crohn's disease. N Engl J Med. 1999;340:1398–1405.

23. Ehrenpreis ED, Kane SV *et al*. Thalidomide therapy for patients with refractory Crohn's disease: an-open-label trial. Gastroenterology. 1999;117:1271–7.

24. Vasiliauskas EA, Kam LY *et al*. An-open-label pilot study of low dose thalidomide in chronically active steroid dependent Crohn's disease. Gastroenterology. 1999;117:1278–87.

25. Sandborn WJ, Targan SR *et al*. A randomized, controlled trial of CDP 571, a humanized antibody to TNF alpha in moderately to severely active Crohn's disease. Gastroenterology. 2000;A655.

26. Sandborn WJ. A preliminary report on the use of oral tacrolimus (FK506) in the treatment of complicated proximal small bowel and fistulizing Crohn's disease. Am J Gastroenterol. 1997;92:876–9.

Section II
Disease states and therapeutic problems in inflammatory bowel diseases

6
Chronic active and steroid-refractory inflammatory bowel disease: definition

C. GASCHÉ

INTRODUCTION

Inflammatory bowel diseases have been separated into two distinct forms, known as ulcerative colitis and Crohn's disease. The natural course of disease is defined by episodes of acute illness ('active disease') and periods with no or only few symptoms ('remissions'). Fortunately, effective glucocorticoid therapy had been found to shorten the time of acute suffering[1,2]. With the failure of steroids in some patients, new subgroups have been defined: chronic active and steroid-refractory disease were separated out and discovered to be an area for alternative (mostly immunosuppressive or experimental) therapies[3]. At the turn of the century we may question whether this separation is still valid.

The term 'chronic active diseases' might be better understood as steroid-dependent diseases. Steroid-dependent and steroid-refractory conditions may occur in both Crohn's disease and ulcerative colitis. In general, steroid dependency means that patients who had primarily responded to steroids cannot taper them off. At each and every attempt to reduce the prednisone dose to below a certain limit, steroid-dependent patients experience a flare in disease activity. On the other hand, steroid-refractory patients do not respond to steroids in the first place. This means that, despite high doses of steroid treatment, disease activity does not decrease. Steroid dependency is found more often in patients with Crohn's disease, and the term 'steroid-refractory disease' has been used mostly in severe ulcerative colitis (Table 1). However, both conditions can occur in both types of inflammatory bowel diseases.

When defining the distinct response profiles to steroids there are always three important variables to consider: (a) what is the adequate steroid dose; (b) what is the appropriate treatment duration; and (c) what is the treatment goal that can be achieved by steroid treatment. In regard to the latter we need to consider different treatment outcome measurements, which most of the time focus on disease

Table 1 Frequency

	Crohn's disease	Ulcerative colitis
Steroid-dependent (chronic active)	$+++$	$+/-$
Steroid-refractory	$+$	$++$

activity. Before defining steroid-dependent or steroid-refractory inflammatory bowel diseases we need to pay attention to these three variables. We should move forward only after giving distinct definitions of the appropriate prednisone dose, treatment duration (steroid tapering scheme) and therapeutic goal. Fortunately, others have already found a consensus on some of these issues.

GUIDELINES

The working party for the recent World Congresses of Gastroenterology had evaluated the response to steroids as a potential phenotypic marker of Crohn's disease subgroups. The following three categories were defined and prospectively evaluated in a series of 500 patients: (a) *steroid resistance*: no satisfactory improvement of clinical symptoms after 4 weeks of steroid treatment with a minimum starting dose of 40 mg prednisolone/day orally; (b) *steroid dependence*: inability to taper steroids to zero after 4 months of treatment (or longer) without recurrence of symptoms or relapse within 1 month after stopping steroid treatment; (c) *steroid responsiveness*: previous clinical response to steroid treatment. The result of this prospective multicentre effort showed that 16% of patients had never been treated with steroids (Figure 1). Due to potential referral bias the size of this group could actually be higher. One should also note that the number of patients who do not respond to corticosteroid therapy exceeds the number of patients who do.

The German Society of Gastroenterology has made attempts to better define chronic active Crohn's disease. In their guidelines for the treatment of Crohn's disease[4], a chronic active disease course was defined as persistence of symptoms over 6 months with a concomitant increase in laboratory measurements. Steroid dependence was considered when 10 mg per day or more of prednisone was used to maintain a stable remission and tapering efforts had failed twice (Table 2). Steroid-refractory Crohn's disease was regarded as continuous disease activity despite high steroid doses over 6 weeks. Similar definitions for ulcerative colitis have not yet been published, but are being studied. Since steroids are not considered to be a first-line therapy, and thus are less frequently used in ulcerative colitis, the definitions of steroid-dependent and steroid-refractory ulcerative colitis might differ slightly from Crohn's disease. This is especially true for steroid-refractory ulcerative colitis. This term has been used mostly for patients with severe colitis who did not respond to maximal treatment with oral steroids (40–60 mg prednisone per day) plus concomitant oral and topical aminosalicylates within 7–10 days. Since sulphasalazine or an alternative aminosalicylate form the backbone of ulcerative colitis therapy, maximal oral and topical use of

Table 2 Possible definitions for Crohn's disease

	Prednisone	*Duration*	*Current activity*	*Therapeutic goal**
Steroid-dependent	>0 mg	4 months	Remission (CDAI < 150)	Taper steroids and keep remission
Steroid-refractory	20–75 mg	6 weeks	Active (CDAI > 200)	Remission (CDAI < 150)

*That cannot be achieved despite steroid treatment.

Table 3 Possible definitions for ulcerative colitis

	Prednisone	*Duration*	*Current activity*	*Therapeutic goal**
Steroid-dependent	>0 mg	4 months	Remission (no visible blood)	Taper steroids and keep remission
Steroid-refractory	40–60 mg	7–10 days	Highly active	Improvement

*That cannot be achieved despite steroids and maximal concomitant treatment with sulphasalazine (or an alternative aminosalicylate) and topical therapy.

these compounds is presumed when considering steroid dependency. The definition of steroid-dependent ulcerative colitis could look much the same as that for Crohn's disease (Table 3). No visible blood is the best indicator of being in remission for patients with ulcerative colitis.

The American College of Gastroenterology has also published practice guidelines on the management of Crohn's disease and ulcerative colitis in adults[5,6]. These guidelines place little emphasis on the terms 'chronic active', 'steroid-dependent' or 'steroid-refractory'. The working definitions rather included the concepts of mild-to-moderate, moderate-to-severe, and severe-to-fulminant disease. Is this a failure or a smart move, not to touch on this sensitive and controversial issue? There are also more open questions such as: Do we now need to adjust definitions after the introduction of topical steroids, i.e. budesonide[7,8]? Or is it better to create new definitions such as budesonide-resistant or budesonide-refractory disease? What about other new drugs such as anti-TNF antibodies (infliximab)? Do we need to define response profiles for these as well? We could play this game indefinitely. In my opinion we should start to reconsider whether we need such definitions at all.

LESSONS LEARNED FROM CLINICAL TRIALS

The question is whether these definitions are relevant for daily practice. Until now these distinct conditions were important in the design, comparison and understanding of clinical trials. Since a broad variety of substances had been tested in clinical trials by different investigators, it is not surprising to find that a variety of definitions had been used in the past. I will give some examples from recently published trials.

In 1994 cyclosporin was officially introduced for the treatment of severe ulcerative colitis refractory to steroids[9]. Patients were eligible to enter the study if they had no response to intravenous corticosteroids (300 mg of hydrocortisone) therapy after 7 or more days. In addition, patients with a relapse of active disease after a recent hospitalization, during which they had responded to intravenous and then oral corticosteroid therapy, were also eligible if they had no response to an additional 60 h of intravenous corticosteroid therapy. In their 1995 paper on the use of oral cyclosporin in chronic active Crohn's disease, Stange and co-workers included patients with either active or inactive disease who had treated with prednisone ≥ 10 mg per day for the last 2 months before study entry[10]. Patients in remission had to have a history of steroid requirement with at least one relapse after reduction of steroid dose during the previous 6 months ('steroid-dependent'). Patients with active disease were characterized by persistent activity despite a prednisone dose ≥ 10 mg per day for the last 2 months before entry ('steroid-refractory'). Despite using the same drug (cyclosporin), the group of patients under investigation was quite different in both trials. Especially the steroid-refractory Crohn's disease subgroup has a completely different clinical profile than did the steroid-refractory patients with severe ulcerative colitis. The Crohn's disease study group for interleukin-10 defined their steroid-refractory patients by having a CDAI between 200 and 350, despite treatment with prednisone in a dose ranging from 10 to 40 mg per day for more than 2 months[11]. These studies clearly demonstrate that definitions used in clinical trials might vary a lot from clinical practice or guidelines.

In the same year Targan and co-workers defined patients to have moderate-to-severe Crohn's disease that was resistant to treatment when the patients met the following criteria: a CDAI between 220 and 400 and any of the following medications: mesalamine for 8 or more weeks, with the dose remaining stable during the 4 weeks before screening; a maximum of 40 mg of corticosteroids per day for 8 or more weeks, with the dose remaining stable during the 2 weeks before screening; and mercaptopurine or azathioprine for 6 or more months, with the dose remaining stable during the 8 weeks before screening[12]. Some clinical investigators criticized this trial for its unusual definitions of active disease (CDAI between 220 and 400), and for lumping aminosalicylate, steroid, mercaptopurine,

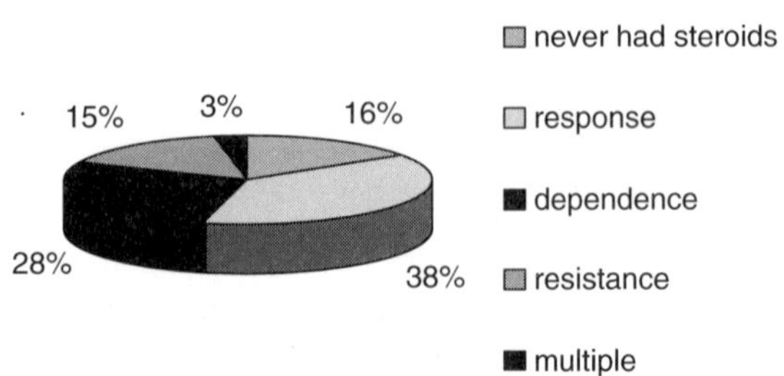

Figure 1 Response to steroids in referral patients with Crohn's disease. Five hundred Crohn's disease patients were prospectively assigned according to their response pattern to steroids. Interestingly, a rather high proportion had never received steroids (16%); 43% of patients were steroid-resistant or -dependent and 38% responded to steroids. For definitions see text

and azathioprine resistance. After being published the trial became the basis for the FDA approval of infliximab in the United States.

The same group of researchers defined chronically active, steroid-dependent Crohn's disease in their thalidomide study in 1999 as CDAI > 250, despite concomitant therapy with prednisone 20 mg or above for at least 1 month and having failed to respond to, or being intolerant to, high-dose mesalamine, mercaptopurine, azathioprine, methotrexate or cyclosporin[13]. This example shows that definitions regarding steroid-dependent or steroid-refractory Crohn's disease are not even consistently used within the same group of investigators. It is a fact that each tested drug might want to target a specific group of patients. Last but not least, Neurath and co-workers found patients eligible for their randomized trial of mycophenolate mofetil vs azathioprine for the treatment of chronic active Crohn's disease, when they had a minimum of three acute flares within the previous 3 years and the CDAI was above 150[14]. This is an example of the different ways in which the term 'chronic active' might be used in the literature. Patients who were enrolled in this trial must have received no steroids at all.

WHAT IS THE TRUE BIOLOGY?

Let us return to the question from above: are these definitions relevant for clinical practice? Since it is obvious from the current literature that strict definitions of what is steroid-dependent or steroid-refractory inflammatory bowel diseases do not exist, there is no reason to invent such definitions for use in clinical practice. The lack of a consensus originates in discordant understanding of what is disease activity (see ongoing disputes about CDAI), what is the appropriate steroid dose, duration and tapering scheme. By bringing up those examples of how these terms were used in different ways, I wanted to make an argument that the definitions of chronic active and steroid-refractory IBD are highly artificial and have very little to do with the biology of the underlying disease. Such definitions help to enroll patients in clinical trials but are generally worthless in clinical practice when dealing with the individual. The time is ripe to start searching for a better understanding of our patients' actual problems.

There might be a physiological mechanism of steroid-dependence/-resistance that still needs to be discovered. Other therapeutic options such as azathioprine or 6-MP have already challenged the central role of glucocorticoids in the treatment of IBD. Instead of defining various subgroups in terms of how they respond to a more or less relevant drug, we might want to start recognizing biological subgroups defined by their disease phenotype. The Vienna classification of Crohn's disease has been credited for stepping into this vacuum[15]. The adjustment of specific therapies by biological markers (for example TNF haplotypes for anti-TNF therapy) might follow.

There are some things which can already be done. For example, when facing the common clinical problem of a steroid-refractory Crohn's disease patient, we might start to look behind the façade. Here is a typical case: a 32-year-old male construction worker with a 10-year history of terminal ileitis, who had undergone resective surgery three times in the past, was referred with intense pain in the right lower quadrant that did not respond to 50 mg of prednisone. The review of the pathological reports from his previous operations revealed that he had been suffering from internal fistulas (a so-called A1/L1/B3 type of Crohn's disease[15]). The physical examination shows subfebrile temperatures and tenderness of the right lower quadrant. Based on this information it is not surprising that this patient did not respond to steroid treatment. Isn't it likely that the same type of disease recurred after surgery[16]? Indeed, transabdominal bowel sonography revealed a complicated fistulous tract arising from the neoterminal ileum. Prednisone treatment was switched to antibiotics and azathioprine was initialized. Within the next couple of weeks the patient improved continuously. There are no data available in the literature that support the use of steroids for treatment of fistulas. In contrast, some studies imply that steroids could even potentially cause the formation of fistulous tracts[17]. If the disease subgroup had been considered in the first place, another steroid-refractory patient could have been avoided.

Besides the B3 subgroup there are also other phenotypic Crohn's disease subgroups, which certainly should not be treated with steroids. The National Cooperative Crohn's Disease Study[1] showed that steroids may be effective with small bowel diseases, and also had some effects in ileocolonic disease; however, steroids appeared to be ineffective in Crohn's colitis. This excludes the L2 subgroup from steroid treatment. The best way, however, to prevent steroid-dependent and steroid-refractory disease is to avoid steroids as treatment of first choice, at least in mild to moderately active cases. Rather than automatically prescribing systemic steroids to our help-seeking patients with inflammatory bowel diseases, physicians should start to adjust their treatment to the actual biological problem, to disease subgroups.

References

1. Summers RW, Switz DM, Sessions JTJ et al. National Cooperative Crohn's Disease Study: results of drug treatment. Gastroenterology. 1979;77:847–69.
2. Malchow H, Ewe K, Brandes JW et al. European Cooperative Crohn's Disease Study (ECCDS): results of drug treatment. Gastroenterology. 1984;86:249–66.
3. Munkholm P, Langholz E, Davidsen M, Binder V. Frequency of glucocorticoid resistance and dependency in Crohn's disease. Gut. 1994;35:360–2.
4. Stange EF, Schreiber S, Raedler A et al. [Therapy of Crohn diseases – results of a Consensus Conference of the German Society of Digestive and Metabolic Diseases]. Z Gastroenterol. 1997;35:541–54.
5. Hanauer SB, Meyers S. Management of Crohn's disease in adults. Am J Gastroenterol. 1997; 92:559–66.
6. Kornbluth A, Sachar DB. Ulcerative colitis practice guidelines in adults. American College of Gastroenterology, Practice Parameters Committee. Am J Gastroenterol. 1997;92:204–11.
7. Rutgeerts P, Lofberg R, Malchow H et al. A comparison of budesonide with prednisolone for active Crohn's disease. N Engl J Med. 1994;331:842–5.
8. Greenberg GR, Feagan BG, Martin F et al. Oral budesonide for active Crohn's disease. Canadian Inflammatory Bowel Disease Study Group. N Engl J Med. 1994;331:836–41.
9. Lichtiger S, Present DH, Kornbluth A et al. Cyclosporine in severe ulcerative colitis refractory to steroid therapy. N Engl J Med. 1994;330:1841–5.
10. Stange EF, Modigliani R, Pena AS, Wood AJ, Feutren G, Smith PR. European trial of cyclosporine in chronic active Crohn's disease: a 12-month study. The European Study Group. Gastroenterology. 1995;109:774–82.
11. Van Deventer SJ, Elson CO, Fedorak RN. Multiple doses of intravenous interleukin 10 in steroid-refractory Crohn's disease. Crohn's Disease Study Group. Gastroenterology. 1997;113:383–9.

12. Targan SR, Hanauer SB, Van Deventer SJ *et al*. A short-term study of chimeric monoclonal anti-body cA2 to tumor necrosis factor alpha for Crohn's disease. Crohn's Disease cA2 Study Group. N Engl J Med. 1997;337:1029–35.

13. Vasiliauskas EA, Kam LY, Abreu-Martin MT *et al*. An open-label pilot study of low-dose thalidomide in chronically active, steroid-dependent Crohn's disease. Gastroenterology. 1999;117:1278–87.

14. Neurath MF, Wanitschke R, Peters M, Krummenauer F, Meyer zum Buschenfelde KH, Schlaak JF. Randomised trial of mycophenolate mofetil versus azathioprine for treatment of chronic active Crohn's disease. Gut. 1999;44:625–8.

15. Gasche C, Scholmerich J, Brynskov J *et al*. A simple classification of Crohn's disease: report of the Working Party for the World Congresses of Gastroenterology, Vienna 1998. Inflamm Bowel Dis. 2000;6:8–15.

16. Greenstein AJ, Lachman P, Sachar DB *et al*. Perforating and non-perforating indications for repeated operations in Crohn's disease: evidence for two clinical forms. Gut. 1988;29:588–92.

17. Yamamoto T, Allan RN, Keighley MR. Risk factors for intra-abdominal sepsis after surgery in Crohn's disease. Dis Colon Rectum. 2000;43:1141–5.

7
Mechanisms of refractory disease

G. ROGLER

INTRODUCTION

Glucocorticoids are used for the suppression or reduction of inflammation in a wide variety of diseases such as rheumatoid diseases, allergic diseases, inflammatory bowel disease and in general autoimmune diseases[1,2]. In many of these cases they are still the standard therapy, due to their high efficacy. However, their use is limited by systemic side-effects. The understanding of the mechanisms by which glucocorticoids suppress or reduce inflammation has increased dramatically during recent years[3–7].

Glucocorticoids have also been proven to be the first choice in the treatment of acute flares of inflammatory bowel disease in several major studies[8–16]. The systemic administration of glucocorticoids (oral or intravenous) during the acute exacerbation of Crohn's disease or ulcerative colitis is followed by a multitude of different effects in different body cells. One of the intended effects is the down-regulation of proinflammatory cytokines[17]. This mechanism is part of the feedback system between inflammation-derived cytokines and CNS-adrenal produced corticosteroids with the physiological relevance of balancing the host defence and anti-inflammatory systems of the body. Among the molecules down-regulated by glucocorticoid receptor (GR) action are multiple cytokines and their receptors, chemokines and their receptors, kinins and their receptors, adhesion molecules and inflammation-associated enzymes such as inducible nitric oxide synthase (iNOS) and the inducible cyclooxygenase (COX-2)[2,18].

Most, if not all, of the effects of glucocorticoids on cells are mediated by binding to cytosolic GR, which are present in all body cells. This member of the steroid receptor superfamily consists of 777 amino acids and was cloned in 1985[19–21]. The GR is a member of a superfamily of steroid receptor with a high degree of genetic similarity with 40–90% of identical amino acid sequences[22–24]. There is only a single GR binding glucocorticoids, with no evidence for subtypes of differing affinity in different tissues[2]. A splice variant of GRα, termed GRβ, has been identified that is not able to bind glucocorticoids as it lacks its ligand-binding domain (LBD). This GRβ, however, still binds to DNA and may therefore potentially interfere with the action of glucocorticoids[25]. It has been speculated that GRβ might be an antagonist of GRα action as it blocks DNA-binding sites without suppressing gene transcription[20,25–28].

An important finding is the occurrence of glucocorticoid responders and non-responders. Non-response to glucocorticoids may be mediated by mutations of the receptor, a reduced number of GRs or down-regulation of the receptor[29]. Recent studies demonstrate that primary (hereditary) abnormalities in the GR gene make 2.3% relatively 'resistant'. 'Resistance' to the beneficial clinical effects of glucocorticoid therapy in patients with inflammatory bowel disease, however, is probably rarely related to hereditary glucocorticoid resistance. In the majority of patients with rheumatoid arthritis or asthma the glucocorticoid resistance seems to be acquired and localized to the sites of inflammation, where it reflects high local cytokine production, which interferes with glucocorticoid action[30]. Glucocorticoid levels (B_{max}) and binding affinities (K_d) vary among patients and have been correlated to patient response. A certain threshold level of GRs is necessary for glucocorticoid responsiveness[31]. In rheumatoid arthritis a decrease of systemic GRs in patients' leucocytes has been found[32]. However, the GR density did not correlate with inflammatory disease activity.

Several studies show that 10–20% of all IBD patients are refractory to the treatment with glucocorticoids at some point of their disease. To elucidate the mechanisms causing this steroid-refractory phenotype would be helpful for several reasons: if factors predicting a lack of treatment response were known, screenings for that factor could be performed before the onset of treatment. This would help to avoid frustrating experiences for both the patient and the physician. Complications due to a delayed onset of an effective treatment could be avoided, as well as side-effects of unsuccessful glucocorticoid treatment. On the other hand, knowledge concerning the mechanisms of refractory disease could provide new possibilities of intervention. If antagonistic molecules are identified a pharmacological down-regulation of these antagonists could improve the steroid response.

However, actions of GRs are complex. Regulation of gene expression and GR actions occur on several levels. It is important first to understand the structure of GR and then the molecular mechanisms of glucocorticoid action. Then we will focus on what is already known about alterations in GR function in glucocorticoid-refractory disease. A later section will speculate on which mechanisms might also be involved in refractory disease and should be investigated in the future.

STRUCTURE OF GR

The molecular structure of GR reveals several functionally distinct domains of the protein (Fig. 1). The N-terminal part of GR contains a transactivation domain (activation function 1, AF1) that plays an important role in gene regulation[33–35]. This structure may be especially important during transactivation activity[36–39]. It is not yet clear how AF1 interacts with other proteins to induce transcription. AF1 has been reported to interact with the basal transcriptional machinery[40,41] but also with other adaptors or co-activators[42–45].

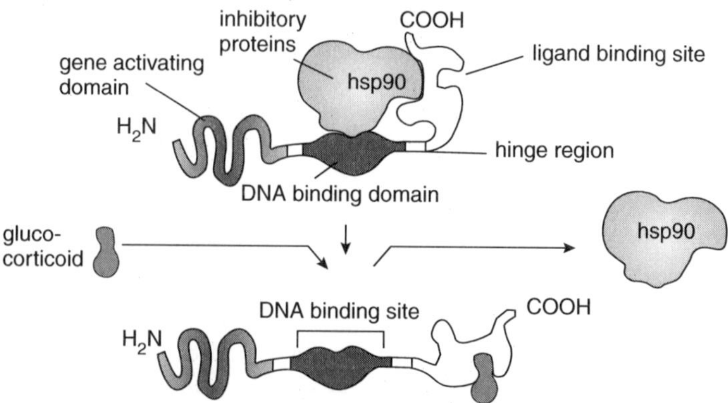

Figure 1 Molecular structure of the glucocorticoid receptor. The N-terminal part of GR contains a transactivation domain that plays an important role in gene regulation. The DNA-binding site (DBD) consists of two zinc-finger domains and contains an invariant pattern of eight cysteins arranged in two groups of four. Between the DBD and the carboxyl-terminal ligand-binding domain (LBD) is a so-called 'hinge region'. This region of the GR protein contains a nuclear localization signal, a binding region for heat-shock protein 90 (hsp90) and a second transactivating domain. The C-terminal LBD not only represents the specific binding sites for glucocorticoids but also serves as a homo-dimerization domain. Additionally it interacts with other proteins regulating GR activity. The inactivated GR is bound to a protein complex of approximately 300 kDa including two molecules of hsp90. The hsp90 proteins cover the nuclear localization site preventing the unliganded GR from localizing to the nuclear compartment. After binding of the specific ligand to the LBD the tertiary structure of the molecule changes, followed by a release of hsp90 from the complex

Like most members of the nuclear receptor superfamily GR contains a DNA-binding site (DBD) consisting of two zinc-finger domains[3]. This area contains an invariant pattern of eight cysteins arranged in two groups of four, so as to coordinate the binding of two zinc atoms[46–48]. This induces the formation of a tertiary structure containing helices that interact with specific DNA sequences organized in GR response elements[49–54]. The DBD is located in the middle of the GR molecule (Fig. 1).

Between the DBD and the carboxyl-terminal ligand binding domain (LBD) is a so-called 'hinge region'. This region of the GR protein contains a nuclear localization signal, a binding region for heat-shock protein 90 (hsp90) and second transactivating domain (activation function 2, AF2)[2].

The C-terminal LBD not only represents the specific binding sites for gluco-corticoids but also serves as a homodimerization domain[3]. Additionally it inter-acts with other proteins regulating GR activity (Fig. 1).

The inactivated GR is bound to a protein complex of approximately 300 kDa. It includes two molecules of hsp90, a 59 kDa immunophilin protein and other inhibitory proteins[2]. The hsp90 proteins cover the nuclear localization site, pre-venting the unliganded GR from localizing the nuclear compartment. After bind-ing of the specific ligand to the LBD the tertiary structure of the molecule changes, followed by a release of hsp90 from the complex (Fig. 1).

The release of hsp90 is followed by an exposure of the nuclear localiza-tion signal, homodimerization and a rapid translocation of the activated

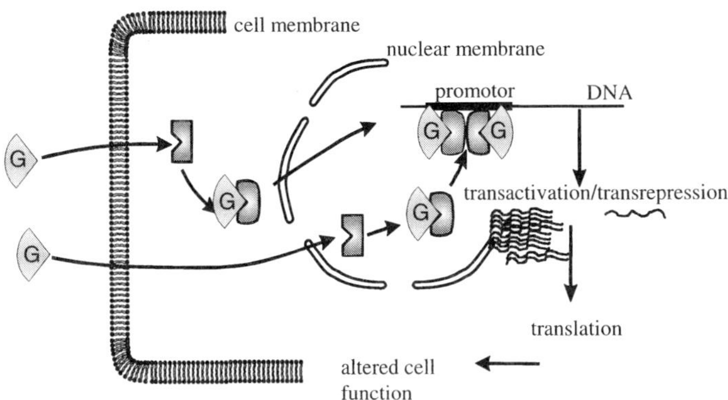

Figure 2 Cellular mechanisms of glucocorticoid receptor action. After binding of glucocorticoids to its receptor hsp90 is released from the complex. This is followed by an exposure of the nuclear localization signal, homodimerization and a rapid translocation of the activated GR/glucocorticoid complex to the nucleus where it can bind its response elements (glucocorticoid response elements, GRE) and mediate transactivation or transrepression of gene transcription

GR/glucocorticoid complex to the nucleus where it can bind its response elements (glucocorticoid response elements, GRE) (Fig. 2).

MECHANISMS OF GR ACTION

Transactivation

Activated and translocated GR can act in two principal ways. It can mediate transactivation of gene transcription or transrepression. Transactivation in general means an induction of transcription of a certain gene. Transrepression is followed by a shutdown or reduction of gene transcripts.

In the nucleus GR can bind to classical GRE to activate transcription of the response gene (Fig. 3A)[55–57]. The GRE has a palindromic motif (consensus sequence: **GGT ACA** NNN **TGT TCT**). GR binds this or similar DNA sequences cooperatively as a homodimer. For homodimerization interaction of a group of five amino acids known as the 'dimerization loop' or 'D-loop' is needed. They are located within the DBD of the GR molecule and are essential for dimerization and transcriptional activation.

A direct transactivation of gene transcription by GR (Fig. 3A) has been described for IL-1 type II receptor that binds IL-1 without induction of signal transduction, thus preventing cells from activation and inflammatory reaction[58–61]. Another important protein whose transcription is transactivated by GR is IκB, the inhibitory protein for the proinflammatory transcription factor NF-κB. GR-mediated transactivation of genes is also involved in the induction of apoptosis in T cells by dexamethasone[62–73].

For other genes a cooperative transactivation involving GR and other transcription factors such as C/EBP has been described (Fig. 3B). In addition to these transactivating actions, which are usually slow and take 12–24 h, GR has more rapid transrepressing activities.

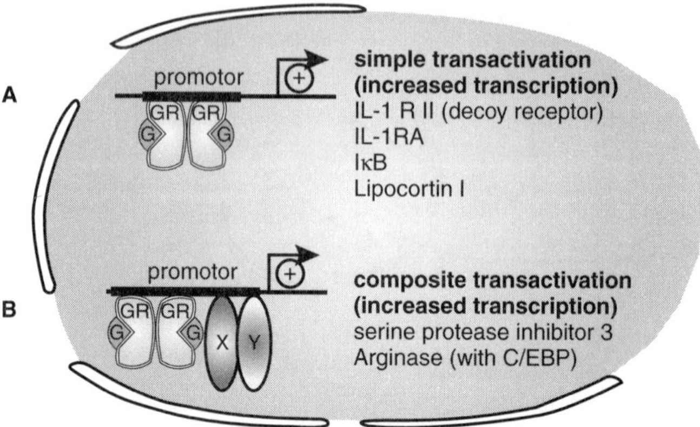

Figure 3 Transactivation of gene transcription by glucocorticoid receptor. A: GR binds as a homodimer to classical GRE to activate transcription of response genes. The GRE has a palindromic motif (consensus sequences: **GGT ACA** NNN **TGT TCT**). A direct transactivation of gene transcription by GR has been described for IL-1 type II, IκB, IL-1RA or lipocortin I. B: For other genes such as serine protease inhibitor 3 or arginase a cooperative transactivation involving GR and other transcription factors such as C/EBP has been described

Transrepression via DNA binding

After characterization of positive transcriptional regulating GRE sequence the existence of negative GRE sites (nGRE) mediating a negative regulation of transcription (transrepression) via glucocorticoids was postulated[57]. However, the concept of a nGRE site is still a matter of discussion, as the consensus-binding site is variable and only described for a few genes[6]. A binding to a promoter sequence and subsequent transrepression by GR has been shown for the pro-opiomelanocortin (POMC) gene, an ACTH precursor allowing a negative feedback circle (Fig. 4C)[74,75]. On the other hand, this may be due not only to a direct effect of GR on transcription of the respective gene, but also to a blockade of the binding of other positive-regulating, transactivating transcription factors[76]. Another promoter containing a nGRE binding site (at -278 to -249 of the promoter) is the corticotropin-releasing hormone (CRH) promoter[77,78].

GR and transactivating transcription factors can compete for binding sites in promoters. The presence of GR can block transactivation of other transcription factors and does not need to actively transrepress transcription itself. In the osteocalcin promoter GR overlaps the TATA box. Activation and nuclear translocation of GR can therefore prevent the binding of the basal transcription factor, TATA-binding protein (TBP), which is necessary for the recruitment of RNA polymerase II and initiation of transcription[79] (competitive transrepression, Fig. 4D).

Transrepression without DNA binding

Besides the competition for binding sites in promoters a transrepression mechanism for GR has been described that *does not involve DNA binding* (Fig. 4E). The promoters of most proinflammatory genes contain binding sites for the

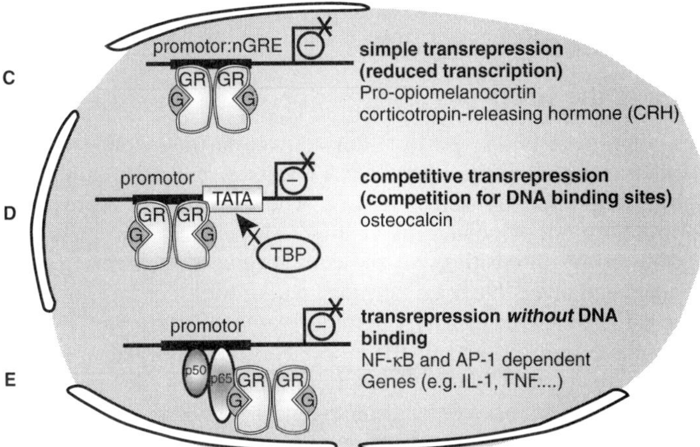

Figure 4 Transrepression of gene transcription by glucocorticoid receptor. C: A binding to a negative glucocorticoid response element (nGRE) and subsequent transrepression by GR has been shown for the pro-opiomelanocortin (POMC) gene, an ACTH precursor and CRH both allowing a negative feedback circle. D: GR and transactivating transcription factors can compete for binding sites in promoters. In the osteocalcin promoter GR overlaps the TATA box. Activation and nuclear translocation of GR can therefore prevent the binding of the basal transcription factor, TATA-binding protein (TBP), which is necessary for the recruitment of RNA polymerase II and initiation of transcription. E: For the p65 subunit of NF-κB and GR a direct physical interaction has been demonstrated, leading to a transrepression of transcription of the NF-κB-dependent gene without DNA binding of GR. This interaction effect does not impair the DNA-binding ability of NF-κB

proinflammatory transcription factors nuclear factor kappa B (NF-κB) or AP-1. In the genes regulated by both factors nGRE are not found. However, glucocorticoids are able to rapidly transrepress AP-1 or NF-κB-induced transcription of these genes. It is not completely clear whether direct protein–protein interactions between GR and AP-1 or NF-κB are sufficient for transrepression[80–82], or whether other mechanisms are involved. However, GR association to AP-1 does not reduce AP-1 DNA binding, as demonstrated by electrophoretic mobility shift assays (EMSA)[81,83]. Similar observations were made for the interaction of NF-κB and GR. For the p65 subunit of NF-κB and GR a direct physical interaction has been demonstrated[7,84–89]. This interaction occurs without impairing the DNA-binding ability of NF-κB[85–87,90–92]. This may indicate that co-activating or co-repressing proteins play a major role for that function.

One of the factors for which proinflammatory transcription factors such as AP-1 and NF-κB and GR could compete is a co-activator molecule called CREB-binding protein (CBP). CBP plays an essential role in the activation of transcription by numerous transcription factors/transcriptional activators[5,88,93–99]. CBP binds and is necessary for coactivation of CREB, AP-1, STATs and NF-κB, as well as nuclear receptors such as GR, progesterone receptor and retinoid receptors[5,99]. It is likely that CBP and the related p300 is not acting as a single co-activator protein, but is present in the nucleus in a complex of proteins[5,99]. CPB and p300 acetylate free histones *in vitro*, which is necessary for successful transcription[5,99]. Other co-activators are p160/SRC, the TRAP/DRIP/ARC complex and the P/CAF complex (for a review see ref. 5).

Regulation of the GR gene

To further complicate this system of transactivation, transrepression *with* DNA binding and transrepression *without* DNA binding, the expression of the GR gene itself is regulated by activated GR. The GR (GRα) represses its own synthesis in a hormone-dependent manner[100]. The reduction in cellular receptor levels is followed by insensitivity of the cells to glucocorticoids. It is dose- and time-dependent and reversible upon hormone withdrawal. For this down-regulation of GR expression by GR itself DNA binding seems to be crucial[101–105].

However, this is not the end of the story. The phosphorylation status of GR may be important for this feedback function. Deletion of phosphorylation sites from the GR protein by site-directed mutagenesis resulted in a GR that cannot repress its own transcription upon binding of glucocorticoids[106,107].

GRβ

In contrast to GRα the shorter GRβ isoform that is generated by alternative splicing lacks a LBD. GRβ is identical to GRα through the first 727 amino acids but differs in the carboxyl-terminus, where it lacks the last 50 amino acids found in GRα but contains an additional 15 non-homologous amino acids[7]. As with GRα, GRβ is widely expressed in adult human tissues, but is primarily localized to the cell nucleus independent of the presence of ligand[7]. GRβ still binds to DNA and may therefore potentially interfere with the action of GRα[25,108,109]. It has been speculated that GRβ might be an antagonist of GRα action as it blocks DNA-binding sites without suppressing gene transcription[20,25–28,108–110]. However, this inhibition seems to require increased GRβ expression relative to GRα. This has been studied mainly in transfection assays with overexpression of the β-isoform. A clear functional role has not yet been confirmed[6].

REGULATION OF GR IN INFLAMMATORY BOWEL DISEASE

The regulation of GR action and the mechanisms involved in its function are complex. Investigations on possible mechanisms of steroid-refractory inflammatory bowel disease are still at the very beginning. The few studies that have focused on the problem in recent years have raised more questions than they answered.

As hsp90 has some features of an inhibitory protein of GR, and is bound to its inactive form, Stange and co-workers studied the expression of human hsp90 in patients with Crohn's disease and ulcerative colitis[111]. They found no differences between patients and controls, making a role of hsp90 in refractory disease unlikely.

Shimada and co-workers determined the number and dissociation constant (K_d) of GR in peripheral blood mononuclear cells of six non-responders of glucocorticoid treatment with ulcerative colitis, five responders and 10 healthy controls[112]. They found a significant increase in the number of binding sites and the dissociation constant in non-responders compared to responders. Surprisingly, the number of binding sites was highest in non-responders. The numbers were comparable in responders and healthy controls. It is important to note that blood samples were drawn before initiation of glucocorticoid therapy to avoid feedback regulation of GR numbers[112].

In our own study GR levels were determined via dexamethasone binding only in the cytosolic fraction, to ensure that only free receptor and not already steroid-associated, translocated receptor molecules could bind [^{3}H]-dexamethasone[113]. The dexamethasone binding in cytosol isolated from peripheral blood mononuclear cells (PBMNCs) of corticosteroid-treated IBD patients was significantly lower compared to controls (59.6 ± 57.1 dpm/mg cytosol protein versus 227.0 ± 90.8 dpm/mg cytosol protein, $p = 0.007$) and not glucocorticoid-treated IBD patients (179.7 ± 171.3 dpm/mg cytosol protein $p = 0.002$). 'Peripheral' GR levels in untreated IBD patients did not differ significantly from those of controls[113]. There was no difference in the binding affinity of patients and controls, with an obvious lower binding maximum indicating a reduced receptor number in the steroid-treated patient group.

In contrast to the findings in PBMNCs mucosal GR levels of IBD patients were significantly decreased in both steroid-treated (18.0 ± 15.5 dpm/mg cytosol protein) and untreated (37.8 ± 30.5 dpm/mg cytosol protein) patients compared to controls (125.6 ± 97.1 dpm/mg cytosol protein; $p = 0.00009$ and $p = 0.0008$, respectively)[113].

The reduced binding of [^{3}H] dexamethasone in cytosol from steroid-treated IBD patients is most likely due to a feedback regulation of GR in the cells by the ligand. This assumption is supported by a number of studies[114–116]. Our data indicated that, in contrast to patients with rheumatoid arthritis or other connective tissue diseases in IBD, there is no difference in systemic GR levels between patients not treated with glucocorticoids and control persons. This means that localized inflammation in the intestinal mucosa is not followed by a generalized depression of glucocorticoid receptor levels in leucocytes. Mucosal GR levels in inflamed areas of the mucosa were decreased independent from therapy in both steroid-treated and untreated patients.

Honda and co-workers recently studied the expression of GRα and GRβ in PBMNCs of patients with ulcerative colitis and controls[117]. They found expression of GRβ in only 9.1% of patients with steroid-sensitive disease, whereas it was present in 83.3% of steroid-resistant patients. The authors conclude that polymerase chain reaction of GRβ could provide a tool to predict steroid responsiveness of UC patients[117].

FUTURE PERSPECTIVE: POSSIBLE ROLE OF COACTIVATORS AND COREPRESSORS

For an efficient transcriptional regulation nuclear receptors such as GR require nuclear receptor coregulators, which can be coactivators or corepressors[5,118,119]. Coactivators are molecules that interact with nuclear receptors such as GR, enhancing their transactivation. Nuclear receptor corepressors are factors that interact with nuclear receptors and lower the transcription rate of target genes. As in refractory disease transactivating functions of GR, responsible for many side-effects, are still present but transrepression seems to be impaired, the study of corepressors may become important for the future. Important corepressor proteins are, for example, the nuclear receptor corepressor NCoR[5,118,119] or the silencing mediator for retinoid and thyroid hormone receptor SMRT[5,118,119]. Transcriptional regulation by nuclear receptors such as GR is a multistep process in which a number of diverse factors have important temporally and spatially distinct functions. Mutations of NCoR and SMRT have already been shown to be involved in diseases; for example hormone-resistant breast cancer. A defect in the interaction of corepressors and GR could explain on the one hand the generalized susceptibility to inflammation and on the other a steroid-refractory state during treatment. In recent years the molecular determinants of nuclear receptor–corepressor interaction have been investigated[120].

On the other hand, as mentioned earlier, proinflammatory transcription factors such as AP-1 or NF-κB and GR compete for coactivator molecules such as CBP[5,95]. As mentioned, CBP binding during transcriptional activation is shared by numerous transcription factors/transcriptional activators such as AP-1, STATs and NF-κB and GR[5,88,93–99]. A strong association of CBP with proinflammatory transcription factors could limit the resources for GR to bind CBP and transactivated genes such as IL-1RII and IκB. Sheppard and co-workers concluded from their studies that the GR-mediated repression of p65-dependent gene expression results from the competition for CBP and the related factor SRC-1[95].

It is intriguing for future research on the mechanisms of steroid refractory IBD to focus on these coactivator and corepressor pathways.

SUMMARY

Despite these few studies, most of the questions regarding the mechanisms of steroid-refractory disease are still unanswered[121]. It is not clear why some patients express GRβ and others do not. It is not clear whether changes in glucocorticoid binding are merely an epiphenomenon or a cause of different disease courses. It is not clear whether GRβ expression or decreased GRα levels are really crucial for the treatment success.

Future studies on GR expression in inflammatory bowel disease need to answer several important questions. Are GR levels at the onset of the disease predictive for the success of glucocorticoid therapy? Are low levels correlated with the development of a steroid-refractory disease? If patients show a rapid down-regulation of GR levels during therapy, is this followed by early relapses? Are GR levels up-regulated during remission and are GR levels in remission predictive for the course of the disease?

The question of whether measurement of GRs in the mucosa can be predictive for success of therapy needs answering for the future management of patients with IBD. If it is, patients with low GR levels could be treated primarily with other drugs such as azathioprine.

Prospective studies investigating GRα and GRβ transcripts, as well as glucocorticoid binding in PBMNCs and in the mucosa at the onset of disease before any treatment, will need to be performed to clarify whether both mechanisms are related to steroid-refractory IBD. A study designed to clarify these questions has been started in the German Kompetenznetz-CED project.

However, the regulation of transrepression by GR is very complex. Further studies on those basic mechanisms will provide us with the knowledge we have to transmit into clinic. Our goal should be not only to ensure the predictability of treatment failures, but to understand the mechanisms of refractory disease in order to develop tools to influence or abolish that state of refractivity.

References

1. Barnes PJ, Adcock I. Anti-inflammatory actions of steroids: molecular mechanisms. Trends Pharmacol Sci. 1993;14:436–41.
2. Barnes PJ. Anti-inflammatory actions of glucocorticoids: molecular mechanisms. Clin Sci (Colch). 1998;94:557–72.
3. Kumar R, Thompson EB. The structure of the nuclear hormone receptor. Steroids. 1999;64:310–19.
4. Webster JC, Cidlowski JA. Mechanisms of glucocorticoid-receptor-mediated repression of gene expression. Trends Endocrinol Metab. 1999;10:396–402.
5. Glass CK, Rosenfeld MG. The coregulator exchange in transcriptional functions of nuclear receptors. Genes Dev. 2000;114:121–41.
6. Newton R. Molecular mechanisms of glucocorticoid action: what is important? Thorax. 2000;55:603–13.
7. McKay LI, Cidlowski JA. Molecular control of immune/inflammatory responses: interactions between nuclear factor-kappa B and steroid receptor-signaling pathways. Endocrinol Rev. 1999;20:435–59.
8. Truelove S, Witts L. Cortisone in ulcerative colitis: preliminary report on a therapeutic trial. Br Med J. 1954;2:375–8.
9. Truelove S, Witts L. Cortisone and corticotrophin in ulcerative colitis. Br Med J. 1959;10:387–94.
10. Jones J, Lennard-Jones J. Corticosteroids and corticotrophin in the treatment of Crohn's disease. Gut. 1966;7:181–7.
11. Roberts G, Naish J. Corticosteroids in Crohn's disease. Gut. 1968;9:736.
12. Lennard-Jones J. Toward optimal use of corticosteroids in ulcerative colitis and Crohn's disease. Gut. 1983;24:177–81.
13. Jewell D. Corticosteroids for the management of ulcerative colitis and Crohn's disease. Gastroenterol Clin N Am. 1989;18:21–34.
14. Routes J, Claman H. Corticosteroids in inflammatory bowel disease. A review. J Clin Gastroenterol. 1987;9:529–35.
15. Hanauer S, Baert F. Medical therapy of inflammatory bowel disease. Med Clin N Am. 1994;78:1413–26.
16. Malchow H, Ewe K, Brandes J *et al.* European Cooperative Crohn's Disease Study (ECCDS): results of drug treatment. Gastroenterology. 1984;86:249–66.
17. Brattsand R, Linden M. Cytokine modulation by glucocorticoids: mechanisms and actions in cellular studies. Aliment Pharmacol Ther. 1996;10(Suppl. 2):81–92.
18. Barnes PJ. Novel approaches and targets for treatment of chronic obstructive pulmonary disease. Am J Respir Crit Care Med. 1999;160:S72–9.
19. Weinberger C, Hollenberg SM, Rosenfeld MG, Evans RM. Domain structure of human glucocorticoid receptor and its relationship to the v-erb-A oncogene product. Nature. 1985;318:670–2.
20. Hollenberg SM, Weinberger C, Ong ES *et al.* Primary structure and expression of a functional human glucocorticoid receptor cDNA. Nature. 1985;318:635–41.
21. Weinberger C, Hollenberg SM, Ong ES *et al.* Identification of human glucocorticoid receptor complementary DNA clones by epitope selection. Science. 1985;228:740–2.
22. Evans R. The steroid and thyroid hormone receptor superfamily. Science. 1988;240:889–95.
23. Arriza JL, Weinberger C, Cerelli G *et al.* Cloning of human mineralocorticoid receptor complementary DNA: structural and functional kinship with the glucocorticoid receptor. Science. 1987;237:268–75.
24. Evans R. Molecular characterization of the glucocorticoid receptor. Recent Prog Horm Res. 1989;45:1–22.
25. Bamberger CM, Bamberger AM, de Castro M, Chrousos GP. Glucocorticoid receptor beta, a potential endogenous inhibitor of glucocorticoid action in humans. J Clin Invest. 1995;95:2435–41.

26. Oakley RH, Webster JC, Sar M, Parker CR, Jr, Cidlowski JA. Expression and subcellular distribution of the beta-isoform of the human glucocorticoid receptor. Endocrinology. 1997;138: 5028–38.

27. Oakley RH, Sar M, Cidlowski JA. The human glucocorticoid receptor beta isoform. Expression, biochemical properties, and putative function. J Biol Chem. 1996;271:9550–9.

28. Oakley RH, Jewell CM, Yudt MR, Bofetiado DM, Cidlowski JA. The dominant negative activity of the human glucocorticoid receptor beta isoform. Specificity and mechanisms of action. J Biol Chem. 1999;274:27857–66.

29. Lamberts S, Koper J, Biemond P, den-Holder F, de Jong F. Cortisol receptor resistance: the variability of its clinical presentation and response to treatment. J Clin Endocrinol Metab. 1992;74: 313–21.

30. Lamberts SW, Huizenga AT, de Lange P, de Jong FH, Koper JW. Clinical aspects of glucocorticoid sensitivity. Steroids. 1996;61:157–60.

31. Okret S, Dong Y, Tanaka H, Cairns B, Gustafsson J. The mechanism for glucocorticoid-resistance in a rat hepatoma cell variant that contains functional glucocorticoid receptor. J Steroid Biochem Mol Biol. 1991;40:353–61.

32. Schlaghecke R, Beuscher D, Kornely E, Specker C. Effects of glucocorticoids in rheumatoid arthritis. Diminished glucocorticoid receptors do not result in glucocorticoid resistance. Arthritis Rheum. 1994;37:1127–31.

33. Giguere V, Hollenberg SM, Rosenfeld MG, Evans RM. Functional domains of the human glucocorticoid receptor. Cell. 1986;46:645–52.

34. Hollenberg SM, Giguere V, Evans RM. Identification of two regions of the human glucocorticoid receptor hormone binding domain that block activation. Cancer Res. 1989;49:2292–4s.

35. Hollenberg SM, Giguere V, Segui P, Evans RM. Colocalization of DNA-binding and transcriptional activation functions in the human glucocorticoid receptor. Cell. 1987;49:39–46.

36. Dahlman-Wright K, Baumann H, McEwan IJ et al. Structural characterization of a minimal functional transactivation domain from the human glucocorticoid receptor. Proc Natl Acad Sci USA. 1995;92:1699–703.

37. Dahlman-Wright K, McEwan IJ. Structural studies of mutant glucocorticoid receptor transactivation domains establish a link between transactivation activity in vivo and alpha-helix-forming potential in vitro. Biochemistry. 1996;35:1323–7.

38. McEwan IJ, Wright AP, Dahlman-Wright K, Carlstedt-Duke J, Gustafsson JA. Direct interaction of the tau 1 transactivation domain of the human glucocorticoid receptor with the basal transcriptional machinery. Mol Cell Biol. 1993;13:399–407.

39. McEwan IJ, Dahlman-Wright K, Almlof T, Ford J, Wright AP, Gustafsson JA. Mechanisms of transcription activation by nuclear receptors: studies on the human glucocorticoid receptor tau 1 transactivation domain. Mutat Res. 1995;333:15–22.

40. Henriksson A, Almlof T, Ford J, McEwan IJ, Gustafsson JA, Wright AP. Role of the Ada adaptor complex in gene activation by the glucocorticoid receptor. Mol Cell Biol. 1997;17:3065–73.

41. Ford J, McEwan IJ, Wright AP, Gustafsson JA. Involvement of the transcription factor IID protein complex in gene activation by the N-terminal transactivation domain of the glucocorticoid receptor in vitro. Mol Endocrinol. 1997;11:1467–75.

42. Guarente L. Transcriptional coactivators in yeast and beyond. Trends Biochem Sci. 1995;20:517–21.

43. Zeiner M, Gehring U. A protein that interacts with members of the nuclear hormone receptor family: identification and cDNA cloning. Proc Natl Acad Sci USA. 1995;92:11465–9.

44. Onate SA, Tsai SY, Tsai MJ, O'Malley BW. Sequence and characterization of a coactivator for the steroid hormone receptor superfamily. Science. 1995;270:1354–7.

45. Chakravarti D, LaMorte VJ, Nelson MC et al. Role of CBP/P300 in nuclear receptor signalling. Nature. 1996;383:99–103.

46. Muller M, Renkawitz R. The glucocorticoid receptor. Biochim Biophys Acta. 1991;1088: 171–82.

47. Muller M, Baniahmad C, Kaltschmidt C, Renkawitz R. Multiple domains of the glucocorticoid receptor involved in synergism with the CACCC box factor(s). Mol Endocrinol. 1991;5: 1498–503.

48. Baniahmad C, Muller M, Altschmied J, Renkawitz R. Co-operative binding of the glucocorticoid receptor DNA binding domain is one of at least two mechanisms for synergism. J Mol Biol. 1991;222:155–65.

49. Baumann H, Paulsen K, Kovacs H *et al.* Refined solution structure of the glucocorticoid receptor DNA-binding domain. Biochemistry. 1993;32:13463–71.
50. Luisi BF, Xu WX, Otwinowski Z, Freedman LP, Yamamoto KR, Sigler PB. Crystallographic analysis of the interaction of the glucocorticoid receptor with DNA. Nature. 1991;352:497–505.
51. Pan T, Freedman LP, Coleman JE. Cadmium-113 NMR studies of the DNA binding domain of the mammalian glucocorticoid receptor. Biochemistry. 1990;29:9218–25.
52. Freedman LP, Luisi BF, Korszun ZR, Basavappa R, Sigler PB, Yamamoto KR. The function and structure of the metal coordination sites within the glucocorticoid receptor DNA binding domain. Nature. 1988;334:543–6.
53. Freedman LP, Yamamoto KR, Luisi BF, Sigler PB. More fingers in hand. Cell. 1988;54:444.
54. Luisi BF, Schwabe JW, Freedman LP. The steroid/nuclear receptors: from three-dimensional structure to complex function. Vitam Horm. 1994;49:1–47.
55. Jantzen HM, Strahle U, Gloss B *et al.* Cooperativity of glucocorticoid response elements located far upstream of the tyrosine aminotransferase gene. Cell. 1987;49:29–38.
56. Beato M, Truss M, Chavez S. Control of transcription by steroid hormones. Ann NY Acad Sci. 1996;784:93–123.
57. Beato M. Gene regulation by steroid hormones. Cell. 1989;56:335–44.
58. Abbinante N, Simpson L, Leikauf G. Corticosteroids increase secretory leukocyte protease inhibitor transcript levels in airway epithelial cells. Am J Physiol. 1995;268:L601–6.
59. Colotta F, Dower SK, Sims JE, Mantovani A. The type II 'decoy' receptor: a novel regulatory pathway for interleukin 1. Immunol Today. 1994;15:562–6.
60. Colotta F, Mantovani A. Induction of the interleukin-1 decoy receptor by glucocorticoids. Trends Pharmacol Sci. 1994;15:138–9.
61. Colotta F, Re F, Muzio M *et al.* Interleukin-1 type II receptor: a decoy target for IL-1 that is regulated by IL-4. Science. 1993;261:472–5.
62. Purton JF, Boyd RL, Cole TJ, Godfrey DI. Intrathymic T cell development and selection proceeds normally in the absence of glucocorticoid receptor signaling. Immunity. 2000;13:179–86.
63. Kofler R. The molecular basis of glucocorticoid-induced apoptosis of lymphoblastic leukemia cells. Histochem Cell Biol. 2000;114:1–7.
64. Hulkko SM, Wakui H, Zilliacus J. The pro-apoptotic protein death-associated protein 3 (DAP3) interacts with the glucocorticoid receptor and affects the receptor function. Biochem J. 2000;349:885–93.
65. Jamieson CA, Yamamoto KR. Crosstalk pathway for inhibition of glucocorticoid-induced apoptosis by T cell receptor signaling. Proc Natl Acad Sci USA. 2000;97:7319–24.
66. Yang Y, Ashwell JD. Thymocyte apoptosis. J Clin Immunol. 1999;19:337–49.
67. Tolosa E, King LB, Ashwell JD. Thymocyte glucocorticoid resistance alters positive selection and inhibits autoimmunity and lymphoproliferative disease in MRL-lpr/lpr mice. Immunity. 1998;8:67–76.
68. Cidlowski JA, King KL, Evans-Storms RB, Montague JW, Bortner CD, Hughes FM, Jr. The biochemistry and molecular biology of glucocorticoid-induced apoptosis in the immune system. Recent Prog Horm Res. 1996;51:457–90.
69. Nieto MA, Gonzalez A, Gambon F, Diaz-Espada F, Lopez-Rivas A. Apoptosis in human thymocytes after treatment with glucocorticoids. Clin Exp Immunol. 1992;88:341–4.
70. Wyllie AH, Morris RG. Hormone-induced cell death. Purification and properties of thymocytes undergoing apoptosis after glucocorticoid treatment. Am J Pathol. 1982;109:78–87.
71. Wyllie AH, Morris RG, Smith AL, Dunlop D. Chromatin cleavage in apoptosis: association with condensed chromatin morphology and dependence on macromolecular synthesis. J Pathol. 1984;142:67–77.
72. Ramdas J, Liu W, Harmon JM. Glucocorticoid-induced cell death requires autoinduction of glucocorticoid receptor expression in human leukemic T cells. Cancer Res. 1999;59:1378–85.
73. Ramdas J, Harmon JM. Glucocorticoid-induced apoptosis and regulation of NF-kappaB activity in human leukemic T cells. Endocrinology. 1998;139:3813–21.
74. Drouin J, Sun YL, Chamberland M *et al.* Novel glucocorticoid receptor complex with DNA element of the hormone-repressed POMC gene. EMBO J. 1993;12:145–56.
75. Charron J, Drouin J. Glucocorticoid inhibition of transcription from episomal proopiomelanocortin gene promotor. Proc Natl Acad Sci USA. 1986;83:8903–7.
76. Murphy EP, Conneely OM. Neuroendocrine regulation of the hypothalamic pituitary adrenal axis by the nurr1/nur77 subfamily of nuclear receptors. Mol Endocrinol. 1997;11:39–47.

77. Malkoski SP, Handanos CM, Dorin RI. Localization of a negative glucocorticoid response element of the human corticotropin releasing hormone gene. Mol Cell Endocrinol. 1997;127:189–99.
78. Malkoski SP, Dorin RI. Composite glucocorticoid regulation at a functionally defined negative glucocorticoid response element of the human corticotropin-releasing hormone gene. Mol Endocrinol. 1999;13:1629–44.
79. Newton R, Barnes P, Adcock I. Transcription factors. In: Barnes PJ, Rodger IW, Thomson NC, editors. Asthma: Basic Mechanisms and Clinical Management. London: Academic Press, 1998:459–74.
80. Schule R, Rangarajan P, Kliewer S et al. Functional antagonism between oncoprotein c-Jun and the glucocorticoid receptor. Cell. 1990;62:1217–26.
81. Jonat C, Rahmsdorf HJ, Park KK et al. Antitumor promotion and antiinflammation: down-modulation of AP-1 (Fos/Jun) activity by glucocorticoid hormone. Cell. 1990;62:1189–204.
82. Yang-Yen HF, Chambard JC, Sun YL et al. Transcriptional interference between c-Jun and the glucocorticoid receptor: mutual inhibition of DNA binding due to direct protein–protein interaction. Cell. 1990;62:1205–15.
83. Konig H, Ponta H, Rahmsdorf HJ, Herrlich P. Interference between pathway-specific transcription factors: glucocorticoids antagonize phorbol ester-induced AP-1 activity without altering AP-1 site occupation in vivo. EMBO J. 1992;11:2241–6.
84. Caldenhoven E, Liden J, Wissink S et al. Negative cross-talk between Re1A and the glucocorticoid receptor: a possible mechanism for the antiinflammatory action of glucocorticoids. Mol Endocrinol. 1995;9:401–12.
85. Ray A, Prefontaine KE. Physical association and functional antagonism between the p65 subunit of transcription factor NF-kappa B and the glucocorticoid receptor. Proc Natl Acad Sci USA. 1994;91:752–6.
86. Ray A, Siegel MD, Prefontaine KE, Ray P. Anti-inflammation: direct physical association and functional antagonism between transcription factor NF-KB and the glucocorticoid receptor. Chest. 1995;107:139S.
87. Scheinman RI, Gualberto A, Jewell CM, Cidlowski JA, Baldwin AS, Jr. Characterization of mechanisms involved in transrepression of NF-kappa B by activated glucocorticoid receptors. Mol Cell Biol. 1995;15:943–53.
88. McKay LI, Cidlowski JA. CBP (CREB binding protein) integrates NF-kappaB (nuclear factor-kappaB) and glucocorticoid receptor physical interactions and antagonism. Mol Endocrinol. 2000;14:1222–34.
89. McKay LI, Cidlowski JA. Cross-talk between nuclear factor-kappa B and the steroid hormone receptors: mechanisms of mutual antagonism. Mol Endocrinol. 1998;12:45–56.
90. Brostjan C, Anrather J, Csizmadia V et al. Glucocorticoid-mediated repression of NFkappaB activity in endothelial cells does not involve induction of IkappaBalpha synthesis. J Biol Chem. 1996;271:19612–16.
91. Wissink S, van Heerde EC, Schmitz ML et al. Distinct domains of the Re1A NF-kappaB subunit are required for negative cross-talk and direct interaction with the glucocorticoid receptor. J Biol Chem. 1997;272:22278–84.
92. Wissink S, van Heerde EC, van der Burg B, van der Saag PT. A dual mechanism mediates repression of NF-kappaB activity by glucocorticoids. Mol Endocrinol. 1998;12:355–63.
93. Kamei Y, Xu L, Heinzel T et al. A CBP integrator complex mediates transcriptional activation and AP-1 inhibition by nuclear receptors. Cell. 1996;85:403–14.
94. Sheppard KA, Rose DW, Haque ZK et al. Transcriptional activation by NF-kappaB requires multiple coactivators. Mol Cell Biol. 1999;19:6367–78.
95. Sheppard KA, Phelps KM, Williams AJ et al. Nuclear integration of glucocorticoid receptor and nuclear factor-kappaB signaling by CREB-binding protein and steroid receptor coactivator-1. J Biol Chem. 1998;273:29291–4.
96. Kurokawa R, Kalafus D, Ogliastro MH et al. Differential use of CREB binding protein–coactivator complexes. Science. 1998;279:700–3.
97. Torchia J, Rose DW, Inostroza J et al. The transcriptional co-activator p/CIP binds CBP and mediates nuclear-receptor function. Nature. 1997;387:677–84.
98. Horvai AE, Xu L, Korzus E et al. Nuclear integration of JAK/STAT and Ras/AP-1 signaling by CBP and p300. Proc Natl Acad Sci USA. 1997;94:1074–9.
99. Glass CK, Rose DW, Rosenfeld MG. Nuclear receptor coactivators. Curr Opin Cell Biol. 1997;9:222–32.

100. Oakley RH, Cidlowski JA. Homologous down regulation of the glucocorticoid receptor: the molecular machinery. Crit Rev Eukaryot Gene Expr. 1993;3:63–88.
101. Burnstein KL, Cidlowski JA. Regulation of gene expression by glucocorticoids. Annu Rev Physiol. 1989;51:683–99.
102. Burnstein KL, Jewell CM, Cidlowski JA. Human glucocorticoid receptor cDNA contains sequences sufficient for receptor down-regulation. J Biol Chem. 1990;265:7284–91.
103. Burnstein KL, Bellingham DL, Jewell CM, Powell-Oliver FE, Cidlowski JA. Autoregulation of glucocorticoid receptor gene expression. Steroids. 1991;56:52–8.
104. Burnstein KL, Cidlowski JA. The down side of glucocorticoid receptor regulation. Mol Cell Endocrinol. 1992;83:C1–8.
105. Burnstein KL, Cidlowski JA. Multiple mechanisms for regulation of steroid hormone action. J Cell Biochem. 1993;51:130–4.
106. Webster JC, Cidlowski JA. Downregulation of the glucocorticoid receptor. A mechanism for physiological adaptation to hormones. Ann NY Acad Sci. 1994;746:216–20.
107. Webster JC, Jewell CM, Bodwell JE, Munck A, Sar M, Cidlowski JA. Mouse glucocorticoid receptor phosphorylation status influences multiple functions of the receptor protein. J Biol Chem. 1997;272:9287–93.
108. Bamberger CM, Else T, Bamberger AM, Beil FU, Schulte HM. Regulation of the human interleukin-2 gene by the alpha and beta isoforms of the glucocorticoid receptor. Mol Cell Endocrinol. 1997;136:23–8.
109. Bamberger CM, Bamberger AM, Wald M, Chrousos GP, Schulte HM. Inhibition of mineralo-corticoid activity by the beta-isoform of the human glucocorticoid receptor. J Steroid Biochem Mol Biol. 1997;60:43–50.
110. Bamberger CM, Schulte HM, Chrousos GP. Molecular determinants of glucocorticoid receptor function and tissue sensitivity to glucocorticoids. Endocrinol Rev. 1996;17:245–61.
111. Stahl M, Ludwig D, Fellermann K, Stange EF. Intestinal expression of human heat shock protein 90 in patients with Crohn's disease and ulcerative colitis. Dig Dis Sci. 1998;43:1079–87.
112. Shimada T, Hiwatashi N, Yamazaki H, Kinouchi Y, Toyota T. Relationship between glucocorticoid receptor and response to glucocorticoid therapy in ulcerative colitis. Dis Colon Rectum. 1997;40:S54–8.
113. Rogler G, Meinel A, Lingauer A et al. Glucocorticoid receptors are down-regulated in inflamed colonic mucosa but not in peripheral blood mononuclear cells from patients with inflammatory bowel disease. Eur J Clin Invest. 1999;29:330–6.
114. Rosewicz S, McDonald AR, Maddux BA, Goldfine ID, Miesfeld RL, Logsdon CD. Mechanism of glucocorticoid receptor down-regulation by glucocorticoids. J Biol Chem. 1988;263:2581–4.
115. Okret S, Poellinger L, Dong Y, Gustafsson JA. Down-regulation of glucocorticoid receptor mRNA by glucocorticoid hormones and recognition by the receptor of a specific binding sequence within a receptor cDNA clone. Proc Natl Acad Sci USA. 1986;83:5899–903.
116. Cidlowski JA, Cidlowski NB. Regulation of glucocorticoid receptors by glucocorticoids in cultured HeLa S3 cells. Endocrinology. 1981;109:1975–82.
117. Honda M, Orii F, Ayabe T et al. Expression of glucocorticoid receptor beta in lymphocytes of patients with glucocorticoid-resistant ulcerative colitis. Gastroenterology. 2000;118:859–66.
118. McKenna NJ, Lanz RB, O'Malley BW. Nuclear receptor coregulators: cellular and molecular biology. Endocrinol Rev. 1999;20:321–44.
119. McKenna NJ, Xu J, Nawaz Z, Tsai SY, Tsai MJ, O'Malley BW. Nuclear receptor coactivators: multiple enzymes, multiple complexes, multiple functions. J Steroid Biochem Mol Biol. 1999;69:3–12.
120. Perissi V, Staszewski LM, McInerney EM et al. Molecular determinants of nuclear receptor–corepressor interaction. Genes Dev. 1999;13:3198–208.
121. Stange EF. Glucocorticoid receptor activity in inflammatory bowel disease: hindsight or foresight? Eur J Clin Invest. 1999;29:278–9.

8
Limitations of standard therapy for inflammatory bowel disease

D. P. B. McGOVERN, T. AHMAD and D. P. JEWELL

INTRODUCTION

Despite considerable advances, in recent years, leading to new and potent therapies available to clinicians treating patients with inflammatory bowel disease (IBD), it remains a sobering fact for the clinicians that:

1. Approximately one in three patients with acute severe attacks of ulcerative colitis (UC) fail standard medical therapy and either require surgery or rescue therapy with cyclosporin.
2. Approximately 70% of all patients with UC in whom surgery is necessary require this as a result of uncontrolled disease.
3. Approximately 60% of patients with Crohn's disease (CD) will require surgery at some time during their lifetime.
4. Commonly used IBD therapies are associated with significant adverse drug reactions.

This chapter will discuss some of the theories and evidence as to why standard therapies for IBD fail. The therapies that will be considered are salicylates, corticosteroids, thiopurines and methotrexate. Reasons for failing medical therapy can be largely categorized into one of four groups: (a) lack of compliance, (b) inappropriate formulation and route of drug administration, (c) inadequate dose of drug, and (d) host/genetic factors causing failure and intolerance.

COMPLIANCE

Lack of compliance (concordance) with medical therapy is a considerable problem faced by clinicians from all branches of medicine. Assessment of compliance of 5-aminosalicylates during clinical trials using pill counting and patient interview estimates that compliance of medication is of the order of 70%[1]. Nevertheless, pill counting cannot necessarily be relied upon, as suggested by a study of bronchodilators in smokers. Approximately 30% of the patients fired their inhalers 100 times or more in a 3-h period (usually just prior to clinic visits) in order to give the impression of compliance[2]. An alternative method of measuring salicylate compliance is measurement of serum metabolites. Serum sulphapyridine concentrations were measured in inpatients taking sulphasalazine for UC. Measurements were then repeated during clinic follow-up, and in over 40% of patients there was a greater than 25% decrease in serum levels compared with those recorded as inpatients[3]. In fact community-based studies have estimated compliance to be in the range of 40–50%[4]. There is little published evidence evaluating whether or not compliance with salicylates is important in preventing relapse. However, there is evidence suggesting that long-term compliance with salicylates may reduce the risk of developing colorectal cancer in UC[5,6]. There are problems with these studies in that they are retrospective, but they do suggest that, even in quiescent disease, those at risk of cancer should be encouraged to continue taking salicylates long-term.

There are few data on compliance with corticosteroid therapy but data from trials (again using pill counting) have shown that, even during active disease, patients may not take their medication. Approximately one in 20 patients were excluded from analysis for lack of compliance with either budesonide or prednisolone[7] in active disease or with budesonide given as prevention of recurrence from CD following surgical resection[8].

Patients obviously have concerns about the long-term safety of immunosuppressants and even under study conditions approximately 3% of paediatric IBD patients do not take 6-mercaptopurine[9], and up to 12% of patients do not comply with prescribed methotrexate[10]. This result is surprisingly high, but may reflect the fact that methotrexate is taken weekly (more difficult to remember?) and is often prescribed as a subcutaneous or intramuscular injection (less acceptable?).

Despite the paucity of evidence evaluating the relationship between outcome and compliance it would appear logical that improved compliance with proven effective therapies would lead to improved outcomes. It is clear that a good, trusting doctor–patient relationship is essential for good communication, which in turn leads to good compliance. Patients do not comprehend discharge plans as well as doctors think they do[11], and in an attempt to overcome this some physicians give patients copies of their discharge summaries/clinic letters. Improved communication will lead to better patient understanding of why they should be compliant with medication and what the consequences of non-compliance might be. The effect of, and adverse events from, medication are one of the major concerns of patients with IBD[12]. Nurse practitioners may have an important role to play in educating/counselling patients about their medication.

Compliance may also improve with more tolerable medication and simplified medical regimens. Patients with IBD prefer taking less tablets[13] and tolerate foam enemas better than liquid enemas[14]. There is also evidence that consuming the daily prescribed salicylate dose in one go is as effective as, and as well tolerated as, multiple smaller doses[15].

In summary, perhaps as little as 40% of prescribed medication for IBD is actually taken as directed. Evidence of the relationship between compliance and outcome in IBD is needed. Improved communication, patient comprehension, drug tolerability and simpler drug regimens may all help to overcome this significant barrier to optimum patient care.

OPTIMAL FORMULATION, ROUTE AND DOSE OF MEDICATION

Salicylates and corticosteroids

The salicylates, probably more than any other treatment for IBD, are a heterogeneous group of drugs, which theoretically require careful correlation between site of disease and route, formulation and dosage of the chosen salicylate. It is important to consider their use in the context of inducing remission in active disease and also in maintaining remission in quiescent disease, as well as examining the appropriate formulation for distal vs extensive disease.

Active distal ulcerative colitis

Safdi *et al.* demonstrated that combination therapy with both oral and topical salicylates is more effective than either alone, and that topical salicylates are more effective, at similar doses, than oral salicylates alone[16]. They randomized 60 patients with distal colitis to receive either mesalamine (mesalazine) rectal enema nocte or oral mesalamine 2.4 g daily, or a combination of the two treatments. At week 6 combination therapy resulted in a greater improvement (-5.2) in total disease activity index (DAI) score than either mesalamine enemas (-4.4) or mesalamine tablets alone (-3.9). Physicians' and patients' ratings of improvement indicated that combination therapy significantly improved disease status, compared with oral mesalamine.

Topical therapy has an important role to play in the management of distal disease but there are significant differences in the pharmacokinetics of the available rectal preparations. Suppositories, once dissolved, coat only the rectum and rectosigmoid[17], whereas less than 10% of liquid enemas remain in the rectum in active disease[18] (the bulk of an enema remains in the sigmoid colon). Foam and liquid enemas also have different pharmacokinetic properties; in healthy volunteers the splenic flexure was reached in seven of eight patients using a 100 ml liquid enema, whereas a foam enema remained in the sigmoid in about 50% of patients[19]. Disease activity does not appear to influence the distribution of enemas[16]. Compliance, as discussed earlier, may be an important determinant of response to therapy, and foam enemas are better tolerated than liquid enemas[14]. A more recent study has suggested that a mesalazine gel preparation is better tolerated than, and is as effective as, equivalently dosed enemas[20]. From this evidence it is apparent that rectal preparations are important in the management of distal UC and that the preparation, where tolerated, should be: (a) suppositories for proctitis, (b) foam enemas for colitis limited to the rectum and sigmoid, and (c) liquid enemas for colitis extending to the splenic flexure.

Given that rectal therapy is important for active distal disease, the question remains as to which of the available therapies is first line. Topical salicylates are more effective than other topical therapies[21] for induction of remission of distal UC with a pooled odds ratio (POR) of 2.03 (95% CI 1.28–3.20) when compared to conventional rectal corticosteroids. The same study also demonstrated that conventional rectal corticosteroids and rectal budesonide are more effective than placebo (POR of 2.42 (95% CI 1.72–3.41) and 1.89 (95% CI 1.29–2.76), respectively). Rectal budesonide and conventional corticosteroids seem to be of equivalent efficacy, but budesonide produced less endogenous cortisol suppression.

It is worth noting that this meta-analysis excluded 50 out of 83 identified trials as a result of poor methodology. There is one further study of note which suggested that the combination of beclomethasone diproprionate (3 mg) and mesalazine (2 mg) in enema form produced better clinical, endoscopic and histological improvement than either therapy alone[22]. Unfortunately such combination therapies are not yet available, but clinicians have extrapolated the results by prescribing corticosteroid enemas mane and 5-ASA enemas nocte.

It is clear that rectal 5-ASAs are more effective than rectal corticosteroids but, in the UK at least, rectal corticosteroids are often the first line of therapy. This is probably due to the high cost of rectal 5-ASA (March 2000 prices for 8 weeks of a steroid enema (prescribed b.d.) is approximately £30–£45 compared to £140–£300 for salicylate enemas), clearly a limiting factor in the use of optimal medical therapy. This price differential is not universal as there is little difference in price between 5-ASA and steroid enemas in Canada[21]. The reason for this price disparity is not clear.

The dose of rectal mesalazine does not appear to be important in the induction of remission of distal UC. No clear dose–response curve (above 1 g/day) has been demonstrated in a number of trials included in a meta-analysis of rectal aminosalicylates[23]. One study examined 113 patients with active distal colitis using 5-ASA enemas at doses of 1 g, 2 g and 4 g, and found that at 4 weeks there was no difference in remission rates (63%, 67% and 72%, respectively)[24]. Therapy with 1 g 5-ASA suppositories once a day appears to be superior to 500 mg 5-ASA suppositories twice a day[25]. In contrast to rectal 5-ASA, there appears to be a dose–response curve for oral salicylate therapy[26]. There are few data comparing the different formulations of oral salicylates in active distal disease, but it would seem reasonable to extrapolate the data which show that azo-bonded salicylates have higher luminal concentrations in the colonic epithelium than those seen in slow-release mesalazine[27].

Occasionally patients fail to respond to oral salicylates and some combination of rectal salicylates and corticosteroids; these patients would normally be treated with a short course of prednisolone. Similarly, on the rare occasions that patients with distal disease become systemically unwell, patients should be managed in an identical manner to patients with more extensive disease.

Extensive ulcerative colitis

Mildly active. There is little doubt that oral therapy is necessary for extensive disease. Some physicians will, however, use rectal preparations as adjunct therapy in this situation.

Oral salicylates are probably the first-line therapy for mildly active extensive UC. The evidence suggests that the dose–response is much more important than the preparation of salicylate in inducing remission, as clearly demonstrated in a meta-analysis by Sutherland *et al.*[28]. They examined eight trials including over 1000 patients comparing oral 5-ASA and placebo for induction of remission. A dose–response trend was apparent: (a) <2 g/day, OR 1.5; 95% CI 0.89–2.6; (b) 2–2.9 g/day, OR 1.9, 95% CI 1.3–2.8; (c) >3 g/day, OR 2.7; 95% CI 1.8–3.9.

Moderate or severely active colitis. Although it is claimed that up to 80% of patients will respond to 2–4.8 g of mesalazine daily[29], oral corticosteroids are the mainstay of treatment for moderately active disease and for those patients who have failed salicylate therapy. Prednisolone is the most commonly used oral corticosteroid in the UK, and there seems to be little difference between prednisolone and other oral glucocorticoid preparations. Budesonide therapy is not appropriate in this setting given its pharmacodynamic profile. Centres in different parts of the world use different doses of prednisolone, but there is only one trial which has examined this issue[30]. Baron *et al.* demonstrated that in active colitis 40 mg of prednisolone was more effective than 20 mg of prednisolone (65% and 30% into remission, respectively) and that there was no added benefit from increasing this dose to 60 mg (though more of these patients had side-effects).

In a severe attack of colitis accompanied by systemic symptoms, patients require hospital admission, close monitoring and liaison between surgeon and physician. Again corticosteroids remain the treatment of choice. Standard regimes include intravenous hydrocortisone 400 mg/day, prednisolone 40–60 mg/day or methylprednisolone 32–48 mg/day. There are no trials comparing oral vs intravenous therapy. There are also no dose–response trials, though one study has suggested that pulsed methylprednisolone (1 g/day) was no more effective than standard hydrocortisone doses[31]. Continuous infusions of corticosteroids may provide constant plasma levels, ease of administration and lower overall costs. Intravenous adrenocorticotropic hormone (ACTH) is an alternative which may be more effective than intravenous hydrocortisone in patients with a severe attack who had not received oral prednisolone prior to admission. However, in patients who have received prior steroids, hydrocortisone is more effective than ACTH[32]. Some centres use rectal corticosteroid preparations in addition to systemic therapy. There are no comparative studies examining the role of rectal treatment in addition to systemic corticosteroids in severe UC.

Maintenance of remission of ulcerative colitis

Distal disease. Rectal salicylates are more effective than oral salicylates in maintaining remission in distal colitis. A meta-analysis clearly demonstrated the benefit of rectal salicylates over placebo, and that rectal salicylates were more effective than oral salicylates (OR 2.41; 95% CI 1.05–5.54)[23]. Furthermore, rectal and oral salicylates are better than oral alone: 72 patients were randomized to receive oral mesalazine 1.6 g/day and either placebo enemas or mesalazine enemas twice a week, over a period of 1 year. Seventy-one per cent of the patients on combination therapy remained in remission compared to 31% in the oral therapy alone group ($p = 0.036$, number needed to treat (NNT) $= 3$)[34]. A major problem with rectal therapy may be compliance as it is unpopular with patients. This problem may be overcome by using intermittent rectal therapy, which is effective, though there may be a 'frequency–response trend' (Table 1)[35]. There does appear to be a dose–response phenomenon as the relapse rate in distal colitis was 10% in those who used twice-daily 400 mg suppositories compared to 30% in those who used the suppositories only once daily (relapse rate on placebo 47%)[36].

There are few trials of oral salicylates specifically looking at maintenance of remission in distal colitis. It would seem logical that azo-bonded salicylates would be the most effective in distal disease, in part confirmed by a study comparing Asacol 1.2 g/day and olsalazine 1.0 g/day in 100 patients with UC. At 12 months

Table 1 Differing regimens of mesalazine enemas for maintenance of remission in distal colitis[35] (percentage in remission)

	Mesalazine enemas (4 g)			Placebo
	Daily	Every other day	Every third day	
6 weeks	89	86	83	68
24 weeks	91	72	65	48

46% of patients on Asacol had relapsed compared to 24% on olsalazine ($p = 0.025$, NNT = 4)[37]. The authors concluded that olsalazine was superior to Asacol, particularly in patients with left-sided disease. Dose of salicylate may be important in distal disease as in 198 patients treated with olsalazine 2 g, 1 g or 0.5 g per day over 12 months, the highest dose was most effective in proctitis[38].

Extensive disease.   Oral therapy is necessary for the maintenance of remission in extensive disease. There appears to be little difference between the different formulations of 5-ASA compounds. Delayed-release mesalazine 0.8 g/day is of equal efficacy to sulphasalazine 2 g/day (relapse rate 38% and 39%, respectively) though reported side-effects were higher in the sulphasalazine group (headache 8% vs 27%, abdominal discomfort 12% vs 32%) (see Table 3 for numbers needed to harm (NNH) for sulphasalazine)[39]. No difference in efficacy was reported between olsalazine (1 g/day) and sulphasalazine (2 g/day)[40] or between balsalazide and mesalazine[41] (though the authors did claim a benefit for balsalazide). A recent meta-analysis comparing sulphasalazine and the newer 5-ASAs showed a slight benefit for sulphasalazine in maintaining remission in UC (OR 1.29, 95% CI 1.06–1.57) and surprisingly there was no increase in adverse events in the sulphasalazine group[42]. Some people have interpreted this study as demonstrating a superiority of sulphasalazine, suggesting that the sulphapyridine ring may have an immunomodulatory effect on the colonic mucosa. However, it should be noted that the sulphasalazine trials included in this analysis included only patients who had been brought into remission by (and were thus known to be tolerant of) sulphasalazine.

There is contradictory evidence regarding the dose–response of salicylates in the maintenance of remission of UC. Azad Khan *et al.* suggested that 2 g/day of sulphasalazine was more effective than 1 g/day in maintaining remission, and that while 4 g/day was slightly more effective than 2 g/day this was more than offset by an increase in adverse events[43]. Other studies have shown that lower doses are equally efficacious to higher doses using Pentasa[44] or balsalazide[45], and in a meta-analysis of 10 studies there was no clear dose–response trend identified[28]. One study has demonstrated that intermittent treatment with 2.4 g/day for the first week of each month is as effective as 1.6 g/day for the whole month (relapse of 29% vs 34%, respectively) and that taking 3 g/day of sulphasalazine at the first sign of relapse results in the same overall relapse rate as regularly taking 2 g/day[46].

Corticosteroids are not routinely used in the maintenance of remission of ulcerative colitis, though one trial has demonstrated that they may be effective when given on alternate days at a dose of 40 mg prednisolone/day[47]. The concern about the side-effects of long-term corticosteroid therapy limits their use in this setting.

Crohn's disease

Active disease. There has been much debate about the role of salicylates in Crohn's disease. The National Cooperative Crohn's Disease Study (NCCDS)[48] demonstrated their potential effectiveness by demonstrating that sulphasalazine at a dose of 15 mg/kg per day (up to a maximum of 5 g/day) induced remission (CDAI < 150) in 43% of patients compared to 30% of those receiving placebo (though the difference did not achieve statistical significance). A total of 310 patients with CD affecting the terminal ileum ($\pm$ the colon) were randomized to receive Pentasa 1 g, 2 g, 4 g or placebo daily[49]. There was no difference in remission rates between placebo and the groups receiving 1 and 2 g of Pentasa daily, but the relapse rate was significantly higher in the placebo group when compared to the group receiving 4 g/day (43% and 18%, respectively, NNT 4). Unfortunately a similarly designed trial failed to show any benefit of Pentasa over placebo[50]. A smaller trial compared Eudragit S coated Asacol (800 mg q.d.s.) in patients with colonic CD ($\pm$ terminal ileal disease) for 16 weeks; 45% of the Asacol group had achieved remission at 16 weeks compared to only 22% of the placebo-treated group (NNT 4)[51]. There are no trials comparing the different 5-ASA preparations in inducing remission in CD. Some studies have suggested that 5-ASAs may be as effective as corticosteroids in achieving remission, but corticosteroids certainly seem to achieve remission more rapidly[52]. Given the delay in inducing remission, and the uncertainty of the efficacy of salicylates, their routine use in CD is not universal. If they are to be used it would seem logical that high doses are required and the 5-ASA preparation should be tailored to disease distribution (slow release for small bowel CD, azo-bonded for colonic disease and probably rectal for distal disease).

For many years corticosteroids have been the mainstay of treatment for active CD. Corticosteroids should be administered orally, systemically or rectally according to disease distribution and severity of activity, in a similar fashion to administration to patients with UC.

A major recent advance in corticosteroid therapy for CD has been the development of potent topical corticosteroids which undergo high hepatic first-pass metabolism. Budenofalk (oral pH-dependent) and Entocort (controlled ileal release) are the commercially available forms of budesonide. Both drugs (at a dose of 9 mg/daily) have been shown to be almost as effective as conventional steroids (6-methylprednisolone 48 mg and prednisolone 40 mg) in achieving remission in terminal ileal and ascending colonic CD[53,54]. These studies did, however, demonstrate that steroid side-effects are markedly reduced in the budesonide groups (e.g. steroid side-effects in patients on 6-methylprednisolone occurred in 69.7% of patients compared to only 28.6% of the Budenofalk group, NNH with methylprednisolone compared to Budenofalk is 2)[53]. Anecdotal evidence suggests that patients with CD who have had previous small bowel resections, an ileostomy or have extensive small bowel disease, do less well on slow-release (enteric-coated) prednisolone, perhaps due to reduced absorption and lower serum levels. For this reason some authorities avoid enteric-coated prednisolone in this setting.

There may be a dose–response curve for corticosteroids in CD. In a multi-centre European study 83% of patients with active CD went into remission at 18 weeks after receiving 48 mg/day of 6-methylprednisolone. The remission rate increased to 92% when patients were prescribed 1 mg/day of the 6-methylprednisolone[55].

Maintenance of remission in CD. Few areas in the therapeutics of IBD have created as much controversy as the role of salicylates in the maintenance of remission in CD. A meta-analysis of trials examining the role of mesalazine as maintenance therapy for patients with medically induced remission found no overall benefit when compared to placebo (pooled risk difference -4.7%, 95% CI -9.6% to 2.8%)[56]. The same meta-analysis examined the role of mesalazine in surgically induced remission; however, a further study has been published since the original meta-analysis[57] and the authors have correspondingly updated their results. These show a pooled risk of further attack of -10% (95% CI -16.9% to -3.2%) which gives a NNT of 10 (i.e. physicians need to treat 10 patients to prevent one relapse)[58]. There is some concern about the methodology of one of the included studies (lack of placebo in control group), and if this study is removed from the analysis the NNT rises to 12[59].

There are no data to support the use of standard corticosteroids as long-term maintenance therapy for CD. There have been a number of studies evaluating the role of budesonide as maintenance therapy but the results of a pooled analysis of these are disappointing[60]. There is a significant delay to relapse in patients treated with 6 mg of budesonide compared to placebo, but at 1 year there was no difference in relapse rates between the two groups.

It remains a sobering fact for clinicians treating patients with CD that cessation of smoking is probably the most effective intervention for improving outcomes. Sutherland *et al.* demonstrated that recurrence, 10 years after surgery, of CD was significantly higher in smokers than non-smokers (70% and 41%, respectively) and that the effect of smoking on recurrence seemed greater for women than men (OR 4.2 (95% CI 2.0–4.2) and 1.5 (0.8–6.0), respectively)[112]. A further study demonstrated that smoking was the only significant predictor of surgical recurrence of CD (hazard ratio 2.0; 95% CI 1.2–3.8)[113]. Given the adverse influence of smoking on CD, as well as cardiovascular and bone disease, all CD patients should be questioned about their smoking habits at each clinic visit. If they continue to smoke then they should be informed of the risks and persuaded to give up.

Thiopurine therapy for IBD

Thiopurines are effective therapies for maintenance of remission in IBD. The evidence suggests that they play no role in acute disease management. However, one study has demonstrated that patients with CD who required prednisolone for acute symptoms required less prednisolone, and achieved better long-term remission rates, when 6-mercaptopurine (6-MP) was started concomitantly[61].

The thiopurines are a heterogeneous group of drugs. Approximately three-quarters of IBD patients intolerant of azathioprine (AZA) tolerated 6-MP[62].

The authors suggest that the imidazole ring cleaved from AZA as it is converted to 6-MP may be responsible for this intolerance. The imidazole ring has potent immunomodulatory properties of its own[63], but there are remarkably few data on the relative efficacies of AZA and 6-MP. Calne *et al.* demonstrated that renal allografts survived longer in dogs treated with AZA compared to those receiving 6-MP[64]. A recent abstract presented data suggesting a greater *in-vitro* suppression of proinflammatory cytokines by AZA than by 6-MP[65]. A multi-centre study comparing the efficacy of AZA and 6-MP in the management of IBD is due to start in the near future. There are significant differences in bioavailability between the different oral preparations of thiopurine[66]. Patients treated with either branded AZA (Imuran) or 6-MP achieved significantly higher erythrocyte 6-thioguanine nucleotide (the cytotoxic metabolites of thiopurines which have been correlated with clinical responsiveness in patients with IBD) levels than patients treated with generic AZA. Another recent abstract suggests that patients intolerant of 6-MP (possibly due to elevated 6-methylmercaptopurine (6-MMP) levels) are able to tolerate thioguanine (6-TG)[67]. 6-TG is a closely related thiopurine compound that is converted to the 6-thioguanine nucleotides by a different pathway than AZA/6-MP, leading to less 6-MMP production.

One of the major problems of thiopurine therapy is the prolonged time (up to 16 weeks) for AZA or 6-MP to exert its full immunomodulatory effect. In an attempt to overcome this Sandborn *et al.* compared a regimen of a high-loading intravenous dose of azathioprine (40 mg/kg) vs placebo, both followed by standard oral azathioprine (2 mg/kg per day)[33]. The loading dose, however, did not decrease the time to response in patients with steroid-treated CD beginning AZA therapy. Another major problem with thiopurine therapy is the side-effects exhibited by up to a quarter of patients[68]; these may be in part overcome by the development of a delayed-release AZA formulation (currently undergoing phase II trials) or a rectal formulation of AZA. Oral AZA has a bioavailability of 47% compared to 7% and 1–5% of the delayed-release and rectal formulations respectively[114].

There are no dose–response studies of thiopurine therapy, though most experts agree that 2 mg/kg per day is the optimum starting dose. There is, however, a positive association between response to 6-MP and cumulative dose (dose multiplied by duration of therapy)[115]. Two studies found that the mean maintenance dose of AZA used in two different hospitals in the UK was approximately 1.5 mg/kg per day[69,70]. This is probably an accurate reflection, certainly in the UK, of the doses of thiopurines that patients are receiving. It may be that gastroenterologists are quick to reduce the dose of thiopurines if bone marrow toxicity or other adverse events occur, but are more reluctant to increase thiopurine doses if there is a poor/incomplete response.

Methotrexate therapy for IBD

There is increasing evidence that methotrexate is effective in inducing[71] and maintaining[72] remission in Crohn's disease (NNT for induction of remission in chronically active CD is 5, NNT for maintenance of remission of CD is 4). These two studies evaluated intramuscular methotrexate as it has been suggested, by some, that oral methotrexate should not be used due to its variable absorption rate[73]. However, one study suggests that orally administered methotrexate is well absorbed in patients with IBD, including those with severe small bowel disease or previous surgical resection[74]. In patients with squamous cell carcinoma the absolute systemic bioavailability of oral methotrexate (tablets) was 36% ($\pm 10\%$) and of intramuscular methotrexate was 93% ($\pm 14\%$) when compared to the bioavailability of intravenous methotrexate[75]. A further study in rheumatological patients demonstrated no significant difference for the bioavailability between tablet and oral methotrexate solution, or between the bioavailability of subcutaneous and intramuscular methotrexate[76]. There are no data comparing the bioavailability or efficacy of oral, subcutaneous or intramuscular methotrexate in IBD. Increasing numbers of clinicians are prescribing methotrexate for CD and many of them are administering it orally, despite the evidence being less convincing. In a trial of 16 mg/week (increasing to 22.5 mg/week if necessary) of oral methotrexate vs placebo in 33 patients with steroid-dependent CD, fewer methotrexate-treated patients (46%) had flares of CD as compared to those in the placebo group (80%), but this difference did not achieve statistical significance ($p < 0.1$)[10].

The only study designed to compare different doses of methotrexate found no difference in remission rates, percentage of patients who showed improvement, or toxicity between patients with steroid-dependent IBD who received either 15 or 25 mg/week of subcutaneous methotrexate[77]. However, in the intramuscular methotrexate study for maintenance of remission[72], of the patients who relapsed while receiving 12.5 mg/week, 54.5% of those retreated with 25 mg of methotrexate plus prednisolone re-entered remission (compared to only 14.3% of those who received other treatments), suggesting there may be a dose–response trend for some patients at high risk of relapse.

HOST FACTORS INFLUENCING RESPONSE AND INTOLERANCE

Salicylates

A considerable proportion of sulphapyridine and some un-split sulphasalazine is absorbed into the systemic circulation where sulphapyridine undergoes acetylation before being excreted in urine[78]. Sulphapyridine acetylation is polymorphic[79] with higher serum sulphapyridine concentrations in slow than in fast acetylators (serum sulphapyridine concentration 18.5 µg/ml (SD ± 8.2) and 7.5 µg/ml (SD ± 4.3), respectively)[80]. Slow acetylators suffer earlier and more pronounced side-effects from sulphasalazine (including nausea, headache and abdominal discomfort)[81] and are more prone to sulphasalazine-induced haemolysis[82]. Serum sulphapyridine concentrations do correlate with clinical response to sulphasalazine in UC[83], and the authors of this study suggest monitoring of sulphapyridine levels will identify acetylator phenotype and monitor compliance. Prevalence studies have demonstrated that, in the American Caucasian and Afro-Carribean population, approximately 60% are slow acetylators and 25% are rapid acetylators[84]. This differs quite markedly from Japanese populations, in which up to 90% of the population are rapid acetylators[85].

The results of using salicylates for treating CD may, in part, be disappointing as a result of the superficial bowel wall penetration of the active 5-ASA moiety.

CD causes transmural inflammation, and salicylates may be effective only in superficial or early CD. There is evidence demonstrating that the risk of recurrence following surgical resection for CD is, in part, determined by mucosal mesalazine concentration[86]. The same group have suggested that, following surgery (despite 5-ASA), recurrence of CD is significantly higher in patients who have had end-to-end anastomoses than those with other types of anastomosis (end-to-side, side-to-side)[87]. This difference may be due to lower 5-ASA mucosal concentrations around the anastomosis site in end-to-end patients due to faster transit through the anastomosis.

In distal UC oral salicylates may, in part, be less effective than rectal preparations due to proximal colonic stasis that results in reduced concentrations of 5-ASA being delivered to the site of inflammation. In some patients there may be delayed oral–caecal and proximal colonic transit associated with, and contrasting to, rapid transit through inflamed distal bowel[88]. Clinical experience, not confirmed with objective data, suggests that some patients with active distal colitis will not respond to therapy unless their proximal constipation is treated.

Corticosteroids

There is no doubt that some patients with IBD are resistant to corticosteroid therapy[89,90], and it would represent a major clinical advance to be able to identify such patients. Clinical heterogeneity may explain some of the differences in response rates. Patients with UC failing to respond to therapy were more likely to have fever, persistent diarrhoea, rectal bleeding, and elevated serum C-reactive protein[90]. Other studies have suggested that patients with left-sided colitis resistant to corticosteroids have a higher frequency of antineutrophil cytoplasmic antibodies with perinuclear staining (pANCA) than treatment-responsive left-sided colitis (90% vs 62%, respectively $(p=0.03)$)[91]. Patients with CD who did not respond to corticosteroids had a high frequency of HLA-DRB1*04[92], and patients who had the TAP2A gene were more likely to respond to corticosteroids[93].

Corticosteroid receptors express either an active α or antagonistic β chain; β chain mRNA was detectable in four of five poor corticosteroid responders compared to none of eight responders of five healthy controls who all expressed the α chain[94]. The *in-vitro* antiproliferative effect of dexamethasone on phytohaemagglutinin-stimulated peripheral blood T lymphocytes was assessed in 18 patients with severe acute UC[95]. The T lymphocyte steroid sensitivity of patients who either failed or were partial responders to corticosteroid treatment was significantly less than those who responded. Similar results have been demonstrated in asthmatics who are resistant to steroids, who are also known not to have defects either in glucocorticoid absorption and clearance or in the hypothalamic/pituitary/adrenal axis[96]. Unfortunately, while these patients are resistant to the inflammatory effects of steroids they are still very much prone to the cushingoid side-effects. Proinflammatory cytokines reversibly increase T cell glucocorticoid resistance[97]; therefore cytokine polymorphisms may play a role in steroid resistance. Inappropriately elevated secondary messenger proteins such as the transcription factor activator protein 1 (AP-1) which bind to and inactivate the glucocorticoid receptor/glucocorticoid complex have also been suggested as possible culprits in steroid resistance[98]. It is worthy of note that T cell corticosteroid responsiveness is highly variable within the general population[99]. It is clear that further study of this phenomenon is needed in order for clinicians to identify high-risk patients who may benefit from early introduction of more potent immunosuppressants or even surgery.

Glucocorticoids are substrates for the P-glycoprotein 170 (Pgp-170) drug efflux pump that is coded for by the multidrug resistance (MDR) gene. A recent study demonstrated that, compared with controls, the peripheral blood lymphocyte MDR expression was significantly elevated in patients with CD who required bowel resection for failed medical therapy (mean 26.7 (SEM $\pm$ 2.8) vs 11.9 ($\pm$ 1.0); $p < 0.0001$) and also in patients with UC who required proctocolectomy for failed medical therapy (20.3 ($\pm$ 2.5) vs 11.9 ($\pm$ 1.0); $p = 0.001$)[100]. It is not clear whether the elevated MDR expression is as a result of exposure to previous immunomodulatory/cytotoxic therapy or whether it is due to an intrinsic defect, perhaps as a result of a genetic mutation. Single nucleotide polymorphisms have recently been described in the MDR gene, including one that has a homozygous frequency of 24% in the general population[101]. Individuals homozygous for this polymorphism had significantly lower duodenal MDR-1 expression and higher plasma digoxin levels than volunteers with wild-type MDR following oral ingestion of similar doses of digoxin. Patients with this mutation should, in theory, be more sensitive to corticosteroids, though they may exhibit more steroid side-effects.

Thiopurines

Host factors predicting response to, and side-effects from, the thiopurines have probably been more thoroughly investigated than any other drug used to treat IBD. This is because thiopurine methyltransferase (TPMT), a key enzyme in the metabolism of AZA and 6-MP, demonstrates marked inter-individual variation. The genetics of TPMT will be covered in more detail elsewhere in this book, but approximately 12% of the Caucasian population are heterozygous for a mutation in the gene coding for TPMT[102]. These heterozygotes have reduced TPMT activity and are prone to bone marrow toxicity[103] when exposed to thiopurines. However, it is important to note that a number of studies have demonstrated that the majority of patients who develop bone marrow toxicity cannot be completely predicted by TPMT genotype/activity[69,104], and there must be other host factors that predispose to marrow toxicity. One study has suggested parvovirus infection in conjunction with AZA therapy may be responsible for marrow toxicity in a number of patients[105].

In other conditions elevated TPMT activity has been associated with low 6-thioguanine nucleotide (6-TGN) concentrations and poor response to AZA/6-MP[103]. Dubinsky *et al.* demonstrated that in patients with IBD clinical response was highly correlated with 6-TGN levels ($p < 0.0001$)[106]. The same study also demonstrated that gastrointestinal intolerance and hepatotoxicity were associated with elevated 6-methylmercaptopurine (6-MMP) levels that probably occur as a consequence of elevated TPMT activity. Some patients exhibit TPMT activity above the 'normal' range, and the reason for this is not clear (these patients are prone to treatment failure and gastrointestinal hepatotoxicity (see above)). Further work is needed to elicit the cause of elevated TPMT activity, including screening for polymorphisms in the TPMT promoter region.

A number of clinicians routinely screen for TPMT mutations in patients prior to commencing thiopurine therapy. This is currently the only example of genetic screening in widespread pharmacological use.

Methotrexate

One of the host factors that may affect response to methotrexate is the variability in bioavailability between individuals following a dose of oral methotrexate[107]. In 10 patients with rheumatoid arthritis the inter-individual variability in bioavailability showed a more than five-fold range following a similar (15 mg) dose of oral methotrexate.

Methotrexate is a folate antagonist that acts by inhibition of the enzyme dihydrofolate reductase (DHFR). Recent applications of new and sensitive molecular biological techniques have made it possible to study the genetic alterations underlying methotrexate resistance in tumours. Methotrexate resistance can occur as a result of alterations at one of three sites in its metabolic pathway:

1. Decreased influx of methotrexate into cells. This can occur as a result of defects in the reduced folate carrier (rfc), and this is the commonest cause of methotrexate resistance in acute lymphocytic leukaemia (ALL)[108].
2. Mutations leading to increased DHFR activity or a DHFR that is resistant to binding with methotrexate. Increased enzyme activity is the second commonest cause of ALL methotrexate resistance[109].
3. Once inside cells methotrexate is polyglutamylated by folypolyglutamate (fpg) synthase. Methotrexate polyglutamates are retained longer in cells than is simple methotrexate, and consequently exert more cytotoxic effects. Defects in this polyglutamic reaction are the commonest cause of methotrexate resistance in acute myeloid leukaemia[110].

There are no data regarding the frequency of defects in these steps of methotrexate metabolism within the general population, and it is therefore not clear whether methotrexate resistance in CD is due to these defects or other mechanisms. Methotrexate is also a substrate for the drug efflux pump encoded for by the MDR gene (see above).

Increasing knowledge of the genetic (and to a lesser extent acquired) factors that influence response to drugs will, as part of the science of pharmacogenetics, radically alter the way we practise medicine in the future[111]. It may be possible, through new molecular and high-throughput DNA microarray technology, to produce DNA chips that can be used by physicians to identify efficacious and potentially harmful drugs on an individual basis. Thus an 'IBD chip' could be produced containing cDNA to help predict response to salicylates, corticosteroids, thiopurines, methotrexate, cyclosporin, etc. This field of human genetics will benefit greatly from the completion of the human genome project and the human SNP consortium in identifying polymorphisms in the enzymes, proteins and receptors involved in drug metabolism.

SUMMARY

The limitations of therapies for UC, and particularly CD, are all too obvious to clinicians who treat patients with these diseases (see Tables 2 and 3). New

Table 2 NNTs for commonly used therapies for IBD; i.e. for every five patients who are treated with 2 g 5-ASA enema daily, compared to prednisolone foam enemas, one will be prevented from suffering persistent active distal UC[16]

Condition (ref.)	Treatment	Duration of treatment	Comparator	Events being prevented	NNT (numbers needed to treat)
Active distal UC[116]	5-ASA 2 g foam enema o.d.	28 days	Prednisolone 20 mg foam enema o.d.	Persisting active distal colitis	5
Maintenance of remission in distal UC[34]	Oral mesalazine 1.6 g/day and twice-weekly mesalazine enemas	1 year	Oral mesalazine alone	Clinical relapse	3
Maintenance of remission in distal UC[36]	500 mg mesalazine suppositories b.d.	1 year	Placebo	Clinical relapse	3
Maintenance of remission in distal UC[36]	500 mg mesalazine suppositories b.d.	1 year	500 mg mesalazine suppository o.d.	Clinical relapse	5
Active colonic ($\pm$ ileal) Crohn's disease[51]	Eudragit S coated asacol (800 mg q.d.s.)	16 weeks	Placebo	Persisting active ileal Crohn's disease	4
Post-surgical resection in Crohn's disease[58]	Mesalazine (various doses)	Various follow-up times	Placebo	Clinical relapse	10
UC quiescent on azathioprine for >6 months[115]	Continuing azathioprine`	1 year	Stopping azathioprine	Clinical relapse	4
Quiescent Crohn's disease[116]	Azathioprine or 6-mercaptopurine	8–52 weeks	Placebo	Clinical relapse	9
Chronically active Crohn's disease[71]	25 mg weekly intramuscular methotrexate	16 weeks	Placebo	Persisting active Crohn's disease	5
Chronically active Crohn's disease patients who had entered remission on intramuscular methotrexate[72]	15 mg weekly intramuscular methotrexate	40 weeks	Placebo	Clinical relapse	4

Table 3 Numbers needed to harm (NNH) for interventions in IBD; i.e. for every nine patients treated with olsalazine, compared to sulphasalazine, one patient will experience diarrhoea[118]

Condition (ref.)	Treatment	Comparator	Duration of treatment	Adverse event	NNH (number needed to harm)
UC[39]	Sulphasalazine 2 g/day	Delayed-release mesalazine 0.8 g/day	48 weeks	Headaches	5
UC[117]	Oral mesalamine	Placebo	8 weeks	Nausea	22
UC[118]	Oral olsalazine 2 g/day	Sulphasalazine 2 g/day	6 months	Diarrhoea	9
Crohn's disease[53]	Methylprednisolone 48 mg (tapering dose)	Oral pH-modified release budesonide 9 mg/day	8 weeks	Steroid side-effects	2
Crohn's disease[117]	AZA or 6-MP	Placebo	Various	Cause one patient to stop taking medication	14
Chronic active Crohn's disease[71]	Intramuscular methotrexate 25 mg/day	Placebo	16 weeks	Cause one patient to stop taking medication	7
Postsurgical resection for Crohn's disease[112]	Smoking	Not-smoking	10 years	Relapse of CD	3

'molecular' therapies may improve our ability to manage patients with refractory disease, but improved therapeutic benefit can already be achieved by: improving compliance, optimum dosing, appropriate formulation, and using the most effective route.

The possibility of 'individualizing' therapies through advances in pharmacogenetics and understanding of host factors that predict response to therapy will enable clinicians to take this process one step further.

References

1. Gendre JP, Mary JY, Florent C et al. Oral mesalamine (Pentasa) as maintenance treatment for Crohn's disease: a multicenter placebo-controlled study. Gastroenterology. 1993;104:435–9.
2. Simmons MS, Nides MA, Rand CS et al. Unpredictability of deception in compliance with physician-prescribed bronchodilator inhaler use in a clinical trial. Chest. 2000;118:290–5.
3. Van Hees PA, van Tongeren JH. Compliance to therapy in patients on a maintenance dose of sulfasalazine. J Clin Gastroenterol. 1982;4:333–6.
4. Horwitz RAH, Horwitz SM. Adherence to treatment and health outcomes. Arch Intern Med. 1993;153:1863–8.
5. Moody GA, Jayanthi V, Probert CS et al. Long-term therapy with sulphasalazine protects against colorectal cancer in ulcerative colitis: a retrospective study of colorectal cancer risk and compliance with treatment in Leicestershire. Eur J Gastroenterol Hepatol. 1996;8:1179–83.
6. Pinczowski D, Ekbom A, Baron J, Yuen J, Adami H. Risk factors for colorectal cancer in patients with ulcerative colitis: a case study. Gastroenterology. 1994;107:117–20.
7. Barr-Meir S, Chowers Y, Lavy A et al. Budesonide vs prednisolone in the treatment of active Crohn's disease. Gastroenterology. 1998;115:835–40.
8. Hellers G, Cortot A, Jewell DP et al. Oral budesonide for prevention of postsurgical recurrence in Crohn's disease. Gastroenterology. 1999;116:294–300.
9. Dubinsky MC, Lamothe S, Yang HY et al. Pharmacogenomics and metabolite measurement for 6-mercaptopurine therapy in inflammatory bowel disease. Gastroenterology. 2000;118:705–13.
10. Arora S, Katkov W, Cooley J et al. Methotrexate in Crohn's disease: results of a randomized, double-blind, placebo-controlled trial. Hepatogastroenterology. 1999;46:1724–9.
11. Calkins D, Davis RB, Reiley P et al. Patient–physician communication at hospital discharge and patients' understanding of the postdischarge treatment plan. Arch Intern Med. 1997;157:1026–30.
12. Drossman DA, Leserman J, Li ZM et al. The rating form of IBD patient concerns: a new measure of health status. Psychosom Med. 1991;53:701–12.
13. Ode HS. 5-Aminosalicylic acid 1,000-mg caplets vs 500-mg tablets, in maintenance of remission in ulcerative colitis. J Clin Gastroenterol. 1997;24:286–8.
14. Campieri M, Paoluzi P, D'Albaiso G et al. Better quality of therapy with 5-ASA colonic foam in active ulcerative colitis: a multicenter comparative trial with 5-ASA enemas. Dig Dis Sci. 1993;38:1843–50.
15. Hussain F, Ajjan R, Trudgill N et al. Single and divided dose delayed-release mesalazine: are traditional dosing regimens in IBD outmoded? Gastroenterology. 1996;110:A928.
16. Safdi M, De Micco M, Sninsky C et al. A double blind comparison of oral vs rectal mesalamine vs combination therapy in the treatment of distal ulcerative colitis. Am J Gastroenterol. 1997;92:1867–71.
17. Williams CN, Haber G, Aquino JA. Double blind, placebo controlled evaluation of 5-ASA suppositories in active distal proctitis and measurement of extent of spread using 99mTc-labelled 5-ASA suppositories. Dig Dis Sci. 1987;32:71–5S.
18. Van Bodegraven AA, Boer RO, Lourens J et al. Distribution of mesalazine enemas in active and quiescent ulcerative colitis. Aliment Pharmacol Ther. 1996;10:327–32.
19. Brown J, Haines S, Wilding IR. Colonic spread of three rectally administered mesalazine (Pentasa) dosage forms in healthy volunteers as assessed by gamma scintigraphy. Aliment Pharmacol Ther. 1997;11:685–91.
20. Gionchetti P, Ardizzone S, Benvenuti ME et al. A new 5-ASA rectal formulation in the treatment of distal ulcerative colitis: a randomized, 5-ASA foam enema controlled multicentre trial. Ital J Gastroenterol Hepatol. 1997;29:A41.

21. Marshall JK, Irvine EJ. Rectal corticosteroids vs alternative treatment in ulcerative colitis: a meta-analysis. Gut. 1997;40:775–81.
22. Mulder CJJ, Fockens P, Meijer JWR *et al.* Beclomethasone diproprionate (3 mg) versus 5-aminosalicylic acid (2 g) vs the combination of both (3 mg/2 mg) as retention enemas in active ulcerative proctitis. Eur J Gastroenterol Hepatol. 1996;8:549–53.
23. Marshall JK, Irvine EJ. Rectal aminosalicylate therapy for distal ulcerative colitis: a meta-analysis. Aliment Pharmacol Ther. 1995;9:293–300.
24. Campieri M, Gionchetti P, Belluzi A *et al.* Optimum dosage of 5-aminosalicylic acid as rectal enemas in patients with active ulcerative colitis. Gut. 1991;32:929–31.
25. Gionchetti P, Rizello F, Venturi A *et al.* Comparison of mesalazine suppositories in proctitis and distal proctosigmoiditis. Aliment Pharmacol Ther. 1997;11:1053–7.
26. Sninsky CA, Cort DH, Shanahan F *et al.* Oral mesalamine (Asacol) for mildly to moderately active ulcerative colitis. A multicentre study. Ann Intern Med. 1991;115:350–5.
27. Christensen LA, Fallingborg J, Jacobsen BA *et al.* Comparative bioavailability of 5-aminosalicylic acid from controlled release preparation and an azo-bond preparation. Aliment Pharmacol Ther. 1994;8:289–94.
28. Sutherland LR, May GR, Shaffer EA. Sulfasalazine revisited: a meta-analysis of 5-aminosalicylic acid in the treatment of ulcerative colitis. Ann Intern Med. 1993;118:540–9.
29. Kornbluth A, Sachar DB. Ulcerative colitis practice guidelines in adults. American College of Gastroenterology, Practice Parameters Committee. Am J Gastroenterol. 1997;92:204–11.
30. Baron JH, Connell AM, Kanaghinis TG *et al.* Out-patient treatment of ulcerative colitis: comparison between three doses of oral prednisolone. Br Med J. 1962;2:441–3.
31. Rosenberg W, Ireland A, Jewell DP. High-dose methylprednisolone in the treatment of active ulcerative colitis. J Clin Gastroenterol. 1990;12:40–1.
32. Meyer S, Sachar DB, Goldberg JD *et al.* Corticotrophin vs hydrocortisone in the intravenous treatment of ulcerative colitis. Gastroenterology. 1983;85:351–7.
33. Sandborn WJ, Tremaine WJ, Wolf DC *et al.* Lack of effect of intravenous administration on time to respond to azathioprine for steroid-treated Crohn's disease. Gastroenterology. 1999;117: 527–35.
34. D'Albasio G, Pacini F, Camarri E *et al.* Combined therapy with 5-aminosalicylic acid tablets and enemas for maintaining remission in ulcerative proctitis: a randomized double-blind study. Am J Gastroenterol. 1997:92:1143–7.
35. Miner P, Daly R, Nester T and the Rowasa Study Group. The effect of varying dose intervals of mesalamine enemas for the prevention of relapse in distal ulcerative colitis. Gastroenterology. 1994;106:A736.
36. D'Albasio G, Paoluzi P, Campieri M *et al.* Maintenance treatment with ulcerative proctitis with mesalazine suppositories: a double-blind placebo controlled trial. The Italian IBD Study Group. Am J Gastroenterol. 1998;93:799–803.
37. Courtney M, Nunes D, Bergin C *et al.* Randomised comparison of olsalazine and mesalazine in prevention of relapses in ulcerative colitis. Lancet. 1992;339:1279–81.
38. Travis SPL, Tysk C, de Silva HJ *et al.* Optimum dose of olsalazine for maintaining remission in ulcerative colitis. Gut. 1994;35:1282–6.
39. Riley SA, Mani V, Goodman MJ *et al.* Comparison of delayed release 5-aminosalicylic acid (mesalazine) and sulfasalazine as maintenance treatment of patients with ulcerative colitis. Gastroenterology. 1988;94:1383–9.
40. Nilsson A, Danielson A, Lofberg R *et al.* Olsalazine vs sulfasalazine for relapse prevention in ulcerative colitis: a multicenter study. Am J Gastroenterol. 1995;90:381–7.
41. Green JR, Lobo AJ, Holdsworth CD *et al.* Balsalazide is more effective and better tolerated than mesalamine in the treatment of acute ulcerative colitis. Gastroenterology. 1998;114:15–22.
42. Sutherland L, Roth D, Beck P *et al.* Alternative to sulfasalazine; a meta-analysis of 5-ASA in the treatment of ulcerative colitis. Inflam Bowel Dis. 1997;3:665–78.
43. Azad Khan AK, Howes DT, Piris J *et al.* Optimum dose of sulphasalazine for maintenance treatment in ulcerative colitis. Gut. 1980;21:232–40.
44. Fockens F, Mulder CJ, Tytgat GN *et al.* Comparison of the efficacy and safety of 1.5 compared with 3.0 g oral slow release mesalazine (Pentasa) in the maintenance treatment of ulcerative colitis. Eur J Gastroenterol Hepatol. 1995;7:1025–30.
45. Green JR, Swan CH, Rowlinson A *et al.* Short report: Comparison of two doses of balsalazide in maintaining ulcerative colitis in remission over 12 months. Aliment Pharmacol Ther. 1992; 6:647–52.

46. Dickinson RJ, King A, Wight DGD *et al.* Is continuous sulfasalazine necessary in the management of patients with ulcerative colitis? Results of a preliminary study. Dis Colon Rectum. 1985; 28:929–30.
47. Powell-Tuck J, Parkins RA. A controlled trial of alternate day prednisolone as a maintenance treatment for ulcerative colitis in remission. Digestion. 1981;22:263–70.
48. Summers RW, Switz DM, Farmer RG *et al.* National Co-operative Crohn's Disease Study: results of drug treatment. Gastroenterology. 1979;77:847–69.
49. Singleton JW, Hanauer SB, Gitnick GL *et al.* Mesalamine capsules for the treatment of active Crohn's disease: results of a 16 week trial. Pentasa Crohn's Disease Study Group. Gastroenterology. 1993;104:1293–301.
50. Singleton JW. Second trial of mesalamine therapy in the treatment of active Crohn's disease. Gastroenterology. 1994;107:632–3.
51. Tremaine WJ, Schroeder KW, Harrison JM *et al.* A randomized, double-blind, placebo-controlled trial of oral mesalamine (5-ASA) preparation, Asacol, in the treatment of symptomatic Crohn's colitis and ileocolitis. J Clin Gastroenterol. 1994;19:278–82.
52. Martin F, Sutherland LR, Beck IT *et al.* Oral 5-ASA vs prednisolone in short term treatment of Crohn's disease: a multicentre controlled trial. Can J Gastroenterol. 1990;4:452–7.
53. Gross V, Andus T, Caesar I *et al.* Oral pH-modified release budesonide vs 6-methylprednisolone in active Crohn's disease. German/Austrian Budesonide Study Group. Eur J Gastroenterol Hepatol. 1996;89:905–9.
54. Rutgeerts P, Lofberg R, Malchow H *et al.* A comparison of budesonide with prednisolone for active Crohn's disease. N Engl J Med. 1994;331:842–5.
55. Modigliani R, Mary JY, Simon JF *et al.* Clinical, biological and endoscopic picture of attacks of Crohn's disease. Evolution of prednisolone. Gastroenterology. 1990;98:811–18.
56. Camma C, Giunta, Rosselli M *et al.* 5-Aminosalicylic acid in the maintenance treatment of Crohn's disease: a meta-analysis adjusted for confounding variables. Gastroenterology. 1997;118:264–73.
57. Lochs H, Mayer M, Fleig WE *et al.* Prophylaxis of postoperative relapse in Crohn's disease with mesalamine: European Cooperative Crohn's Disease Study. VI. Gastroenterology. 2000;118: 264–73.
58. Cottone M, Camma C. Mesalamine and relapse prevention in Crohn's disease. Gastroenterology. 2000;119:597.
59. Sutherland LR. Reply to letter entitled 'Mesalamine and relapse prevention in Crohn's disease' [see ref. 58]. Gastroenterology. 2000;119:597.
60. Feagan B, Greenberg GR, Lofberg R *et al.* Budesonide controlled ileal release prolongs remission in Crohn's disease (CD): a pooled analysis. Gastroenterology. 1997;112:A970.
61. Markowitz J, Rancher KG, Kohn N *et al.* The multicenter pediatric Crohn's disease 6-mercaptopurine trial. Final results. Gastroenterology. 1999;116:A771.
62. McGovern DPB, El Shobowale Bakre M, Duley J, Travis SPL. Early azathioprine intolerance in IBD patients is imidazole related and independent of thiopurine methyltransferase (TPMT) activity. Gastroenterology. 2000;118:A788.
63. Crawford DJ, Maddocks JL, Jones DN *et al.* Rational design of novel immunosuppressive drugs: analogues of azathioprine lacking the 6-mercaptopurine substituent retain or have enhanced immunosuppressive effects. J Med Chem. 1996;39:2690–5.
64. Calne RY, Alexandre GPJ, Murray JE. A study of the effects of drugs in prolonging survival of homologous renal transplant in dogs. Ann NY Acad Sci. 1962;99:743–61.
65. Louis E, Aboul Nasr El Yafi F, Belaiche J *et al.* High doses of azathioprine but not 6-mercaptopurine inhibit the production of pro-inflammatory cytokines in inflammatory bowel diseases: an *in vitro* study. Gastroenterology. 2000;118:A817.
66. Cuffari C, Hunt S, Bayless TM. Enhanced bioavailability of azathioprine compared to 6-mercaptopurine therapy in inflammatory bowel disease: correlation with treatment efficacy. Aliment Pharmacol Ther. 2000;14:1009–14.
67. Dubinsky MC, Hassard PV, Abreu MT *et al.* Thioguanine (6-TG): a therapeutic alternative in a subgroup of IBD patients failing 6-mercaptopurine (6-MP). Gastroenterology. 2000;118:A960.
68. Fraser AG, Orchard TR, Jewell DP. Side-effects of azathioprine treatment. Gut. 2000;46 (Suppl. II):A13.
69. McGovern DPB, Hussain SH, Worthington J *et al.* Clinical and biochemical predictors of efficacy to and intolerance from azathioprine in patients with inflammatory bowel disease. Gut. 2000;46(Suppl. II):A13.

70. Khan ZH, Wicks AC, Mayberry JF *et al.* Retrospective case series analysis of 111 patients with inflammatory bowel disease on azathioprine: a Leicester General Hospital experience. Gut. 1999;44(Suppl. I):A35.

71. Feagan BG, Rochon J, Fedorak *et al.* Methotrexate for the treatment of Crohn's disease. The North American Crohn's Study Group Investigators. N Engl J Med. 1995;332:292–7.

72. Feagan BG, Fedorak RN, Irvine EJ *et al.* A comparison of methotrexate with placebo for the maintenance of remission in Crohn's disease. North American Crohn's Study Group Investigators. N Engl J Med. 2000;342:1627–32.

73. Lebbe C, Beyler C, Gerber NJ *et al.* Intraindividual variability of the bioavailability of low dose methotrexate after oral administration in rheumatoid arthritis. Ann Rheum Dis. 1994;53:475–7.

74. Moshkowitz M, Oren R, Tishler M *et al.* The absorption of low-dose methotrexate in patients with inflammatory bowel disease. Aliment Pharmacol Ther. 1997;11:569–73.

75. Campbell MA, Perrier DG, Dorr RT *et al.* Methotrexate: bioavailability and pharmacokinetics. Cancer Treat Rep. 1985;69:833–8.

76. Jundt JW, Browne BA, Fiocco GP *et al.* A comparison of low dose methotrexate bioavailability: oral solution, oral tablet, subcutaneous and intramuscular dosing. J Rheumatol. 1993;20:1845–9.

77. Egan LJ, Sandborn WJ, Tremaine WJ *et al.* A randomized dose–response and pharmacokinetic study of methotrexate for refractory inflammatory Crohn's disease and ulcerative colitis. Aliment Pharmacol Ther. 1999;13:1597–604.

78. Schroder H, Campbell DES. Absorption, metabolism and excretion of salicylazosulfapyridine in man. Clin Pharmacol Ther. 1972;13:539–51.

79. Das KM, Eastwood MA. Acetylation polymorphism of sulfapyridine in patients with ulcerative colitis and Crohn's disease. Clin Pharmacol Ther. 1975;18:514–20.

80. Azad Khan AK, Nurazzaman M, Trulove SC. The effect of the acetylator phenotype on the metabolism of sulphasalazine in man. J Med Genet. 1983;20:30–6.

81. Schroder H, Evans DAP. Acetylator phenotype and adverse effects of sulphasalazine in healthy subjects. Gut. 1972;13:278–84.

82. Van Hees PA, Van Elferen LW, Van Rossum JM *et al.* Hemolysis during salicylazosulfapyridine therapy. Am J Gastroenterol. 1979;70:501–5.

83. Cowan GO, Das KM, Eastwood MA. Further studies of sulphasalazine metabolism in the treatment of ulcerative colitis. Br Med J. 1977;2:1057–9.

84. Mitchell RS, Bell JC. Clinical implications of isoniazid PAS and streptomycin blood levels in pulmonary tuberculosis. Trans Am Clin Chim Assoc. 1957;69:98–105.

85. Harris HW, Knight RA, Selin KJ. Comparison of isoniazid concentrations in the blood of people of Japanese and European descent. Am Rev Tuberc. 1958;78:944–8.

86. Frieri G, Pimpo MY, Andreoli A *et al.* Prevention of post-operative recurrence of Crohn's disease requires adequate mucosal concentration of mesalazine. Gruppo Italiano per lo Studio del Colon et del Retto. Aliment Pharmacol Ther. 1999;13:577–82.

87. Frieri G, Pimpo MT, Palumbo G *et al.* Anastomotic configuration and mucosal 5-aminosalicylic acid (5-ASA) concentrations in patients with Crohn's disease: a GISC study. Gruppo Italiano per lo Studio del Colon e del Retto. Am J Gastroenterol. 2000;95:1486–90.

88. Rao SSC, Read NW, Brown C *et al.* Studies on the mechanism of bowel disturbance in ulcerative colitis. Gastroenterology. 1987;93:934–40.

89. Munkholm P, Langholz E, Davidsen M *et al.* Frequency of glucocorticoid resistance and dependency in Crohn's disease. Gut. 1994;35:360–2.

90. Lindgreen SC, Flood LM, Kilander AF *et al.* Early predictors of glucocorticosteroid treatment failure in severe and moderately severe attacks of ulcerative colitis. Eur J Gastroenterol Hepatol. 1998;10:831–5.

91. Sandborn WJ, Landers CJ, Tremaine WJ *et al.* Association of antineutrophil cytoplasmic antibodies with resistance to treatment of left-sided ulcerative colitis: results of a pilot study. Mayo Clin Proc. 1996;71:431–6.

92. Heresbach D, Alizadeh M, Bretagne JF *et al.* Investigation of the association of major histocompatibility complex genes, including HLA class I, class II and TAP genes, with clinical forms of Crohn's disease. Eur J Immunogenet. 1996;23:141–51.

93. Heresbach D, Alizadeh M, Bretagne JF *et al.* TAP gene transporter polymorphism in inflammatory bowel diseases. Scand J Gastroenterol. 1997;32:1022–7.

94. Ayabe T, Imai S, Ashida T *et al.* Glucocorticoid receptor beta expression as a novel predictor for therapeutic efficacy of corticosteroid in patients with ulcerative colitis. Gastroenterology. 1998;114:A924.

95. Hearing SD, Norman M, Probert CSJ *et al*. Predicting therapeutic outcome in severe ulcerative colitis by measuring *in vitro* steroid sensitivity of proliferating peripheral blood lymphocytes. Gut. 1999;45:382–8.

96. Corrigan CJ. Glucocorticoid resistant asthma: T-lymphocyte defects. Am J Respir Crit Care Med. 1996;154;S53–4.

97. Kam JC, Szefler SJ, Surs W *et al*. Combination of IL-2 and IL-4 reduces glucocorticoid receptor binding affinity and T cell response to glucocorticoids. J Immunol. 1993;151:3460–6.

98. Adcock IM, Lane SJ, Brown CR *et al*. Abnormal glucocorticoid receptor activator protein 1 interaction in steroid-resistant asthma. J Exp Med. 1995;182:1951–8.

99. Walker KB, Potter JM, House AK. Interleukin 2 synthesis in the presence of steroids: a model of steroid resistance. Clin Exp Immunol. 1987;68:162–7.

100. Farrell RJ, Murphy A, Long A *et al*. High multidrug resistance (P-glycoprotein 170) expression in inflammatory bowel disease patients who fail medical therapy. Gastroenterology. 2000;118:279–88.

101. Hoffmeyer S, Burk O, von Richter O *et al*. Functional polymorphisms of the human multidrug resistance gene: multiple sequence variations and correlation of one allele with P-glycoprotein expression and activity *in vivo*. Proc Natl Acad Sci USA. 2000;97:3473–8.

102. Weishilboum RM, Sladek SL. Mercaptopurine pharmacogenetics: monogenic inheritance of erythrocyte thiopurine methyltransferase activity. Am J Hum Genet. 1980;32:651–62.

103. Lennard L, Lilleyman JS, Van Loon J *et al*. Genetic variation in response to 6-mercaptopurine for childhood acute lymphoblastic leukaemia. Lancet. 1990;336:225–9.

104. Colombel J, Ferrari N, Debuysere H *et al*. Genotypic analysis of thiopurine S-methyltransferase in patients with Crohn's disease and severe myelosuppression during azathioprine therapy. Gastroenterology. 2000;118:1025–30.

105. Higashida K, Kobayashi K, Sugita K *et al*. Pure red blood cell aplasia during azathioprine therapy associated with parvovirus B19 infection. Paediatr Infect Dis J. 1997;16:1093–5.

106. Dubinsky MC, Lamothie S, Ying Yang H *et al*. Pharmacogenomics and metabolite measurement for 6-mercaptopurine therapy in inflammatory bowel disease. Gastroenterology. 2000;118:705–13.

107. Lebbe C, Beyeler C, Gerber NJ *et al*. Intraindividual variability of the bioavailability of low dose methotrexate after oral administration in rheumatoid arthritis. Ann Rheum Dis. 1994;53:475–7.

108. Gorlick R, Goker K, Trippett T *et al*. Intrinsic and acquired resistance to methotrexate in acute leukemia. N Engl J Med. 1996;335:1041–8.

109. Goker E, Waltham M, Kheradpour A *et al*. Amplification of the dihydrofolate reductase gene is a mechanism of acquired resistance to methotrexate in patients with acute lymphoblastic leukemia and is correlated with p53 gene mutations. Blood. 1995;86:677–84.

110. Lin JT, Tong WP, Trippett TM *et al*. Basis for natural resistance to methotrexate in human acute non-lymphocytic leukemia. Leuk Res. 1991;15:1191–6.

111. Wolf CR, Smith G, Smith RL. Pharmacogenetics. Br Med J. 2000;320:987–90.

112. Sutherland L, Ramcharan S, Bryant H *et al*. Effect of cigarette smoking on recurrence of Crohn's disease. Gastroenterology. 1990;98:1123–8.

113. Cottone M, Rosselli M, Orlando A *et al*. Smoking habits and recurrence in Crohn's disease. Gastroenterology. 1994;106:643–8.

114. Van Os EC, Zins BJ, Sandborn WJ *et al*. Azathioprine pharmacokinetics after intravenous, oral, delayed release oral and rectal foam administration. Gut. 1996;39:63–8.

115. Hawthorne AB, Logan RFA, Hawkey CJ *et al*. Randomised controlled trial of azathioprine withdrawal in ulcerative colitis. Br Med J. 1992;305:20–3.

116. Pearson DC, May GR, Fick GH *et al*. Azathioprine and 6-mercaptopurine in Crohn's disease. A meta-analysis. Ann Intern Med. 1995;123:132–42.

117. Hanauer S, Schwartz J, Robinson M *et al*. Mesalamine capsules for treatment of active ulcerative colitis: results of a controlled trial. Am J Gastroenterol. 1993;88:1188–97.

118. Kruis W, Judmaier G, Kayasseh L *et al*. Double-blind dose-finding study of olsalazine vs sulphasalazine as maintenance therapy for ulcerative colitis. Eur J Gastroenterol Hepatol. 1995;7:391–6.

Section III
Standards: azathioprine/ 6-mercaptopurine

9
Azathioprine/6-mercaptopurine: mechanisms of action, pharmacology and toxicology

W. J. SANDBORN

INTRODUCTION

6-Mercaptopurine and its prodrug azathioprine are effective in inducing and maintaining remission in patients with ulcerative colitis and Crohn's disease[1,2]. The metabolism of these drugs is complex, and practising clinicians often use drug regimens that do not make sense based on their clinical pharmacology[3]. This chapter reviews the mechanisms of action, the clinical pharmacology, and the toxicology of azathioprine and 6-mercaptopurine therapy in patients with inflammatory bowel disease.

MECHANISM OF ACTION

The precise mechanism of action of azathioprine and 6-mercaptopurine is not known. The putative active metabolites of azathioprine and 6-mercaptopurine are the 6-thioguanine nucleotides which apparently inhibit the synthesis of proteins, DNA, and RNA by incorporation into DNA followed by alteration in transcription and/or DNA repair[3]. Proposed mechanisms of action include: (a) inhibition of purine nucleotide biosynthesis and interconversion by the intermediate metabolite thioinosinic acid with resulting inhibition of the DNA synthetic phase of the cell cycle[4]; (b) inhibition of the mixed lymphocyte reaction via interference of antigenic triggering of lymphocytes (azathioprine > 6-mercaptopurine)[5,6]; (c) reduction in natural killer and K cell cytotoxicity[7]; (d) reduction in plasma cells in the rectal lamina propria and a fall in the peripheral lymphocyte count[7,8].

METABOLISM OF AZATHIOPRINE AND 6-MERCAPTOPURINE

Azathioprine is a prodrug that is converted to 6-mercaptopurine via a non-enzymatic nucleophilic attack by sulphydryl-containing compounds such as glutathione present in erythrocytes and other tissues[9,10]. 6-Mercaptopurine is then degraded by thiopurine methyltransferase to 6-methylmercaptopurine or by xanthine oxidase to 6-thiouric acid[3,11]. Alternatively, 6-mercaptopurine may be activated via a multistep enzymatic pathway beginning with the enzyme hypoxanthine phosphoribosyl transferase followed by inosine monophosphate dehydrogenase and guanosine monophosphate synthetase (Fig. 1)[3,11]. The enzyme activity of thiopurine methyltransferase is under genetic control and will be discussed in more detail below[12].

PHARMACOKINETICS OF AZATHIOPRINE AND 6-MERCAPTOPURINE

The median oral bioavailability of azathioprine is 47% (range 27–83%)[13]. The time of maximal concentration for 6-mercaptopurine following azathioprine administration is 2 h, and the half-life is approximately 1 h. The oral bioavailability of 6-mercaptopurine is even lower, approximately 16%[14]. Parent azathioprine and 6-mercaptopurine are not therapeutically active[3]. The putative active metabolites, the 6-thioguanine nucleotides, have a half-life of several days or more[11]. Steady-state concentrations of the 6-thioguanine nucleotides occur after 2–4 weeks of oral dosing with azathioprine 2.0 mg/kg per day[15]. Approximately 88% of azathioprine is converted to 6-mercaptopurine[16]. Azathioprine is 55% 6-mercaptopurine by molecular weight. Thus, a conversion factor of 2.08 will convert a dose of 6-mercaptopurine to azathioprine. This conversion does not account for potential differences in oral bioavailability or efficacy between the two drugs.

GENETIC CONTROL OF THIOPURINE METHYLTRANSFERASE ENZYME ACTIVITY

The enzymatic activity of thiopurine methyltransferase (as determined by radioimmunoassay) is genetically determined[12]. There is a trimodal distribution

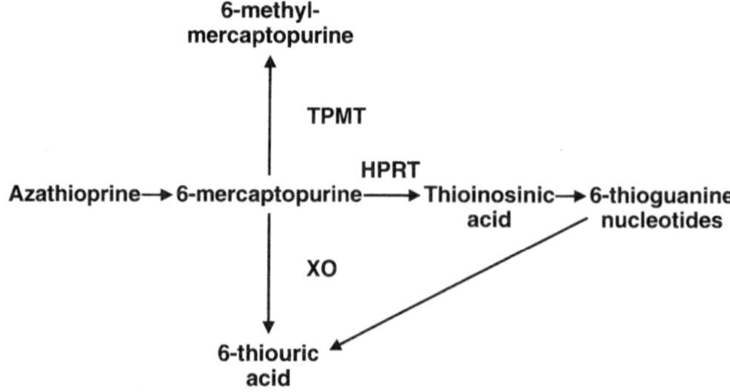

Figure 1 Metabolism of azathioprine and 6-mercaptopurine (TPMT = thiopurine methyltransferase; HPRT = hypoxanthine phosphoribosyl transferase; XO = xanthine oxidase). Reprinted with permission from ref. 11

of thiopurine methyltransferase activity in the general population: homozygous low activity ($<$5.0 U/ml RBC) occurs at a frequency of 0.3%; heterozygous or intermediate activity (5.0–13.7 U/ml RBC) occurs at a frequency of 11.1%; and homozygous high or normal activity (13.8–25.1 U/ml RBC) occurs at a frequency of 88.6% (Fig. 2)[12]. This distribution is consistent with monogenic inheritance. The thiopurine methyltransferase gene has been localized to the short arm of chromosome six[17]. A total of 10 variant alleles for thiopurine methyltransferase have been associated with decreased enzyme activity (*2, *3A, *3B, *3C, *3D, *4, *5, *6, *7, *10) (Fig. 3)[18–20]. The frequency distributions of variant alleles in a large series of patients submitting blood to a clinical laboratory, and in a group of patients with absent thiopurine methyltransferase activity, are shown in Tables 1 and 2[18].

Patients with low or intermediate thiopurine methyltransferase enzyme activity shunt 6-mercaptopurine away from the 6-methylmercaptopurine metabolite and towards the 6-thioguanine nucleotides. Excess concentrations of 6-thioguanine nucleotides have been associated with leukopenia[21,22]. Thus, a baseline determination of thiopurine methyltransferase activity (phenotype) or genotype could be clinically useful to 'customize' the drug dose with the goal of reducing the frequency of leukopenia. Several studies have suggested that this strategy can be effective. One study prospectively determined thiopurine methyltransferase genotypes in 67 consecutive patients with rheumatological disease who were initiating azathioprine therapy at a dose of 2–3 mg/kg per day[23]. The thiopurine methyltransferase genotypes were determined for the *3A, *3C, and *2 variant allele. Six of 67 patients (9%) were heterozygous for thiopurine methyltransferase activity, all six had the *3A allele. Five of six heterozygous patients with intermediate thiopurine methyltransferase activity discontinued therapy within 1 month because of leukopenia, and the sixth patient did not adhere to therapy. The median duration of therapy was 2 weeks (range 2–4 weeks) in the group

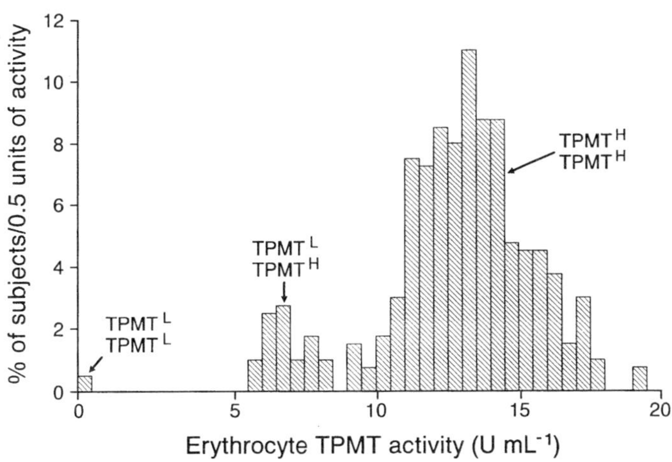

Figure 2 Frequency distribution of red blood cell (RBC) thiopurine methyltransferase activity in a randomly selected population of 298 adult blood donors. Reprinted with permission from ref. 12

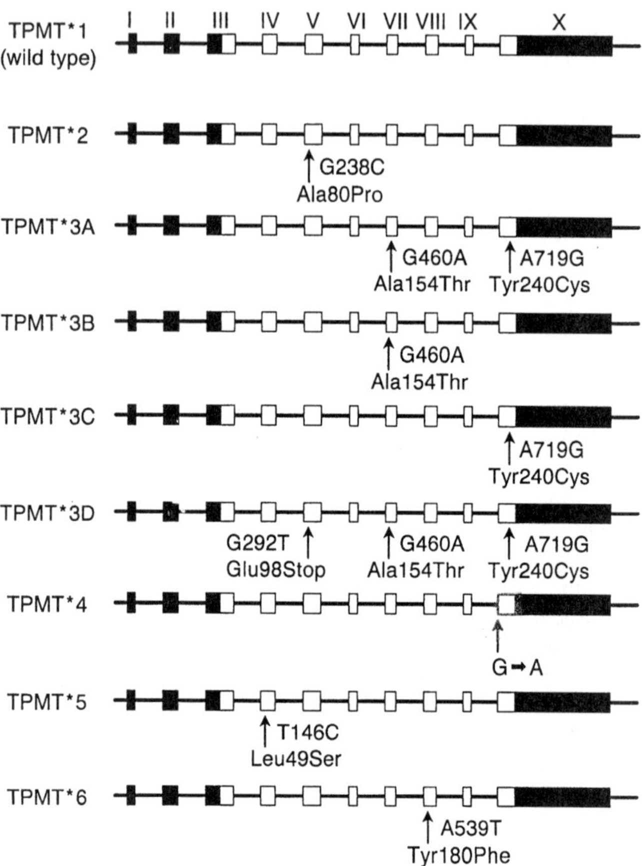

Figure 3 Thiopurine methyltransferase (TPMT) alleles. The figure depicts schematically the 'wild-type' allele for TPMT (TPMT*1) and eight variant alleles for low enzyme activity. Black rectangles represent exons that encode open reading frame (ORF) sequence; white rectangles represent exons or portions of exons that encode untranslated region sequence. Roman numerals are exon numbers. Exon sizes are proportional to their relative lengths, but introns vary greatly in length even though they have been depicted as being equal. Reprinted with permission from ref. 18

with heterozygous thiopurine methyltransferase activity, and 39 weeks (6–180 weeks) in the group with wild-type thiopurine methyltransferase activity. In a second study, 41 patients with Crohn's disease who had developed severe myelo-suppression (white blood cell count < 3000 or platelet count < 100 000) during treatment with azathioprine or 6-mercaptopurine were evaluated for thiopurine methyltransferase genotype[20]. The thiopurine methyltransferase genotypes were determined for the *2, *3A, *3B, *3C, *3D, *4, *5, *6, *7, and *10 variant alleles. Four of 41 patients (10%) had low activity and seven of 41 (17%) had intermediate activity. Early leukopenia was noted in the subjects with low or intermediate thiopurine methyltransferase activity, whereas normal thiopurine methyltransferase activity was noted in patients with late leukopenia. Taken

Table 1   Thiopurine methyltransferase variant allele frequencies in clinical laboratory samples

Allele	No.	Frequency among variant alleles	Frequency in population
*2	1	0.032	0.0018
*3A	17	0.548	0.0300
*3B	2	0.065	0.0035
*3C	4	0.129	0.0071
*3D	1	0.032	0.0018
*4	0	0.000	0.0000
*5	1	0.032	0.0018
?	5	0.161	0.0088

Frequency values were calculated on the basis of the assumption that all 29 samples with intermediate activity were heterozygous, whereas the one sample with very low activity was homozygous for an allele or alleles for low activity, resulting in a total of 31 variant alleles in 30 samples. The frequencies listed as 'among variant alleles' have been calculated on the basis of the 31 variant alleles. The 'population' frequencies are based on proportions of all 566 alleles present in 283 clinical samples studied. Reprinted with permission from ref. 18.

Table 2   Thiopurine methyltransferase (TPMT) genotypes of 18 subjects with very low or absent red blood cell TPMT activity

TPMT genotype	Number of subjects
*3A *3A	12
*3A *3C	4
*3A *4	1
*3A *2	1

Reprinted with permission from ref. 18.

together, these studies suggest that baseline determination of thiopurine methyltransferase activity (phenotype) or genotype can predict the occurrence of early leukopenia in patients with rheumatological diseases or Crohn's disease treated with azathioprine. This observation has led to the recommendation that patients with normal thiopurine methyltransferase activity receive standard doses of azathioprine (2–2.5 mg/kg per day) or 6-mercaptopurine (1.0–1.5 mg/kg per day); and that patients with intermediate thiopurine methyltransferase enzyme activity have their dose of azathioprine or 6-mercaptopurine reduced by 50%[24,25]. Patients with low thiopurine methyltransferase activity should not be treated with azathioprine or 6-mercaptopurine, due to a high mortality from leukopenia and sepsis[26].

THERAPEUTIC DRUG MONITORING

Several studies have reported that patients with inflammatory bowel disease treated with azathioprine or 6-mercaptopurine who respond to therapy have higher median concentrations of the 6-thioguanine nucleotides than patients who fail to respond to therapy[27,28]. One recent study in 93 patients with inflammatory bowel disease reported that the median concentration of 6-thioguanine nucleotides in erythrocytes in responding patients was $312 \, pmol/8 \times 10^8$ RBCs compared to a median concentration of 199 in patients who fail to respond (Table 3)[28]. There was no difference in the median concentrations of 6-methylmercaptopurine between the two patient groups. The breakpoint between the lower two quartiles and the higher two quartiles of 6-thioguanine nucleotide concentrations was $235 \, pmol/8 \times 10^8$ RBCs (Fig. 4a). Sixty-five per cent of responding patients had an erythrocyte 6-thioguanine nucleotide concentration >235 as compared to only 27% of patients failing therapy (Fig. 4b).

Table 3 Values of 6-thioguanine and 6-methylmercaptopurine at designated clinical evaluation points corresponding to therapeutic efficacy

Group	No.	Median 6-thioguanine nucleotide	Median 6-methyl mercaptopurine
Remission	103	312	2683
Relapse	70	199	1739
p-Value		<0.0001	0.37

Reprinted with permission from ref. 28.

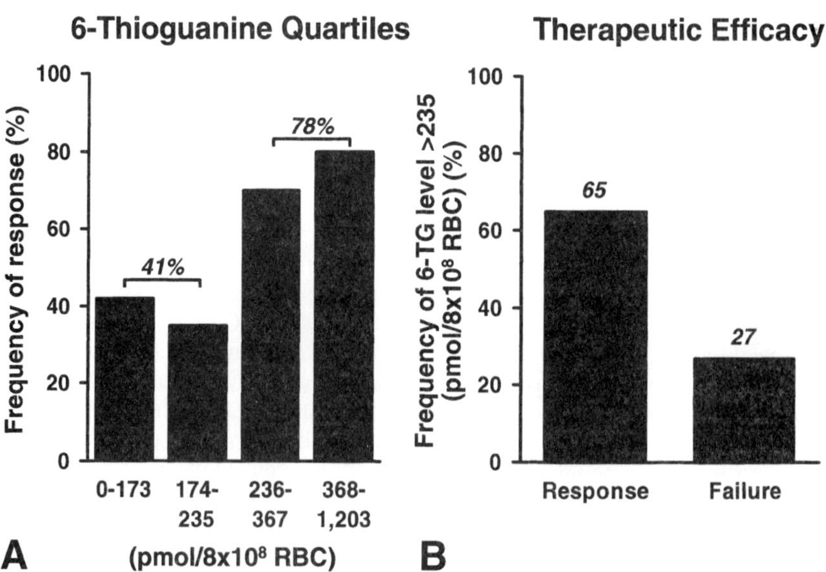

Figure 4 A: Correlation of quartile 6-mercaptopurine metabolite levels with clinical response in inflammatory bowel disease. The frequency of clinical response was significantly higher within the upper 6-thioguanine quartiles ($>235 \, pmol/8 \times 10^8$ RBC), $p<0.001$. B: Frequency of 6-thioguanine levels >235 (pmol/8 × 10⁸ RBC) at clinical evaluation points corresponding to therapeutic response, compared with points of therapeutic failure. $p<0.001$. Reprinted with permission from ref. 28

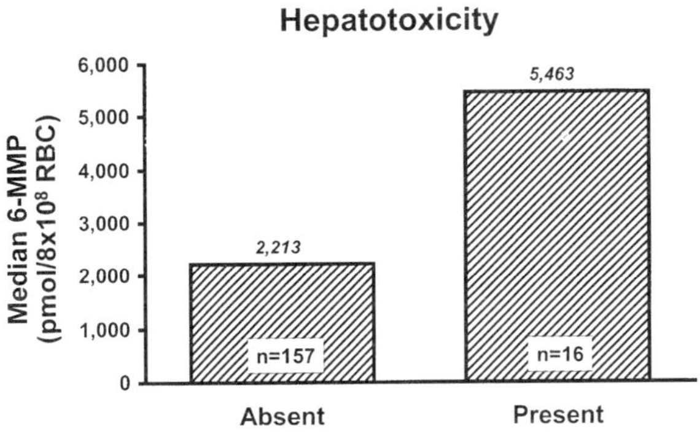

Hepatotoxicity

Figure 5 Correlation of erythrocyte 6-mercaptopurine metabolite levels with drug-related side-effects in inflammatory bowel disease. Correlation of 6-methylmercaptopurine levels with hepatotoxicity. Hepatotoxic events were associated with higher median 6-methylmercaptopurine levels. $p < 0.5$. Reprinted with permission from ref. 28

Thus, the authors suggested that clinicians should adjust azathioprine or 6-mercaptopurine doses to achieve erythrocyte 6-thioguanine nucleotide concentrations > 235 pmol/8 $\times$ 10^8 RBCs. The authors also reported that hepatotoxicity (defined as liver enzymes more than twice normal) occurred in 16 patients, and that the median erythrocyte 6-methylmercaptopurine concentrations were 5463 pmol/8 $\times$ 10^8 RBCs in patients with hepatotoxicity compared to only 2213 pmol/8 $\times$ 10^8 RBCs in patients without hepatotoxicity (Fig. 5)[28]. These findings have not been universally confirmed[15,29]. One recent abstract showed no relationship between disease activity and whole blood 6-thioguanine nucleotide concentrations in 170 patients with inflammatory bowel disease treated with azathioprine or 6-mercaptopurine[29].

TOXICOLOGY

Toxicity associated with azathioprine or 6-mercaptopurine can generally be divided into two types of reactions: allergic-type reactions and non-allergic-type reactions[2]. Allergic-type reactions often occur within 3–4 weeks of initiating therapy, and rechallenge will almost universally lead to recurrent symptoms within one or two doses, and sometimes within minutes to hours. Examples of allergic reactions include pancreatitis, fever, rash, malaise, worsening diarrhoea, and some cases of hepatitis[30–33]. These reactions are probably immunologically mediated and do not appear to be dose-dependent. Non-allergic-type reactions include leukopenia thrombocytopenia, infections, malignancy, and some cases of hepatitis. Elevated concentrations of 6-thioguanine nucleotides are thought to correlate with leukopenia and thrombocytopenia (these would occur more frequently in patients with low or intermediate thiopurine methyltransferase activity), whereas elevated concentrations of 6-methylmercaptopurine are thought to correlate with some cases of hepatitis[21,22,28]. Non-allergic-type reactions are typically dose-dependent. The frequency of adverse reactions in one large series of

396 patients with inflammatory bowel disease treated with 6-mercaptopurine was as follows: overall toxicity 15%; pancreatitis 3.3%, depression 2–5%, allergic reactions 2%; drug hepatitis 0.3%; infectious complications 7.4%; malignant neoplasms 3.1%[30]. The frequency of infectious complications and neoplasms was thought to be similar to the background population, although one patient had herpes virus encephalitis and one patient had a non-Hodgkin's lymphoma involving the central nervous system (both of which could reasonably have been attributed to immune modifier therapy). Other studies have suggested that the frequency of bone marrow suppression is more in the range of 5–10%[34,35]. One large study with over 700 patients did not report an increasing in neoplasms in patients with inflammatory bowel disease treated with azathioprine[36].

NOVEL AZATHIOPRINE DELIVERY SYSTEM

Studies have demonstrated that direct administration of azathioprine to the terminal ileum or colon using delayed-release delivery systems (Eudragit-coated capsules) or rectal foam enemas can markedly reduce the systemic absorption of azathioprine and 6-mercaptopurine[13,37]. The bioavailability of azathioprine administered to the rectum or to the ileum/caecum is 5–10%[13,37]. Thus, 'topical delivery' of azathioprine has the potential to significantly improve the safety profile of azathioprine therapy in patients with inflammatory bowel disease. A double-blind, placebo-controlled dose-ranging trial of delayed-release oral azathioprine in patients with active Crohn's disease is under way in the United States.

CONCLUSIONS

The precise mechanism of action for azathioprine and 6-mercaptopurine is unknown. The oral bioavailability of azathioprine is 50% and for 6-mercaptopurine is 16%. Low thiopurine methyltransferase activity leads to greater concentrations of 6-thioguanine nucleotides, and thiopurine methyltransferase activity is genetically regulated. Patients with low thiopurine methyltransferase activity are at risk for dose-related toxicity associated with azathioprine or 6-mercaptopurine therapy. Some but not all studies have indicated that therapy drug monitoring with erythrocyte 6-thioguanine nucleotides may be clinically useful. The toxicity associated with azathioprine and 6-mercaptopurine is acceptable for selected patients, but may not be acceptable for first-line therapy. Delayed-release oral azathioprine reduces systemic exposure to 6-mercaptopurine, and this should translate into an improved safety profile; however, placebo-controlled efficacy trials are needed.

References

1. Pearson DC, May GR, Fick GH, Sutherland LR. Azathioprine and 6-mercaptopurine in Crohn's disease. A meta-analysis. Ann Intern Med. 1995;123:132–42.
2. Sandborn WJ. A review of immune modifier therapy for inflammatory bowel disease: azathioprine, 6-mercaptopurine, cyclosporine, and methotrexate [See comments]. Am J Gastroenterol. 1996;91:423–33.

3. Lennard L. The clinical pharmacology of 6-mercaptopurine. Eur J Clin Pharmacol. 1992;43: 329–39.
4. Bach JF. The mode of action of immunosuppressive agents. Front Biol. 1975;41:1–374.
5. Szawlowski PW, Al Safi SA, Dooley T, Maddocks JL. Azathioprine suppresses the mixed lymphocyte reaction of patients with Lesch–Nyhan syndrome. Br J Clin Pharmacol. 1985;20: 489–91.
6. Elion GB. Immunosuppressive agents. Transplant Proc. 1977;9:975–9.
7. Campbell AC, Skinner JM, Maclennan IC et al. Immunosuppression in the treatment of inflammatory bowel disease. II. The effects of azathioprine on lymphoid cell populations in a double blind trial in ulcerative colitis. Clin Exp Immunol. 1976;24:249–58.
8. Campbell AC, Skinner JM, Hersey P, Roberts-Thomson P, Maclennan IC, Truelove SC. Immunosuppression in the treatment of inflammatory bowel disease. I. Changes in lymphoid sub-populations in the blood and rectal mucosa following cessation of treatment with azathioprine. Clin Exp Immunol. 1974;16:521–33.
9. Chalmers AH. Studies on the mechanism of formation of 5-mercapto-1-methyl-4-nitroimidazole, a metabolite of the immunosuppressive drug azathioprine. Biochem Pharmacol. 1974;23:1891–901.
10. de Miranda P, Beacham LM III, Creagh TH, Elion GB. The metabolic fate of the methylnitroimidazole moiety of azathioprine in the rat. J Pharmacol Exp Ther. 1973;187:588–601.
11. Chan GL, Erdmann GR, Gruber SA, Matas AJ, Canafax DM. Azathioprine metabolism: pharmacokinetics of 6-mercaptopurine, 6-thiouric acid and 6-thioguanine nucleotides in transplant patients. J Clin Pharmacol. 1990;30:358–63.
12. Weinshilboum RM, Sladek SL. Mercaptopurine pharmacogenetics: monogenic inheritance of erythrocyte thiopurine methyltransferase activity. Am J Hum Genet. 1980;32:651–62.
13. van Os EC, Zins BJ, Sandborn WJ et al. Azathioprine pharmacokinetics after intravenous, oral, delayed release oral and rectal foam administration. Gut. 1996;39:63–8.
14. Zimm S, Collins JM, Riccardi R et al. Variable bioavailability of oral mercaptopurine. Is maintenance chemotherapy in acute lymphoblastic leukemia being optimally delivered? N Engl J Med. 1983;308:1005–9.
15. Sandborn WJ, Tremaine WJ, Wolf DC et al. Lack of effect of intravenous administration on time to respond to azathioprine for steroid-treated Crohn's disease. North American Azathioprine Study Group. Gastroenterology. 1999;117:527–35.
16. Elion GB. The comparative metabolism of Imuran and 6-mercaptopurine in man. Proc Am Assoc Cancer Res. 1969;21.
17. Lee D, Szumlanski C, Houtman J et al. Thiopurine methyltransferase pharmacogenetics. Cloning of human liver cDNA and a processed pseudogene on human chromosome 18q21.1. Drug Metab Dispos. 1995;23:398–405.
18. Otterness D, Szumlanski C, Lennard L et al. Human thiopurine methyltransferase pharmacogenetics: gene sequence polymorphisms. Clin Pharmacol Ther. 1997;62:60–73.
19. Yates CR, Krynetski EY, Loennechen T et al. Molecular diagnosis of thiopurine S-methyltransferase deficiency: genetic basis for azathioprine and mercaptopurine intolerance [See comments]. Ann Intern Med. 1997;126:608–14.
20. Colombel JF, Ferrari N, Debuysere H et al. Genotypic analysis of thiopurine S-methyltransferase in patients with Crohn's disease and severe myelosuppression during azathioprine therapy. Gastroenterology. 2000;118:1025–30.
21. Lennard L, Van Loon JA, Weinshilboum RM. Pharmacogenetics of acute azathioprine toxicity: relationship to thiopurine methyltransferase genetic polymorphism. Clin Pharmacol Ther. 1989;46:149–54.
22. Lennard L, Rees CA, Lilleyman JS, Maddocks JL. Childhood leukaemia: a relationship between intracellular 6-mercaptopurine metabolites and neutropenia. Br J Clin Pharmacol. 1983;16:359–63.
23. Black AJ, McLeod HL, Capell HA et al. Thiopurine methyltransferase genotype predicts therapy-limiting severe toxicity from azathioprine. Ann Intern Med. 1998;129:716–18.
24. Snow JL, Gibson LE. The role of genetic variation in thiopurine methyltransferase activity and the efficacy and/or side effects of azathioprine therapy in dermatologic patients [See comments]. Arch Dermatol. 1995;131:193–7.
25. Snow JL, Gibson LE. A pharmacogenetic basis for the safe and effective use of azathioprine and other thiopurine drugs in dermatologic patients. J Am Acad Dermatol. 1995;32:114–16.
26. Anstey A, Lennard L, Mayou SC, Kirby JD. Pancytopenia related to azathioprine – an enzyme deficiency caused by a common genetic polymorphism: a review. J R Soc Med. 1992;85:752–6.

27. Cuffari C, Theoret Y, Latour S, Seidman G. 6-Mercaptopurine metabolism in Crohn's disease: correlation with efficacy and toxicity. Gut. 1996;39:401–6.
28. Dubinsky MC, Lamothe S, Yang HY *et al.* Pharmacogenomics and metabolite measurement for 6-mercaptopurine therapy in inflammatory bowel disease. Gastroenterology. 2000;118:705–13.
29. Lowry PW, Franklin CL, Weaver AL *et al.* Cross-sectional study of IBD patients taking azathioprine (AZA) or 6-mercaptopurine (6-MP): lack of correlation between disease activity and 6-thioguanine nucleotide (6-TGN) concentration. Gastroenterology. 2000;118:A788.
30. Present DH, Meltzer SJ, Krumholz MP, Wolke A, Korelitz BI. 6-Mercaptopurine in the management of inflammatory bowel disease: short- and long-term toxicity. Ann Intern Med. 1989;111:641–9.
31. Haber CJ, Meltzer SJ, Present DH, Korelitz BI. Nature and course of pancreatitis caused by 6-mercaptopurine in the treatment of inflammatory bowel disease. Gastroenterology. 1986;91:982–6.
32. Sturdevant RA, Singleton JW, Deren JL, Law DH, McCleery JL. Azathioprine-related pancreatitis in patients with Crohn's disease. Gastroenterology. 1979;77:883–6.
33. Cox J, Daneshmend TK, Hawkey CJ, Logan RF, Walt RP. Devastating diarrhoea caused by azathioprine: management difficulty in inflammatory bowel disease. Gut. 1988;29:686–8.
34. Connell WR, Kamm MA, Ritchie JK, Lennard-Jones JE. Bone marrow toxicity caused by azathioprine in inflammatory bowel disease: 27 years of experience. Gut. 1993;34:1081–5.
35. Kirschner BS. Safety of azathioprine and 6-mercaptopurine in pediatric patients within inflammatory bowel disease. Gastroenterology. 1998;115:813–21.
36. Connell WR, Kamm MA, Dickson M, Balkwill AM, Ritchie JK, Lennard-Jones JE. Long-term neoplasia risk after azathioprine treatment in inflammatory bowel disease. Lancet. 1994;343:1249–52.
37. Zins BJ, Sandborn WJ, McKinney JA *et al.* A dose-ranging study of azathioprine pharmacokinetics after single-dose administration of a delayed-release oral formulation. J Clin Pharmacol. 1997;37:38–46.

10
Azathioprine and 6-mercaptopurine in Crohn's disease: acute and chronic active

L. R. SUTHERLAND

INTRODUCTION

Over the past two decades one of the major trends in the therapy of inflammatory bowel disease has been the growing utilization of azathioprine and 6-mercaptopurine (6-MP) by the practice community. At the beginning of the 1990s the use of azathioprine was restricted to only a few centres across North America. By the end of the decade usage of both azathioprine and 6-MP had increased markedly[1]. In particular both medications are being introduced into the therapy of the disease at a much earlier stage. This chapter will review the randomized controlled trials of both azathioprine and 6-MP in the induction and maintenance of remission for Crohn's disease. The mechanism of action, pharmacology and role of monitoring drug levels will be covered by Sandborn (Chapter 9). Pregnancy and azathioprine/6-MP therapy will be reviewed in the chapter on the topic by Dignass (Chapter 26).

INDUCTION OF REMISSION FOR CROHN'S DISEASE

The first isolated case reports of the use of azathioprine for induction of remission in patients with Crohn's disease appeared in the early 1970s. It was not until several years later that the first randomized trials of azathioprine therapy were reported. As was typical of the time, the original trials can be characterized as being both underpowered and including a heterogeneous group of patients. Initially there was confusion regarding the duration of therapy required to induce remission. For example, one trial assessed patients after only 8 weeks of therapy[2]. It was not until the late 1970s and early 1980s that large trials of azathioprine or 6-MP became available[3,4].

In a recent update[5] of the meta-analysis of the use of azathioprine for the induction of remission[6] eight trials involving 425 patients were identified[2-4,7-13]. When the initial analysis was performed significant heterogeneity was encountered. This was not surprising as the duration of therapy ranged from 8 to 52 weeks. It was found that most of the heterogeneity could be explained by creating a new variable representing the cumulative dose (dose/day × duration of trial). The possibility of entering remission increased with increasing cumulative dose. With this adjustment the analysis suggested that patients receiving azathioprine or 6-MP were three times as apt to enter remission compared to those receiving placebo. The number needed to treat (NNT) is 4. Four patients will have to be treated in order to induce one remission with azathioprine.

What other lessons can we learn from the meta-analysis? In reviewing the clinical trials it is striking that the trials in which the majority of patients were not on steroids at the time of initiation of azathioprine therapy generally failed. On the other hand trials in which the azathioprine or 6-MP was given concurrently with steroids were successful. Trials which reported a duration of therapy of ⩽17 weeks generally failed to demonstrate efficacy. Trials of longer than 17 weeks were more often positive. The analysis also demonstrated a steroid-sparing effect of azathioprine.

One of the drawbacks of azathioprine therapy has been the long duration of time required prior to the onset of action. Sandborn and associates proposed that the onset of action could be accelerated by giving a loading dose of azathioprine for the rapid induction of remission. Despite an encouraging open series[11], a large randomized, placebo-controlled trial of intravenous azathioprine failed to demonstrate efficacy[12].

Markowitz has performed a randomized placebo-controlled trial of azathioprine in the paediatric Crohn's disease population and reports impressive results[13]. Fifty-five children were randomly assigned to receive 40 mg of prednisone daily and either 6-MP (1.5 mg/kg per day) or placebo. Remission rates were the same for both groups (89%) at the 3-month assessment, but at the 6-month follow-up there were significant differences between the two groups in terms of the number of children in remission (Fig. 1). In this study the 6-MP appeared to add little benefit in the induction of remission but had superior remission-sustaining properties compared to placebo.

Oren and colleagues reported a randomized controlled trial of methotrexate (12.5 mg/week p.o.), 6-MP (50 mg/day) compared to placebo in a group of patients requiring steroids on a regular basis[14]. The proportion of patients entering remission and the proportion of patients who relapsed following induction of remission did not differ between groups. However, the trial involved only a small number of patients and lacked statistical power to detect small differences in efficacy.

The key message in the use of azathioprine in the induction of remission of Crohn's disease is to be sure that the patient receives an adequate dose of therapy. Many of the patients I see that have been characterized as azathioprine failures have not received an adequate dose (2.0–2.5 mg/kg per day) or duration of therapy (at least 6 months). While it appears that it is not necessary to induce leukopenia in order to induce remission, experienced clinicians do not abandon azathioprine therapy until a degree of leukopenia is reached[15].

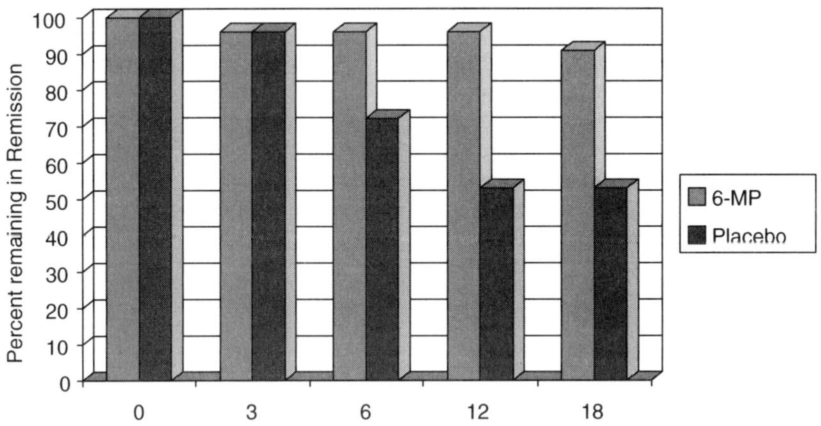

Figure 1   Effect of 6-MP on maintenance of remission in children with Crohn's disease

MAINTENANCE OF REMISSION IN CROHN'S DISEASE

While the induction of remission is important both to physicians and patients, an even more crucial issue is the potential for either azathioprine or 6-MP either to maintain a medically induced remission or to prevent postoperative recurrence. The search for effective maintenance therapy continues. At this point in time the use of mesalamine as maintenance therapy in Crohn's disease remains a source of controversy. There is little support for the use of corticosteroids as maintenance therapy. What role does azathioprine have to play in maintenance therapy of Crohn's disease?

In a recent meta-analysis of azathioprine for maintenance of remission in Crohn's disease patients, six trials involving 319 patients were identified[4,7,10,16,17]. For this analysis there was no evidence of heterogeneity. The odds ratio of staying in remission for all azathioprine-treated patients compared to placebo-treated controls was 2:1 and the NNT was 7. The range of doses of azathioprine varied from 1.0 to 2.5 mg/kg per day. When the data are arranged by daily dose of azathioprine or 6-MP there is a suggestion that the same dose of azathioprine given for induction of remission is also the most effective for maintenance of remission (2.5 mg/kg per day).

Modigliani, in a recent review of the issue of duration of therapy, posed three questions (although he admitted that there was no clear answer to any of the three)[18]. The issues included the relapse risk after discontinuation of therapy, the risks related to continuing the therapy and finally whether or not a previous response to therapy predicted success for subsequent courses of azathioprine.

A major question to be answered is the optimal duration of azathioprine therapy. Investigators in France have reviewed their experience with azathioprine given for a longer duration of time. In their retrospective review they concluded that the risk of relapse after discontinuation of 6-MP was high after 1 and 3 years' therapy. However, there was little additional benefit to be gained if the patient had remained in remission for more than 4 years after the initiation of therapy[19]. A similar survey conducted by American investigators failed to confirm the report from France, but methodological differences between the two studies may explain the differences[20]. The question may be answered by a new clinical trial. A new randomized controlled withdrawal trial for patients who are in remission on azathioprine is currently under way in France. To be eligible, patients have to be in remission for 48 months. The results are expected in 2001.

Present and colleagues have reported their personal experience with almost 400 patients receiving 6-MP[21]. Mean follow-up was approximately 5 years. Recognized complications included pancreatitis (3%), myelosuppression (2%), infections (7%), allergic reactions (2%), hepatitis (2%), and malignancy (3%).

Another group of patients who might benefit from azathioprine/6-MP therapy are patients who have just undergone resection for Crohn's disease. In a large multicentre trial 6-MP was shown to have superior maintenance-sustaining properties compared to either the mesalamine- or placebo-treated patients. It is also important to note that the difference between azathioprine treatment and placebo was essentially nil. The relatively low response rate to 6-MP may all have been related to the low dose of 6-MP given. The dose chosen in this investigator-initiated trial may have been to minimize adverse events rather than maximize efficacy[22].

Immunomodulation has now become an accepted therapy for Crohn's disease. The importance of this approach is recognized by this symposium, which represents a coming-of-age of azathioprine and 6-MP as standard therapy for patients with active or chronic-active Crohn's disease.

References

1. Meuwissen SG, Ewe K, Gassull MA *et al*. IOIBD questionnaire on the clinical use of azathioprine, 6-mercaptopurine, cyclosporin A and methotrexate in the treatment of Crohn's disease. Eur J Gastroenterol Hepatol. 2000;12:13–18.
2. Rhodes J, Bainton D, Beck P, Campbell H. Controlled trial of azathioprine in Crohn's disease. Lancet. 1971;2:1273–6.
3. Present DH, Korelitz BI, Wisch N, Glass JL, Sachar DB, Pasternack BS. Treatment of Crohn's disease with 6-mercaptopurine (6-MP) a long-term, randomized, double blind study. N Engl J Med. 1980;302:981–7.
4. Summers RW, Switz DM, Sessions JT Jr *et al*. National Cooperative Crohn's Disease Study: Results of drug treatment. Gastroenterology. 1979;77:847–69.
5. Sandborn W, Sutherland L, Pearson D, May G, Modigliani R, Prantera C. Azathioprine or 6-mercaptopurine for inducing remission of Crohn's disease (Cochrane Review). In: The Cochrane Library Issue 3 2000 Oxford. Update Software.
6. Pearson DC, May GR, Fick GH, Sutherland LR. Azathioprine and 6-mercaptopurine in Crohn disease. A meta-analysis. Ann Intern Med. 1995;123:132–42.
7. Willoughby JMT, Kumar PJ, Beckett J, Dawson AM. Controlled trial of azathioprine in Crohn's disease. Lancet. 1971;2:944–6.
8. Klein M, Binder HJ, Mitchell M, Aaronson R, Spiro H. Treatment of Crohn's disease with azathioprine: a controlled evaluation. Gastroenterology. 1974;66:916–22.
9. Ewe K, Press AG, Singe CC *et al*. Azathioprine combined with prednisolone or monotherapy with prednisolone in active Crohn's disease. Gastroenterology. 1993;105:367–72.
10. Candy S, Wright J, Gerber M, Adams G, Gerig M, Goodman R. A controlled double-blind study of azathioprine in the management of Crohn's disease. Gut. 1995;37:674–8.
11. Sandborn WJ, Van Os EC, Zins BJ, Tremaine WJ, Mays DC, Lipsky JJ. An intravenous loading dose of azathioprine decreases the time to response in patients with Crohn's disease. Gastroenterology. 1995;109:1808–17.
12. Sandborn WJ, Tremaine WJ, Wolf DC *et al*. Lack of effect of intravenous administration on time to respond to azathioprine for steroid-treated Crohn's disease. Gastroenterology. 1999;117:527–35.

13. Markowitz JF. The multicenter pediatric Crohn's disease 6 mercaptopurine trial: final results. Gastroenterology. 1998;114:1032 (abstract).
14. Oren R, Moshkowitz M, Odes S *et al*. Methotrexate in chronic active Crohn's disease: a double-blind, randomized, Israeli multicenter trial. Am J Gastroenterol. 1997;92:2203–9.
15. Colonna T, Korelitz BI. The role of leukopenia in the 6-mercaptopurine-induced remission of refractory Crohn's disease. Am J Gastroenterol. 1994;89:362–6.
16. Rosenberg JL, Levin B, Wall A, Kirsner JB. A controlled trial of azathioprine in Crohn's disease. Dig Dis. 1975;20:721–6.
17. O'Donoghue DP, Dawson AM, Powell-Tuck J, Bown RL, Lennard-Jones JE. Double-blind withdrawal trial of azathioprine as maintenance treatment for Crohn's disease. Lancet. 1978;2:955–7.
18. Modigliani R. Immunosuppressors for inflammatory bowel disease: how long is long enough? Inflam Bowel Dis. 2000;6:251–7.
19. Bouhnik Y, Lémann M, Mary JY *et al*. Long-term follow-up of patients with Crohn's disease treated with azathioprine or 6-mercaptopurine. Lancet. 1996;347:215–19.
20. Kim PS, Zlatanic J, Korelitz B, Gleim GW. Optimum duration of treatment with 6-mercaptopurine for Crohn's disease. Am J Gastroenterol. 1999;94:3254–7.
21. Present DH, Meltzer SJ, Krumholz MP, Wolke A, Korelitz BI. 6-Mercaptopurine in the management of inflammatory bowel disease: short and long term toxicity. Ann Intern Med. 1989;111:641–9.
22. Korelitz B, Hanauer S, Rutgeerts P, Present D, Peppercorn M. Post-operative prophylaxis with 6MP, 5-ASA or placebo in Crohn's disease: A 2 year multicenter trial. Gastroenterology. 1998;114:A1011 [Abstract].

11
Azathioprine/6-mercaptopurine for the treatment of ulcerative colitis: evidence-based standards for therapy

J. F. MARION

INTRODUCTION

The use of immunomodulators for the treatment of ulcerative colitis (UC) has grown in recent years; however, these agents remain underused. Treating patients with UC with azathioprine (AZA) or 6-mercaptopurine (6-MP) was for many years controversial. Most practising clinicians did not accept chronic medical therapy for what is widely considered a 'surgically remediable' condition. Lack of long-term safety data, and fears about cancer risk, prevented many physicians from recommending the therapy. Wide acceptance of corticosteroid use for maintenance therapy, and frustration over the slow onset of action of immunomodulators, further hindered their use. Finally, early controlled trials, either by faulty design or inadequate dosing, using AZA/6-MP for UC, were disappointing.

Several factors contributed to the increased acceptance of AZA/6-MP in the treatment of UC. First, these drugs were established as therapy for Crohn's disease. Secondly, gathering evidence showing the lack of benefit of corticosteroids for maintenance therapy in UC disillusioned many clinicians. Furthermore, increasing patient and clinician dissatisfaction with the 'curative' proctocolectomy and ileal pouch–anal anastomosis motivated the development of more aggressive colon-salvaging regimens. Finally, long-term safety data accumulated over 40 years, showing AZA/6-MP to be safe, have significantly expanded the use of these drugs.

The controlled and uncontrolled data regarding the use of AZA/6-MP for UC, while limited, offer several insights into their proper role. This chapter will review this accumulated experience and discuss several areas. Which ulcerative colitis patients should be offered AZA/6-MP? When should therapy be started? When should the medications be stopped? Questions regarding monitoring of patients taking these medicines, and discussion of ongoing trials, will be addressed.

UNCONTROLLED TRIALS

Several uncontrolled trials influenced the evolution of the acceptance of these agents. The uncontrolled studies examining the use of AZA/6-MP for UC offer several lessons in dosing, efficacy and safety. The first published trial, Bean in 1962[1], used 6-MP at an induction dose of 300 mg/day, which was subsequently reduced to 50–100 mg/day. An excellent response without significant toxicity was observed. As a result of this pioneering use of these agents we are now entering our fifth decade of use of AZA/6-MP for UC. Furthermore, this study raises the issue of the value of using a higher induction dose. The study was largely ignored, and further clinical trials were not started for another decade.

Controlled trials were published in the 1970s, which will be discussed later in the chapter.

The next uncontrolled series, published by Adler in 1990, reviewed their group's 18-year experience of using 6-MP for UC in steroid-refractory patients[2]. The population is not uniform in either severity or its use of concomitant medications, further no information is available as to the number of patients in the intent-to-treat category, nevertheless the study warrants notice. The group demonstrated a steroid-sparing effect of 61% and 'remission' in 56%. It is not clear how these patients were selected over the 18-year period described.

George and co-workers published a retrospective series of 105 patients with UC treated with 6-MP; again the majority (85%) was taking a mean dose of 30 mg/day of prednisone. A remission rate with complete withdrawal of steroids was described for 65% of patients[3]. Of interest was an observed relapse rate of 87% once 6-MP was withdrawn compared to a relapse rate of 32% for patients maintained on 6-MP. Toxicities were reversible but three colonic neoplasms (high-grade dysplasia (one), Dukes A (one) and Dukes C (one) carcinoma) were observed. The Dukes C carcinoma was found in a patient with 22 years of UC.

The increasing acceptance of colon-salvaging therapies has been blunted by concerns about the efficacy and safety of using either corticosteroids or cyclosporin in the long term. Replacement of remission-inducing but toxic therapies with safer, long-term maintenance therapies motivated our group to retrospectively examine the effect of 6-MP following response to intravenous cyclosporin for severe, steroid-refractory UC. The relapse rate following response to intravenous cyclosporin was disappointing. Any patients taking AZA/6-MP were excluded from the original controlled trial of cyclosporin. Furthermore, there was considerable trepidation about using triple immunosuppressive therapy (corticosteroid, cyclosporin and AZA/6-MP). This group of patients had never received AZA/6-MP, and thus could be compared to patients who were given these agents.

The initial response rate to intravenous cyclosporin was 83% (29/35); 18/29 responders received 6-MP upon discharge; 67% (12/18) had avoided colectomy as at 5.4 years follow-up compared to 27% (3/11) in the non-6-MP group.

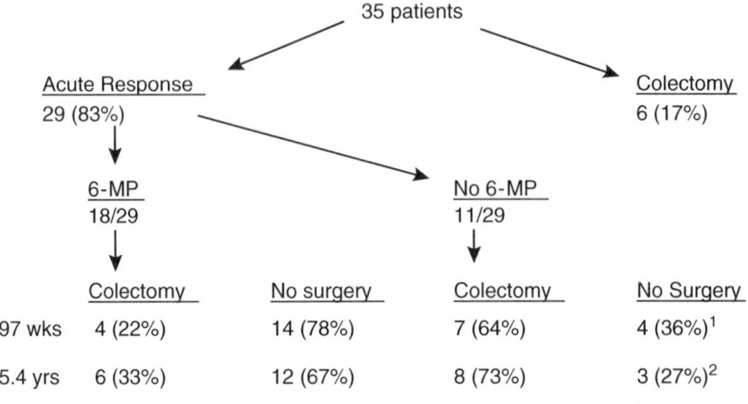

Figure 1   6-MP/AZA in ulcerative colitis – following IV CSA response

Two in the 6-MP group have had relapses requiring additional intravenous cyclosporin therapy during this follow-up period (unpublished data) (See Figure 1).

The toxicity of this regimen is significant, and precludes this colon-salvaging regimen anywhere but at a medical centre with physicians and staff experienced in the protocol. *Pneumocystis carinii* pneumonia is a potentially fatal complication and occurred in four patients in this series. One death occurred, a gastrointestinal bleed, in this group. Careful monitoring including physical examination, complete blood counts with differential white blood cell, blood urea nitrogen/creatinine, liver function tests and urine analysis should be done the week after discharge, and monthly until corticosteroids have been withdrawn.

CONTROLLED TRIALS

The controlled literature regarding AZA/6-MP for UC is disappointing, but offers some important lessons in the use of these agents. The Oxford experience using AZA in a placebo-controlled trial demonstrated a reduced relapse rate among patients with established disease at the time of enrolment. There was no clinical observed benefit during the initial month following a relapse and there was no benefit during the first year among patients having their first attack at the time of enrolment[4].

Rosenberg *et al.* performed a double-blind, placebo-controlled trial using AZA for corticosteroid-dependent UC. While no clinical benefit was seen some steroid-sparing effect was observed in the AZA group in the 6-month trial.[5] Kirk and Lennard-Jones published a double-blind placebo-controlled 6-month trial using AZA in 44 patients with steroid-refractory UC. A steroid-sparing effect and decreased disease activity was seen. Three of 14 in the placebo group but none in the AZA group required colectomy. No significant toxicities were observed.[6] They concluded that 'azathioprine may have a role in the treatment of a few patients with troublesome chronic colitis for whom conventional drug treatment is ineffectual, or for whom continuous corticosteroid treatment is needed to control symptoms, and for whom surgical treatment is inappropriate'.

Despite the relatively disappointing results of the controlled trials the use of these agents gradually increased. Hawthorne *et al.* raised the question of duration of immunomodulatory therapy in an AZA/placebo withdrawal study. Patients were followed for 1 year after randomization, and relapse as an endpoint was defined clinically and endoscopically. AZA was clearly beneficial in patients who had achieved remission on the drug. Withdrawal nearly doubles the risk of relapse and strongly argues in favour of indefinite therapy for these patients[7].

Currently we are enrolling patients in a double-blind placebo-controlled trial using AZA following intravenous corticosteroid or cyclosporin response in UC patients.

CONCLUSIONS

The controlled and uncontrolled literatures both demonstrate the safety and efficacy of AZA/6-MP for steroid-refractory UC. Inability to predict future natural history, and lack of sound clinical data, preclude recommending these agents prior to initial steroid requirement. These agents do not appear to play a role in the acute setting or in the induction of remission.

The duration of therapy with these agents is not known. However, when used in chronically active, steroid-requiring patients the risk of relapse appears high when these medications are withdrawn. Stopping AZA/6-MP in patients who have achieved remission on the agents greatly increases their risk of relapse, and patients should be made aware of that risk. There is no evidence of significant long-term toxicities to recommend against indefinite use. There appears to be no significant benefit in using one agent over the other.

Dosing of AZA/6-MP in these trials consisted of two primary strategies. Initially high induction dosing was later adjusted downward and did not appear to increase either toxicity or efficacy. Starting with a lower dose and increasing the dose to 2–2.5 mg/kg (AZA) or 1–1.5 mg/kg (6-MP) predominated the uncontrolled literature. No clear benefit of either approach was demonstrated.

Monitoring of patients of AZA/6-MP varied considerably between the controlled and uncontrolled literature. A complete blood count with white blood cell (WBC) differential biweekly until a stable dose is achieved, and then every 2–4 months thereafter, is sufficient. Liver function tests should be obtained at least every 6 months. A target WBC range of 3000–5000 should be achieved if no response is seen within 6 months. The use of 6-MP metabolite levels to guide therapy has not been shown to improve efficacy or reduce the number of adverse events. Attempts to wean steroids should be made only *after* 3 months of AZA/6-MP therapy.

Severe adverse reaction (pancreatitis, allergic reaction) preclude rechallenging or trial of sister drug.

When used in conjunction with cyclosporin and corticosteroids extreme caution must be used, and frequent monitoring is essential. *Pneumocystis carinii* prophylaxis is imperative in these patients. Only centres experienced in the use of these agents simultaneously should use them.

If you are unable to wean a patient from steroids, or fail to see any response to AZA/6-MP within 6 months, the agents should be considered ineffective and other treatments should be considered. On the other hand, should a patient respond to these agents, long-term follow-up must be reinforced. The likelihood of colectomy for responding patients appears considerably lower in responders, and as a result their risk of colonic neoplasia is considerably higher. Colonoscopic surveillance for colon cancer prevention is crucial in patients who are successfully maintained on immunomodulatory therapy.

Wider use of these agents can be expected over the coming years. When our ability to predict the natural history of UC in certain patients improves, we can better target those who are likely to require or be refractory to steroids. Currently there are no data to support using AZA/6-MP prior to initial steroid requirement. Patients who require steroids for their UC should be considered candidates for these therapies.

References

1. Bean *et al.* 6-Mercaptopurine in the treatment of ulcerative colitis. Med J Austr. 1962;2:592.
2. Adler DJ, Korelitz BI. The therapeutic efficacy of 6-mercaptopurine in refractory ulcerative colitis. Am J Gastroenterol. 1990;85:717.
3. George J *et al.* The long-term outcome of ulcerative colitis treated with 6-mercaptopurine. Am J Gastroenterol. 1996;91:1711.
4. Jewel DP, Truelove SC. Azathioprine in ulcerative colitis: final report on controlled therapeutic trial. Br Med J. 1974;4:627.
5. Rosenberg JL *et al.* A controlled trial of azathioprine in the management of chronic ulcerative colitis. Gastroenterology. 1975;69:96.
6. Kirk AP, Lennard-Jones JE. Controlled trial of azathioprine in chronic ulcerative colitis. Br Med J. 1982;284:1291.
7. Hawthorne AB *et al.* Randomised controlled trial of azathioprine withdrawal in ulcerative colitis. Br Med J. 1992;305:20.

Section IV
Standards: methotrexate

12
Methotrexate: mechanisms of action, pharmacology and toxicology

A. SCHNABEL

Over the past decade methotrexate (MTX) evolved to be the leading disease-modifying agent for rheumatoid arthritis of high and intermediate activity (reviewed in ref. 1). Due to its high anti-inflammatory potency and favourable risk/benefit ratio, MTX largely replaced parenteral and oral gold compounds, D-penicillamine and also azathioprine. Given its proven advantages over other agents in rheumatoid arthritis, it is being increasingly used in other inflammatory conditions. These include collagen vascular diseases, systemic vasculitides, psoriasis including psoriatic arthritis, steroid-dependent asthma, sarcoidosis as well as chronic inflammatory bowel diseases[1–6]. Although experimental verification of its clinical value in the latter conditions is still fragmentary, the clinical impression is that appropriately selected patients experience at least a steroid-saving effect with MTX and that the scope of low-dose MTX treatment goes well beyond rheumatoid arthritis.

Chemically, MTX is an analogue of dihydrofolic acid. Substitution of one hydroxyl group by an amino residue and insertion of a further methyl group into the folic acid molecule results in the MTX molecule (Fig. 1). This competes with dihydrofolic acid for its binding site on dihydrofolate reductase, which is a key enzyme in the generation of tetrahydrofolic acid (THF). THF is the parent

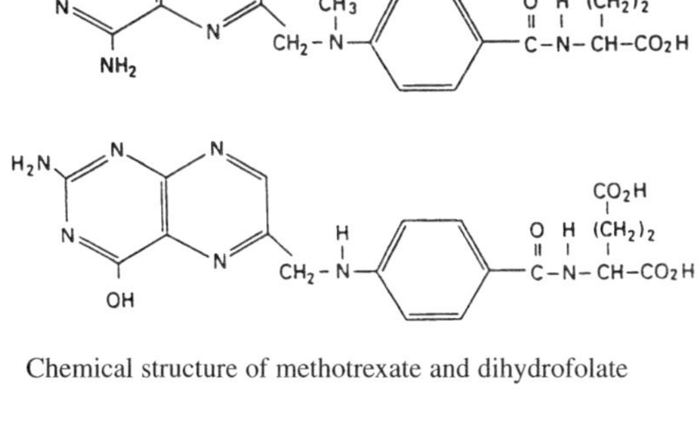

Figure 1 Chemical structure of methotrexate and dihydrofolate

compound for a number of cofactors for pyrimidine and purine synthesis and for the generation of methionine from homocysteine (reviewed in ref. 7). THF depletion due to high doses of MTX leads to the depletion of nucleic acid constituents and thereby has an antiproliferative effect. The same effect is enhanced by methionine depletion. Rapidly growing tumour cells are commonly more susceptible to MTX than are normal cells, and this is the basis of the protocols using high doses of MTX for antiproliferation and subsequent rescue of normal cells by commensurate doses of folic acid[8].

While the mechanism of action of high doses of MTX is thus quite straightforward, the mechanisms underlying the anti-inflammatory effect of low doses of MTX are still being explored. By all standards, low-dose MTX has no cytotoxic or antiproliferative effects, but it is rather an immune modulator (Table 1). It inhibits various neutrophil functions, suppresses the generation of TNF-α, IL-6 and IL-8, inhibits the binding of IL-1 to its target cells and elevates serum levels of IL-10, which can have anti-inflammatory and immunosuppressive properties (reviewed in ref. 9).

An attractive concept accounting for these effects is the adenosine hypothesis. Partial blockade of purine synthesis and of homocysteine methylation by MTX results in a sequence of metabolic changes which ultimately lead to the accumulation of adenosine and AMP and increased extracellular adenosine levels[9]. Adenosine has anti-inflammatory properties by interfering with the accumulation of neutrophils and by deactivating a spectrum of inflammatory cells via the adenosine A2 receptor. Many of the effects elicited by adenosine *in vitro* parallel the effects of MTX *in vivo*[9], but definitive proof of the adenosine hypothesis is still missing. An important element of proof would be to elaborate other stimulators of adenosine A2 receptors and demonstrate that these mimic the anti-inflammatory effects of MTX; but such studies are missing.

Table 2 shows selected pharmacokinetic data of MTX. Current dosage ranges are between 10 and 25 mg once a week. The bioavailability of enteral MTX

Table 1 Immunomodulating effect of MTX

Neutrophil migration/activation	⇓
TNF-α	⇓
IL-6	⇓
IL-8	⇓
IL-1 activity	⇓
IL-10	⇑

Table 2 Low Dose MTX – pharmacology

Dosing	10–25 mg once per week
Bioavailability	45–100% of oral dose
Initial/terminal half-life	1.5–3.5/8–15 h
Elimination	Renal excretion (glomerular + tubular)
Enhanced MTX toxicity with:	Cotrimoxazole, acetylsalicylic acid, some non-steroidal anti-inflammatory agents, probenecid, other organic acids

varies individually between 45% and 100%[7], and this causes many rheumatologists to administer MTX only intravenously. The initial (distribution) half-life is 1.5–3.5 h, the terminal (elimination) half-life is 8–15 h. Intracellularly MTX is mainly present in the form of polyglutamates, and these are retained much longer than the parent compound[7]. Elimination occurs mainly through renal excretion, and renal insufficiency proved to be the preeminent risk factor for side-effects[10]. MTX accumulation becomes clinically significant when the glomerular filtration rate drops to less than 50% of normal, i.e. when the serum creatinine level exceeds the upper limit of normal. A number of drugs can interfere with the excretion of MTX; the most important are acetylsalicylic acid, certain non-steroidal anti-inflammatory agents, cotrimoxazole, probenecid and other organic acids[7].

Fortunately, the combination of MTX with sulphasalazine proved to be safe[11,12]. Firstly, sulphasalazine has also a weak anti-folate effect, which might enhance the same effect of MTX. Moreover, due to its sulphone structure, it may theoretically interfere with the tubular secretion or reabsorption of MTX. In practice, however, the combination of these two agents proved to have additive therapeutic effects (sulphasalazine is also a disease-modifying agent for rheumatoid arthritis), but they are not additive with respect to side-effects[11,12]. Combinations of MTX with other disease-modifying agents are being used increasingly in patients who respond poorly to MTX monotherapy. An additive therapeutic effect in the absence of added toxicity was also demonstrated for combinations of MTX with antimalarials[13], cyclosporin A[14] and for triple therapy with MTX/sulphasalazine/hydroxychloroquine[15]. Promising preliminary observations are also available for MTX plus leflunomide[16] (Table 3).

Withdrawal of MTX due to side-effects amounts to 15% during the first year of treatment; thereafter to less than 5% per year[17,18]. In rheumatoid arthritis patients, elevated transaminase levels comprise the most common adverse event during the first year (Fig. 2). This can be largely avoided by omitting other hepatotoxic medications (e.g. non-steroidal anti-inflammatory agents)[1]. Long-term monitoring of liver histology disclosed that MTX can cause some degree of hepatic fibrosis, but this is usually functionally irrelevant (reviewed in ref. 19). On the other hand, repeated elevation of the transaminases above three times normal values is associated with substantial risk of progressive hepatic injury, and in these patients MTX should be withdrawn. Liver cirrhosis is distinctly rare

Table 3 Therapeutic effect of combinations of MTX with other anti-inflammatory agents

MTX + sulphasalazine (SSZ)	Additive
MTX + antimalarials	Additive
MTX + SSZ + hydroxychloroquine	Additive
MTX + cyclosporin A	Additive
MTX + leflunomide	(Additive)
MTX + azathioprine	Non-additive
MTX + parenteral/oral gold	Non-additive

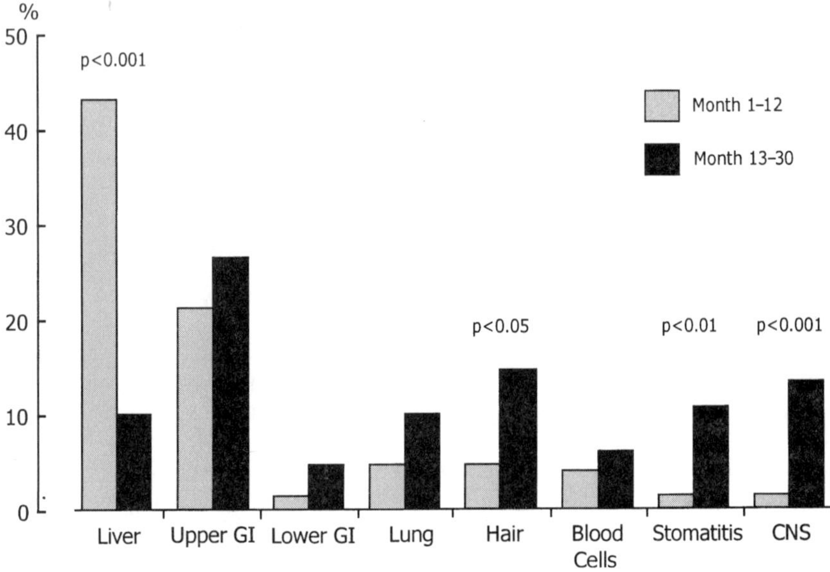

Figure 2 Annual incidence of MTX side effects during and beyond the first year of treatment

in rheumatoid arthritis patients treated with MTX, but is somewhat more common in psoriatics. Regular alcohol consumption appears to greatly enhance the prevalence of MTX-associated liver disease[19].

Gastrointestinal discomfort and inappetence are the most common MTX side-effects in the long run, but in few patients are these troublesome enough to cause cessation of treatment[18]. Stomatitis occurs episodically in up to 10% of patients. MTX-induced diarrhoea is very rare. Gastrointestinal side-effects can mostly be avoided or mitigated by folic or folinic acid supplementation (reviewed in ref. 7). Haemocytopenia is rarely a dose-limiting problem in low-dose MTX treatment, but failure to interrupt treatment in the event of leuko-cytopenia of other origin (e.g. virally induced) can result in protracted and life-threatening agranulocytosis[1]. A rare but life-threatening pulmonary side-effect is MTX-induced pneumonitis. Occurring in less than 5% of patients it can hit early as well as late in the course of treatment[1]. It is an immunologically mediated condition which needs to be distinguished from infectious pneumonia. It requires definitive discontinuation of MTX.

MTX treatment appears to result in a somewhat diminished resistance against infections. These involve mainly conventional bacterial agents[20]. Opportunistic infections are dominated by herpes zoster[1]. It is common practice to interrupt the MTX treatment for 1–2 weeks in the event of a major infection. MTX is highly teratogenic. Accidental MTX treatment during pregnancy resulted in a high rate of central nervous system and limb abnormalities[21].

Side-effects are mostly controlled by (1) eliminating concomitant medications that interfere with MTX (e.g. non-steroidal anti-inflammatory agents), (2) short-term interruption of MTX treatment or (3) dose reduction[1]. A major part of the gastrointestinal side-effects, including transaminase elevation, and of haematological side-effects, appear to originate from the anti-folate effect of MTX. Many of these can be prevented or mitigated by appropriately dosed folic or folinic acid supplements given timely spaced from MTX. Dosing schedules that reduce toxicity without interfering with the anti-inflammatory effect to any major extent comprise either a single dose of folinic acid administered 24 h after MTX, or small doses of folic acid administered several-fold per week, but sparing the MTX day[7] (Table 4).

On balance, MTX is the best-examined disease-modifying antirheumatic agent in current use; no other agent has been examined so extensively with respect to efficacy, long-term safety, prevention and treatment of side-effects and range of applicability. This does not, of course, mean that MTX is the ideal anti-inflammatory agent. Some of the still-viable problems encountered with MTX are listed in Table 5. However, this means that MTX treatment given by an experienced physician and monitored closely – including laboratory checks with blood cell count, liver and kidney values every 2–4 weeks – has a favourable risk/benefit ratio. A further important aspect of MTX is that it can be combined with other anti-inflammatory agents. This offers the opportunity to keep patients who respond poorly to single-agent therapy on a treatment with well-tolerated combinations. In many cases this obviates the need to advance to high-risk treatment modalities or to leave the patient suboptimally treated.

Table 4 Prevention of MTX side-effects with folic/folinic acid

Folic acid:
  5–10 mg on 5–6 days per week (except MTX day)

Folinic acid:
  mg FNA = mg MTX, administered 24 h after MTX

→ *Diminished stomatitis, gastrointestinal and hepatic side-effects*

Table 5

Pro MTX	Contra MTX
Best-studied DMAR	
High efficacy combined with favourable risk/benefit ratio	Significant hepatic, renal, myeloid disease precludes MTX treatment
Favourable long-term tolerability	Patients tend to become weary of MTX
Many side-effects amenable to prevention	Strict surveillance is required throughout treatment
Combination with other DMARs enhances efficacy	Monotherapy not universally effective

DMAR = disease-modifying antirheumatic drug.

References

1. Schnabel A, Gross WL. Low-dose methotrexate in rheumatic diseases – efficacy, side effects, and risk factors for side effects. Semin Arthritis Rheum. 1994;23:310–27.
2. Kipen Y, Littlejohn GO, Morand EF. Methotrexate use in systemic lupus erythematosus. Lupus. 1997;6:385–9.
3. Pachman LM, Hayford JR, Chung A et al. Juvenile dermatomyositis at diagnosis: clinical characteristics of 79 children. J Rheumatol. 1998;25:1198–204.
4. de Groot K, Mühler M, Reinhold-Keller E, Paulsen J, Gross WL. Induction of remission in Wegener's granulomatosis with low-dose methotrexate. J Rheumatol. 1998;25:492–5.
5. Matthew GM. Low-dose methotrexate spares steroid usage in steroid-dependent asthmatic patients – a metaanalysis. Chest. 1997;112:29–33.
6. Baughman RP, Winget DB, Lower EE. Methotrexate is steroid sparing in acute sarcoidosis: results of a double blind, randomized trial. Sarcoidosis Vasc Diffuse Lung Dis. 2000;17:60–6.
7. van Ede AE, Laan RFJM, Blom HJ, De Abreu RA, van de Putte LBA. Methotrexate in rheumatoid arthritis: an update with focus on mechanisms involved in toxicity. Semin Arthritis Rheum. 1998;27:277–92.
8. Hardman JG, Limbird LE, Molinoff PB, Ruddon RW, Goodman Gillman A. The Pharmacological Basis of Therapeutics. New York: McGraw-Hill, 1996:1243–7.
9. Kremer JM. Methotrexate and leflunomide: biochemical basis for combination therapy in the treatment of rheumatoid arthritis. Semin Arthritis Rheum. 1999;29:14–26.
10. Felson DT, Chernoff M, Anderson JJ et al. The effect of age and renal function on the efficacy and toxicity of methotrexate in rheumatoid arthritis. J Rheumatol. 1995;22:218–23.
11. Haagsma CJ, van Riel PLCM, de Jong AJL, van de Putte LBA. Combination of sulphasalazine and methotrexate versus the single components in early rheumatoid arthritis: a randomized, controlled, double-blind, 52 week clinical trial. Br J Rheumatol. 1997;36:1082–8.
12. Boers M, Verhoeven AC, Markusse HM, van de Laar MAFJ et al. Randomised comparison of combined step-down prednisolone, methotrexate and sulphasalazine with sulphasalazine alone in early rheumatoid arthritis. Lancet. 1997;350:309–18.
13. Ferraz MB, Pinheiro GRC, Helfenstein M et al. Combination therapy with methotrexate and chloroquine in rheumatoid arthritis. Scand J Rheumatol. 1994;23:231–6.
14. Tugwell P, Pincus T, Yocum D et al. Combination therapy with cyclosporine and methotrexate in severe rheumatoid arthritis. N Engl J Med. 1995;333:137–41.
15. O'Dell JR, Haire CE, Erikson N et al. Treatment of rheumatoid arthritis with methotrexate alone, sulfasalazine and hydroxychloroquine, or a combination of all three medications. N Engl J Med. 1996;334:1287–91.
16. Weinblatt ME, Kremer JM, Coblyn JS et al. Pharmacokinetics, safety, and efficacy of combination treatment with methotrexate and leflunomide in patients with active rheumatoid arthritis. Arthritis Rheum. 1999;42:1322–8.
17. Schnabel A, Reinhold-Keller E, Willmann V, Gross WL. Tolerability of methotrexate starting with 15 or 25 mg/week for rheumatoid arthritis. Rheumatol Int. 1994;14:33–8.
18. Schnabel A, Herlyn K, Burchardi C, Reinhold-Keller E, Gross WL. Long-term tolerability of methotrexate at doses exceeding 15 mg per week in rheumatoid arthritis. Rheumatol Int. 1996;15:195–200.
19. Kremer JM. Liver toxicity does not have to follow methotrexate therapy of patients with rheumatoid arthritis. Am J Gastroenterol. 1997;92:194–6.
20. Schnabel A, Burchardi C, Gross WL. Major infections during methotrexate treatment for rheumatoid arthritis. Semin Arthritis Rheum. 1996;25:357–9.
21. Lloyd ME, Carr M, McElhatton P, Hall GM, Hughes RA. The effects of methotrexate on pregnancy, fertility and lactation. Q J Med. 1999;92:551–63.

13
Methotrexate therapy for Crohn's disease

B. G. FEAGAN

INTRODUCTION

Despite many recent advances, significant limitations exist in the medical management of patients with Crohn's disease. Although glucocorticoids are highly effective for the induction of remission[1,2], their chronic use is characterized by the frequent occurrence of side-effects. Accordingly treatment alternatives are required for patients who are refractory to glucocorticoid therapy. Methotrexate is an effective and safe treatment for glucocorticosteroid-dependent patients in other chronic inflammatory diseases such as psoriasis and rheumatoid arthritis (RA)[3-7]. Thus, it is logical that methotrexate was also evaluated as a therapy for inflammatory bowel disease.

Methotrexate has been used clinically for over 40 years. The development of this drug as a treatment for leukaemia was based on determination of the three-dimensional structure of the enzyme dihydrofolate reductase. Since this enzyme requires folic acid as a cofactor for activity methotrexate was synthesized as a competitive antagonist of folic acid. Thus methotrexate is one of the earliest examples of a 'designer drug'. Inhibition of dihydrofolate reductase by high-dose methotrexate interferes with DNA synthesis, which ultimately results in the death of leukaemic cells[8]. During an initial experience with methotrexate in oncology it was serendipitously recognized that children with leukaemia, who had concomitant psoriasis or RA, showed improvement of these conditions. This observation led to the evaluation of low-dose (5–25 mg weekly) methotrexate as a treatment for a number of autoimmune diseases. Over the past decade clinical trials have shown that methotrexate has an emerging role for the treatment of Crohn's disease and other inflammatory conditions.

PHARMACOLOGY

Methotrexate is administered by the oral, subcutaneous, intramuscular or intravenous route[9]. The drug is highly bioavailable at doses of 15 mg or less; however, absorption may be erratic with high oral doses[10].

Following absorption, methotrexate is concentrated in the liver, kidneys, and synovium with a steady-state volume of distribution of approximately 1 L/kg. The parent molecule is transported into cells by an energy-dependent process. The enzyme hepatic aldehyde converts methotrexate to a primary metabolite, 7-hydroxymethotrexate. The drug is subsequently eliminated from the body through glomerular filtration; tubular secretion and reabsorption also occur. Organic acids such as acetylsalicylic acid (ASA) and some non-steroidal anti-inflammatory drugs may interfere with renal tubular secretion and thus increase serum methotrexate levels. As a consequence clinically significant drug interactions have been reported in patients with RA. Therefore methotrexate should be used cautiously in patients with renal impairment. Therapeutic drug monitoring has not been shown to be useful in patients with RA[11].

Although the mechanism of the anti-inflammatory effect of methotrexate is poorly understood, it is not likely through the inhibition of dihydrofolate reductase, since folate supplementation does not reduce clinical efficacy in patients with RA[12]. Although the mechanism of action remains unknown several immunosuppressive properties have been demonstrated *in vitro*, including suppression of proinflammatory molecules, a decrease in cytotoxic T cell function, and reduction in neutrophil activity[13]. Inhibition of adenosine metabolism does not seem to be an important mechanism of action in patients with inflammatory bowel disease (IBD).

Adverse event profile

Low-dose methotrexate was first identified as an effective treatment for severe psoriasis in the early 1960s[4]. The dose used as treatment for psoriasis and other autoimmune diseases is approximately 1/40 of that used in oncology. Despite impressive efficacy an unacceptably high incidence of hepatic toxicity was noted in psoriatic patients who had received chronic treatment with methotrexate. In the series by Malatjalian *et al.*, of 104 patients who were treated for a mean duration of 3.38 years with doses of 20–25 mg/week, 23.1% showed significant pathological changes (cirrhosis and/or active hepatitis) on liver biopsy[14]. These findings might have led to the abandonment of methotrexate as treatment for autoimmune disease if not for subsequent pharmacokinetic investigations which demonstrated that continuous (daily) drug administration results in high hepatic methotrexate concentrations[15]. This finding is explained by the observation that polyglutamic folic acid is concentrated intrahepatically. Since methotrexate is a folate analogue the drug likewise accumulates in the liver and causes toxicity. However, high intrahepatic concentrations of methotrexate do not occur if sufficient time is allowed between doses for the drug to be excreted by the kidney[16]. This understanding of the pharmacokinetics of methotrexate led to the development of once-weekly dosing schedules, which in turn resulted in a significant reduction in the incidence of hepatic toxicity. However, the rate of methotrexate hepatic toxicity may also relate to the underlying disease state as the incidence of this complication is higher in psoriasis and low in RA. This may reflect differences among populations in the prevalence of risk factors (alcohol use, diabetes mellitus, and obesity) for methotrexate toxicity. Only limited data are available to assess the potential risk of methotrexate-associated hepatic fibrosis in IBD.

Other important adverse effects of methotrexate include nausea[17], bone marrow suppression[18], and hypersensitivity pneumonitis[19]. Methotrexate must not be given to women of childbearing potential, due to the risk of teratogenicity[20].

METHOTREXATE AS A THERAPY FOR CROHN'S DISEASE

Munkholm and colleagues have documented the natural history of active Crohn's disease in Copenhagen County. The majority of patients who are treated with a course of conventional glucocorticoid therapy become either steroid-dependent (36%) or steroid-resistant (20%)[21]. Thus only a minority (44%) of patients experience a durable treatment response to glucocorticoid therapy. Patients who require chronic steroid therapy experience considerable morbidity and are at risk for disease-related mortality. Although surgery is an important treatment option, Crohn's disease frequently recurs following a bowel resection.

Patients who require chronic steroid therapy are appropriate candidates for immunosuppressive drug therapy. The greatest experience has been with the purine antimetabolites 6-mercaptopurine (6-MP) and azathioprine. Although early studies demonstrated conflicting results as to the efficacy of these drugs[1], data from two randomized placebo-controlled trials[22,23] and a meta-analysis[24] indicate that they are effective both for the induction of remission and for maintenance therapy in Crohn's disease. However, the onset of action of azathioprine is relatively slow (3–6 months)[24,25], which may be a consequence of individual variability in the time required to obtain a steady-state concentration of immunosuppressive drug metabolites. Moreover, less than half of patients who receive maintenance therapy with the purine antimetabolites remain free of a relapse over 1 year[22,23]. Although the purine metabolites are relatively well tolerated as chronic therapy, serious toxicity can occur[26], most notably pancreatitis, leukopenia and infection. Therefore alternative medical treatments are desirable.

In 1989 Kozarek and colleagues[27] first reported the use of methotrexate for the treatment of IBD in 21 patients (14 with Crohn's disease, seven with ulcerative colitis) with chronically active disease. Methotrexate was administered intramuscularly at a dose of 25 mg once-weekly with conversion to a maintenance dose of 15 mg orally in patients who responded to therapy. Approximately two-thirds of patients showed improvement in symptoms in this uncontrolled study, and a steroid-sparing effect was also demonstrated. Notably one-third of the Crohn's patients demonstrated endoscopic improvement, whereas no such beneficial effect was seen in the patients with ulcerative colitis. On the basis of these promising results several randomized controlled trials were subsequently conducted.

Four randomized, double-blind, placebo-controlled trials of methotrexate in chronic active, steroid-dependent Crohn's disease have been reported. In the largest study the North American Crohn's Study Group (NACSG) investigators[17] assigned 141 patients with chronically active steroid-dependent disease to 25 mg of intramuscular methotrexate weekly or a placebo. Following 16 weeks of treatment, 39.4% of methotrexate-treated patients were in remission without prednisone, compared with 19.1% in the placebo arm ($p = 0.025$). Beneficial effects of methotrexate treatment were seen for disease activity, quality of life, and

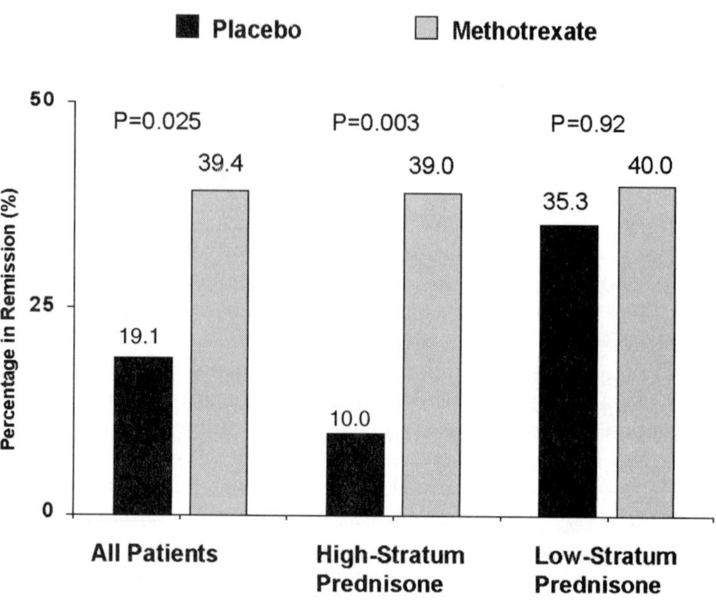

Figure 1 Percentages of patients in remission at week 16, according to study group and stratum of daily prednisone dose before entry into the study (from ref. 17)

prednisone utilization. The effect of treatment was greatest in those patients who had required greater than 20 mg of prednisone per day to control their symptoms.

Although withdrawal from therapy for adverse events occurred more frequently in the methotrexate group (17% vs 2%, $p = 0.012$) the majority of withdrawals were protocol-defined and were attributable to asymptomatic elevations of hepatic enzymes. On the basis of these results the investigators concluded that methotrexate was an effective treatment for induction of remission in glucocorticoid-dependent patients (Fig. 1).

A second trial, performed by Oren and colleagues in Israel[28], compared oral methotrexate (12.5 mg weekly), and 6-MP (50 mg once daily), to a placebo in 84 patients with chronically active steroid-dependent disease. Patients were also allowed treatment with 5-aminosalicylates. Remission was defined as the occurrence of a Harvey–Bradshaw score of <4 without steroid use at the end of 9 months of treatment. The proportion of patients who met this criterion in the three treatment groups was: 12/26 (46%) of patients who received placebo, 13/32 (41%) of patients assigned to 6-MP, and 10/26 (38%) of patients who received methotrexate ($p > 0.05$). Similarly, no significant differences were demonstrated among treatment groups in the time required to enter remission, mean Harvey–Bradshaw scores or the average monthly steroid dose. In subgroup analyses the methotrexate-treated patients showed a significant improvement in general well-being and reduction in abdominal pain relative to the other two groups. This negative trial has been criticized because of the relatively low doses of 6-MP and methotrexate which were chosen for evaluation.

A third trial recently published by Arora and colleagues[29] compared oral methotrexate 15–22.5 mg weekly to placebo in 33 Crohn's disease patients who were treated for 1 year. Fewer methotrexate-treated patients experienced disease-related exacerbations during the follow-up period (46% vs 80%) but this difference was not statistically significant. Similarly a non-significant trend towards an increased number of side-effects in the methotrexate-treated patients (33% vs 0%, $p < 0.2$) was observed.

Data from a recently completed maintenance study[30] show that low-dose methotrexate is effective as a maintenance therapy in patients with quiescent disease. In this study 76 patients were randomly assigned to receive maintenance therapy with 15 mg weekly of intramuscular methotrexate or placebo. Prior to entry into the trial, all of the patients had been documented with chronically active steroid-dependent disease and then had been successfully treated with a methotrexate induction regimen (16–24 weeks of 25 mg weekly by intramuscular injection). The efficacy of treatment was compared by analysing the proportion of patients who remained free of a relapse (CDAI increase > 100 points or need for treatment of active Crohn's disease) over 40 weeks of follow-up. At the end of the study 26 patients (65%) had remained in remission over the entire duration of follow-up in the methotrexate group, compared with 14 patients (38.9%) in the placebo group ($p = 0.015$). Accordingly individuals who received methotrexate were less likely to require prednisone therapy (11 of 40, 27.5%, vs 21 of 36, 58.3%, $p = 0.007$) and had lower disease activity (mean $\pm$ SE CDAI scores 135 ± 16 compared with 196 ± 18, $p = 0.001$). Moreover, over half of the patients who relapsed were successfully retreated with the induction regimen of

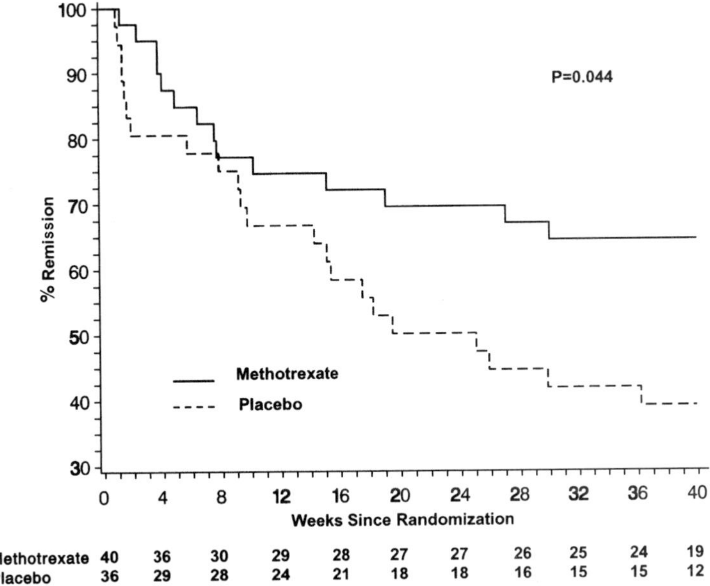

Figure 2 Kaplan–Meier estimates of the time to relapse in the methotrexate and the placebo groups (from ref. 30)

methotrexate (25 mg weekly), were free of prednisone and in remission at the end of the trial. An interesting finding was the relatively high rate of remission observed in the placebo group (38.9%); based on previous trials of azathioprine and/or glucocorticoids a response rate of no greater than 20% was anticipated. One possible explanation is the possibility that the induction regimen of methotrexate which patients had received prior to randomization resulted in healing of mucosal ulceration and a durable clinical response. Although no serious adverse events were observed in this study, the participants were selected for tolerance of methotrexate.

What conclusions can be drawn from these clinical trials? The largest studies have provided rigorous evidence which supports the efficacy of methotrexate both in active disease and for maintenance therapy. However, several points should be made regarding the methotrexate regimens which were utilized. First, in the NACSG trial[17] methotrexate was used at a relatively high dose (25 mg weekly) in conjunction with prednisone. Thus the efficacy of methotrexate monotherapy for induction of remission is unknown. Second, methotrexate was given by intramuscular injection. Using this route of administration 15 mg of methotrexate was also shown to be effective for maintenance therapy. In contrast, Oren and colleagues[28], who used a methotrexate dose of 12.5 mg orally for induction or remission, could not demonstrate a beneficial effect of methotrexate (or low-dose 6-MP) in comparison to placebo. Finally, although the trial of Arora and colleagues[29] had limited statistical power, a beneficial response was suggested using a higher oral dose than that used in the Israeli study (15–22.5 mg weekly). Collectively, these data may mean that the dose–response curve for methotrexate therapy in Crohn's disease is shifted to the right in comparison to RA, where oral methotrexate doses as low as 7.5 mg/week are effective. If drug doses greater than 15 mg/week are required for efficacy then oral administration may be suboptimal due to incomplete drug absorption from the gastrointestinal tract. Intramuscular injection is inconvenient for patients and relatively costly if administration by health-care personnel is required. One potential solution to this problem is the use of subcutaneous administration of the drug. This approach has been utilized in RA with good results[11]. In our experience patients can easily be taught to self-inject methotrexate subcutaneously.

Important questions remain regarding the potential clinical applications of methotrexate in Crohn's disease. No data from controlled trials are currently available regarding the use of the drug for the treatment of fistulas. An initial uncontrolled experience suggests that methotrexate is effective for this indication[31] in patients who have been refractory to therapy with purine antimetabolites. Similarly, our anecdotal experience is that methotrexate is effective for some extraintestinal manifestations of the disease including arthralgias and arthritis, erythema nodosum and pyoderma gangrenosum. Additional experience with these syndromes is needed.

Ulcerative colitis

The majority of patients with ulcerative colitis are successfully managed with 5-ASA and brief courses of glucocorticoids. Patients with refractory disease, as defined by the need for chronic glucocorticoid therapy to control symptoms, often undergo colectomy, since many clinicians are reluctant to consider the use of chronic immunosuppression in a disease which can be treated surgically and has a time-dependent, increased risk of colon cancer[32]. Thus it is not surprising that far fewer data are available to assess the efficacy of immunosuppressive drugs in this condition as compared with Crohn's disease.

Although no large randomized controlled trials have evaluated the use of the purine antimetabolites in patients with chronically active ulcerative colitis, Hawthorne and colleagues[33] have performed a withdrawal study which evaluated the efficacy of azathioprine in 79 patients who entered remission after receiving azathioprine therapy. Patients who were assigned to withdraw from azathioprine had a greater rate of relapse at 1 year compared to those who remained on drug therapy (59% vs 35%, $p = 0.04$).

Only one randomized, double-blind, placebo-controlled trial of methotrexate in chronic active ulcerative colitis has been performed. In this study Oren and colleagues[16,34] compared oral methotrexate (12.5 mg weekly) to placebo for 9 months in 67 patients who had received steroids and/or immunosuppressive drugs for at least 4 of the 12 preceding months. No statistically significant differences were demonstrated among the treatment groups in the proportion of patients achieving remission, the time required to achieve remission, or the proportion of patients experiencing a relapse after a remission had been obtained.

Thus no good data from controlled trials exist to support the use of methotrexate as a therapy for ulcerative colitis. A research priority should be to evaluate the efficacy of a higher dose of methotrexate than 12.5 mg weekly in this disease.

CONCLUSIONS

Over the past decade methotrexate has emerged as a new treatment for chronically active Crohn's disease. Notwithstanding the data described previously, the purine antimetabolites remain the most frequently prescribed drug for these patients. This practice is based on the results of three relatively small, randomized controlled trials which utilized an adequate dose of either 6-MP or azathioprine[22,23,26]. In RA methotrexate has superseded azathioprine as a therapy due to superior efficacy and long-term tolerability. In the absence of good comparative data, clinicians must decide whether methotrexate or the purine antimetabolites is the preferred treatment for Crohn's disease[35,36]. Extensive long-term experience exists with the purine antimetabolites, whereas the risk of liver disease from methotrexate remains an issue. However, the risk of significant hepatic toxicity in RA is low and surveillance liver biopsy is no longer recommended. In the absence of biopsy data from patients with Crohn's disease the American Rheumatology Association guidelines regarding surveillance for hepatic toxicity should be followed[37].

The emergence of infliximab as a new therapy for patients with refractory Crohn's disease[38,39] should also focus additional attention on the use of methotrexate as an alternative to the purine antimetabolites. In patients with RA concomitant treatment with methotrexate has been shown to enhance the response to infliximab therapy. Furthermore, patients who are receiving methotrexate are less likely to develop human antichimaeric antibodies[40]. These antibodies, which may block the beneficial action of infliximab or cause adverse effects, are a significant limitation to the long-term use of this form of treatment. Thus, a strong rationale exists to consider methotrexate–infliximab combination therapy in Crohn's disease.

Although controlled trials to compare the relative efficacy and safety of azathioprine and methotrexate in therapy-resistant patients are desirable, in my opinion these studies will be difficult, if not impossible, to conduct because of the relatively small differences in potency and tolerability between these agents. A more productive area for future investigation will be to explore the use of these drugs in combination with infliximab and other biological treatments.

References

1. Summers RW, Switz DM, Sessions JT Jr et al. National Cooperative Crohn's Disease Study: results of drug treatment. Gastroenterology. 1979;77:847–69.
2. Rutgeerts P, Lofberg R, Malchow H et al. A comparison of budesonide with prednisolone for active Crohn's disease. N Engl J Med. 1994;331:842–5.
3. Klippel JH, Decker JL. Methotrexate in rheumatoid arthritis. N Engl J Med. 1985;312:853–4.
4. Black RL, O'Brien WM, Van Scott EJ, Auerback R, Eisen AZ, Bunim JJ. Methotrexate therapy in psoriatic arthritis: double-blind study on 21 patients. J Am Med Assoc. 1964;189:743–7.
5. Willkens RF, Sharp JT, Stablein D, Marks C, Wortmann R. Comparison of azathioprine, methotrexate, and the combination of the two in the treatment of rheumatoid arthritis. A forty-eight-week controlled clinical trial with radiologic outcome assessment. Arthritis Rheum. 1995;38:1799–806.
6. Weinstein GD, Jeffes E, McCullough JL. Cytotoxic and immunologic effects of methotrexate in psoriasis. J Invest Dermatol. 1990;95:49–52S.
7. Weinblatt ME, Coblyn JS, Fox DA. Efficacy of low-dose methotrexate in rheumatoid arthritis. N Engl J Med. 1985;312:818–22.
8. Goodman LS, Gilman A. The Pharmacological Basis of Therapeutics. New York: McGraw-Hill, 1996.
9. Jundt JW, Browne BA, Fiocco GP, Steele AD, Mock D. A comparison of low dose methotrexate bioavailability: oral solution, oral tablet, subcutaneous and intramuscular dosing. J Rheumatol. 1993;20:1845–9.
10. Hillson JL, Furst DE. Pharmacology and pharmacokinetics of methotrexate in rheumatic disease. Practical issues in treatment and design. Rheum Dis Clin N Am. 1997;23:757–78.
11. Bannwarth B, Pehourcq F, Schaeverbeke T, Dehais J. Clinical pharmacokinetics of low-dose pulse methotrexate in rheumatoid arthritis. Clin Pharmacokinet. 1996;30:194–210.
12. Morgan SL, Baggott JE, Vaughn WH et al. Supplementation with folic acid during methotrexate therapy for rheumatoid arthritis. Ann Intern Med. 1994;121:833–41.
13. Cronstein BN, Naime D, Ostad E. The antiinflammatory mechanism of methotrexate. J Clin Invest. 1993;92:2675–82.
14. Malatjalian DA, Ross JB, Williams CN, Colwell SJ, Eastwood BJ. Methotrexate hepatotoxicity in psoriatics: report of 104 patients from Nova Scotia, with analysis of risks from obesity, diabetes and alcohol consumption during long term follow-up. Can J Gastroenterol. 1996;10:369–75.
15. Hall PD, Jenner MA, Ahern MJ. Hepatotoxicity in a rat model caused by orally administered methotrexate. Hepatology. 1991;14:906.
16. Lewis JH, Schiff EAC. Methotrexate-induced chronic liver injury: guidelines for detection and prevention. Am J Gastroenterol. 1988;88:1337–45.
17. Feagan BG, Rochon J, Fedorak RN et al. Methotrexate for the treatment of Crohn's disease. N Engl J Med. 1995;332:292–7.
18. Al-Awadhi A, Dale P, McKendry R. Pancytopenia associated with low dose methotrexate therapy. A regional survey. J Rheumatol. 1993;20:1121–5.
19. Searles G, McKendry RJ. Methotrexate pneumonitis in rheumatoid arthritis: potential risk factors: four case reports and a review of the literature. J Rheumatol. 1987;14:1164–71.
20. Kozlowski RD, Steinbrunner JV, MacKenzie AH, Clough JD, Wilke WS, Segal AM. Outcome of first-trimester exposure to low-dose methotrexate in eight patients with rheumatic disease. Am J Med. 1990;88:589–92.

21. Munkholm P, Langholz E, Davidsen M, Binder V. Frequency of glucocorticoid resistance and dependency in Crohn's disease. Gut. 1994;35:360–2.
22. O'Donaghue DP, Dawson AM, Powell-Tuck J, Bown RL, Lennard-Jones JE. Double-blind withdrawal trial of azathioprine as maintenance treatment for Crohn's disease. Lancet. 1978;2:955–7.
23. Candy S, Wright J, Gerber M, Adams G, Gerig M, Goodman R. A controlled double blind study of azathioprine in the management of Crohn's disease. Gut. 1995;37:674–8.
24. Pearson DC, May GR, Fick GH, Sutherland LR. Azathioprine and 6-mercaptopurine in Crohn's disease: a meta-analysis. Ann Intern Med. 1995;122:132–42.
25. Present DH, Korelitz BI, Wisch N, Glass JL, Sachar DB, Pasternack BS. Treatment of Crohn's disease with 6-mercaptopurine. N Engl J Med. 1980;302:981–7.
26. Present DH, Meltzer SJ, Krumholz MP, Wolke A, Korelitz BI. 6-Mercaptopurine in the management of inflammatory bowel disease: short- and long-term toxicity. Ann Intern Med. 1989; 111:641–9.
27. Kozarek RA, Patterson DJ, Geland MD, Botoman VA, Ball TJ, Wilske KR. Methotrexate induces clinical and histologic remission in patients with refractory inflammatory bowel disease. Ann Intern Med. 1989;110:353–6.
28. Oren R, Moshkowitz M, Odes S *et al*. Methotrexate in chronic active Crohn's disease: a double-blind, randomized, Israeli multicenter trial. Am J Gastroenterol. 1997;92:2203–9.
29. Arora S, Katkoc W, Cooley J *et al*. Methotrexate in Crohn's disease: results of a randomized double-blind, placebo-controlled trial. Hepatogastroenterology. 1999;46:1724–9.
30. Feagan BG, Fedorak RN, Irvine EJ *et al*. A comparison of methotrexate with placebo for the maintenance of remission in Crohn's disease. *N Engl Med* 2000:342(22):1627–32.
31. Mahadevan U, Marion JF, Present DH. The place for methotrexate in the treatment of refractory Crohn's disease. AGA Abstract A1031, 1997.
32. Ekbom A. Cancer risk in inflammatory bowel disease. Can J Gastroenterol. 1995;9:23–6.
33. Hawthorne AB, Logan RFA, Hawkey CJ *et al*. Randomized controlled trial of azathioprine withdrawal in ulcerative colitis. Br Med J. 1992;305:20–2.
34. Oren R, Arber N, Odes S *et al*. Methotrexate in chronic active ulcerative colitis: a double-blind, randomized, Israeli multicenter trial. Gastroenterology. 1996;110:1416–21.
35. Korelitz BI, Present DH. Methotrexate for Crohn's disease. N Engl J Med. 1995;333:600–1.
36. Feagan BG, McDonald JWD. Methotrexate for Crohn's disease. N Engl J Med. 1995;333: 600–1.
37. Kremer JM, Alarcon GS, Lightfoot RW Jr *et al*. Methotrexate for rheumatoid arthritis. Suggested guidelines for monitoring liver toxicity. American College of Rheumatology. Arthritis Rheum. 1994;37:316–28.
38. Targan SR, Rutgeerts P, Hanauer SB *et al*. A multicenter trial of anti-tumor necrosis factor (TNF) antibody (cA2) for treatment of patients with active Crohn's disease. Gastroenterology. 1995;110:A1026.
39. Present DH, Rutgeerts P, Targan S *et al*. Infliximab for the treatment of fistulas in patients with Crohn's disease. N Engl J Med. 1999;340:1398–405.
40. Maini RN, Breedveld FC, Kalden JR *et al*. Therapeutic efficacy of multiple intravenous infusion of anti-tumor necrosis factor alpha monoclonal antibody combined with low-dose weekly methotrexate in rheumatoid arthritis. Arthritis Rheum. 1998;41:1552–63.

14
Methotrexate therapy for ulcerative colitis

T. GILAT, M. MOSHKOWITZ and R. OREN

The number of useful therapies for chronic active ulcerative colitis (UC), as well as for the maintenance of remission, is quite limited. Existing therapies either have severe potential side-effects or are of low efficacy. Therefore the suggestion that methotrexate (MTX) might be effective[1] in these situations aroused considerable interest. MTX has been used for many years in rheumatoid arthritis with relatively good results and few side-effects. The problem with evaluating the efficacy of MTX in UC is the paucity of studies, particularly controlled double-blind studies. Table 1 summarizes the few existing uncontrolled studies[1-3]. This shows that there were few patients in each of these studies, and the dose of MTX, as well as the mode of its administration, differed between the studies. Therefore no therapeutic conclusions can be derived from these studies; indeed, as shown in Table 2, the results were not impressive.

Table 1 Methotrexate in UC – uncontrolled studies

	No.	*Dose (mg)*	*Route*	*Duration (months)*
Kozarek *et al.* 1989[1]	7	25	i.m	3
Baron *et al.* 1993[2]	8	15	Oral	4
Egan *et al.* 1999[3]	14	15/25	s.c.	4

Table 2 Uncontrolled studies – response to methotrexate

	No.	*Clinical response (%)*		*Sigmoidoscopic (%)*	*Steroid reduction (%)*	
		Partial	*Complete*		*Partial*	*Complete*
Kozarek *et al.* 1989[1]	7	70	0	0	71	14
Baron *et al.* 1993[2]	8	37	0	37	37	0
Egan *et al.* 1999[3]	14	33	17	–		15

To date only one controlled randomized double-blind study has been published[4]. This included 67 patients (37 placebo, 30 MTX) treated for 9 months. All patients had chronic active UC as evidenced by a Mayo Clinic Score of $\geqslant 7$ and the use of steroids and/or immunosuppressives for over 4 months in the preceding 12 months. Patients continued with their conventional therapy and received in addition oral MTX 12.5 mg/week or placebo. Steroids were tapered and could be raised or reintroduced as clinically indicated (see Tables 3–5). Patients were seen at 1-month intervals and sigmoidoscopy was performed at 0, 3, 6 and 9 months. The study protocol is shown in Table 3. Twenty-five patients receiving placebo and 23 receiving MTX completed the 9 months of the study. The proportions of dropouts, treatment failures and those with side-effects (all mild) are given in Table 4. The proportion of patients entering remission, the mean Mayo Clinic score and the mean monthly steroid dose throughout the 9 months of study were not significantly different between the MTX and placebo groups. The proportion of patients relapsing after entering remission, the time until first remission and the percentage of the total study time in remission (Table 5) were again not significantly different between the two groups[4].

Table 3 Study protocol

Chronic active UC
Mayo Clinic score $\geqslant 7$
Steroids/immunosuppressives $> 4/12$ months
MTX 12.5 mg/week vs placebo 9 months
5-ASA continued, steroids tapered
Follow-up: Clinical 1 × month, sigmoidoscopy 0, 3, 6, 9 months

Table 4 Follow-up (9 months)

	Placebo	*MTX*
Completed	25	23
Dropouts	9	2
Treatment failure	2	3
Side-effects	1	2

Table 5 Study outcome

	Placebo	*MTX*	*p*
Percentage entering first remission	48.6	46.7	n.s.
Time to remission (months)	3.4	4.1	n.s.
Percentage relapsing after remission	44.4	64.3	n.s.
Percentage time in remission	41.1	36.9	n.s.

Thus the only large-scale controlled, randomized study did not show any advantage of MTX over placebo in chronic active UC. There was no effect on induction of remission or on maintenance of remission, and this over a period of 9 months. When combined with the meagre results of the small-scale uncontrolled studies it can be concluded that at present there is no evidence that MTX is effective or useful in UC. This conclusion is subject to several caveats. One relates to dose. The dose used in the first study of Kozarek *et al.*[1] was 25 mg/week intramuscularly. The dose used in the controlled study was 12.5 mg/week orally. A higher dose might be more effective. Egan *et al.*[3] did not find any significant difference between doses of 25 mg and 15 mg/week given subcutaneously to patients with active IBD. The second caveat relates to the route of administration. MTX given parenterally produced higher blood levels and higher tissue levels as compared to an equal oral dose. In rheumatoid arthritis, however, in which MTX has been used for years, oral therapy is perfectly effective and much used. The question was raised whether, in inflammatory bowel disease, oral methotrexate might be poorly absorbed. A comparison of MTX blood levels in patients with UC, rheumatoid arthritis and Crohn's disease after a single oral dose of MTX showed no differences[5]. The last caveat relates to the paucity of studies. One large-scale controlled study and three small uncontrolled studies provide an insufficient basis for judging the effects of a new therapy. More studies are required.

References

1. Kozarek RA, Patterson DJ, Gelfand MD, Botoman VA, Ball TJ, Wilske KR. Methotrexate induces clinical and histologic remission in patients with refractory inflammatory bowel disease. Ann Intern Med. 1989;110:353–6.
2. Baron TH, Truss CD, Elson CO. Low-dose oral methotrexate in refractory inflammatory bowel disease. Dig Dis Sci. 1993;38:1851–6.
3. Egan LJ, Sandborn WJ, Tremaine WJ *et al.* A randomized dose–response and pharmacokinetic study of methotrexate for refractory inflammatory Crohn's disease and ulcerative colitis. Aliment Pharmacol Ther. 1999;13:1597–604.
4. Oren R, Arber N, Odes S *et al.* Methotrexate in chronic active ulcerative colitis: a double-blind, randomized, Israeli multicenter trial. Gastroenterology. 1996;110:1416–21.
5. Moshkowitz M, Oren R, Tishler M *et al.* The absorption of low-dose methotrexate in patients with inflammatory bowel disease. Aliment Pharmacol Ther. 1997;11:569–73.

Section V
New developments: mycophenolate mofetil

15
Mycophenolate mofetil – an introduction to its pharmacology

K. FELLERMANN

INTRODUCTION

Mycophenolate mofetil (MMF) is an immunosuppressive agent which has entered clinical practice recently. It was isolated from *Penicillium* strains at the beginning of the 1900s and fomerly known for its antimicrobial activity. The immunosuppressive properties became apparent in the late 1960s[1] and the first clinical trials were performed in autoimmune disease[2]. Later the interest shifted to transplantation medicine, where it was shown to be superior to azathioprine in decreasing the incidence of acute renal allograft rejection and treatment. It is now implemented in many transplantation protocols in combination with other immunomodulatory drugs.

PHARMACODYNAMIC PROPERTIES

MMF is the prodrug of the active compound mycophenolic acid (MPA). It is a non-competitive, reversible inhibitor of type II inosine monophosphate dehydro-genase (IMPDH). MPA blocks the *de-novo* synthesis of guanosine nucleotides in eukaryotic cells, thereby diminishing the substrates for DNA and RNA synthe-sis[3]. B and T lymphocytes are especially affected as they depend on the *de-novo* synthesis[4]. Other cells, e.g. granulocytes, can utilize a salvage pathway catalysed by hypoxanthine–guanine phosphoribosyltransferase (HGPRT) which bypasses the depletion of guanosine nucleotides.

In-vitro data revealed that it inhibits mitogen- and antigen-stimulated B and T cell proliferation, antibody formation[5] as well as mixed lymphocyte responses[6]. The exposure to MPA decreases the pools of guanosine triphosphates and deoxyguanosine triphosphates in lymphocytes but not in neutrophils, evidence for the cell-specific action[7]. Another interesting feature is the reduced incorporation of mannose and fucose in glycoproteins[8,9]. It was demonstrated that MMF-treated monocytes have a decreased adhesion to endothelial cells or extracellular matrix proteins. This may have the consequence of an impaired homing of lymphocytes and monocytes to sites of inflammation. Early cytokine responses such as IL-1 and IL-2 signalling remain unaffected[5]. The antigen- or mitogen-stimulated expression of IL-2R is reduced or unchanged[5,10,11]. In summary, MMF is more selective than azathioprine and acts at a later stage compared to cyclosporin or steroids.

The efficacy in the prevention of allograft rejection has been observed in several animal models, and is reviewed elsewhere[12].

PHARMACOKINETIC PROPERTIES

MMF is rapidly absorbed and hydrolysed to MPA by plasma esterases in the blood stream. The oral bioavailability exceeds 90% in healthy volunteers. However, in the immediate post-transplantation period it is decreased by approximately 50% due to an excessive clearance. Maximum plasma levels are obtained within 1–2 h after administration. About 97% of MPA are bound to albumin. MPA is subsequently glucuronidated in the liver to MPAG, an inactive compound. Ninety-three per cent of the drug is eliminated in the urine, mostly as the glucuronidated metabolite (87%), but a considerable amount undergoes enterohepatic circulation, which prolongs the apparent half-life to 18 h.

Drugs such as aciclovir competing with renal tubular secretion potentially inhibit the elimination of MPAG. Bile acid sequestrants and antibiotics interfere with enterohepatic circulation and reduce the AUC of MPA. Antacids impair the oral absorption of MMF, whereas food consumption reduces peak plasma levels only[13].

CLINICAL TRIALS IN RENAL TRANSPLANTATION

Three large comparative multicentre trials[14–16] have been conducted to evaluate the clinical efficacy and safety of MMF in renal transplantation. In the prevention of rejection MMF has been combined with cyclosporin and steroids, with or without antithymocyte globulin for induction. The instituted dose was 2 or 3 g MMF per day. In one trial MMF resulted in a decreased frequency of biopsy-proven rejection or treatment failure (30.3% on 2 g, 38.8% on 3 g) compared to placebo (56%) within 6 months[16]. The higher dose was less well tolerated and responsible for an increased treatment failure rate despite fewer rejections. Full courses of immunosuppressive therapy for acute rejection episodes were necessary in 28.5% and 24.4% on 2 and 3 g MMF compared to 51.8% on placebo, though not significant. No differences were observed in terms of graft loss or patient survival.

The other studies were conducted in comparison to azathioprine including 1002 patients[14,15]. A lower proportion of patients treated with MMF than with azathioprine experienced a biopsy-proven acute rejection (19.7% and 19.8% on 2 g MMF, 15.9% and 17.5% on 3 g MMF, 35.5% and 38% on 100–150 mg azathioprine). The incidence of treatment failure including rejection was similarly reduced with MMF (38.2% and 31.1% on 2 g MMF, 34.8% and 31.3% on 3 g MMF, 50% and 47.6% on 100–150 mg azathioprine). Antilymphocyte therapy tended to be less often necessary in the MMF-treated groups. As in the placebo-controlled trial, graft loss or patient survival was similar in all groups at the end of 6 months. One of these trials including 503 patients has been extended to 3 years[17] and resembles the initial findings. Graft and patient survival exceeded 80% in all treatment groups (intention-to-treat analysis 81.9% and 84.8% on 2 and 3 g MMF, respectively vs 80.2% on azathioprine). Mortality was comparable in all three groups. A dose-related adverse event profile is seen in the cumulative analysis of the two comparative trials with azathioprine[14,15]. They mostly comprised the gastrointestinal system (e.g. diarrhoea, nausea and vomiting), and lymphatic and haematopoietic disorders (e.g. leucopenia and anaemia). Patients were withdrawn in 13.9% on placebo and in 17.6% and 25.6% on 2 and 3 g MMF, respectively. Azathioprine resulted in a withdrawal rate of 7.9% due to adverse events, while 9.1% and 13.9% terminated the study on 2 and 3 g MMF. The most common side-effect was diarrhoea. This was most often observed in the 3 g MMF group (36.1%). The level with 2 g MMF (31%) was still above that with azathioprine (20.9%). Whether this side-effect is related to high mucosal levels due to enterohepatic circulation is currently unknown. Except for an increased frequency of leucopenia in the 3 g MMF group (34.5% vs 23.2% and 24.8% on 2 g MMF and azathioprine, respectively), the haematological and lymphatic adverse events were similar in all treatment groups. A slight increase in cytomegalovirus infections was notified upon MMF. However, the proportion of patients with other opportunistic infections was equally distributed among the treatment groups. The overall frequency of neoplasms was 5.4% and 4.0% in those patients receiving 2 and 3 g MMF, respectively, compared to 4.5% on azathioprine and 1.8% on placebo. At 3 years lymphoproliferative disorders were diagnosed in 1.2% and 1.8% on 2 and 3 g MMF, respectively, and 0.8% on azathioprine in a single trial[17]. However, the observation time is clearly too short to draw any final conclusion regarding the incidence of malignancies.

Apart from transplantation medicine, beneficial effects of MMF in auto-immune diseases have been reported for the therapy of psoriasis[18,19], as well as rheumatoid arthritis[20]. Some patients refractory to conventional therapy had been treated for as long as 13 years with doses ranging from 2 to 7 g per day, and experienced significant improvement. No serious side-effects were observed.

Whether drug monitoring is of any value is currently unknown. A high-performance liquid chromatography-based analysis and an enzyme-multiplied immunoassay technique assay are available at specialized facilities.

CONCLUSION

The results of the trials with MMF published to date are encouraging, and have expanded the pharmacological armoury in prevention and treatment of allograft rejection. MMF is an elegant drug due to its selective mode of action in the late stage of the immune response. Autoimmune diseases may be future targets.

References

1. Mitsui A, Suzuki S. Immunosuppressive effect of mycophenolic acid. J Antibiot. 1969;22: 358–63.

2. Gomez EC, Menendez L, Frost P. Efficacy of mycophenolic acid for the treatment of psoriasis. J Am Acad Dermatol. 1979;1:531–7.

3. Franklin TJ, Cook JM. The inhibition of nucleic acid synthesis by mycophenolic acid. Biochem J. 1969;113:515–24.

4. Allison AC, Hovi T, Watts RWE, Webster AD. Immunological observations on patients with the Lesch–Nyhan syndrome, and on the role of *de-novo* purine synthesis in lymphocyte transformation. Lancet. 1975;2:1179–83.

5. Eugui EM, Almquist AJ, Muller CD, Allison AC. Lymphocyte-selective cytostatic and immunosuppressive effects of mycophenolic acid *in vitro*: role of deoxyguanosine nucleotide depletion. Scand J Immunol. 1991;33:161–73.

6. Burlingham WJ, Grailer AP, Hullett DA, Sollinger HW. Inhibition of both MLC and *in vitro* IgG memory response to tetanus toxoid by RS-61443. Transplant. 1991;51:545–7.

7. Allison AC, Almquist AJ, Muller CD, Eugui EM. *In vitro* immunosuppressive effects of mycophenolic acid and an ester prodrug, RS-61443. Transplant Proc. 1991;23:10–14.

8. Allison AC, Kowalski WJ, Muller CD, Waters RV, Eugui EM. Mycophenolic acid and brequinar, inhibitors of purine and pyrimidine synthesis, block the gylcosylation of adhesion molecules. Transplant Proc. 1993;25:67–70.

9. Sokoloski JA, Sartorelli AC. Effects of the inhibitors of IMP dehydrogenase, tiazofurin and mycophenolic acid, on glycoprotein metabolism. Mol Pharmacol. 1985;28:567–73.

10. Weaver JL, Pine AS, Aszalos A. Comparison of the *in vitro* and biophysical effects of cyclosporine A, FK-506, and mycophenolic acid on human peripheral blood lymphocytes. Immunopharmacol Immunotoxicol. 1991;13:563–76.

11. Woo J, Zeevi A, Yao GZ, Strednak J, Todo S, Thomson AW. Effects of FK 506, mycophenolic acid, and bredinin on OKT-3-, PMA-, and alloantigen-induced activation molecule expression on cultured CD4[+] and CD8[+] human lymphocytes. Transplant Proc. 1991;23:2939–40.

12. Fulton B, Markham A. Mycophenolate mofetil. A review of its pharmacodynamic and pharmakokinetic properties and clinical efficacy in renal transplantation. Drugs. 1996;51:278–98.

13. Hoffmann-La Roche. CellCept, monography. 1995; Grenzach-Whylen, Germany.

14. Tricontinental Mycophenolate Mofetil Renal Transplantation Study Group. A blinded, randomized clinical trial of mycophenolate mofetil for the prevention of acute rejection in cadaveric renal transplantation. Transplant. 1996;61:1029–37.

15. Sollinger HW. Mycophenolate mofetil for the prevention of acute rejection in primary cadaveric renal allograft recipients. US Renal Transplant Mycophenolate Mofetil Study Group. Transplant. 1995;60:225–32.

16. European Mycophenolate Mofetil Cooperative Study Group. Placebo-controlled study of mycophenolate mofetil combined with cyclosporin and corticosteroids for prevention of acute rejection. Lancet. 1995;345:1321–5.

17. Mathew TH. A blinded, long-term, randomized multicenter study of mycophenolate mofetil in cadaveric renal transplantation: results at three years. Tricontinental Mycophenolate Mofetil Renal Transplantation Study Group. Transplant. 1998;65:1450–4.

18. Marinari R, Fleischmeyer R, Schragger AH, Rosenthal AL. Mycophenolic acid in the treatment of psoriasis. Arch Dermatol. 1977;113:930–2.

19. Epinette WW, Parker CM, Jones EL, Greist MC. Mycophenolic acid for psoriasis. J Am Acad Dermatol. 1987;17:962–71.

20. Goldblum R. Therapy of rheumatoid arthritis with mycophenolate mofetil. Clin Exp Rheumatol. 1993;11:S117–19.

16
Mycophenolate mofetil in Crohn's disease

W. PETRITSCH

INTRODUCTION

The thiopurines 6-mercaptopurine and the prodrug azathioprine (AZA) have been used for decades in a variety of mainly autoimmune diseases and in transplantation medicine; they have also become the standard first-line immunosuppressive agents in the treatment of Crohn's disease. They are now generally accepted when moderate to severe Crohn's disease is refractory to steroids or when steroid tapering is not possible[1,2]. Unfortunately, in about 40% of all patients AZA is either ineffective or must be stopped because of side-effects[3-6]. Moreover, it does not show an effect before 3 months. New immunosuppressive agents would thus be highly desirable, and mycophenolate mofetil (MMF) could be such a drug. MMF has been shown to be superior to AZA for prevention and treatment of acute rejection following allograft transplantation in renal and cardiac transplantation[7-12]. MMF or its active metabolites inhibit the *de-novo* pathway of purine synthesis in T and B lymphocytes. Moreover, it was recently shown that MMF inhibits intestinal smooth muscle cell growth and the synthesis of fibronectin *in vitro*[13]. This may be useful in preventing smooth muscle hyperplasia and stricture formation in inflammatory bowel disease (IBD).

CLINICAL STUDIES

Up to now nine publications have reported the use of MMF in IBD (Table 1). Half of them describe the use of MMF in Crohn's disease alone. In the first study, by Horgan[14], which is available only as an abstract, prednisolone could be markedly reduced in two patients and clinical improvement was achieved in one patient with fistulas. In 1998 two further studies were published. Florin reported a favourable clinical response in all three patients with perianal disease and a symptomatic improvement, defined as decrease of greater than 100 points in CDAI, in two of three patients with chronic active disease[15]. None of the six

Table 1 Publications on mycophenolate mofetil in IBD

Reference	Design	Crohn's disease	Follow-up (months)	Response (%)
Horgan et al. 1997[14]	Case report*	3/5	0.8–6	75
Florin 1998[15]	Case report	6/8	6–12	100
Fickert et al. 1998[16]	Case report	6/6	6–12	100
Neurath et al. 1999[17]	Randomized prospective MMF vs AZA	70/70	6	Advantage in subgroup
Hassard et al. 2000[18]	Case report	11/11	5–26	27
Fellermann et al. 2000[19]	Open prospective	11/24	3–6	9
Skelly et al. 2000[20]	Case report*	6/11	0.8–7	0
Wenzl et al. 2000[21]	Open retrospective*	20/20	36	20
Miehsler et al. 2000[22]	Open retrospective*	15/15	12	60

*Only abstract available.

patients tolerated AZA or 6-mercaptopurine, or showed any response. In our first study we treated two patients with highly active Crohn's disease and four with perianal disease, all intolerant to AZA[16]. Within an observation period of 6–12 months all patients improved as measured by the PDAI (decrease from 13.0 to 9.0) or CDAI (mean decrease from 437 to 228). Neurath et al. published the only randomized controlled study so far comparing 15 mg/kg MMF versus 2.5 mg/kg AZA in active Crohn's disease[17]. None of the patients was on immunosuppression before. This study found that, in patients with moderate disease (CDAI 150–300), MMF treatment was as effective as AZA (both in combination with steroids). In highly active disease (CDAI > 300) MMF led to an earlier reduction in CDAI (Fig. 1). At the end of the 6-month study there was no longer any statistical difference between the two treatment groups. However, it should be emphasized that the study was not blinded. Both the investigator and the patient were informed about treatment. Moreover, there was a maintenance treatment with prednisolone of 5 mg throughout the whole study period. In the report by Hassard et al. only 7/11 patients could continue treatment longer than 8 weeks[18]. However, in contrast to the previous study, the patient group was very inhomogeneous. Patients were either intolerant or resistant to AZA therapy. The results were disappointing. Only one patient achieved a complete remission longer than a year, and two were considered as partial responders (decline in Harvey–Bradshaw index by > 25% compared with baseline and a reduction in steroid use). Fellerman et al. treated 11 patients with active Crohn's disease with MMF and steroids in a tapered pattern in an open-label study[19]. At the end of the 6-month study period remission (defined as induction and maintenance of remission with a CDAI < 150) was maintained only in one patient. In a small study Skelly et al. could not find any improvement in six patients with Crohn's disease and intolerant or without response to AZA at a dosage of 1 g/day[20]. Long-term follow-up of 36 months by our group showed at the end that only 4/20 patients

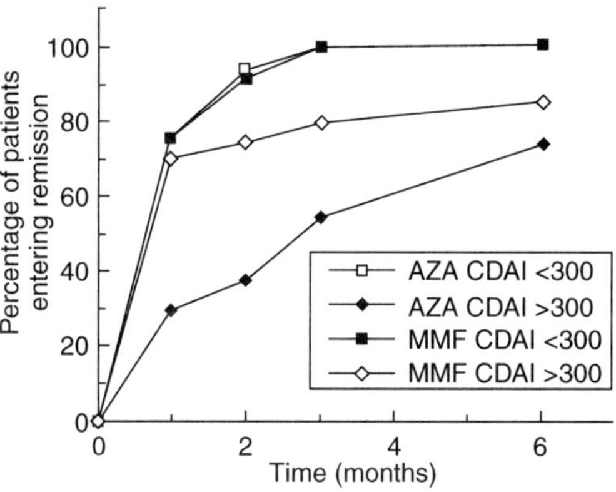

Figure 1 Cumulative percentage of patients entering remission at indicated time points. From ref. 17, with permission

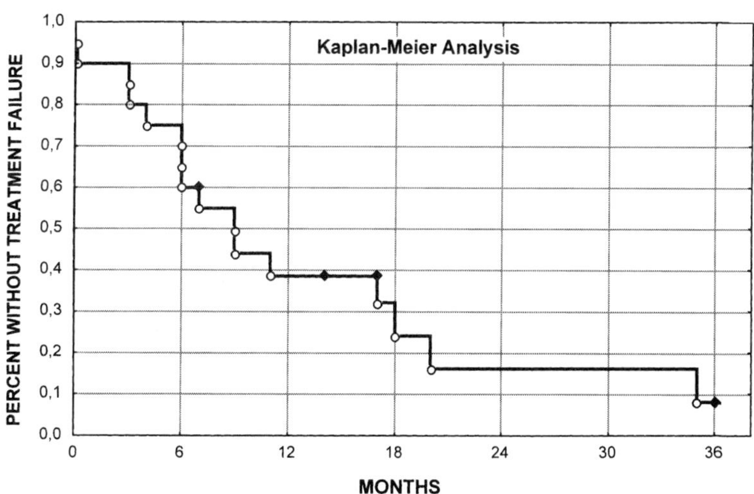

Figure 2 Cumulative probability of relapse in 20 Crohn's disease patients treated with mycophenolate mofetil

were not treatment failures (Fig. 2)[21]. Treatment failure was defined very strictly as lack of response (no clinical remission without steroids achieved) or relapse after initial response or discontinuation of MMF for any reasons. Finally Miehsler and colleagues from Vienna reported in a retrospective study that after 12 months a remission could be achieved in 9/15 patients under MMF, all of whom were intolerant to AZA[22]. Prednisolone tapering was possible at an earlier stage in comparison to an AZA-matched group. Flare-ups, however, were higher in the MMF groups.

TOLERABILITY

In transplantation MMF has generally demonstrated an acceptable safety profile. The principal adverse events described in transplant patients are diarrhoea, leukopenia and infections (generally cytomegalovirus, CMV). Rates of treatment discontinuation because of adverse events were higher with MMF 3 g/day and, to a lesser extent, with MMF 2 g/day than with placebo (26% and 18% vs 14%)[23]. Side-effects in transplantation were similar comparing MMF vs AZA (13% for MMF 2 g/day and 15% for MMF 3 g/day vs 14–16% for AZA)[8,12]. Overall MMF 2 g/day was better tolerated than 3 g/day in patients undergoing transplantation[7,8,23]. Gastrointestinal side-effects play a major role. Most common are diarrhoea, abdominal pain, nausea and vomiting. Nevertheless gastrointestinal tract ulceration, haemorrhage or perforation occurred in a small number (< 1–5%) of transplant patients treated with MMF[7,12,23,24]. Concomitant infections such as CMV may be responsible for these rare adverse gastrointestinal reactions. Side-effects with MMF in patients with IBD are summarized in Table 2. Overall the adverse rate seems to be rather high (50/146, 34%). As far as noted in 11 patients the side-effects were severe, and treatment had to be stopped. Some side-effects such as arthralgia may be due to the underlying disease itself, and others are difficult to judge, as all reports are open-label trials without a placebo arm. Nevertheless it is remarkable that Neurath *et al.*, using the lowest dose (15 mg/kg, 1.5 g/day) and new patients, also described the lowest adverse event rate[17]. On the other hand MMF was well tolerated in most of the patients intolerant to previous AZA therapy[15,16,22].

Table 2 Adverse events reported in 146 patients with IBD treated with mycophenolate mofetil[14–22]

Gastrointestinal	Diarrhoea	7
	Nausea and vomiting	6
	Severe colonic ulceration	2
	Elevated liver enzymes	2
Rheumatological	Arthralgia	9
Dermatological	Rash, erythema	7
Others	Infections	3
	Anaemia	1
	Headache	2
	Depression	1
	Sleeplessness	1
	Sweating	1
	Hypertension	1
	Blurred vision	1
	Flu-like symptoms	1
	Unknown	3

DISCUSSION

On the basis of the available studies MMF seems not to be significantly superior to AZA in Crohn's disease patients in comparison to the first transplantation studies. The only controlled trial in Crohn's disease which compared MMF head-to-head with AZA was unblinded, and showed an advantage for MMF only in a subgroup of patients. In our long-term follow-up study after 36 months only 20% were in remission without any steroids. Even if this is not directly comparable, the probability of relapse in Crohn's disease patients treated with AZA was only 22% in a major French study after 3 years[25]. In long-term follow-up studies (3 years) comparing MMF vs AZA in renal and cardiac transplantation MMF is, however, slightly superior (approximately 5%) to AZA[26]. There could be a number of reasons for the quite different results in the IBD case reports and Neurath *et al.*'s controlled trial. Indications for treatment and definition of response were rather different. In most reports there was a subgroup of IBD patients who were intolerant to AZA or who did not respond to it. Only the two German studies used MMF as a first-line drug[17,19]. No study was blinded and dosages differed; nevertheless, most investigators used 2 g/day. This dose seems to be the most suitable one when efficacy and tolerance are compared in transplantation studies. With the increasing number of published cases and the prolonged observation time tolerance and rate of efficacy of MMF have decreased. A controlled double-blind study would be necessary to definitively determine the role of MMF in the treatment of Crohn's disease. Unfortunately, a randomized double-blind multicentre trial comparing MMF and AZA that had been planned and implemented was stopped for undisclosed reasons by the sponsoring company (Roche, Basel, Switzerland), although slow recruitment at the beginning and the development of other new drugs (for example tumour necrosis factor antibodies) could have been involved in the decision to discontinue the study[27]. In absence of a controlled double-blind trial the importance of MMF in treatment of Crohn's disease remains open. At the moment MMF cannot be recommended for regular use outside of clinical studies for the treatment of Crohn's disease. Nevertheless it is an alternative for patients who need basic immunosuppression and do not tolerate or respond to AZA or 6-MP, and for whom methotrexate for whatever reason is not an option.

SUMMARY

Mycophenolate mofetil (MMF) is a new immunosuppressive agent which inhibits DNA synthesis leading to suppression of B and T cells. In transplantation it is superior to azathioprine with regard to allograft rejection. Experience with MMF in Crohn's disease is limited. Open-label reports are inconsistent concerning tolerance and efficacy. The only controlled trial is unblinded and shows that MMF is superior to azathioprine in highly active disease within 6 months. The overall adverse event rate reported in all patients with IBD treated with mycophenolate mofetil is 34%. At the moment MMF cannot be recommended for regular use outside of clinical studies or selected cases for the treatment of Crohn's disease.

References

1. Stange EF, Schreiber S, Raedler A *et al*. Therapie des Morbus Crohn – Ergebnisse einer Konsensuskonferenz der Deutschen Gesellschaft für Verdauungs- und Stoffwechselkrankheiten. Z Gastroenterol. 1997;35:541–54.
2. Pearson DC, May GR, Fick GH, Sutherland LR. Azathioprine and 6-mercaptopurine in Crohn's disease. A meta-analysis. Ann Intern Med. 1995;122:132–42.
3. Present DH, Meltzer SJ, Krumholz MP, Wolke A, Korelitz BI. 6-Mercaptopurine in the management of inflammatory bowel disease: short- and long-term toxicity. Ann Intern Med. 1989; 111:641–9.
4. Present DH, Burton IK, Wisch N, Glass JL, Sachar DB, Pasternack BS. Treatment of Crohn's disease with 6-mercaptopurine. N Engl J Med. 1980;302:981–7.
5. O'Brien JJ, Bayless TM, Bayless JA. Use of azathioprine or 6-mercaptopurine in the treatment of Crohn's disease. Gastroenterology. 1991;101:39–46.
6. Korelitz BI, Adler DJ, Mendelsohn RA, Sacknoff AL. Long-term experience with 6-mercaptopurine in the treatment of Crohn's disease. Am J Gastroenterol. 1993;88:1198–205.
7. Sollinger HW, US Renal Transplant Study Group. Mycophenolate mofetil for the prevention of acute rejection in primary cadaveric renal allograft recipients. Transplantation. 1995;60:225–32.
8. Tricontinental MMRTSG. A blinded, randomized clinical trial of mycophenolate mofetil for the prevention of acute rejection in cadaveric renal transplantation. Transplantation. 1996;61: 1029–37.
9. US Mycophenolate Mofetil Study Group. Mycophenolate mofetil for the prevention of acute rejection of primary cadaveric kidney transplants: status of the MYC 1866 study at 1 year. Transplant Proc. 1997;29:348–9.
10. US Renal Transplant Mycophenolate Mofetil Study Group. Mycophenolate mofetil in cadaveric renal transplantation. Am J Kidney Dis. 1999;34:296–303.
11. Mathew TH, Tricontinental MMRTSG. A blinded, long-term, randomized multicenter study of mycophenolate mofetil in cadaveric renal transplantation: results at three years. Transplantation. 1998;65:1450–4.
12. Kobashigawa J, Miller L, Renlund D *et al*. A randomized active-controlled trial of mycophenolate mofetil in heart transplant recipients. Transplantation. 1998;66:507–15.
13. Zeeh JM, Riley NE, Hoffmann P, Goebel H, Gerken G. Mycophenolate mofetil inhibits growth and expression of extracellular matrix in human intestinal and rate colonic smooth muscle cells. Gastroenterology. 1999;111:A948.
14. Horgan K. Initial experience with mycophenolate mofetil in the treatment of severe inflammatory bowel disease. Gastroenterology. 1997;112:A999.
15. Florin THJ. Treatment of steroid refractory inflammatory bowel disease (IBD) with mycophenolate mofetil (MMF). Aust NZ J Med. 1998;28:344–5.
16. Fickert P, Hinterleitner TA, Wenzl HH, Aichbichler BW, Petritsch W. Mycophenolate mofetil in patients with Crohn's disease. Am J Gastroenterol. 1998;93:2529–32.
17. Neurath MF, Wanitschke R, Peters M *et al*. Randomised trial of mycophenolate mofetil versus azathioprine for treatment of chronic active Crohn's disease. Gut. 1999;44:625–8.
18. Hassard PV, Vasiliauskas EA, Kam LY, Targan SR, Abreui MT. Efficacy of mycophenolate mofetil in patients failing 6-mercaptopurine or azathioprine therapy for Crohn's disease. Inflamm Bowel Dis. 2000;6:6–20.
19. Fellermann K, Steffen M, Stein J *et al*. Mycophenolate mofetil: lack of efficacy in chronic active inflammatory bowel disease. Aliment Pharmacol Ther. 2000;14:171–6.
20. Skelly MM, Curtis H, Jenkins D, Hawkey CJ, Logan RF. Toxicity of mycophenolate mofetil (MMF) in patients with inflammatory bowel disease (IBD). Gastroenterology. 2000;118:A789.
21. Wenzl HH, Hinterleitner TA, Fickert P *et al*. Low efficacy of long-term treatment with mycophenolate mofetil in patients with Crohn's disease. Gastroenterology. 2000;118:A790.
22. Miehsler W, Reinisch W, Moser G, Gangl A, Vogelsang H. Ist Mycophenolate Mofetil eine Alternative zu Azathioprin bei chronisch aktiven Mb. Crohn. Z Gastroenterol. 2000;38:437.
23. European Mycophenolate Mofetil Cooperative Study Group. Placebo-controlled study of mycophenolate mofetil combined with cyclosporin and corticosteroids for prevention of acute rejection. Lancet. 1995;345:1321–5.
24. Hoffmann-La Roche F. Mycophenolate mofetil prescribing information. Nutley (NJ), USA, 1998.

25. Bouhnik Y, Lemann M, Mary JY *et al.* Long-term follow-up of patients with Crohn's disease treated with azathioprine or 6-mercaptopurine. Lancet. 1996;347:215–19.
26. Hosenpud JD, Bennett LE. Mycophenolate mofetil compared to azathioprine improves survival in patients surviving the initial cardiac transplant hospitalization: an analysis of the joint UNOs/ISHLT thoracic registry. AST Chicago, 13–17 May 2000, Abstract 743.
27. Rampton DS, Neurath MF, Almer S, D'Haens G, Petritsch W, Stange EF. Mycophenolate mofetil in Crohn's disease. Lancet. 2000;356:163–4.

17
Mycophenolate mofetil in ulcerative colitis: acute and chronic

K. FELLERMANN

As the use of azathioprine and 6-mercaptopurine is limited by frequent adverse side-effects[1], and trials with methotrexate have been disappointing in ulcerative colitis (UC)[2], alternative treatment options are clearly warranted. The immuno-suppressant mycophenolate mofetil (MMF), which is equally effective compared to azathioprine in preventing graft rejection after organ transplantation, may be a novel choice. Beneficial effects have been reported in psoriasis[3,4] and rheuma-toid arthritis[5]. Moreover, a more rapid action than azathioprine has been claimed[6].

Only limited, open-label experience is available in UC at present. Initial reports claimed a benefit in patients who relapsed or were intolerant to azathio-prine and were switched to MMF, mostly in conjunction with steroids. The insti-tuted dose ranged from 1 to 2 g/day. Horgan[7] reported on two UC patients, one steroid-refractory and one steroid-dependent. Both had entered remission by 3 months and experienced a decreased steroid demand. Florin et al.[8] treated two patients of whom one reached remission with 1 g MMF/day. With the same dose one UC patient showed clinical improvement and a decreased steroid demand[9] but another five failed to achieve remission[10]. Moreover, atypical colonic ulcera-tions occurred in one patient, which has already been described in renal trans-plant recipients, as well as one case of major lower gastrointestinal bleeding.

In a first larger cohort MMF was tested in chronic active UC defined as a steroid demand $\geqslant 10$ mg prednisone per day in the preceding 2 months and mod-erate to severe activity according to Truelove[11]. Thirteen patients were treated with 2 g/day and a tapering steroid protocol for 6 months, starting with 60 mg prednisolone equivalent. The primary endpoint was remission induction by 3 months and maintenance after 6 months. Whereas six patients achieved remis-sion by 3 months, none maintained the remission over the whole study period. A small subset of patients with a partial response by 3 months were continued, but all stopped the drug eventually. Another study investigated the response to 20 mg/kg MMF/day compared to 2 g azathioprine/day and a standardized steroid-tapering regimen in active UC (CAI $\geqslant 6$)[12]. The observation lasted 12 months and, by the end, seven of eight patients (88%) in the MMF and all 12 patients (100%) in the azathioprine group were in remission. At each interim analysis remission rates were higher in patients on azathioprine, e.g. at 6 months 92% on azathioprine vs 67% on MMF. Not all patients were able to completely withdraw steroids at the end after 1 year (azathioprine 58%, MMF 38%). Besides the extraordinarily high therapeutic gain of azathioprine in this trial, the result with 1.5 g MMF/day is still impressive, and contrasts with the former study. On the other hand, this is reminiscent of a previously published study with MMF in Crohn's disease, in which it proved to be at least equally effective compared to azathioprine[13].

Due to the inconsistent results of MMF in UC to date, prescription cannot be recommended. Further controlled investigations are clearly warranted to clarify its role in UC.

References

1. Sandborn WJ. A review of immune modifier therapy for inflammatory bowel disease: azathioprine, 6-mercaptopurine, cyclosporine, and methotrexate. Am J Gastroenterol. 1996;91:423–33.
2. Oren R, Arber N, Odes S *et al.* Methotrexate in chronic active ulcerative colitis: a double-blind, randomized, Israeli multicenter trial. Gastroenterology. 1996;110:1418–21.
3. Marinari R, Fleischmeyer R, Schragger AH, Rosenthal AL. Mycophenolic acid in the treatment of psoriasis. Arch Dermatol. 1977;113:930–2.
4. Epinette WW, Parker CM, Jones EL, Griest MC. Mycophenolic acid for psoriasis. J Am Acad Dermatol. 1987;17:962–71.
5. Goldblum R. Therapy of rheumatoid arthritis with mycophenolate mofetil. Clin Exp Rheumatol. 1993;11:S117–19.
6. Schiff MH, Goldblum R, Rees MMC. 2-Morpholino-ethyl mycophenolic acid (ME-MPA) in the treatment of refractory rheumatoid arthritis (RA). Arthritis Rheum. 1990;33:s155.
7. Horgan K. Initial experience with mycophenolate mofetil in the treatment of severe inflammatory bowel disease. Gastroenterology. 1997;112:A999.
8. Florin TH, Roberts RK, Watson MR, Radford-Smith GL. Treatment of steroid refractory inflammatory bowel disease (IBD) with mycophenolate mofetil. Aust NZ J Med. 1998;28:344–5.
9. Nehme OS, Overley CA, O'Brien JJ. The role of mycophenolate mofetil in the management of refractory inflammatory bowel disease (IBD). Gastroenterology. 1998;114:A1049.
10. Skelly MM, Curtis H, Jenkins D, Hawkey CJ, Logan RF. Toxicity of mycophenolate mofetil (MMF) in patients with inflammatory bowel disease (IBD). Gastroenterology. 2000;118:A818.
11. Fellermann K, Steffen M, Stein J *et al.* Mycophenolate mofetil: lack of efficacy in chronic active inflammatory bowel disease. Aliment Pharmacol Ther. 2000;14:171–6.
12. Orth T, Peters M, Schlaak JF *et al.* Mycophenolate mofetil versus azathioprine in patients with chronic active ulcerative colitis: a 12-month pilot study. Am J Gastroenterol. 2000;95:1201–7.
13. Neurath MF, Wanitschke R, Peters M, Krummenauer F, Meyer zum Büschenfelde K-H, Schlaak JF. Randomised trial of mycophenolate mofetil versus azathioprine for treatment of chronic active Crohn's disease. Gut. 1999;44:625–8.

Section VI
New developments: cyclosporin/tacrolimus

18
Cyclosporin and tacrolimus in acute and chronic Crohn's disease

J. BRYNSKOV

INTRODUCTION

It is now 16 years since the first case report on cyclosporin treatment of Crohn's disease was published[1]. This was followed by numerous uncontrolled studies[2], and later a series of placebo-controlled clinical trials. Cyclosporin has continued to attract interest in the field of inflammatory bowel disease, and there are several reasons for this. First, cyclosporin was the first immunosuppressive drug with a rather selective effect on T-lymphocyte-mediated immune responses[3]. Second, cyclosporin acts by inhibiting the transcription and production of interleukin-2 and interferon-γ, an effect which is consistent with the emerging view that Crohn's disease is a T-helper-1-type disease[4]. Third, the dramatic short-term response to high-dose intravenous cyclosporin treatment in severe ulcerative colitis has served to maintain a continued interest in this drug[5].

Unfortunately, cyclosporin treatment is associated with a well-established risk of side-effects. These include renal function impairment, hypertension, hypertrichosis, tremor/paraesthesias, liver dysfunction, gingival hyperplasia, and dyspepsia[3]. Another increasing matter of concern is the risk of life-threatening side-effects, including opportunistic infections such as *Pneumocystis carinii* pneumonia, which may occur as a result of the use of multiple immunosuppressive agents[6–10]. The aim of this overview is primarily to clarify the role of cyclosporin treatment in Crohn's disease, but the limited clinical experience with tacrolimus/FK-506, a similar immunosuppressive drug, will also be addressed.

CONTROLLED TRIAL EXPERIENCE

For safety reasons all clinical trials in Crohn's disease, except one, have been performed using a low daily oral dosage of cyclosporin (~5 mg/kg per day). In two trials subgroups of patients were included in order to address whether cyclosporin maintains remission or prevents worsening. As shown in Table 1, both these trials clearly showed that cyclosporin provides no benefit in terms of preventing a flare-up. Therefore, oral low-dose cyclosporin has no role in the long-term management of patients with inactive or low-active disease[11,12].

The effect of addition of oral cyclosporin to ongoing treatment in active Crohn's disease has been studied in four trials. Three of these trials showed no significant benefit of low-dose cyclosporin ($\sim$5 mg/kg per day)[11-13]. In the last study a higher average daily dosage was used, which may explain the demonstration of a transient, but significant, effect in several independent measures of Crohn's disease activity[14,15] (Table 2). Taken together these data show that oral low-dose cyclosporin treatment has no consistent effect in patients with active Crohn's disease, but suggest a dose–response relationship. This notion is supported by the remarkable short-term efficacy of high-dose intravenous cyclosporin in ulcerative colitis[5]. In this setting cyclosporin is typically administered in a dosage of 4 mg/kg per day, which is equivalent to an oral dosage of $\sim$16 mg/kg per day, or three-fold that administered in the majority of clinical trials in Crohn's disease.

Table 1 Final response rates to oral low-dose cyclosporin treatment in patients with inactive or low-active Crohn's disease

	Cyclosporin	Placebo	P-Value
Stange et al.[11]			
Response	16/56 (29%)	16/62 (26%)	
Failure	40/56 (71%)	46/62 (74%)	n.s.
Feagan et al.[12]			
Failure/worsening	64/99 (65%)	47/94 (50%)	n.s.

*n.s. = Not significant.

Table 2 Final response rates to oral cyclosporin treatment in patients with active Crohn's disease

	Cyclosporin	Dosage (mg/kg per day)	Placebo	P-Value
Stange et al.[11]				
Response	2/33 (6%)	5	3/31 (10%)	
Failure	31/33 (94%)		28/31 (90%)	n.s.
Feagan et al.[12]				
Failure/worsening	27/52 (52%)	5	33/60 (55%)	n.s.
Jewell et al.[13]				
Response	26/72 (36%)	5	32/74 (43%)	
Failure	46/72 (64%)		42/74 (57%)	n.s.
Brynskov et al.[14]				
Response	22/37 (59%)	8	11/34 (32%)	
Failure	15/37 (41%)		23/34 (68%)	0.03

*n.s. = Not significant.

INTRAVENOUS CYCLOSPORIN TREATMENT: UNCONTROLLED EXPERIENCE

Cyclosporin is rather poorly absorbed from the gastrointestinal tract, although a more favourable absorption fraction can be obtained with a newer microemulsion formulation[16]. The absorption of cyclosporin follows zero-order kinetics, and both the extent and rate of bioavailability have been found to be decreased in patients with Crohn's disease and apparent drug malabsorption as judged from blood levels[17]. These issues, and the demonstration that colonic mucosal cyclosporin levels are ten-fold higher after intravenous compared to oral administration[18], have raised interest in the therapeutic potential of intravenous high-dose cyclosporin in severe inflammatory[19–22] or fistulizing Crohn's disease[20,23,24]. At present this therapeutic approach has not been tested in controlled trials, and part of the existing clinical experience has been published only in abstract form. The result obtained in a number of representative studies in inflammatory disease are summarized in Table 3 and in fistulizing disease in Table 4. The initial response rate in these series is comparable to that observed in ulcerative colitis (~75%) with about half of the patients remaining better after transferring to oral cyclosporin. However, more prolonged follow-up shows that only one in five patients achieves a long-term benefit from this treatment. It is currently unresolved whether better long-term efficacy can be obtained if cyclosporin is combined with azathioprine[20], and at least in patients with fistulizing disease,

Table 3 Response rates during intravenous and subsequent oral cyclosporin treatment in patients with severe inflammatory Crohn's disease

Reference	Intravenous	Oral	Follow-up
Santos et al.[19]	6/8	5/8	0/8
Egan et al.[20]	4/9	4/9	0/9
Gurudu et al.[21]	6/6	4/6	0/6
Hermida-Rodriguez et al.[22]	6/8*	—	4/8
Total	22/31 (71%)	12/23 (52%)	6/31 (19%)

* Only intravenous cyclosporin.

Table 4 Response rates during intravenous and subsequent oral cyclosporin treatment in patients with fistulizing Crohn's disease

Reference	Intravenous	Oral	Follow-up
Hanauer and Smith[23]	10/12*	6/12*	—
Present and Lichtiger[24]	14/16	9/16	—
Egan et al.[20]	7/9	5/9	2/9[†]
Total	31/37 (83%)	20/37 (54%)	2/9 (22%)

* Number of fistulas in five patients.
[†] Maintained on cyclosporin and azathioprine.

anti-tumour necrosis factor (TNF)-α treatment (infliximab) appears to represent a better therapeutic option[25]. At present the lack of controlled data indicates that high-dose intravenous cyclosporin remains an experimental option in Crohn's disease.

TACROLIMUS/FK-506

Tacrolimus/FK-506 is a macrolide immunosuppressant with an effect similar to that of cyclosporin. Tacrolimus has a greater potency and a more favourable absorption profile than cyclosporin, and it has been used successfully in liver transplantation[26]. The clinical experience with oral tacrolimus treatment in Crohn's (and ulcerative colitis) is very limited[27–30]. However, a small study in patients with fistulizing Crohn's disease showed an initial complete response in seven of 11 patients, which was maintained in five[30]. The remaining four patients also experienced some improvement, but oral tacrolimus has a side-effect profile similar to that of cyclosporin, and controlled data are not available to support the use of this treatment.

Interestingly, tacrolimus has been shown to be rather effective in certain inflammatory skin disorders, and a recent pilot study using a home-made tacrolimus ointment suggested that topical treatment is useful in oral manifestations of Crohn's disease as well as in perianal ulcerations. There was no evidence of systemic absorption, and this approach deserves further evaluation[31]. Likewise, uncontrolled data and clinical experience suggest that cyclosporin also may benefit skin complications of inflammatory bowel disease, such as pyoderma gangrenosum[32–34], probably reflecting the distribution kinetics of this drug[17].

CONCLUSION

Addition of oral low-dose cyclosporin has no relapse-preventing effect in patients with inactive or low-active Crohn's disease. Likewise, oral low-dose cyclosporin treatment has no consistent effect in active Crohn's disease. Uncontrolled trials suggest a short-term effect of high-dose intravenous cyclosporin treatment in severe inflammatory or fistulizing Crohn's disease, but most patients relapse. Since intensive cyclosporin treatment is associated with a risk of severe side-effects, in particular if combined with other immunosuppressive agents, this treatment remains an experimental approach. The same applies to the use of oral tacrolimus treatment, although a recently devised ointment for oral or perianal Crohn's disease deserves further evaluation.

References

1. Allison MC, Pounder RE. Cyclosporin for Crohn's disease. Lancet. 1984;1:1242.
2. Brynskov J. The role of cyclosporin therapy in Crohn's disease. A review. Dig Dis. 1991; 9:236–44.
3. Brynskov J. Cyclosporin in Crohn's disease. Therapeutic and pathogenetic implications. Dan Med Bull. 1994;41:332–44.
4. Romagnani S. Th1/Th2 cells. Inflamm Bowel Dis. 1999;5:285–94.

5. Lichtiger S, Present D, Kornbluth A *et al.* Cyclosporin in severe ulcerative colitis refractory to steroid therapy. N Engl J Med. 1994;330:1841–5.
6. Haslam N, Hearing SD, Probert CS. Audit of cyclosporin use in inflammatory bowel disease: limited benefits, numerous side effects. Eur J Gastroenterol Hepatol. 2000;12:657–60.
7. Van Gossum A, Schmit A, Adler M *et al.* Short- and long-term efficacy of cyclosporin administration in patients with severe ulcerative colitis. Belgian IBD Group. Acta Gastroenterol Belg. 1997;60:197–200.
8. Quan VA, Saunders BP, Hicks BH, Sladen GE. Cyclosporin treatment for ulcerative colitis complicated by fatal *Pneumocystis carinii* pneumonia. Br Med J. 1997;314:363–4.
9. Smith MB, Hanauer SB. *Pneumocystis carinii* pneumonia during cyclosporin treatment for ulcerative colitis. N Engl J Med. 1992;327:497–8.
10. Santos J, Baudet S, Casellas F *et al.* Efficacy of intravenous cyclosporine for steroid-refractory attacks of ulcerative colitis. J Clin Gastroenterol. 1995;20:285–9.
11. Stange EF, Modigliani R, Peña AS *et al.* European trial of cyclosporine in chronic active Crohn's disease. Gastroenterology. 1995;109:774–82.
12. Feagan BG, McDonald JWD, Rochon J *et al.* Low-dose cyclosporine for the treatment of Crohn's disease. N Engl J Med. 1994;330:1846–51.
13. Jewell DP, Lennard-Jones JE and the Cyclosporin Study Group of Great Britain and Ireland. Oral cyclosporin for chronic active Crohn's disease: a multicentre controlled trial. Eur J Gastroenterol Hepatol. 1994;6;499–505.
14. Brynskov J, Freund L, Nørby Rasmussen S *et al.* A placebo-controlled, double-blind, randomized trial of cyclosporine therapy in chronic active Crohn's disease. N Engl J Med. 1989;321:845–50.
15. Brynskov J, Freund F, Nørby Rasmussen S *et al.* Final report on a placebo-controlled, double-blind, randomised, multicentre trial of cyclosporin treatment in active chronic Crohn's disease. Scand J Gastroenterol. 1991;26:689–95.
16. Actis GC, Volpes R, Rizzetto M. Oral microemulsion cyclosporin to reduce steroids rapidly in chronic active ulcerative colitis. Eur J Gastroenterol Hepatol. 1999;11:905–8.
17. Brynskov J, Freund L, Campanini MC, Kampmann JP. Cyclosporin pharmacokinetics after intravenous and oral administration in patients with Crohn's disease. Scand J Gastroenterol. 1992;27:961–7.
18. Sandborn WJ, Strong RM, Forland SC, Chase RE, Cutler RE. The pharmacokinetics and colonic tissue concentrations of cyclosporin after IV, oral, and enema administration. J Clin Pharmacol. 1991;31:76–80.
19. Santos JV, Baudet JA, Casellas FJ *et al.* Intravenous cyclosporine for steroid-refractory attacks of Crohn's disease. J Clin Gastroenterol. 1995;20:207–10.
20. Egan LJ, Sandborn WJ, Tremaine WJ. Clinical outcome following treatment of refractory inflammatory and fistulizing Crohn's disease with intravenous cyclosporine. Am J Gastroenterol. 1998;93:442–8.
21. Gurudu SR, Griffel LH, Gialanella RJ, Das KM. Cyclosporine therapy in inflammatory bowel disease: short-term and long-term results. J Clin Gastroenterol. 1999;29:151–4.
22. Hermida-Rodriguez C, Cantero Perona J, Garcia-Valriberas R, Pajared Garcia JM, Mate-Jimenez J. High-dose intravenous cyclosporine in steroid refractory attacks of inflammatory bowel disease. Hepato-Gastroenterology. 1999;46:2255–68.
23. Hanauer SB, Smith MB. Rapid closure of Crohn's disease fistulas with continuous intravenous cyclosporin A. Am J Gastroenterol. 1993;88:646–9.
24. Present DN, Lichtiger S. Efficacy of cyclosporin in treatment of fistula in Crohn's disease. Dig Dis Sci. 1994;39:374–80.
25. Present DH, Rutgeerts P, Targan S *et al.* Infliximab for the treatment of fistulas in patients with Crohn's disease. N Engl J Med. 1999;340:1398–405.
26. Peters DH, Fitton A, Plosker GL, Faulds D. Tacrolimus: a review of its pharmacology and therapeutic potential in hepatic and renal transplantation. Drugs. 1993;46:756–94.
27. Bousvaros A, Wang A, Leichtner AM. Tacrolimus (FK-506) treatment of fulminant colitis in a child. J Ped Gastroenterol Nutr. 1996;23:329–33.
28. Sandborn WJ. Preliminary report on the use of oral tacrolimus (FK-506) in the treatment of complicated proximal small bowel and fistulizing Crohn's disease. Am J Gastroenterol. 1998; 93:1860–6.
29. Fellerman K, Ludwig D, Stahl M, David-Walek T, Stange EF. Steroid-unresponsive acute attacks of inflammatory bowel disease: immunomodulation by tacrolimus (FK506). Am J Gastroenterol. 1998;93:1860–6.

30. Lowry PW, Weaver AL, Tremaine WJ, Snadborn WJ. Combination therapy with oral tacrolimus (FK506) and azathioprine or 6-mercaptopurine for treatment-refractory Crohn's disease perianal fistulae. Inflamm Bowel Dis. 1999;5:239–45.
31. Casson DH, Eltumi M, Tomlin S, Walker-Smith JA, Murch SH. Topical tacrolimus may be effective in the treatment of oral and perianal Crohn's disease. Gut. 2000;47:436–40.
32. Bardazzi F, Guidetti MS, Passarini B, Spetoli E. Cyclosporin A in metastatic Crohn's disease. Acta Derm Venerol (Stockh). 1995;75:324–5.
33. Futami H, Kodaira M, Furuta T, Hanai H, Kaneko E. Pyoderma gangrenosum complicating ulcerative colitis: successful treatment with methylprednisolone pulse therapy and cyclosporine. J Gastroenterol. 1998;33:408–11.
34. Carp JM, Onuma E, Das K, Gottlieb ABB. Intravenous cyclosporine therapy in the treatment of pyoderma gangrenosum secondary to Crohn's disease. Cutis. 1997;60:135–8.

19
Cyclosporin – what have we learned in the past 15 years?

S. LICHTIGER

INTRODUCTION

Cyclosporin, a potent immunosuppressant of interleukin-2 (IL-2), is obtained by extraction of the soil fungus *Tolypocladium infatum*. Its mechanism of action is by inactivating calcineurin, which prevents the transcription of messenger-RNA encoding for IL-2 and its receptor. Other hypothesized theories concerning the mechanism of action of cyclosporin include suppression of activating factors by helper T cells. Cyclosporin acts only on lymphocytes; not on granulocytes, monocytes, or macrophages. Since the T cell plays a pivotal role in mucosal inflammation, the rationale for the use of the drug in these diseases is obvious. Given that the immunological pathway in active inflammatory bowel disease is similar to the pathway of transplant rejection, it made sense to study cyclosporin in the setting of both ulcerative colitis and Crohn's disease. When we began studying the medication in inflammatory bowel disease we had also the advantage of knowing that it was effective in pyoderma gangrenosum, psoriasis, and uveitis, as well as knowing its effect on peripheral arthritis, be it rheumatoid in origin or other inflammatory arthritides. The successful use of cyclosporin in each of these conditions laid the foundation that precipitated the study of cyclosporin in ulcerative colitis. We also realized that we needed a drug that worked quickly, as patients with severe ulcerative colitis, and who have failed steroid treatment, have little time before colectomy becomes necessary.

PATIENT SELECTION

Initially, we studied patients who failed at least 10 days of parenteral steroids. Although the European literature states that 5 days without response is sufficient reason for colectomy, it was felt that patients should be given a longer time on intravenous steroids, and in the mid-1980s we waited a full 10 days. We have learned that this is unnecessary, as failure to respond by 7 days gives sufficient time to consider the addition of cyclosporin A (CsA). Inclusion required an objective score on a defined index in which seven categories were delineated. This index, which takes into account objective as well as subjective criteria, has remained effective in defining severe colitis.

Several of the exclusion criteria have been redefined, including the initial creatinine clearance that was established at greater than 100 ml/min in 1985. Because of the paucity of problems with both hypertension and renal insufficiency, this has been revised to more than 75 ml/min. Other revisions in the exclusion criteria include accepting patients who have blood pressure of up to 140 systolic and 90 diastolic. In the initial pilot, as well as in a double-binded trial, our definition was a systolic over 120 and a diastolic over 85. In the early studies, patients with toxic megacolon were not eligible for entry. In the second 7 years of cyclosporin use, four patients with toxic megacolon have been entered, all of whom were treated successfully. In the years from 1985 to 1992 pregnant women were not entered into the study; however, since 1993 five women have been treated with CsA during pregnancy, and although two of the five required colectomy, there were no maternal or fetal abnormalities in this subgroup of patients.

METHODS

When cyclosporin was initially used for autoimmune indications in the early 1980s, several papers studying pharmacokinetics showed the necessity of blood levels being therapeutic. The unique problem that we had was administering cyclosporin to patients who had poor absorptive capacity, recognizing that the therapeutic effect was contingent upon therapeutic blood levels. There were data published showing that diarrhoea, anaemia, and abnormal small bowel motility contributed to subtherapeutic levels. Therefore, when cyclosporin was used in ulcerative colitis, we administered it intravenously. This assured therapeutic levels for a span of 7–14 days, sufficient time for parameters such as diarrhoea and anaemia to be corrected. CsA was given by continuous infusion and we published data proving that steady, therapeutic, blood levels were reached. The initial dose borrowed from the transplant population was 4 mg/kg per day, and the duration of treatment was anywhere from 7 to 14 days. We monitored blood levels of drug and renal function every other day until success, as defined by our objective criteria, was reached. There is debate within the literature as to the starting dose. Several Italian studies that have proved 2 mg/kg per day to be effective; however, there is no study that compares the therapeutic effect of 4 mg vs 2 mg. Unless people have renal insufficiency, or are on other drugs that interact with CsA, our starting dose remains 4 mg/kg per day. Our initial inclusion criteria necessitated a patient failing 10 days of intravenous steroids. We have learned that failure on steroids after 5–7 days is an indication of inclusion. What we have also learned is that failure of intravenous CsA at 8–10 days is a harbinger of failure when the duration of treatment is extended.

Our initial blood-drawing every day was overzealous, and at present we check renal function, CsA levels and complete blood count every 2–3 days. Hypertension is an early-warning sign of nephrotoxicity, and a blood pressure of 140/90 is followed by decreasing the dose by 33%. The present goal of avoiding colectomy in the acute or intravenous phase has not changed. Once a patient is deemed a success he/she is transferred to oral CsA with a starting dose between 6 and 8 mg/kg per day. As opposed to the initial 7 years of studies, we do not consider 6 months to be the endpoint of the oral phase. The patient is usually on CsA for a total of 2 months, and withdrawal of cyclosporin is performed in a gradual manner. Blood levels are studied within 1 week of discharge, and a pharmacokinetic profile is determined. The oral drug is given twice daily, and 6-mercaptopurine is added at approximately 2–4 weeks. Our aim in the oral phase has been to achieve steroid withdrawal, clinical remission as defined by our index, and colonoscopic healing. These three criteria still remain, and serve as the basis to treat. However, these criteria are not subject to a full 6 months, and at present the quicker we can get patients off CsA, the better it is.

Demographics were compared between 1987 and 1993, and were compared to the demographics used from 1993 to 2000. In each group 75 patients' charts were reviewed and the mean age, male to female ratio, and extent of disease were very similar. Sixty-five per cent had universal colitis and approximately 35% had left-sided disease. What changed during this time period was that, in 1987–1993, the mean duration of disease was 5.8 years, whereas in 1993–2000 the mean duration was 7.4 years. This probably reflects our confidence in treating patients who were older, as well as the lack of any data suggesting that either dysplasia or carcinoma would arise in patients who have longer histories of ulcerative colitis. In 1993 the mean duration of treatment with intravenous steroids prior to the initiation of cyclosporin was 8.4 days, as opposed to 6.8 days through the year 2000. As mentioned earlier in this chapter, this reflected the efficacy as well as the modicum of adverse effects noted in the pilot study.

CYCLOSPORIN LEVELS

As mentioned earlier in this chapter, it was clear that patients improved only when the drug level was within therapeutic range. This was easily interpreted from the pilot study, in which patients who flared while on intravenous cyclosporin had subtherapeutic blood levels of the drug. What was not clear at the time was the association between higher therapeutic levels and clinical response. Response was independent of the actual blood level. Patients who had a blood level of 400 μg did just as well as patients who had blood levels of 600 μg. What was observed was the fact that, on the same dosage of CsA, blood levels would be within 10% of each other on an every-other-day basis. It was the change from intravenous to oral CsA at which blood levels become relatively erratic. Although each patient had a pharmacokinetic profile, change in steroid dose, haemoglobin, weight, and oral absorption all contributed to inconsistent blood levels. In the majority of patients who broke through the oral cyclosporin it was very difficult to reinstate remission.

What was clear from the first few years of using CsA was that adverse effects were correlated with higher blood levels. Incidents of hypertension as well as renal insufficiency reflected a blood level of 600 μg or greater. There was no significant difference in mean intravenous or oral CsA levels between long-term success or failures. The mean cyclosporin level in responders during the intravenous phase was approximately 600, whereas the mean level in failures was approximately 525. In the oral phase the mean level in successes was approximately 500, whereas the mean level in failures was 550.

Over recent years there has been debate as to whether the tissue level of CsA is a greater factor in prediction than is blood level of the drug. There have been several studies that correlate the tissue level of CsA with actual response. Tissue concentration of the drug is higher in colonic cells than in small bowel cells, which may explain the fact that Crohn's disease is not as responsive to cyclosporin as is ulcerative colitis. Because of the cost, as well as burden of measuring tissue levels, it is unlikely that this premise will be proven, and at present blood levels continue to be the gold standard.

RESULTS OF STUDIES USING CsA IN ULCERATIVE COLITIS

Series of studies were reviewed in order to compare our data with data from other medical centres. Despite the aforementioned suggestion of beginning treatment with intravenous CsA, four papers were published on the use of oral CsA in patients with severe ulcerative colitis. There were 46 patients entered into the studies and the initial oral dose ranged from 4 to 15 mg/kg per day. Response varied in each of the studies with 0 response at 3 weeks in one study, and 80% response at the same time period in a smaller series. When these patients were followed for 3 months there was a 14–34% response rate at that time. It is clear that oral medication should not be initial treatment, and erratic blood levels are probably the reason for that. In the 46 patients who were on oral CsA, six patients had reversible nephrotoxicity. Five of the six patients had erratically high cyclosporin blood levels.

The next study reviewed was published in *The Journal of Clinical Gastroenterology* by Actis *et al*. In this study the starting dose of intravenous cyclosporin was 2 mg/kg per day in a total of eight patients, all of whom had failed intravenous steroids. One of the eight underwent immediate colectomy; two of the eight failed in the oral phase, and five of the eight responded as defined by clinical and endoscopic healing. Despite their initial dose of 2 mg/kg per day, all patients had therapeutic blood levels, and adverse effects seemed to be less frequent, albeit this was a small study. Two of the initial eight patients developed reversible nephrotoxicity, and 25% were higher than in our patients who were started on 4 mg/kg per day. There has been no report of a large series of adult patients who were started on this lower dose; however, there is some paediatric literature that suggests its effectiveness. At this time we continue to recommend the initial dose of 4 mg/kg per day, with titration of the dose to therapeutic blood levels.

In a large retrospective study from the University of Chicago, 42 patients were entered on CsA with a starting dose of 4 mg/kg per day. Of the initial 42, six patients underwent an immediate colectomy. Ten of the remaining 46 were advanced to the oral phase; however they required colectomy within several months. Twenty-six of the original 42 patients did well both on the intravenous and oral phase of CsA. Of the responding 26, 20 were placed on 6-mercaptopurine (6-MP); however, each was placed on 6-MP at a different time. The review concluded with the suggestion that CsA is effective in severe ulcerative colitis, and that the long-term response is better when patients were given 6-MP. Toxicity included a single patient with seizures, and another patient who had *Pneumocystis carinii*.

In reviewing my data on 150 patients who have received CsA, I split the responses of those treated from 1987 through 1993, as opposed to patients treated from 1993 through 2000. All patients were begun on 4 mg/kg per day, and of the 75 patients entered from 1987 through 1993, 16 underwent immediate colectomy in the acute phase of the study. Fifty-nine of the 75 (79%) were considered successes on the intravenous CsA and were entered into the chronic phase of the study, which at that time was defined as 6 months on oral CsA. The mean response time to the intravenous medication was 5.7 days. Of the successful 59.17 (29%) underwent colectomy, with 12 of the 17 having surgery within 1 month. In most of these 17 patients the response to intravenous CsA was not as rapid or definitive as the response of those who were successful in the oral phase, and 12 of the 17 had subtherapeutic blood values early in the oral phase. Of the 42 patients who continued to do well at 6 months, all of this subgroup were off CSA and steroids. Twenty-six of the 42 were on 6-MP, and all patients were on some form of acetylsalicylic acid. These patients have been followed, with a mean follow-up of 9.2 years. Twenty-four of the original 75 (45%) have continued to do well long-term, and most of these patients have been off an immunomodulator at some point in their responsive years.

Contrasting that subgroup to patients who were treated from 1993 through 2000, only 11 (15%) underwent colectomy while on parenteral CsA. Of the remaining 64 (85%), 11 patients underwent colectomy, seven of the 11 within 3 months. There were several factors that contributed to the greater success in the latter 7 years, including earlier institution of 6-MP, maintaining patients on a higher dose of oral CsA until the 6-MP was effective, and more frequent pharmacokinetic profiling during the initial month on oral cyclosporin. Fifty-eight of the 64 entered into the chronic phase were placed on 6-MP at 2–3 weeks after hospital discharge. Fifty-three of the 64 who entered the chronic phase were doing well at 3 months, which over the past 7 years has become our endpoint of the chronic phase. Forty-seven of the original 75 (63%) are at present well, and have been in clinical and endoscopic remission with a mean follow-up of 4.3 years.

What lessons have we learned in the past 15 years? CsA is a drug that induces but does not maintain response. The starting dose of parenteral CsA should be 4 mg/kg per day; however, in the elderly, the hypertensive, or in patients with renal disease, the dose can start at 2 mg/kg per day. Maximum duration of treatment is 10 days and, if successful, oral dosage of 6–8 mg/kg per day should be started. 6-MP should be added early in the CsA oral phase, as long-term remission on 6-MP is greater than on CsA alone. The duration of the chronic phase should be 3 months. Pharmacokinetics should be checked periodically as factors such as weight, anaemia, and concurrent medication are always changing.

TOXICITY – CYCLOSPORIN IN ULCERATIVE COLITIS

In 1983, when we began using the drug, the toxicity reported was in the transplant population. Since most of the transplant population were recipients of kidneys, the data were skewed as to patients who had renal dysfunction. Thus, we had little background in terms of predicting toxicity; however, we are careful to select young patients with normal renal function who were not on concomitant drugs that may affect renal functions (even to the point of excluding patients on high doses of non-steroidal anti-inflammatory agents). In our pilot study published in the *Lancet* there was a modicum of nephrotoxicity and all reactions were reversible. A single patient developed renal failure and eventually died from complications relating to it. However, she was taking a much higher dose than we instructed her to take.

Of the 150 patients whose charts were reviewed for this study, the most common complication was paraesthesias. Fifty-three had mild paraesthesias that did not necessitate a dosage change and the one patient who developed moderate paraesthesias responded to decreasing the dose. Hypertension as defined by a blood pressure of greater than 140 systolic or 90 diastolic was seen in 20% of patients, most of whom responded to lowering of the dose. Ten of the 34 who developed hypertension responded to the addition of verapamil. Headache was noted in 18% of patients, and dyspepsia was noted in 15%. Four of the 150 patients developed infectious complications including herpes zoster in two of them. The aforementioned patient who developed renal failure from CsA eventually died of *Klebsiella* sepsis. One developed a grand-mal seizure, was taken off the drug and underwent colectomy. One woman developed breast carcinoma 7 years after stopping the CsA, and one patient developed a non-Hodgkin's lymphoma 13 years after receiving CsA. The two cancers were probably not a result of the immunosuppression, as they appeared many years after the cyclosporin treatment. We have learned that careful monitoring of blood urea nitrogen (BUN), and creatinine, cyclosporin blood levels is necessary to minimize complications. The onset of hypertension should be followed by a decrease of 33% in the dosage of CsA.

Intravenous cyclosporin is rapidly effective in the treatment of severe ulcerative colitis. Colectomy is avoided in 80% of patients in the acute phase. Oral cyclosporin maintains response in 48% of patients initially treated with parenteral CsA. In order to improve long-term remission, 6-MP/azathioprine should be added within the first month of CsA treatment. Although it is not known exactly when to add it, our usual approach in these patients is to add 6-MP 2 weeks after discharge from hospital. Use of careful monitoring of blood pressure, BUN, and creatinine, minimizes significant adverse effects. Cyclosporin level should be therapeutic, and although response is not directly a reflection of blood level, adverse effects are. Further investigation involves discovering the ideal time for adding cyclosporin to steroids. Should one wait until intravenous steroids fail, prior to initiating CsA treatment? Is 2 mg/kg per day as effective as 4 mg/kg per day? Are there further precautions that can be taken in order to minimize either hypertension or renal insufficiency? Clearly, CsA should play a role in treatment of severe ulcerative colitis. Retrospective quality-of-life studies in patients who have had colectomy and ileoanal pull-through suggest that those treated successfully with medical therapy do better on an objective quality-of-life scale. The answers to all the aforementioned questions will come from further retrospective analysis, as well as future research.

Section VII
New developments: anti-TNF antibodies

20
Inhibition of tumour necrosis factor alpha as a therapeutic strategy in Crohn's disease

S. J. H. VAN DEVENTER

INTRODUCTION

Tumour necrosis factor alpha (TNF-α) is a molecule consisting of three non-covalently linked 17 kDa proteins that is mainly produced by monocytes and lymphocytes in response to various proinflammatory stimuli[1-4]. Initially identified as a circulating endogenous inflammatory mediator, important activities of TNF-α in immune-mediated inflammation have subsequently been recognized. TNF has a wide range of proinflammatory activities on a wide range of cells, including induction of secondary cytokines and chemokines; up-regulation of cell adhesion molecules; activation of the coagulation as well as fibrinolytic systems; induction of iNOS; increase of the synthesis of prostaglandins, leukotrienes and platelet-activating factor; and induction as well as inhibition of apoptosis[5-8]. Innate immunity is importantly dependent on TNF-α, and administration of TNF-α-neutralizing antibodies renders animals extremely sensitive to a wide range of infections, in particular those caused by intracellular organisms. On the other hand, in several animal models the tissue damage caused by overwhelming systemic infections is in part mediated by TNF-α, and the efficacy of TNF antagonism has been investigated in large controlled clinical trials. The results of these investigations indicated that neutralization of TNF-α did not improve the survival of patients with severe sepsis, but with one exception (see below) such interventions did not increase mortality either[9]. In the past decade it has become clear the TNF-α is also importantly involved in compartmentalized chronic inflammatory reactions, and in these conditions serum concentrations are not informative. In a still-increasing list of diseases – including rheumatoid arthritis, Crohn's disease, Behcet's disease and spondylitis – TNF-α is believed to have a central role in initiating and perpetuating inflammation. These findings have made therapeutic inhibition of the synthesis, release or biological activity of TNF an attractive therapeutic strategy. This chapter reviews the scientific rationale and the current status of TNF-targeting therapies in Crohn's disease.

TRANSCRIPTION, TRANSLATION, AND POST-TRANSLATIONAL PROCESSING OF TNF-α

The TNF-α gene in humans is located in the short arm of chromosome 6, between the HLA class I and II loci, and close to the lymphotoxin-α gene. Various stimuli – including bacterial endotoxins, osmotic shock, reactive oxygen radicals, PAF, and T-cell receptor activation – lead to increased transcription of the TNF-α gene. These stimuli signal TNF transcription through two partly linked transcription pathways, i.e. activation of NF-κB and the MAP (p38) kinase cascade (which also regulates translation), and TNF-α transcription is inversely correlated with the intracellular concentration of cAMP[10–12]. TNF-α mRNA is rapidly degraded by RNA-ses that target the 5′-untranslated region, and corticosteroids (negative) and IFN-γ (positive) increase TNF production at the post-transcriptional level[13,14]. Finally, elements with the TNF-α 3′-UTR inhibit translation at ribosomal levels. Hence, the cellular production of TNF-α is tightly controlled at the transcriptional and translational levels, presumably in order to prevent uncontrolled release of this highly inflammatory protein. TNF-α is translated as a propeptide that contains an unusually long signal peptide that remains retained within the cell membrane. This signal peptide does not include domains that are known to induce intracellular signalling, but does contain a nuclear localization sequence that may be involved in 'reverse signalling'. Membrane-bound TNF-α is biologically active as a homotrimer, and activates the p75 TNF receptor (TNFRII) in cell-to-cell contacts[15]. Release of biologically active TNF-α is dependent on the activity of a membrane-associated metalloproteinase called TNF-α converting enzyme (TACE)[16–19]. Soluble TNF-α is biologically active as a homotrimer, and exerts autocrine, paracrine and endocrine effects through activation of the p55 TNF receptor (TNFRI, which is expressed by a wide range of cells) or the p75 TNF receptors (TNFRII, mainly expressed by white blood cells)[6,20–22]. Significant concentrations of soluble TNFRI and TNFRII circulate in healthy humans, and various inflammatory conditions cause further shedding of both TNF receptors. Because TNF receptors can bind and neutralize TNF-α, this is considered an endogenous TNF-α blocking system, and TNF-α/TNF receptor complexes can be cleared by the kidney[23].

Binding of trimeric TNF-α to its specific receptors causes trimerization and a conformational change, which initiates intracellular signalling[24]. Although both TNFRI and TNFRII bind TNF-α with a high affinity, and both are capable of intracellular signalling, it is believed that most proinflammatory effects are a consequence of activation of TNFRI, TNFRII being able to bind and transfer TNF-α to TNFRI ('ligand passing'). Moreover, apoptosis induction is exclusively signalled by TNFRI[25]. The intracytoplasmic tail of TNFRI contains at least three domains that are involved in signal transduction. The first domain has been implicated in release of ceramide, the second domain (known as the death domain) induces apoptosis through activation of caspase 8, and the third domain activates NF-κB via TRAF-2, thereby causing transcription of a wide range of proinflammatory genes[26–28]. It has recently been recognized that NF-κB induction protects against apoptosis, and TNF-α therefore signals both pro- and anti-apoptotic pathways[29].

TNF INHIBITORS

The production of TNF can be therapeutically affected at the transcriptional, post-transcriptional and post-translational levels. Membrane-bound and soluble TNF can be neutralized using high-affinity antibodies or TNF receptor fusion proteins.

Phosphodiesterase inhibitors, including the methylxanthine group of drugs (pentoxifyllin, oxpentifyllin), rolipram (specific for PDE4), and thalidomide analogues, increase intracellular cAMP concentrations which, presumably through a CREB-dependent mechanism, leads to reduced transcription of several genes including the TNF-α gene[30–34]. In animal models, including primate endotoxaemia and various models of experimental bowel disease, reduction of TNF production has been demonstrated *in vivo*. However, oxpentifyllin treatment of patients with active Crohn's disease did not have therapeutic effects, despite a demonstrated reduction of TNF-α production by peripheral blood monocytes[35,36]. Two uncontrolled studies suggested therapeutic benefit of thalidomide treatment of patients with active Crohn's disease, but it remains uncertain whether this was a result of a reduction of TNF-α production[37,38]. In AIDS and tuberculosis thalidomide did not alter TNF-α production *in vivo*[39,40].

TACE is a zinc-dependent metalloproteinase, and more or less specific inhibitors have been synthesized. In animal models, metalloproteinase inhibitors did reduce the severity of experimental colitis, but this effect seemed to be mediated by non-specific inhibition of various metalloproteinases, because TNF production was not changed by the treatment[41].

Various high-affinity TNF-binding monoclonal antibodies have been generated and tested in Crohn's disease. The first generation of these antibodies consisted of human–mouse chimaeric antibodies, which were followed by 'humanized', and recently completely human antibodies. Infliximab is a first-generation mouse–human chimaeric antibody that effectively neutralizes human TNF-α[42,43]. At a single dose of 5 mg/kg infliximab induces therapeutic responses (a reduction of the Crohn's disease activity index) in two-thirds of patients and complete remissions (a reduction of the CDAI below 150) in half of (therapy-refractory) patients with active Crohn's disease[44]. It also causes complete closure of all perianal fistulas in 55% of patients[45]. A small study suggested that repeated dosing (every 8 weeks) may maintain therapeutic responses for a period of 44 weeks, and large controlled studies are ongoing to investigate the maintenance efficacy and potential steroid-sparing effects[46].

CDP571 is a humanized anti-TNF-α antibody that induced remissions in about 50% of patients with active Crohn's disease[47,48]. It has been recently shown that repeated CDP571 administration maintains remission, and may be steroid-sparing. D2E7 is a completely human anti-TNF-α antibody that is currently being tested for efficacy in Crohn's disease, but results have not yet been reported[49].

In general, the short-term toxicity of anti-TNF antibodies is mild and consists mainly of headache, a slight increase of upper respiratory infections, and infusion-related allergic reactions. After infliximab infusion about 13% of patients develop low-titre antibodies (human anti-chimaeric antibodies – HACAs) and low-titre anti-dsDNA antibodies occur in a minority of patients following infliximab and CDP571 treatment. It remains to be seen whether anti-TNF therapies increase the long-term risk of lymphomas or carcinomas, but these have been reported in anti-TNF-treated patients. About 20% of patients that were treated with the early infliximab formulation developed a delayed hypersensitivity syndrome consisting of fever, and (sometimes) severe muscle and joint aches, which is related to induction of high-titre HACAs. Such patients respond well to treatment with NSAIDs or steroids, but are not eligible for further infliximab treatment, because the high-titre HACAs interfere with therapeutic efficacy. Anecdotal reports have listed striking effects of infliximab treatment on extra-intestinal manifestations, on spondylitis, on Crohn's lesions within ileoanal pouches, and in Behcet's disease[50–52].

Etanercept is a high-affinity TNF-α-binding fusion protein consisting of two TNFRII receptors that are 'grafted' on a IgG1 tail. It has been demonstrated to be effective in rheumatoid arthritis, and controlled clinical trials in Crohn's disease have been initiated[53–55].

ANTI-TNF THERAPIES AND IMMUNOSUPPRESSIVE DRUGS

Many patients treated with anti-TNF antibodies also used azathioprine or methotrexate, but a systemic analysis of potential advantages or disadvantages of combination therapy has not been performed. Nonetheless, there are several indications that combination therapy improves efficacy and possibly reduces the incidence of side-effects of anti-TNF-α antibodies. A retrospective analysis of infliximab-treated patients showed that the remission duration was much longer in patients who were using azathioprine[46]. It is also documented that the incidence of HACAs is lower in patients who are using immunosuppressives. Finally, methotrexate seems to increase the therapeutic efficacy of infliximab and etanercept in rheumatoid arthritis patients[56].

ANTI-TNF AND THE THERAPEUTIC REPERTOIRE IN CROHN'S DISEASE

All TNF-targeting trials have been conducted in (therapy-refractory) active Crohn's disease patient groups, and virtually all patients used mesalamine, prednisone, immunosuppressives, or combinations of these drugs. Most trials have been designed to demonstrate remission induction, and preliminary data indicate potential for remission maintenance and steroid-sparing effects. To date, in view of the uncertainty concerning long-term safety and the high costs of treatment, anti-TNF-α is generally considered a third-line therapy in Crohn's disease. Although appropriate trials need to be conducted, in view of several lines of circumstantial evidence it seems logical to combine anti-TNF-α therapies with immunosuppressive therapies (azathioprine or methotrexate). It is also not known whether TNF-targeting therapies should be instituted early, or whether treatment should be restricted to patients with therapy-refractory disease. In rheumatoid arthritis, TNF-neutralizing drugs prevent joint destruction and are considered disease-modifying. It is conceivable that similar effects may result from early anti-TNF treatment of Crohn's disease, but the clinical studies have not yet been performed. Finally, only one small trial has investigated the long-term (44-week) effect of repeated infliximab administration, and two large clinical trials have been initiated to confirm the long-term efficacy of Crohn's disease.

In summary, TNF-neutralizing therapies have initiated a paradigm shift in the treatment of Crohn's disease. However, many questions concerning long-term safety, efficacy and potential synergism with immunosuppressive drugs remain to be answered.

References

1. Idriss HT, Naismith JH. TNF alpha and the TNF receptor superfamily: structure–function relationship(s). Microsc Res Tech. 2000;50:184–95.
2. Tang P, Hung MC, Klostergaard J. Human pro-tumor necrosis factor is a homotrimer. Biochemistry. 1996;35:8216–25.
3. Hlodan R, Pain RH. The folding and assembly pathway of tumour necrosis factor TNF alpha, a globular trimeric protein. Eur J Biochem. 1995;231:381–7.
4. Beutler B, Greenwald D, Hulmes JD et al. Identity of tumour necrosis factor and the macrophage-secreted factor cachectin. Nature. 1985;316:552–4.
5. Tracey KJ, Cerami A. Tumor necrosis factor: an updated review of its biology. Crit Care Med. 1993;21:S415–22.
6. Liu ZG, Hsu H, Goeddel DV, Karin M. Dissection of TNF receptor 1 effector functions: JNK activation is not linked to apoptosis while NF-kappaB activation prevents cell death. Cell. 1996;87:565–76.
7. Wang CY, Mayo MW, Korneluk RG, Goeddel DV, Baldwin AS Jr. NF-kappaB antiapoptosis: induction of TRAF1 and TRAF2 and c-IAP1 and c-IAP2 to suppress caspase-8 activation. Science. 1998;281:1680–3.
8. Kitson J, Raven T, Jiang YP et al. A death-domain-containing receptor that mediates apoptosis. Nature. 1996;384:372–5.
9. Abraham E. Why immunomodulatory therapies have not worked in sepsis. Intens Care Med. 1999;25:556–66.
10. Lee JC, Kumar S, Griswold DE, Underwood DC, Votta BJ, Adams JL. Inhibition of p38 MAP kinase as a therapeutic strategy. Immunopharmacology. 2000;47:185–201.
11. Han J, Lee JD, Bibbs L, Ulevitch RJ. A MAP kinase targeted by endotoxin and hyperosmolarity in mammalian cells. Science. 1994;265:808–11.
12. van der Poll T, Calvano SE, Kumar A, Coyle SM, Lowry SF. Epinephrine attenuates down-regulation of monocyte tumor necrosis factor receptors during human endotoxemia. J Leukocyte Biol. 1997;61:156–60.
13. Caput D, Beutler B, Hartog K, Thayer R, Brown-Shimer S, Cerami A. Identification of a common nucleotide sequence in the 3′-untranslated region of mRNA molecules specifying inflammatory mediators. Proc Natl Acad Sci USA. 1986;83:1670–4.
14. Han J, Brown T, Beutler B. Endotoxin-responsive sequences control cachectin/tumor necrosis factor biosynthesis at the translational level [Published erratum appears in J Exp Med. 1990;171:971–2]. J Exp Med. 1990;171:465–75.
15. Kriegler M, Perez C, DeFay K, Albert I, Lu SD. A novel form of TNF/cachectin is a cell surface cytotoxic transmembrane protein: ramifications for the complex physiology of TNF. Cell. 1988;53:45–53.

16. Moss ML, Jin SL, Becherer JD *et al.* Structural features and biochemical properties of TNF-alpha converting enzyme (TACE). J Neuroimmunol. 1997;72:127–9.

17. Moss ML, Jin SL, Milla ME *et al.* Cloning of a disintegrin metalloproteinase that processes precursor tumour-necrosis factor-alpha [Published erratum appears in Nature. 1997;386:738]. Nature. 1997;385:733–6.

18. Black RA, Rauch CT, Kozlosky CJ *et al.* A metalloproteinase disintegrin that releases tumour-necrosis factor-alpha from cells. Nature. 1997;385:729–33.

19. Killar L, White J, Black R, Peschon J. Adamalysins. A family of metzincins including TNF-alpha converting enzyme (TACE). Ann NY Acad Sci. 1999;878:442–52.

20. Sherry B, Cerami A. Cachectin/tumor necrosis factor exerts endocrine, paracrine, and autocrine control of inflammatory responses. J Cell Biol. 1988;107:1269–77.

21. Tartaglia LA, Ayres TM, Wong GH, Goeddel DV. A novel domain within the 55 kd TNF receptor signals cells death. Cell. 1993;74:845–53.

22. Tartaglia LA, Pennica D, Goeddel DV. Ligand passing: the 75-kDa tumor necrosis factor (TNF) receptor recruits. TNF for signaling by the 55-kDa TNF receptor. J Biol Chem. 1993;268:18542–8.

23. Bemelman FJ, Jansen J, Van der Poll T, Van Deventer SJH, Ten Berge RJM. Increase of sTNF receptor levels in acute renal allograft rejection after treatment with OKT3. Nephrol Dial Transplant. 1994;9:1786–90.

24. Vandevoorde V, Haegeman G, Fiers W. Induced expression of trimerized intracellular domains of the human tumor necrosis factor (TNF) p55 receptor elicits TNF effects. J Cell Biol. 1997;137:1627–38.

25. Tartaglia LA, Rothe M, Hu YF, Goeddel DV. Tumor necrosis factor's cytotoxic activity is signaled by the p55 TNF receptor. Cell. 1993;73:213–16.

26. Kronke M. Involvement of sphingomyelinases in TNF signaling pathways. Chem Phys Lipids. 1999;102:157–66.

27. Strelow A, Bernardo K, Adam-Klages S *et al.* Overexpression of acid ceramidase protects from tumor necrosis factor-induced cell death. J Exp Med. 2000;192:601–12.

28. Song HY, Regnier CH, Kirschning CJ, Goeddel DV, Rothe M. Tumor necrosis factor (TNF)-mediated kinase cascades: bifurcation of nuclear factor-kappaB and c-jun N-terminal kinase (JNK/SAPK) pathways at TNF receptor-associated factor 2. Proc Natl Acad Sci USA. 1997;94:9792–6.

29. Beg AA, Baltimore D. An essential role for NF-kappaB in preventing TNF-alpha-induced cell death [See comments]. Science. 1996;274:782–4.

30. Levi M, Ten Cate H, Bauer KA *et al.* Inhibition of endotoxin-induced activation of coagulation and fibrinolysis by pentoxifylline or by a monoclonal anti-tissue factor antibody in chimpanzees. J Clin Invest. 1994;93:114–20.

31. Moreira AL, Kaplan G, Villahermosa LG *et al.* Comparison of pentoxifylline, thalidomide and prednisone in the treatment of ENL [Letter]. Int J Lepr Other Mycobact Dis. 1998;66:61–5.

32. MacKenzie SJ, Houslay MD. Action of rolipram on specific PDE4 cAMP phosphodiesterase isoforms and on the phosphorylation of cAMP-response-element-binding protein (CREB) and p38 mitogen-activated protein (MAP) kinase in U937 monocytic cells. Biochem J. 2000;347:571–8.

33. Neuner P, Klosner G, Schauer E *et al.* Pentoxifylline *in vivo* down-regulates the release of IL-1 beta, IL-6, IL-8 and tumour necrosis factor-alpha by human peripheral blood mononuclear cells. Immunology. 1994;83:262–7.

34. Ross SE, Williams RO, Mason LJ *et al.* Suppression of TNF-alpha expression, inhibition of Th1 activity, and amelioration of collagen-induced arthritis by rolipram. J Immunol. 1997;159:6253–9.

35. Bauditz J, Ruckert Y, Raedler A, Nikolaus S, Lochs H, Schreiber S. Tumour necrosis factor inhibition by oxpentifylline and intestinal inflammation in Crohn's disease [Letter; comment]. Lancet. 1995;345:1445.

36. Bauditz J, Haemling J, Ortner M, Lochs H, Raedler A, Schreiber S. Treatment with tumour necrosis factor inhibitor oxpentifylline does not improve corticosteroid dependent chronic active Crohn's disease [See comments]. Gut. 1997;40:470–4.

37. Vasiliauskas EA, Kam LY, Abreu-Martin MT *et al.* An open-label pilot study of low-dose thalidomide in chronically active, steroid-dependent Crohn's disease. Gastroenterology. 1999;117:1278–87.

38. Ehrenpreis ED, Kane SV, Cohen LB, Cohen RD, Hanauer SB. Thalidomide therapy for patients with refractory Crohn's disease: an open-label trial. Gastroenterology. 1999;117:1271–7.
39. Haslett PA, Klausner JD, Makonkawkeyoon S et al. Thalidomide stimulates T cell responses and interleukin 12 production in HIV-infected patients. AIDS Res Hum Retroviruses. 1999;15:1169–79.
40. Bekker LG, Haslett P, Maartens G, Steyn L, Kaplan G. Thalidomide-induced antigen-specific immune stimulation in patients with human immunodeficiency virus type 1 and tuberculosis. J Infect Dis. 2000;181:954–65.
41. Sykes AP, Bhogal R, Brampton C et al. The effect of an inhibitor of matrix metalloproteinases on colonic inflammation in a trinitrobenzenesulphonic acid rat model of inflammatory bowel disease. Aliment Pharmacol Ther. 1999;13:1535–42.
42. Siegel SA, Shealy DJ, Nakada MT et al. The mouse/human chimeric monoclonal antibody cA2 neutralizes TNF in vivo and protects transgenic mice from cachexia and TNF lethality in vivo. Cytokine. 1995;7:251–9.
43. Knight DM, Trinh H, Le J et al. Construction and initial characterization of a mouse–human chimeric anti-TNF antibody. Cytokine. 1995;7:15–25.
44. Targan SR, Hanauer SB, Vandeventer SJH et al. A short-term study of chimeric monoclonal antibody Ca2 to tumour necrosis factor alpha for Crohn's disease. N Engl J Med. 1997; 337:1029–35.
45. Present DH, Rutgeerts P, Targan S et al. Infliximab for the treatment of fistulas in patients with Crohn's disease. N Engl J Med. 1999;340:1398–405.
46. Rutgeerts P, D'Haens G, Targan S et al. Efficacy and safety of retreatment with anti-tumor necrosis factor antibody (infliximab) to maintain remission in Crohn's disease. Gastroenterology. 1999;117:761–9.
47. Dhainaut JF, Vincent JL, Richard C et al. CDP571, a humanized antibody to human tumor necrosis factor-alpha: safety, pharmacokinetics, immune response, and influence of the antibody on cytokine concentrations in patients with septic shock. CPD571 Sepsis Study Group. Crit Care Med. 1995;23:1461–9.
48. Stack WA, Mann SD, Roy AJ et al. Randomised controlled trial of CDP571 antibody to tumor necrosis factor-alpha in Crohn's disease [See comments]. Lancet. 1997;349:521–4.
49. Kempeni J. Update on D2E7: a fully human anti-tumour necrosis factor alpha monoclonal antibody [In process citation]. Ann Rheum Dis. 2000;59:144–5.
50. Ricart E, Panaccione R, Loftus EV, Tremaine WJ, Sandborn WJ. Successful management of Crohn's disease of the ileoanal pouch with infliximab. Gastroenterology. 1999;117:429–32.
51. Sheldon DG, Sawchuk LL, Kozarek RA, Thirlby RC. Twenty cases of peristomal pyoderma gangrenosum: diagnostic implications and management. Arch Surg. 2000;135:564–8; discussion 568–9.
52. Brandt J, Haibel H, Cornely D et al. Successful treatment of active ankylosing spondylitis with the anti-tumor necrosis factor alpha monoclonal antibody infliximab [In process citation]. Arthritis Rheum. 2000;43:1346–52.
53. Moreland LW, Margolies G, Heck LW Jr et al. Recombinant soluble tumor necrosis factor receptor (p80) fusion protein: toxicity and dose finding trial in refractory rheumatoid arthritis. N Engl J Med. 1996;335:1607–8; discussion 1608–9.
54. Moreland LW, Baumgartner SW, Schiff MH et al. Treatment of rheumatoid arthritis with a recombinant human tumor necrosis factor receptor (p75)-Fc fusion protein [See comments]. N Engl J Med. 1997;337:141–7.
55. Moreland LW, Schiff MH, Baumgartner SW et al. Etanercept therapy in rheumatoid arthritis. A randomized, controlled trial. Ann Intern Med. 1999;130:478–86.
56. Weinblatt ME, Kremer JM, Bankhurst AD et al. A trial of etanercept, a recombinant tumor necrosis factor receptor: Fc fusion protein, in patients with rheumatoid arthritis receiving methotrexate [See comments]. N Engl J Med. 1999;340:253–9.

21
Anti-tumour necrosis factor antibodies in Crohn's disease and ulcerative colitis

B. E. SANDS

INTRODUCTION

The release of infliximab (chimaeric monoclonal anti-tumour necrosis factor (TNF) antibody) onto the American market over 2 years ago provided a categorically new agent for the treatment of Crohn's disease. This provided the first biological response modifier indicated for Crohn's disease. Since approval of the drug in first the American, and later Canadian and European markets, the drug has become widely used. Although clinical experience has grown large, available data from randomized controlled trials remain relatively limited. The current approach to the use of infliximab in Crohn's disease is based on this relatively limited set of data, as well as new observations in the course of clinical care. Other anti-TNF agents continue to be investigated.

EARLY STUDIES OF INFLIXIMAB IN CROHN'S DISEASE

Early, open-label trials of infliximab, then called cA2, provided encouraging results. Beginning with case reports of excellent responses in patients with otherwise refractory Crohn's disease and ulcerative colitis, van Dullemen *et al.* reported their experience with 10 patients with refractory Crohn's disease, each of whom received a single infusion of infliximab[1]. Eight patients received 10 mg/kg, while two additional patients received 20 mg/kg of the drug. Although open-label studies in Crohn's disease are generally fraught with the possibility of placebo response and over-estimation of effect, abrupt and prolonged drops in Crohn's disease activity index (CDAI) scores were seen in all but one patient. This response was observed within 2 weeks of a single infusion and the duration of this effect extended in most cases to 8 weeks or more. These observations in the clinic were accompanied by marked improvement in endoscopic appearance, with observations of rapid healing of even deep, serpiginous ulcers within 4 weeks.

The first North American study, performed by McCabe *et al.*[2], extended the open-label experience with this medication and explored a wider range of doses. Patients with active Crohn's disease, not responding to other therapies, were given a single infusion of infliximab in escalating dosing cohorts of 1, 5, 10, and 20 mg/kg. Clinical responses (decrease in CDAI by 70 points or more) were observed over 12 weeks and endoscopic responses were scored using the *Crohn's Disease Endoscopic Index of Severity*. Doses of 5 mg and higher all proved efficacious, with concomitant documentation of improved endoscopic appearance. It is notable that many patients receiving 1 mg/kg had a clinical response, albeit of a relatively brief duration. To date this remains the only reported experience in doses ranging below 5 mg/kg in Crohn's disease, and all subsequent controlled trials in Crohn's disease focused on doses of 5 mg and higher as effective doses.

RANDOMIZED CONTROLLED TRIALS OF INFLIXIMAB IN CROHN'S DISEASE

In 1997 Targan *et al.*[3] reported the results of a randomized controlled trial of infliximab for patients with active Crohn's disease not responding to other therapies. Patients were permitted on trial if they had active symptoms of Crohn's disease as defined by a CDAI of 220 to as high as 450. Concomitant therapy with 5-aminosalicylates, corticosteroids, 6-mercaptopurine, or azathioprine was permitted. Adequate washout periods for these medications and stable doses while on study were required by the protocol. Patients were randomized in a blinded fashion to receive an infusion of placebo, or infliximab at 5, 10, or 20 mg/kg. Clinical response was observed, and patients failing to demonstrate a decrease in CDAI of 70 or more points by week 4 were permitted to receive an open-label infusion of infliximab 10 mg/kg.

Overall, patients receiving infliximab had an initial response rate of 64% compared to 17% among patients treated with placebo. Patients who failed to respond to an initial infusion of infliximab who then received an open-label infusion of the drug were half as likely to respond as those who responded to an initial infusion. Individually, each dose level of infliximab proved significantly better in achieving clinical response and clinical remission than placebo. The highest response rate, however, was observed among patients receiving 5 mg/kg of infliximab, with an observed response rate of 81% compared to 50% and 64% for patients treated with 10 and 20 mg/kg, respectively.

A second phase of study, reported by Rutgeerts *et al.*[4], provides the only available clinical trial data regarding repeating dosing in Crohn's disease. Patients who displayed a response to either the initial, blinded infusion, or to a subsequent open-label infusion, and who maintained a response at 8 weeks post-infusion, were eligible to begin receiving repeated dosing. Eligible patients were re-randomized at week 12 to receive either placebo or infliximab 10 mg/kg every 8 weeks for four additional infusions. A trend towards maintenance of clinical response at week 48 was observed among treated patients compared to placebo.

Applying the more stringent criteria of clinical remission, defined as CDAI less than 150 and a decrease in CDAI from baseline of 70 or more points, a statistically significant difference was observed between treated and untreated patients at week 48. In addition, health-related quality of life, as denoted by total score on the IBDQ, was significantly different among the two treated groups. A steady increase in C-reactive protein was observed over the duration of the study of placebo-treated patients, while patients who remained on therapy continued to have low and flat levels of C-reactive protein. Upon discontinuation of repeated dosing the proportion of patients in clinical response appeared to taper off, indicating loss of response as the interval from last treatment increased.

Serendipitous observations of healing of fistula among patients treated in earlier studies led to a randomized controlled trial for healing of fistulas in Crohn's disease. Present et al.[5] reported the results of what to date remains the only randomized control trial of the healing of fistulas in Crohn's disease. Patients with enterocutaneous fistula (primarily perianal fistula) were randomized to receive either placebo or infliximab at 5 or 10 mg/kg given as infusions at week 0, 2, and 6. The major endpoint of the study was closure of 50% or more of fistula for a given individual over two successive visits, 1 month apart. Closure was defined as a lack of drainage despite gentle compression of the skin around the fistula orifice. A complete response was defined as closure of all fistulas over a 1-month interval.

Applying these endpoints, infliximab was found to be superior to placebo in achieving both a clinical response and a complete response. Sixty-two per cent of patients receiving infliximab achieved a clinical response, compared to 26% among patients receiving placebo. Forty-six per cent of infliximab-treated patients achieved a complete response, compared to only 13% among patients given placebo. These results conclusively demonstrated the short-term benefits of infliximab for healing a perianal fistula. However, without additional therapy it has been observed that all patients eventually had relapse of their fistulas, with median duration of responses approximating 12 weeks. Studies of maintenance dosing for both inflammatory and fistulizing Crohn's disease are ongoing.

PAEDIATRIC CROHN'S DISEASE AND INFLIXIMAB

Baldassano et al.[6] have reported results of a randomized control trial in children with Crohn's disease. Results were obtained similar to or superior to those seen in adult patients. Preliminary observations show a slightly higher dose of 10 mg/kg to be more efficacious in achieving remission in children.

PREDICTORS OF CLINICAL RESPONSE TO INFLIXIMAB

Post-hoc analysis of data from clinical trials has failed to reveal patient characteristics predictive of clinical response to infliximab. Regardless of prior treatment, duration of disease, or severity of symptoms, the overwhelming factor in clinical improvement on trial has been whether or not the patient received active drug as opposed to placebo. Conflicting results have been obtained regarding the utility of identifying specific TNF genotypes as markers for responsiveness to infliximab. Marion *et al.*[7] have reported that the TNF microsatellite marker TNFa2b1c2d4e1 does not predict responsiveness to infliximab in patients with inflammatory or fistulizing disease, contradicting earlier reports. Variations at position -308 in the TNF promoter have been shown to contribute to the regulation of TNF production, and carriers of allele 2 at this site produce high amounts of TNF. Vermeire *et al.*[8] have shown a significant association between carriage of allele 1 (either as TNF-α-308*1,1 or TNF-α-308*1,2) and response to infliximab. The presumed mechanism of resistance among homozygous carriers of allele 2 is production of TNF in excess of the binding capacity of standard doses of infliximab.

LOSS OF RESPONSE TO INFLIXIMAB

Shortly prior to the release of infliximab on the American market, patients previously enrolled in clinical trials in the United States were eligible again to receive infliximab in an open-label protocol. Ten of 40 patients treated in this way were observed to have a delayed hypersensitivity reaction[9]. Clinical manifestations of this reaction included myalgias, fever, joint aches, and oedema. Among patients for whom serum was available, these reactions were shown to be accompanied by the expression of human antichimaeric antibodies. Furthermore, all such patients experienced loss of response to infliximab. The two key factors in the occurrence of these events appeared to include the long interval between treatments (approximately 2 years for most of these patients) and perhaps lack of concomitant immunosuppressive therapy during the initial treatment. In addition, most patients who experienced delayed hypersensitivity reactions had been treated with a liquid formulation, different from the lyophilized preparation currently marketed. These observations have informed the subsequent approach to clinical care of patients given infliximab, and suggest that therapy should be undertaken with the understanding that intermittent treatment over long intervals may be particularly conducive to host responses against this chimaeric antibody.

HUMANIZED ANTI-TNF ANTIBODY CDP571 IN CROHN'S DISEASE

A humanized anti-TNF antibody, CDP571, has been investigated as a treatment of Crohn's disease, with the hope of less antigenicity than infliximab. An initial placebo-referenced trial in active Crohn's disease demonstrated a significant decrease in CDAI from baseline among patients receiving a single infusion[10]. This has led to two recently reported clinical trials, one in moderately to severely active Crohn's disease, and a second in patients with steroid-dependent Crohn's disease. Patients with moderately to severely active Crohn's disease (CDAI 220–450) received an initial CDP571 dose of 10 or 20 mg/kg or placebo. At week 2 there was a significant difference in clinical response (CDAI decrease by 70 or more) among patients receiving 10 mg/kg (54%) compared to placebo (27%) (see Fig. 1). The proportion of responders among patients treated with 20 mg/kg (37%) was not significantly different from placebo. Groups were further subdivided to receive CDP571 at 10 mg/kg or placebo every 8 weeks for

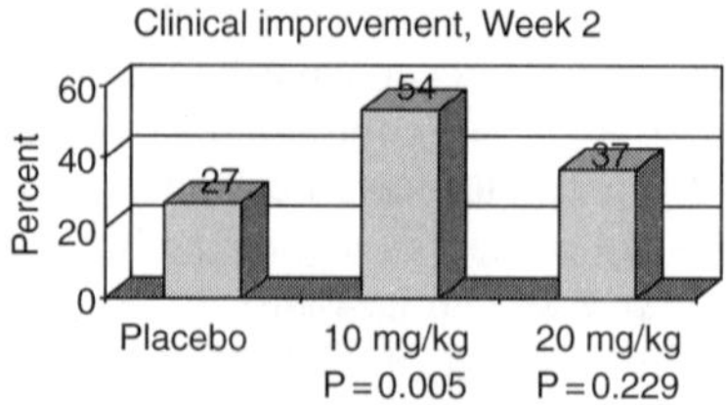

Figure 1 Humanized anti-TNF antibody CDP571 in moderately to severely active Crohn's disease. Clinical improvement was defined as a reduction from baseline CDAI by 70 or more points. Data from ref. 11

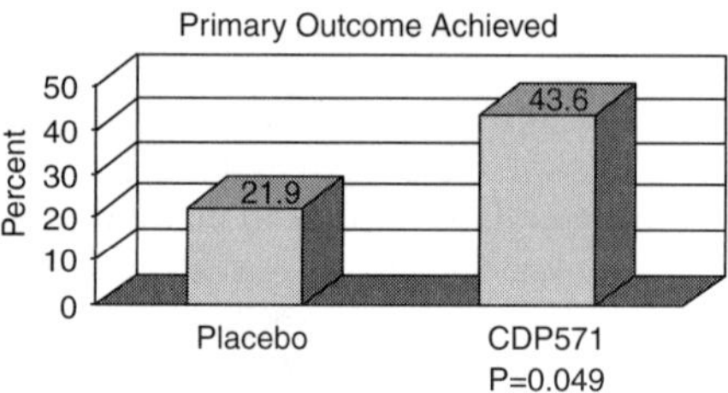

Figure 2 Humanized anti-TNF antibody CDP571 in steroid-dependent Crohn's disease. Primary outcome was discontinuation of corticosteroids at week 40, and no flare in symptoms. Data from ref. 12

two additional infusions, or an additional infusion of CDP571 at 10 mg/kg or placebo at week 12. Time to withdrawal was significantly longer for the 10 mg/kg dosed at 12-week intervals compared to placebo[11].

In a second study, patients with steroid-dependent Crohn's disease received either 20 mg/kg CDP571 followed by 10 mg/kg at week 8, or received placebo at weeks 0 and 8. Steroid-dependence was defined as meeting the following characteristics: (1) inactive symptoms (CDAI < 150); (2) prednisone dose of 15–40 mg/day or budesonide 9 mg/day for more than 8 weeks; and (3) inability to taper corticosteroid despite an attempt to do so within the previous 8 weeks. Steroids were tapered according to a predefined regimen. Among patients assigned to CDP571, 43.6% had successfully tapered at week 40 without flare of disease, compared to 21.9% among patients assigned to placebo ($p = 0.049$, see Fig. 2)[12]. This study provides clear evidence of the steroid-sparing effect of CDP571 in Crohn's disease.

ETANERCEPT (TNF RECEPTOR FUSION PROTEIN) IN CROHN'S DISEASE

Etanercept, a recombinant fusion protein of the p75 TNF receptor with an IgG_1 backbone, is available for treatment of rheumatoid arthritis. No data from randomized controlled trials are available regarding the safety and efficacy of etanercept in Crohn's disease. A pilot study from D'Haens et al.[13] explored the efficacy and safety of etanercept in patients with moderately to severely active Crohn's disease, as defined by a CDAI between 220 and 450. Patients received etanercept 25 mg subcutaneously twice weekly for 12 weeks. At week 2, six of 10 patients experienced a decrease in CDAI by at least 70 points. The median CDAI was lower at week 2 (166, range 107–392) compared to baseline (305, range 294–418). Significantly decreased serum C-reactive protein levels were observed. These data provide justification for additional study of this agent in IBD.

ANTI-TNF ANTIBODIES IN ULCERATIVE COLITIS

To date few data are available on the potential of anti-TNF antibodies for the treatment of ulcerative colitis. Evans et al.[14] reported their open-label experience in treating patients with mild to moderate ulcerative colitis with CDP571. Fifteen patients received a single infusion of 5 mg/kg CDP571 and were followed for 8 weeks. Eleven patients had left-sided disease, four had universal colitis, and six were steroid-refractory. A significant reduction in Powell–Tuck scores from 6.7 to 4.6 was observed at week 1 ($p = 0.023$). At week 2 the difference was no longer significant, with a mean Powell–Tuck score of 5.5. Sands et al.[15] reported limited experience with infliximab in 11 patients enrolled in a study of this agent as a treatment for severe, steroid-refractory ulcerative colitis. Eight of the 11 received infliximab as a single infusion of 5, 10, or 20 mg/kg, and three received placebo. The response rate among patients receiving active treatment was approximately 50%. The response seemed best among patients treated with a relatively high dose of 20 mg/kg. None of the patients who received placebo improved. No definite conclusions may be drawn from this study, due to the limited number of patients who completed the protocol before its premature termination.

FUTURE DIRECTIONS

Studies currently under way will provide a basis for ongoing treatment with repeated doses of anti-TNF antibody in Crohn's disease. It is likely that small molecule inhibitors of TNF, including inhibitors of phosphodiesterase IV and thalidomide homologues, will also be examined. The specific clinical indications for anti-TNF antibody in Crohn's disease will probably be expanded to roles in postsurgical prophylaxis and as early treatment for new-onset disease.

References

1. van Dullemen HM, van Deventer SJ, Hommes DW et al. Treatment of Crohn's disease with anti-tumor necrosis factor chimeric monoclonal antibody (cA2). Gastroenterology. 1995;109:129–35.
2. McCabe RP, Woody J, van Deventer S et al. A multicenter trial of cA2 anti-TNF chimeric monoclonal antibody in patients with active Crohn's disease. Gastroenterology. 1996;110:A962.
3. Targan SR, Hanauer SB, van Deventer SJH et al. A short-term study of chimeric monoclonal antibody cA2 to tumor necrosis factor α for Crohn's disease. N Engl J Med. 1997;337:1029–35.
4. Rutgeerts P, D'Haens G, Targan SR et al. Efficacy and safety of retreatment with anti-tumor necrosis factor antibody (infliximab) to maintain remission in Crohn's disease. Gastroenterology. 1999;117:761–9.

5. Present DH, Rutgeerts P, Targan S *et al*. Infliximab for the treatment of fistulas in patients with Crohn's disease. N Engl J Med. 1999;340:1398–405.
6. Baldassano R, Vasiliauskas E, Braegger CP *et al*. A multicenter study of infliximab (anti-TNFα antibody) in the treatment of children with active Crohn's disease. Gastroenterology. 1999;116:A665.
7. Marion JF, Bodian C, Toy L, Chapman ML, Scherl EJ, Present DH. TNF microsatellite polymorphism does not predict response to infliximab in patients with Crohn's disease. Gastroenterology. 2000;118:A654.
8. Vermeire S, Monsuur F, Groenen P, Peeters M, Vlietinck R, Rutgeerts P. Response to anti-TNFα treatment is associated with the TNFα-308*1 allele. Gastroenterology. 2000;118:A654.
9. Hanauer SB, Rutgeerts PJ, D'Haens G *et al*. Delayed hypersensitivity to infliximab (Remicade) re-infusion after 2–4 year interval without treatment. Gastroenterology. 1999;116:A731.
10. Stack WA, Mann SD, Roy AJ *et al*. Randomised controlled trial of CDP571 antibody to tumor necrosis factor-alpha in Crohn's disease. Lancet. 1997;349:521–4.
11. Sandborn WJ, Targan SR, Hanauer SB *et al*. A randomized controlled trial of CDP571, a humanized antibody to TNFα, in moderately to severely active Crohn's disease. Gastroenterology. 2000;118:A655.
12. Feagan B, Sandborn WJ, Baker JP *et al*. A randomized, double-blind, placebo-controlled, multicenter trial of the engineered human antibody to TNF (CDP571) for steroid sparing and maintenance of remission in patients with steroid-dependent Crohn's disease. Gastroenterology. 2000;118:A655.
13. D'Haens G, Swijsen C, Noman M, Lemmens L, Geboes K, Rutgeerts P. Etanercept (TNF receptor fusion protein, Enbrel) is effective and well tolerated in active refractory Crohn's disease: results of a single center pilot trial. Gastroenterology. 2000;118:A656.
14. Evans RC, Clarke L, Heath P, Stephens S, Morris AI, Rhodes JM. Treatment of ulcerative colitis with an engineered human anti-TNF alpha antibody CDP571. Aliment Pharmacol Ther. 1997;11:1031–5.
15. Sands BE, Podolsky DK, Tremaine WJ *et al*. Chimeric monoclonal anti-tumor necrosis factor antibody (cA2) in the treatment of severe, steroid-refractory ulcerative colitis. Gastroenterology. 1996;110:A1008.

Section VIII
Future trends: molecular therapy

22
Development of antisense to intercellular adhesion molecule-1 (ISIS 2302) for inflammatory bowel disease therapy

B. R. YACYSHYN

ISIS 2302 (ANTISENSE TO ICAM-1)

ISIS 2302 is 20-base phosphorothioate oligodeoxynucleotide that inhibits intercellular adhesion molecule-1 (ICAM-1) expression through an antisense mechanism of action[1,2]. ISIS 2302 is designed to specifically hybridize to a sequence in the 3'-untranslated region of the human ICAM-1 message. The heterodimer formed serves as a substrate for RNase H, with subsequent cleavage of the m-RNA, down-regulation of intracellular specific message content, and inhibition of specific protein synthesis. RNase H is a family of ubiquitous enzymes whose functions have not been fully defined, but among its functions appears to be the degradation of Okazaki fragments generated during normal DNA replication.

ICAM-1, a member of the immunoglobulin superfamily, is an inducible transmembrane glycoprotein constitutively expressed at low levels on vascular endothelial cells and on a subset of leucocytes[3–5]. In response to proinflammatory mediators many cell types up-regulate expression of ICAM-1 on their surface. The primary counterligands for ICAM-1 are the beta-2 integrins, LFA-1 and Mac-1, expressed on leucocytes[6–8].

ICAM-1 serves multiple functions in the propagation of inflammatory processes, the best characterized being facilitation of leucocyte emigration from the intravascular space in response to inflammatory stimuli[9–11]. ICAM-1 also appears to provide an important secondary signal during antigen presentation and to play an important role in cytotoxic T-cell, NK cell, and neutrophil-mediated target cell damage[12–17]. Any or all of the above functions makes ICAM-1 a theoretically attractive therapeutic target for inflammatory disease. As an oligonucleotide ISIS 2302 is non-immunogenic and therefore does not suffer from the same limitation in the treatment of chronic disease as the murine

ICAM-1 antibody. As an antisense inhibitor of ICAM-1, ISIS 2302 provides a tool to investigate the pathogenic significance of ICAM-1 in the maintenance of a spectrum of inflammatory diseases and in the induction of acute organ transplant rejection.

PHARMACOLOGY

ISIS 2302 is a 20-base phosphorothioate oligodeoxynucleotide, with a sequence of 5' GCCCAAGCTGGCATCCCTCA 3' and a molecular weight of 6781.24 amu. ISIS 2302 selectively inhibits cytokine-induced ICAM-1 expression on a wide variety of human cells *in vitro*[18-20]. Functional effects of ICAM-1 down-regulation can also be demonstrated *in vitro*: inhibition of leucocyte adherence to human endothelial cells and intestinal fibroblasts, and decreased T-cell proliferation to IL-4/GM-CSF-treated monocytes (dendritic cells, Isis Pharmaceuticals, unpublished data)[1,21,22]. A murine analogue, ISIS 3082, has been shown to be active in multiple models of inflammation including prolongation of cardiac allograft survival, carrageenan-induced neutrophil infiltration (Isis Pharmaceuticals, unpublished data), dextran sulphate-induced colitis, endotoxin-induced neutrophil migration, and collagen-induced arthritis (Isis Pharmaceuticals, unpublished observations)[23-25]. In each study, control oligonucleotides failed to demonstrate pharmacological activity, suggesting that the anti-inflammatory activity of ISIS 3082 was due to inhibition of ICAM-1 expression. Baker *et al.*, from Isis, recently reported the benefit of antisense to TNF-A (ISIS 2302) in the chronic dextran sulphate sodium model of colitis[26]. In the endotoxin pneumonitis and the dextran sulphate-induced colitis models, down-regulation of either ICAM-1 message or protein in involved tissue was sought and demonstrated. A rat analogue, ISIS 9125, was also effective in the prevention of rat cardiac and renal allograft rejection[27]. Antisense to ICAM-1 has recently been evaluated in the HLA-B27 transgenic rat model by our laboratory with similar, corroborative findings (manuscript submitted).

As an antisense drug, ISIS 2302 inhibits *de-novo* synthesis of ICAM-1, and pharmacological activity must therefore await turnover of already expressed protein. In animal models of disease, therapeutic activity was generally seen with doses ranging from 0.03 to 10 mg/kg, depending upon the model, administered three times weekly to daily over 1–2 weeks. Down-regulation of ICAM-1 message, protein, or function was also demonstrated in target tissue from the models in which it was investigated. In humans, doses of 0.5–2 mg/kg have provided evidence of therapeutic effect in phase 2 studies in rheumatoid arthritis and Crohn's disease. A dose-responsive, qualitative reduction in mucosal ICAM-1 expression was also observed in the Crohn's study.

CLINICAL EFFICACY – PHASE 2a TRIALS

Phase 2a trials were initiated in several clinical indications including Crohn's disease and ulcerative colitis. These Phase 2a trials were therefore designed as fixed-dose, within-patient, dose-escalation studies, generally beginning at 0.5 mg/kg and escalating to 1 and 2 mg/kg every other day intravenously in successive cohorts. These studies enrolled refractory patients, with efficacy being assessed by standard, well-accepted outcome measures. All but the psoriasis trial were/are double-blinded, placebo-controlled, and randomized (3 : 1; study drug : placebo), and all but the renal transplant study involve a 4-week treatment period. Treatment in the renal transplant study is for 2 weeks. In addition, the renal transplant study differs from the other studies by specifying two additional lower dose groups of 0.05 and 0.1 mg/kg and by providing for a phase 1 and a phase 2 segment. In each study 17–52 patients were enrolled at one or two centres. Patients were followed for up to 6 months after the treatment period, or until disease relapsed or failed to respond to study drug.

CROHN'S DISEASE

This study was a 20-patient, double-blinded, placebo-controlled, randomized (3 : 1; study drug : placebo), single-centre study that enrolled steroid-dependent patients with moderately active Crohn's disease despite background corticosteroids ($\leqslant 40$ mg prednisone or equivalent/day)[28]. Four patients each were assigned to the 0.5 and 1 mg/kg dose group, the remaining 12 patients to the 2 mg/kg dose group, and all patients received 13 intravenous infusions of ISIS 2302 or placebo over 26 days. Patients were then followed for a total of 6 months. Moderately active was defined as a Crohn's Disease Activity Index (CDAI) $\geqslant 200$ and $\leqslant 350$. Background 5-ASA drugs in stable dosage were also permitted. Corticosteroids were to remain stable during the 26-day treatment period. The primary efficacy measures were the CDAI. Endoscopic Index of Severity (EIS) and the Inflammatory Bowel Disease Questionnaire, a quality of life measure, were also followed.

The CDAI is a validated clinical instrument[29,30] that is widely accepted as the 'gold standard' in evaluating clinical disease activity and response. It is a composite score based upon patient diaries and more objective measures, and can range from 0 to approximately 600. A CDAI of < 150 is widely accepted as defining disease remission, and a decrease of 70–100 points as a response. Over the investigated dose range of 0.5–2 mg/kg there was no consistent evidence of a dose response for clinical measures, and data are therefore presented for the combined ISIS 2302 group as compared to placebo. At the end of the treatment period, seven of 15 (47%) ISIS 2302-treated and one of five placebo-treated patients, a patient already in remission at baseline though with active disease at screening, were in remission. At the end of month 6, five of the seven ISIS 2302-treated remitters were still in remission, and a sixth patient had a CDAI of 156.

Supportive trends favouring ISIS 2302 over placebo were also observed for other clinical (EIS and IBDQ) and pharmacological measures. Mucosal biopsies from the same area of the intestine were obtained at baseline and day 26, immunohistochemically stained for ICAM-1, and qualitatively assessed by a blinded pathologist as to whether ICAM-1 expression had increased, remained constant, or decreased. Statistically significant reductions in ICAM-1 expression were observed in the ISIS 2302 group as compared to the placebo group ($p = 0.033$); ICAM-1 was judged to be reduced in seven of nine patients receiving the 2 mg/kg dose as compared to one of the five placebo patients.

Two patients with upper gastrointestinal obstructive symptoms due to gastro-duodenal Crohn's disease experienced resolution of these symptoms, and the two patients with an open enterocutaneous fistula at baseline experienced closure; all four patients received ISIS 2302.

By amendment to the protocol, upon disease relapse after completion of the original trial, patients were offered open-label treatment with ISIS 2302 at their originally assigned schedule[28]. Seven patients availed themselves of retreatment some 7–13 months after their original therapy: four of these patients (responders) had experienced sustained remission (three) or response (one), two patients (non-responders) had experienced only short-lived responses to original treatment with ISIS 2302, and the one placebo-treated patient had experienced a late and short-lived remission. During the retreatment protocol all four previous responders again experienced a sustained remission or response that lasted at least through the 6-month retreatment trial, as did the previously placebo-treated patient. As expected, the two previous non-responders only experienced short-lived improvements in their disease activity. ISIS 2302 continued to be well tolerated upon retreatment. These data, though open-label and limited, suggest that retreatment with ISIS 2302 is both safe and effective in previous responders.

Based upon the encouraging safety and efficacy profile of ISIS 2302 in the pilot study, a 300-patient pivotal trial exploring the steroid-sparing and remission-inducing qualities of ISIS 2302 was initiated, as well as two smaller studies investigating short duration (5-day) intravenous and low-dose (0.5 mg/kg) subcutaneous administration. Complete evaluation and analysis of these studies is nearing conclusion.

ULCERATIVE COLITIS

An enema study in distal ulcerative colitis is currently under way in Europe. ISIS 2302 by enema is taken up in mg/g concentrations by intestinal epithelium in experimental animals and is well tolerated. At this time it is not known whether a topical approach with ISIS 2302 will be effective in this disease, but an antisense to NF-κB administered by enema was reported to be effective in treating established colitis in two mouse models: IL-10-deficient mice and TNBS-induced colitis[31].

PHASE 2b CROHN'S DISEASE

A 300-patient, randomized, double-blinded, placebo-controlled, 6-month study in steroid-dependent (10–40 mg/day of prednisone or equivalent for at least 3 months), active Crohn's disease (CDAI 200–350) has been fully recruited. Beginning on day 8, patients in the high-dose corticosteroid stratum (20–40 mg/day) were assigned to 20 mg/day of prednisone and tapered by 2.5 mg/day per week thereafter as tolerated, so that patients would have the opportunity to be at a dosage of zero at the beginning of week 10. Patients in the low-dose stratum (10–19 mg/day) remained on their entry level of prednisone and began tapering dosage by 2.5 mg/day per week on the same protocol day that a patient entering in the high-dose stratum would taper to a lower dosage. In this way all patients had the opportunity to be completely weaned from corticosteroids on the same protocol day. A 4- and a 2-week regimen of 2 mg/kg intravenously three times weekly during months 1 and 3 are being compared to placebo. The primary endpoint in this trial is complete clinical remission at the end of week 14, defined as a CDAI < 150 and a steroid dose of zero. Completion of data analysis of this study is nearly finished.

Antisense technology offers the potential for rapid and highly efficient drug discovery with absolute target specificity. This, together with the wide therapeutic index in the treatment of a broad spectrum of human diseases, will allow antisense therapeutics a considerable horizon in the future of human inflammatory diseases.

References

1. Bennett CF, Condon T, Grimm S, Chan H, Chiang MY. Inhibition of endothelial cell-leukocyte adhesion molecule expression with antisense oligonucleotides. J Immunol. 1994;152:3530–40.
2. Chang JY, Sehgal SN, Bansbach CC. FK506 and rapamycin: novel pharmacological probes of the immune response. Trends Pharmacol Sci. 1991;12:218.
3. Dustin ML, Rothlein R, Bhan AK, Dinarello CA, Springer TA. Induction by IL 1 and interferon gamma: tissue distribution, biochemistry, and function of a natural adherence molecule (ICAM-1). J Immunol. 1986;137:245–54.
4. Rothlein RM, Dustin L, Marlin SD, Springer TA. A human intercellular adhesion molecule (ICAM-1) distinct from LFA-1. J Immunol. 1986;137:1270–4.
5. Simmons DM, Makgoba W, Seed B. ICAM, an adhesion ligand of LFA-1, is homologous to the neural cell adhesion molecule NCAM. Nature. 1988;331:624–7.
6. Marlin SD, Springer TA. Purified intercellular adhesion molecule-1 (ICAM-1) is a ligand for lymphocyte function associated antigen-1 (LFA-1). Cell. 1987;51:813–19.
7. Diamond MS, Staunton DE, deFougerolles AR *et al*. ICAM-1 (CD54): a counter-receptor for Mac-1 (CD11b/CD18). J Cell Biol. 1990;111:3129–39.
8. Diamond MS, Staunton DE, Marlin SD, Springer TA. Binding of the integrin Mac-1 (CD11b/CD18) to the third immunoglobulin-like domain of ICAM-1 (CD54) and its regulation by glycosylation. Cell. 1991;65:961.
9. Butcher EC. Leukocyte–endothelial cell recognition: three (or more) steps to specificity and diversity. Cell. 1991;67:1033–6.
10. Furie MB, Tancinco MCA, Smith CW. Monoclonal antibodies to leukocyte integrins CD11a/CD18 and CD11b/CD18 or intercellular adhesion molecule-1 inhibit chemoattractant-stimulated neutrophil transendothelial migration *in vitro*. Blood. 1991;78:2089–97.
11. Oppenheimer-Marks N, Davis LS, Bogue DT, Ramberg J, Lipsky PE. Differential utilization of ICAM-1 and VCAM-1 during the adhesion and transendothelial migration of human T lymphocytes. J Immunol. 1991;147:2913–21.
12. Altmann DM, Hogg N, Trowsdale J, Wilkinson D. Contransfection of ICAM-1 and HLA-DR reconstitutes human antigen-presenting cell function in mouse L cells. Nature 1989;338:512–14.
13. Van Seventer GA, Shimizu Y, Horgan KJ, Shaw S. The LFA-1 ligand ICAM-1 provides an important costimulatory signal for T cell receptor-mediated activation of resting T cells. J Immunol. 1990;144:4579–86.
14. Kuhlman P, Moy VT, Lollo BA, Brian AA. The accessory function of murine Intercellular Adhesion Molecule-1 in T lymphocyte activation. J Immunol. 1991;146:1773–82.
15. Makgoba MW, Sanders ME, Luce GEG *et al*. Functional evidence that intercellular adhesion molecule-1 (ICAM-1) is a ligand for LFA-1-dependent adhesion in T cell-mediated cytotoxicity. Eur J Immunol. 1988;18:637–40.
16. Allavena P, Paganin C, Martin-Padura I *et al*. Molecules and structures involved in the adhesion of natural killer cells to vascular endothelium. J Exp Med. 1991;173:439–48.
17. Entman MI., Youker K, Shoji T *et al*. Neutrophil induced oxidative injury of cardiac myocytes. J Clin Invest. 1992;90:1335–45.

18. Bennett CF, Crooke ST. Regulation of endothelial cell adhesion molecule expression with anti-sense oligonucleotides. Adv Pharmacol. 1994;28:1–43.
19. Miele ME, Bennett CF, Miller BE, Welch DR. Enhanced metastatic ability of TNF-a treated malignant melanoma cells is reduced by intercellular adhesion molecule-1 (CD54) antisense oligonucleotides. Exp Cell Res. 1994;214:231–41.
20. Nestle F, Mitra RS, Bennett CF, Nickoloff BJ. Cationic lipid is not required for uptake and inhibitory activity of ICAM-1 phosphorothioate antisense oligonucleotide in keratinocytes. J Invest Dermatol. 1994;103:569–75.
21. Rivera MT, Fisher PJ, Stein DJ et al. Antisense oligonucleotides, but not steroids, inhibit human intestinal microvascular endothelial cell (HIMEC) adhesion molecule expression and leukocyte binding: a novel therapeutic strategy in intestinal inflammation. Gastroenterology. 1999;116: G2916.
22. Musso A, Condon TF, Bennett CF, Levine AD, Fiocchi C. ICAM-1 antisense disrupts intestinal fibroblast–T-cell interaction: implications for modulation of intestinal inflammation. Gastroen-terology. 1998;114:G4284.
23. Stepkowski SM, Tu Y, Condon TP, Bennett CF. Blocking of heart allograft rejection by ICAM-1 antisense oligonucleotides alone or in combination with other immunosuppresive modalities. J Immunol. 1994;153:5336–46.
24. Bennett CF, Kornbrust D, Henry S et al. An ICAM-1 antisense oligonucleotide prevents and reverses dextran sulfate sodium-induced colitis in mice. J Pharmacol Exp Ther. 1997;280: 988–1000.
25. Kumasaka T, Quinlan WM, Doyle NA et al. The role of ICAM-1 in endotoxin-induced pneumo-nia evaluated using ICAM-1 antisense oligonucleotides, anti-ICAM-1 monoclonal antibodies, and ICAM-1 mutant mice. J Clin Invest. 1996;97:2362–9.
26. Baker B, Murthy S, Flanigan A, Siwikowski A, Butler M, Dean N. Dose-dependent reduction of chronic dextran sulfate sodium (DSS)-induced colitis in mice treated with TNF-A antisense oligonucleotide (ISIS 25302). Gastroenterology. 2000;118:A2980.
27. Stepkowski S, Wang M, Condon TP. Protection against allograft rejection with intercellular adhesion molecule-1 antisense oligodeoxynucleotides. Transplant. 1998;66:699–707.
28. Yacyshyn B, Bowen-Yacyshyn MB, Jewell L et al. A placebo-controlled trial of ICAM-1 anti-sense oligonucleotide in the treatment of Crohn's disease. Gastroenterology. 1998;114:1133–42.
29. Best WR, Bectel JM, Singleton JW, Kern F. Development of a Crohn's disease activity index: National Cooperative Crohn's Disease Study. Gastroenterology. 1976;70:439–44.
30. Best WR, Bectel JM, Singleton JW. Rederived values of the eight coefficients of the Crohn's Disease Activity Index. Gastroenterology. 1979;77:483–6.
31. Neurath MF, Petterson S, Meyer KH. Local administration of antisense phosphorothioate oligonucleotides to the p65 subunit of NF-kB abrogates established experimental colitis in mice. Nat Med. 1996;2:998–1004.

23
NF-κB: a key transcription factor in chronic intestinal inflammation

M. F. NEURATH

Crohn's disease and ulcerative colitis are the two major forms of inflammatory bowel diseases (IBD) in humans. In spite of various intensive studies in the past, the aetiology and immunopathogenesis of IBD is still poorly understood. However, it has become clear that dysregulated cytokine production and signalling mechanisms by epithelial cells, mucosal lymphocytes and macrophages are important in the pathogenesis of both Crohn's disease and ulcerative colitis[1]. This is underlined by studies over recent years in various murine models of chronic intestinal inflammation resembling IBD. These models have provided important clues as to the nature of such dysregulation and to its possible cytokine-based treatment[2]. Thus, in studies of several of the models most closely resembling Crohn's disease, it was found that production of large amounts of Th1-type cytokines (e.g. IFN-γ and TNF) whose promoters are regulated by NF-κB, is a major and essential feature of the inflammation[3]. Finally, it has been shown that the Th1 cytokine production in these models is triggered by macrophages via increased production of IL-12, a cytokine that plays a major role in driving T cell differentiation and whose expression is also at least partially triggered by NF-κB.

NF-κB designates a group of transcription factors defined in part by their ability to bind a specific DNA sequence first identified in the enhancer of the immunoglobulin κ light-chain gene[4-6]. In mammals the NF-κB family consists of several proteins including NF-κB1 (p50), NF-κB2 (p52), p65 (RelA), c-Rel (Rel), and RelB which share the so-called Rel homology domain. NF-κB can be found in the cytoplasm of most cells as an inactive complex with unprocessed precursor proteins (e.g. p105) or IκB (e.g. IκBα) proteins[4-6]. Activation of cells with various stimuli then initiates a signalling cascade that finally leads to the disruption of the inactive complex and the release of NF-κB (Figs 1 and 2). In lymphocytes NF-κB can be released by stimulating cells with various agents such as LPS, PMA, PHA, immunoglobulin receptor-crosslinking, interleukin-2, and crosslinking of surface CD3 or CD28. However, another important mechanism to activate NF-κB involves the receptor of advanced glycation end-products

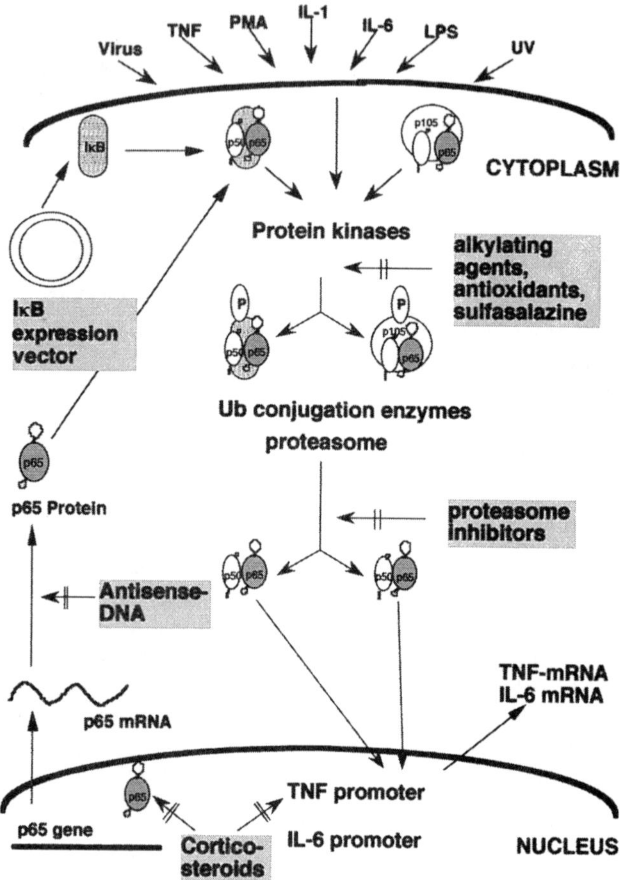

Figure 1 Activation process of NF-κB and strategies to inhibit NF-κB function in IBD. While alkylating agents, sulphasalazine and antioxidants may block protein kinases, antisense DNA can inhibit translation of p65. In addition, corticosteroids lead to blockade of p65 and adenoviral expression vectors could deliver genes whose products inactivate NF-κB

(RAGE). In contrast to cytokine-dependent activation of NF-κB, RAGE has been shown to mediate long-term activation of NF-κB (Fig. 3). Upon activation, NF-κB translocates into the nucleus and binds to DNA. The prototypical NF-κB is a heterodimer composed of the p50 and p65 subunits and the latter is the most frequent component of active NF-κB in humans.

NF-κB is a key regulator of the inducible expression of many genes associated with immune function in the gut. For instance, NF-κB plays an essential role in the transcriptional regulation of many cytokine genes (e.g. interleukin (IL)-1, IFN-γ, IL-2, IL-6, IL-8, IL-12p40) in lymphocytes, epithelial cells and monocytes[4–6]. However, the potential role of NF-κB in immune modulation in the gut

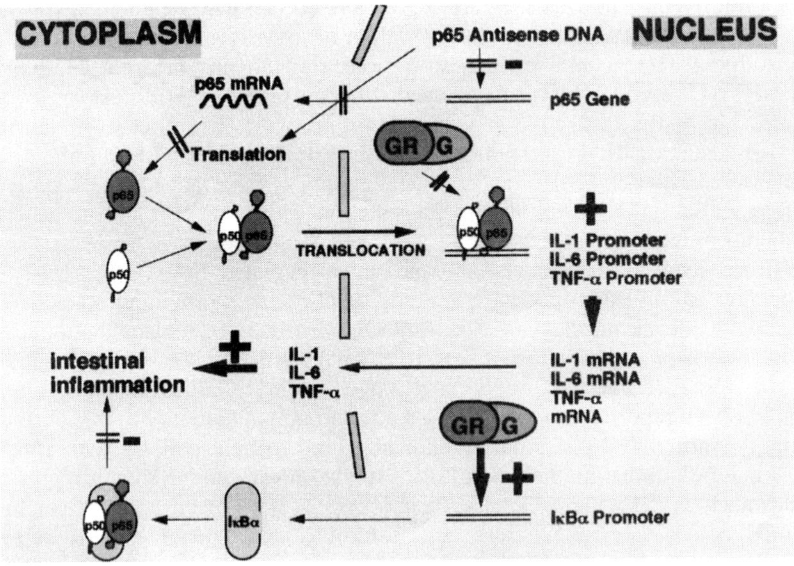

Figure 2 Mechanisms of NF-κB inactivation by corticosteroids. Corticosteroids can activate IκB gene transcription leading to increased IκB levels. The major pathway of blocking NF-κB, however, is mediated by direct complex formation between corticosteroids (G) and p65 (Modified according to ref. 18)

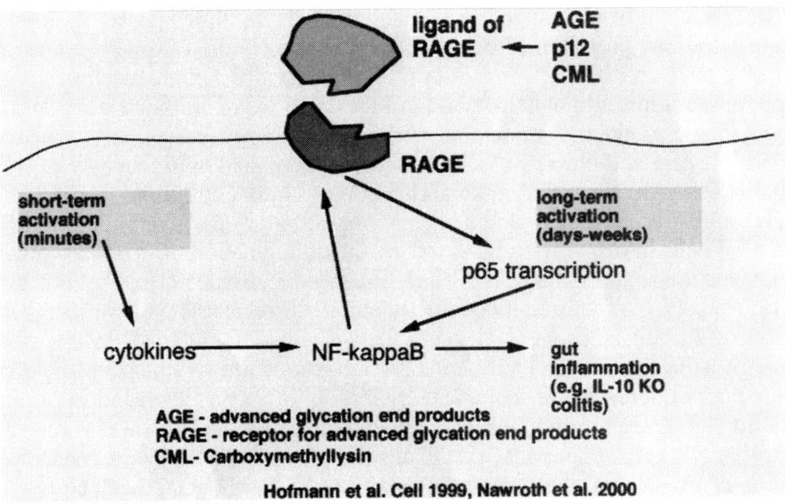

Figure 3 A role for RAGE in long-term activation of NF-κB in intestinal inflammation. RAGE seems to activate p65 gene transcription upon binding of specific ligands such as AGE, p12 and CML

is not limited only to cytokine gene regulation. NF-κB has been demonstrated to have an important function in the regulation of a variety of genes encoding for transcription factors and cell adhesion molecules. For instance, the binding of NF-κB, ATF-2 and HMG-I(Y) to the E-selectin promoter is necessary for the expression of the respective gene. Furthermore, it has been demonstrated that NF-κB regulates the expression of genes for the TAP-transporter (TAP-1), the proteasome subunit LMP-1 and the MHC class II invariant chain[7–8], proteins with essential functions for antigen presentation. Thus, NF-κB seems to be a key regulator of immune cell function.

NF-κB itself is extensively up- and down-regulated by a wide variety of exogenous stimuli that modulate immune function, thus providing a positive or negative feedback mechanism. For instance, NF-κB transactivates the inducible NO-synthase promoter in response to LPS, giving rise to increased production of NO, a substance that is strongly up-regulated in the inflamed intestine[9] that in turn has been reported to inhibit NF-κB activation in endothelial cells[10–11]. Interestingly, various other substances clinically used to treat patients with chronic intestinal inflammation, including IL-10, sulphasalazine and immunosuppressive drugs such as cyclosporin A and glucocorticoids, have been reported to inhibit NF-κB activation[12–17]. Whereas corticosteroids have been shown to repress NF-κB activity by inducing IκBα protein production and complex formation with NF-κB p65, the inhibitory mechanism of IL-10 on NF-κB activation is based on blockade of the inhibitor of κB kinase[23]. The importance of this function is highlighted by the fact that IL-10 knockout mice with chronic intestinal inflammation have been shown to have activated NF-κB p65[18].

The above data encouraged studies on the identification of signalling pathways and transcription factors that govern cytokine gene transcription in IBD. Although some NF-κB family members are apparently important in preventing inflammatory responses (e.g. RelB), it was found that nuclear NF-κB levels are increased in IBD patients. In particular, the p65 subunit was highly activated in epithelial cells and lamina propria macrophages from patients with active Crohn's disease and ulcerative colitis[18,19,24]. In addition, it was recently demonstrated that a specific p65 antisense oligonucleotide can block p65 expression and proinflammatory cytokine production by lamina propria macrophages in patients with active Crohn's disease and ulcerative colitis[18]. Furthermore, in a murine model of colitis p65, antisense treatment led to an abrogation of chronic intestinal inflammation. Interestingly, recent data by Jobin and co-workers showed activation of NF-κB in epithelial cells in response to IL-1 and an altered regulation of IκBα degradation in native colonic epithelial cells[19]. Such enhanced resistance of epithelial cells to IκBα proteolysis suggested a potentially increased responsiveness to therapeutic blockade. Indeed, adenoviral-mediated delivery of a mutant NF-κB-repressing IκBα protein resulted in inhibition of IL-8 production by intestinal epithelial cells. Furthermore, pharmacological inhibition of IκBα degradation strongly reduced IL-8 secretion by intestinal epithelial cells. Finally, recent evidence suggests that NF-κB is important in regulating ICAM-1 expression in the intestine[20]. Preliminary data from the same group also showed a beneficial therapeutic effect of proteasome inhibitors (that block NF-κB activation) in experimental colitis.

Inhibition of NF-κB activity has recently been suggested as a major component of the anti-inflammatory activity of glucocorticoids that are frequently used

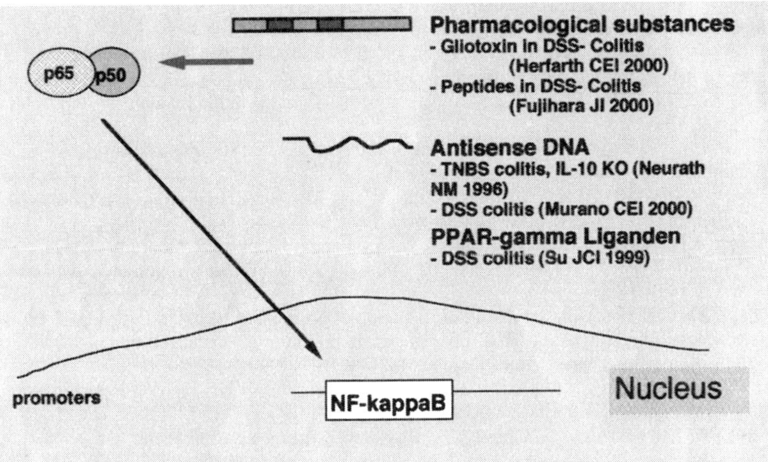

Figure 4   Targeting of the NF-κB activation pathway in intestinal inflammation. In animal models of intestinal inflammation gliotoxin, specific peptides, antisense DNA and PPAR-γ ligands have been successfully used to suppress NF-κB activity and intestinal inflammation

for treatment of chronic intestinal inflammation in humans[21–22]. Although activation of NF-κB p65 is not specific for patients with IBD, its perpetuated activation makes it a very attractive target for therapeutic intervention. Thus, down-regulation of NF-κB activity emerges as a potential key event in the control of chronic intestinal inflammation in humans, and strategies to inhibit NF-κB activity more specifically are desirable. Such strategies include antioxidants, proteasome inhibitors, inhibition of NF-κB by adenoviral IκB expression vectors, and antisense DNA targeting of NF-κB p65 (Figs 3 and 4). Thus, the above data suggest that targeting of NF-κB may be a novel molecular approach for the treatment of patients with IBD that could lead to the design of new treatment strategies that have added specificity but reduced toxicity compared to standard immunosuppressive therapy.

In summary, NF-κB is a pleiotropic transcription factor with key functions in the intestinal immune system. NF-κB family members control transcriptional activity of various promoters of proinflammatory cytokines, cell surface receptors, transcription factors and adhesion molecules that are involved in intestinal inflammation. The perpetuated activation of NF-κB in patients with active IBD suggests that regulation of NF-κB activity is a very attractive target for therapeutic intervention. Such strategies include antioxidants, proteasome inhibitors, inhibition of NF-κB by adenoviral IκB expression vectors, and antisense DNA targeting of NF-κB. These approaches will hopefully permit the design of new treatment strategies for chronic intestinal inflammation.

References

1. Strober W, Neurath MF. Immunological diseases of the gastrointestinal tract. In: Rich RR, editor. Clinical Immunology. St Louis: Mosby, 1995;1401–28.

2. Elson CO, Sartor RB, Tennyson GS, Riddell RH. Experimental models of inflammatory bowel disease. Gastroenterology. 1995;109:1344–67.
3. Strober W, Kelsall BL, Fuss I *et al*. Reciprocal IFN-γ and TGF-β responses regulate the occurrence of mucosal inflammation. Immunol Today. 1997;18:61–4.
4. Baeuerle P, Henkel T. Function and activation of NF-kappa B in the immune system. Annu Rev Immunol. 1994;12:141–53.
5. Baldwin AS. The NF-kappa B and I kappa B proteins: new discoveries and insights. Annu Rev Immunol. 1996;14:649–62.
6. Ryseck RP, Bull P, Takamiya M *et al*. RelB, a new Rel family transcription activator that can interact with p50-NF-kappa B. Mol Cell Biol. 1992;12:674–83.
7. Wright KL, White LC, Kelly A, Beck S, Trowsdale J, Ting JP. Coordinate regulation of the human TAP1 and LMP2 genes from a shared bidirectional promoter. J Exp Med. 1995;181:1459–68.
8. Brown AM, Linhoff MW, Stein B *et al*. Function of NF-kappa B/Rel binding sites in the major histocompatibility complex class II invariant chain promoter is dependent on cell-specific binding of different NF-kappa B/Rel subunits. Mol Cell Biol. 1994;14:2926–36.
9. Xie QW, Kashiwabara Y, Nathan C. Role of transcription factor NF-kappa B/Rel in induction of nitric oxide synthase. J Biol Chem. 1994;269:4705–14.
10. Zeiher AM, Fisslthaler B, Schray UB, Busse R. Nitric oxide modulates the expression of monocyte chemoattractant protein 1 in cultured human endothelial cells. Circ Res. 1995; 76:980–92.
11. Peng HB, Libby P, Liao JK. Induction and stabilization of I kappa B alpha by nitric oxide mediates inhibition of NF-kappa B. J Biol Chem. 1995;270:14214–21.
12. Mukaida N, Morita M, Ishikawa Y *et al*. Novel mechanism of glucocorticoid-mediated gene repression. Nuclear factor-kappa B is target for glucocorticoid-mediated interleukin 8 gene repression. J Biol Chem. 1994;269:13289–96.
13. Wang P, Wu P, Siegel MI, Egan RW, Billah MM. Interleukin (IL)-10 inhibits nuclear factor kappa B (NF kappa B) activation in human monocytes. IL-10 and IL-4 suppress cytokine synthesis by different mechanisms. J Biol Chem. 1995;270:9558–64.
14. Frantz B, Nordby EC, Bren G *et al*. Calcineurin acts in synergy with PMA to inactivate I kappa B/MAD3, an inhibitor of NF-kappa B. EMBO J. 1994;13:861–72.
15. Chen D, Rothenberg EV. Interleukin 2 transcription factors as molecular targets of cAMP inhibition: delayed inhibition kinetics and combinatorial transcription roles. J Exp Med. 1994;179:931–9.
16. Neumann M, Grieshammer T, Chuvpilo S *et al*. RelA/p65 is a molecular target for the immunosuppressive action of protein kinase A. EMBO J. 1995;14:1991–2003.
17. van Deventer SJH, Elson CO, Fedorak RN. Multiple doses of intravenous interleukin-10 in steroid-refractory Crohn's disease. Gastroenterology. 1997;113:383–9.
18. Neurath MF, Pettersson S, Meyer zum Büschenfelde KH, Strober W. Local administration of antisense phosphorothioate oligonucleotides to the p65 subunit of NF-κB abrogates experimental colitis in mice. Nature Med. 1996;2:998–1004.
19. Jobin C, Haskill S, Mayer L, Panja A, Sartor BR. Evidence for altered regulation of IκBα degradation in human colonic epithelial cells. J Immunol. 1997;158:226–34.
20. Morise Z, Brand S, Komatsu S, Russell JM, Granger DN, Grisham MB. Inhibition of ICAM-1 expression and mucosal injury by a selective proteasome inhibitor in a model of NSAID-induced gastropathy: role of NF-kappaB. Gastroenterology. 1997;A775.
21. Scheinman RI, Cogswell PC, Lofquist AK, Baldwin AS. Role of transcriptional activation of IκBα in mediation of immunosuppression by glucocorticoids. Science. 1995;270:283–6.
22. Auphan N, DiDonato JA, Rosette C, Helmberg A, Karin M. Immuno-suppression by glucocorticoids: inhibition of NF-κB activity through induction of IκBα synthesis. Science. 1995;270:286–90.

24
Cellular and molecular mechanisms of anti-interleukin-12 therapy in the treatment of inflammatory bowel disease

I. FUSS, M. BOIRIVANT, T. MARTH, W. STROBER
and M. F. NEURATH

Studies in experimental models of mucosal inflammation have led to major new insights into the abnormalities present in their counterpart human diseases (inflammatory bowel diseases; IBD) as well as exciting new approaches to the therapy of these diseases[1–3]. One such approach, the administration of anti-IL-12, has been shown to be effective in both the prevention and treatment of experimental mucosal inflammation[4,5]. At first sight the mechanism underlying the therapeutic effect of this antibody appears to be due to its ability to neutralize a key cytokine responsible for the inflammation, during its inductive phase (IL-12). However, recent work has disclosed that the mechanisms involved are more profound[6] in that anti-IL-12 not only neutralizes IL-12, but affects the survival of $CD4^+$ T cells mediating the inflammation, so that the main action of the antibody is on the cells inducing or producing cytokines, rather than the cytokines themselves. These findings have important implications for the design of more effective cytokine-based treatments of both IBD and other inflammatory states having a similar pathogenesis.

Immune responses in the mucosa are frequently characterized by major expansions of antigen-specific T cells having potent effector functions[1,7]. While this may be important for host defence it may lead to cell populations with substantial autoreactivity and the capacity to cause mucosal inflammation. To deal with this latter possibility the mucosal immune system has evolved several strategies for the control of mucosal immune responses. Among these is the regulation of programmed cell death or apoptosis, either that occurring via an active mechanism following TCR stimulation (activation-induced cell death) or that occurring via a passive mechanism following lymphokine (e.g. IL-2) withdrawal[8,9]. The active mechanism involves death receptors such as Fas and TNF-RI and/or their ligands (FasL and TNF-α), whereas the passive mechanisms do not. To understand how these forms of apoptosis operate within the mucosal immune system at a molecular level we need first to describe the major signalling events occurring during death-receptor-mediated apoptosis and how it interacts with apoptosis mechanisms mediated by mitochondria.

Death-receptor-induced apoptosis comprises signalling processes via Fas (CD95, APO-1), or a number of other receptors such as TNF-R1, TRAIL-R1 and 2, and DR3 or DR6[8,10]. Upon triggering of Fas the adaptor molecule FADD (Fas-associated death-domain-containing protein) and pro-caspase-8 are recruited to the Fas receptor, thereby forming a death-induced signalling complex (DISC) (Fig. 1)[8,11,12]. Recruitment of pro-caspase-8 leads to its autoproteolytic activation and release of active enzyme caspase-8 (FLICE) into the cytosol where it can trigger two signalling pathways. The first pathway is activated by small amounts of caspase-8 and involves the cleavage of the pro-apoptotic BID molecules followed by the release of cytochrome-*c* from mitochondria into the cytoplasm[11]; the cytochrome-*c* then binds to Apaf-1 forming a complex that, in turn, binds to caspase-9 and causes its autoactivation; finally, activated caspase-9 activates other proteases including caspase-3, which thus leads to the cleavage of multiple substrates and the apoptotic death of the cell. The second pathway of Fas-mediated apoptosis is activated by large amounts of caspase-8, which directly activates caspase-3, thereby bypassing the mitochondria. Since only apoptotic activities of mitochondria are inhibited by Bcl-2 and Bcl-x_L, the first pathway is inhibited by these anti-apoptotic proteins[10], whereas the second pathway is not so inhibited. Passive forms of apoptosis, on the other hand, are generally due to proteins that act exclusively via mitochondrial mechanisms; thus passive apoptosis due to lymphokine withdrawal is strongly inhibited by Bcl-2 and Bcl-x_L.

Returning now to apoptosis in mucosal tissue *per se*, we find that, in the normal (uninflamed) lamina propria, lamina propria T cells (LP-T cells) consist of CD45RO memory cells with constitutively high-level Fas expression (but not TNF-R1/R2 expression). In the unstimulated state, i.e. prior to stimulation with anti-CD2/anti-CD28, LP-T cells exhibit increased susceptibility to Fas-mediated apoptosis as compared to unstimulated peripheral blood T cells due to an as-yet-unknown downstream change in the Fas signalling pathway. In addition, these cells exhibit increased spontaneous apoptosis, i.e. non-activation-induced, non-Fas-mediated apoptosis, compared to peripheral blood cells, probably due to a passive apoptotic mechanism associated with IL-2 withdrawal, since this apoptosis is diminished by addition of IL-2, and enhanced by addition of anti-IL-12. Finally, in the stimulated state, i.e. after stimulation with anti-CD2/anti-CD28, LP-T cell apoptosis is further augmented compared to stimulated peripheral blood T cells[13]. This increased apoptosis is entirely due to activation-induced apoptosis involving death receptors, since it is seen when the cells are activated via CD2 rather than CD3 activation pathways and the former are more effective means of activating LP-T cells[14]. In addition, this apoptosis is extinguished by antibodies that block Fas and is unaffected by addition of IL-2 or anti-IL-2[13].

A very different picture obtains with respect to LP-T cells derived from areas of mucosal inflammation, i.e. from colons obtained from patients with Crohn's disease or ulcerative colitis, as well as other forms of colonic inflammation. In this case, while LP-T cells express similar spontaneous apoptosis as do cells

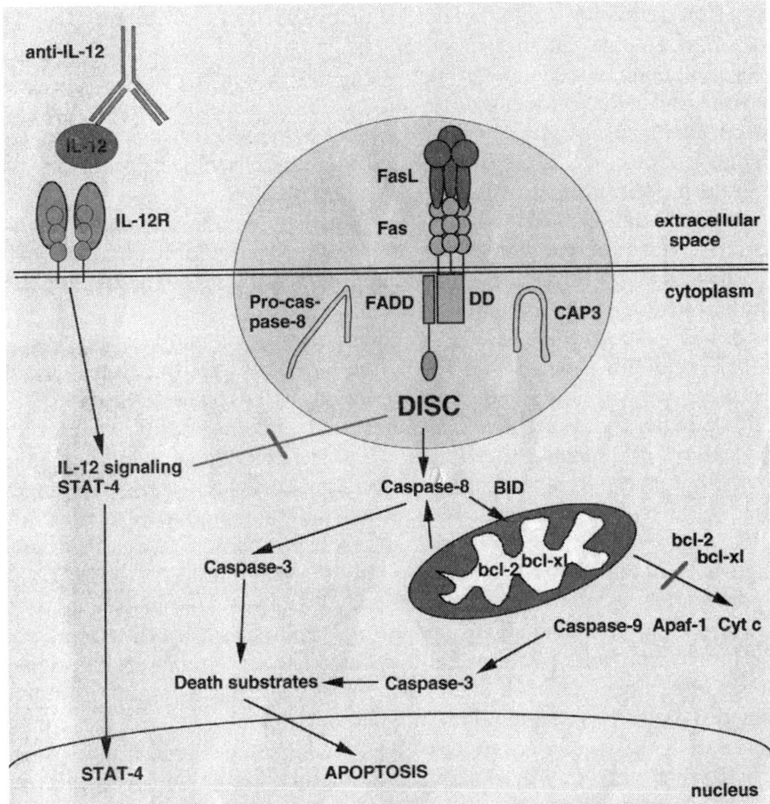

Figure 1 Apoptosis of mucosal T cells via the Fas/FasL system and suppression of Fas-mediated apoptosis by IL-12. Activation of Fas by FasL leads to formation of the DISC (death-induced signalling complex) and activation of caspase-8 (FLICE). The latter, in turn, leads to either direct activation of caspase-3 or indirect activation of caspase-3 via BID and mitochondrial proteins (see text)[8]. IL-12 suppresses these events by unknown mechanisms downstream of the formation of the DISC. Susceptibility to Fas-mediated cell death is increased in LP-T cells from normal (uninflamed) mucosa, whereas in LP-T cells from inflamed mucosa this increased susceptibility is diminished, presumably because of the presence of increased amounts of IL-12. Antibodies to TNF-α which have been shown to be effective in the treatment of Crohn's disease may also induce apoptosis, possibly by blocking an anti-apoptosis pathway initiated via the TNF-α receptor

from uninflamed tissues, the cells exhibit decreased activation-induced apoptosis compared to cells from uninflamed tissues[15]. Moreover, this resistance of LP-T cells to apoptosis (at least in patients with Crohn's disease) is not restricted to death receptor-induced apoptosis, since T cells from Crohn's disease patients grow more rapidly in response to IL-2 than do control T cells, and are more resistant to IL-2 deprivation-induced apoptosis and apoptosis mediated by nitric oxide[16]. Two possible mechanisms may contribute to this broad resistance to apoptosis. One relates to the fact that T cells in inflamed tissues express increased levels of Bcl-2 which then may inhibit apoptotic mechanisms that involve mitochondria. Another relates to the anti-apoptotic effects of IL-12 discussed below. The latter mechanism, however, applies only to Th1 T cell-mediated mucosal inflammation characterized by increased IL-12 secretion. Overall, the picture that emerges is that in uninflamed mucosal tissues T cells manifest increased apoptosis mediated by the Fas pathway which places a limit on the expansion of T cells following direct stimulation by specific antigen. In contrast, in inflamed mucosal tissue, T cells manifest increased resistance to apoptosis: they thus exhibit prolonged survival and increased cytokine production which may, in turn, significantly aggravate the inflammation.

The above relationship of LP-T cells to apoptosis in the normal and inflamed mucosa provides the background for the finding that administration of various antibodies, such as antibodies to IL-12, appears to suppress experimental intestinal inflammation by the induction of T cell apoptosis[6].

First, with respect to IL-12, it was shown that administration of a neutralizing anti-IL-12 antibody to mice with TNBS colitis, a Th1 T cell-mediated inflammation replete with cells producing large amounts of IL-12 and IFN-γ and TNF-α, is followed after 2 days by the appearance of apoptotic (TUNEL+) CD4$^+$ cells at the site of inflammation in the colon[6]. This induction of T cell apoptosis is followed by the rapid resolution of the inflammatory state, and may explain the dramatic and rapid suppression of intestinal inflammation after treatment with anti-IL-12 antibodies[4,15,17]. The anti-IL-12-induced apoptosis was a Fas-mediated phenomenon in that the cells being lost were preferentially Fas-bearing cells[6]. In addition, the therapeutic effect of the antibody was greatly diminished in MRL/lpr mice, mice that cannot mediate apoptosis via the Fas pathway, or in normal (SJL/J) mice who were administered Fas-Fc, an agent that blocks Fas signalling via Fas-L, but does not itself signal via Fas[6]. These results strongly imply that activated Th1 cells producing inflammatory cytokines require the continued presence of IL-12 if they are to avoid a Fas-mediated death. The mechanism by which IL-12 counteracts the Fas pathway in such cells is not yet fully understood, although it is known that it does not involve the induction of the anti-apoptotic proteins, Bcl-2 or Bcl-x$_L$, nor the formation of the DISC; it may thus act on mitochondria-independent post-DISC formation events (Fig. 1).

Thus, apoptosis mechanisms appear to play a significant role in the down-regulation of mucosal immune responses and the elimination of self-reactive clones in that normal LP-T cells exhibit an enhanced susceptibility to Fas-mediated apoptosis[13]. However, in Crohn's disease (and in other types of mucosal inflammation) LP-T cells manifest a resistance to apoptosis induced via death receptor pathways and, in at least the case of Crohn's disease, by other apoptotic pathways also[15,16]. Such defective apoptosis is likely to contribute to the inappropriate T cell accumulation that occurs in chronic mucosal inflammation. Treatment modalities such as anti-IL-12 antibodies mediate their rapid beneficial effects on mucosal inflammation at least in part by causing the apoptosis of T cells mediating the inflammation. In so doing, these antibodies effectively override the increase in resistance to apoptosis associated with mucosal inflammation.

The relevance of these findings to human IBD or, indeed, to other human Th1 or Th2 T cell-mediated inflammations, is varied. Thus, as shown in Fig. 2, in a Th1 T cell-mediated inflammation such as Crohn's disease[18,19], the provision of an IL-12 inhibitor such as anti-IL-12 not only results in resolution of disease because of neutralization of the cytokines that initiate the Th1 T cell pathway of inflammation, but such treatment also results in the death of induced CD4$^+$

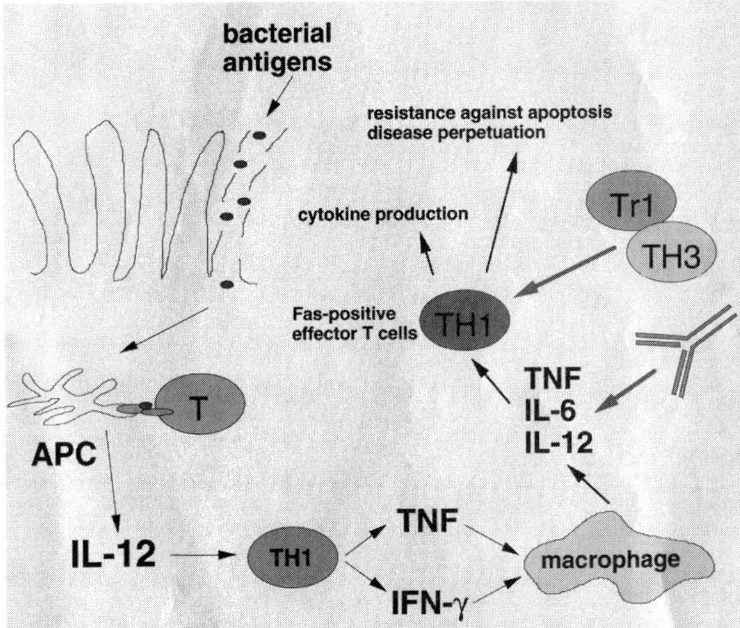

Figure 2 Mechanisms underlying the therapeutic effects of anti-IL-12 in murine models of mucosal inflammation and possibly in IBD. In many of these models (and in human Crohn's disease) bacterial antigens in the gut are thought to induce T cell activation and Th1 T cell differentiation via IL-12[22–24]. Mediator substances secreted by Th1 T cells such as TNF-α and IFN-γ then activate macrophages to release IL-6 and IL-12 that, in turn, induce T cell resistance to apoptosis and prolonged cytokine production by Fas-expressing Th1 effector T cells. Production of TNF-α, IL-6, and IL-1β by activated macrophages leads to accumulation of inflammatory cells and tissue damage by activation of matrix-metalloproteinase[25]. This can be arrested by antibodies such as anti-IL-12 and anti-TNF-α, which induce Th1 T cell apoptosis. Thus these antibodies, alone or in combination, provide an attractive new approach to the therapy of IBD

effector Th1 T cells. Anti-TNF-α, another antibody that interacts with an important cytokine in the Th1 pathway, and is now being used with considerable success to treat patients with Crohn's disease, has also been reported to act by inducing apoptosis of Th1 T cells[20] (personal communication, S. van Deventer). The mechanism of such activation is still unknown, but it should be noted that the TNF receptors have both pro-apoptotic and anti-apoptotic effects, so that the anti-TNF-α being used may selectively induce the latter[10].

Finally, it has been shown that induction of Fas-mediated apoptosis with a small molecule can be used to treat T cell-mediated autoimmune diseases[21]. While these data support the approach summarized here with respect to IBD, one should not lose sight of the fact that the use of anticytokines (or anticytokine receptors) may prove to be the superior approach. This follows from the fact that therapeutic antibodies have long half-lives and, in the case of anti-IL-12 and anti-TNF-α, induce T cell death by largely independent or possibly synergistic mechanisms. Thus, the future of therapy for many types of inflammation may lie in combination anticytokine/anticytokine receptor therapy.

References

1. Elson CO, Sartor RB, Tennyson GS, Riddell RH. Experimental models of inflammatory bowel disease. Gastroenterology. 1995; 109:1344–67.
2. Strober W, Kelsall B, Fuss I et al. Reciprocal IFN-gamma and TGF-beta responses regulate the occurrence of mucosal inflammation. Immunol Today. 1997;18:61–4.
3. Duchmann R, Zeitz M. Crohn's Disease in Handbook of Mucosal Immunology (Ogra P and Strober W, eds.), Academic Press; 1998.
4. Neurath MF, Fuss I, Kelsall BL, Stuber E, Strober W. Antibodies to interleukin-12 abrogate established experimental colitis in mice. J Exp Med. 1995;182:1280–9.
5. Simpson SJ, Shah S, Comiskey M et al. T cell-mediated pathology in two models of experimental colitis depends predominantly on the interleukin-12/signal transducer and activator of transcription (stat)-4 pathway, but not conditional on interferon gamma expression by T cells. J Exp Med. 1998;187:1225–34.
6. Fuss IJ, Marth T, Neurath MF et al. Anti-interleukin 12 treatment regulates apoptosis of Th1 T cells in experimental colitis in mice. Gastroenterology. 1999;117:1078–88.
7. Groux H, Powrie F. Regulatory T cells and inflammatory bowel disease. Immunol Today. 1999;20:442–6.
8. Scaffidi C, Kirchhoff S, Krammer PH, Peter ME. Apoptosis signaling in lymphocytes. Curr Opin Immunol. 1999;11:277–85.
9. Zheng L, Fisher G, Miller RE et al. Influence of apoptosis in mature T cells by tumour necrosis factor. Nature. 1995;377:348–51.
10. Lenardo M, Chan F, Hornung F et al. Crucial role for p80 TNF-R2 in amplifying p60 TNF-R1 apoptosis signals in T lymphocytes. Annu Rev Immunol. 1999;17:221–53.
11. Scaffidi C, Fulda S, Srinivasan A et al. Two CD95 (APO-1/Fas) signaling pathways. EMBO J. 1998;17:1675–87.
12. Zhang J, Cado D, Chen A, Kabra NH, Winoto A. Fas-mediated apoptosis and activation-induced T-cell proliferation are defective in mice lacking FADD/MORT 1. Nature. 1998;392:296–300.
13. Boirivant M, Pica R, DeMaria R et al. Stimulated human lamina propria T cells manifest enhanced Fas-mediated apoptosis. J Clin Invest. 1996;98:2616–22.
14. Targan SR, Deem RL, Liu M, Wang S, Nel A. Definition of a lamina propria T cell responsive state. Enhanced cytokine responsiveness of T cells stimulated through the CD2 pathway. J Immunol. 1995;154:664–75.
15. Boirivant M, Marini M, Di-Felice G et al. Lamina propria T cells in Crohn's disease and other gastrointestinal inflammation show defective CD2 pathway-induced apoptosis. Gastroenterology. 1999;116:557–65.
16. Ina K, Itoh J, Fukushima K et al. Resistance of Crohn's disease T cells to multiple apoptotic signals is associated with a BCL-21 BAX mucosal imbalance. J Immunol. 1999;163:1081–90.
17. Davidson NJ, Hudak SA, Lesley RE et al. IL-12, but not IFN-gamma, plays a major role in sustaining the chronic phase of colitis in IL-10 deficient mice. J Immunol. 1998;161:3143–49.
18. Plevy SE, Landers CJ, Prehn J et al. A role for TNF-alpha and mucosal T helper-1 cytokines in the pathogenesis of Crohn's disease. J Immunol. 1997;159:6276–82.
19. Fuss I, Neurath MF, Boirivant M et al. Disparate CD4 + lamina propria lymphokine secretion profiles in inflammatory bowel disease. J Immunol. 1996;157:1261–70.
20. Targan SR, Hanauer SB, Deventer SJV et al. A short term study of chimeric monoclonal antibody CA2 to tumor necrosis factor alpha for Crohn's disease. New Engl J Med. 1997;337:1029–35.
21. Zhou T, Song L, Yang P et al. Bisindolymaleimide VIII facilitates Fas-mediated apoptosis and inhibits T cell-mediated autoimmunity. Nature Med. 1999;5:42–8.
22. Sartor R. Post-operative recurrence of Crohn's disease: the enemy is within the fecal stream. Gastroenterology. 1998;114:398–400.
23. Monteleone G, Biancone L, Marasco R et al. Interleukin-12 is expressed and actively released by Crohn's disease intestinal lamina propria mononuclear cells. Gastroenterology. 1997;112:1169–78.
24. Cong Y, Brandwein SL, McCabe RP et al. CD4 + T cells reactive to enteric bacterial antigens in spontaneously colitic C3H/HeJBir mice: increased T helper cell type 1 response and ability to transfer disease. J Exp Med. 1998;187:855–64.
25. Pender SL, Fell JM, Chamow SM, Ashkenazi A, MacDonald TT. A P55 TNF receptor immunoadhesin prevents T cell-mediated intestinal injury by inhibiting matrix metalloproteinase production. J Immunol. 1998;160: 4098–103.

25
Interleukin-2-related strategies in experimental models of inflammatory bowel disease

A. STALLMACH

INTRODUCTION

The aetiology of inflammatory bowel disease (IBD), Crohn's disease and ulcerative colitis, remains poorly understood[1,2]. The development of these diseases may be a result of uncontrolled or inadequately down-regulated cellular immune responses in the intestinal mucosa towards a hitherto unknown agent, probably a constituent of the luminal content[3]. CD4[+] T cells seem to play an important role in the pathogenesis of IBD[2]. In IBD patients an expansion of the CD4[+] T-cell pool has been observed both in the mucosa and in peripheral blood[4,5]. Furthermore, CD4[+] T cells have been shown to play a central role in a number of animal models of IBD[6,7]. These observations place CD4[+] T cells as central players in the field of IBD research. In recent years increasing evidence has supported the concept that polarized Th1-type and Th2-type responses in humans could play an important role in certain diseases. Th1-like cells produce proinflammatory cytokines such as interleukin (IL)-2, interferon (IFN)-γ and tumour necrosis factor (TNF)-α, whereas Th2-like cells produce regulatory substances such as IL-4, IL-5 and IL-10[8]. A third group of Th3-like cells, which produce transforming growth factor beta (TGF-β), is induced upon low-dose oral antigen administration, provides mucosal T helper function and down-regulates Th1 cell function[9]. Although the Th1/Th2 paradigm oversimplifies the intricacies of the immune system, it offers a useful concept for understanding chronic inflammation. In general, Crohn's disease is thought to be a Th1-like disease, whereas ulcerative colitis is thought to be a Th2-like disease (for review see ref. 10).

Current concepts for the treatment of severe IBD rely on the efficacy of drugs such as corticosteroids, azathioprine, and cyclosporin that interfere with the immune response by abrogating cytokine production and cell proliferation[11]. Side-effects and dose-limiting toxicity are the result of their limited specificity for dysregulated immune responses in IBD. Remarkable and more specific immunosuppressive effects can be achieved by monoclonal antibody (mAB) treatment. Since 1991, mouse anti-human CD4 mAB had been used for immuno-suppression in severe Crohn's disease or ulcerative colitis[12]. Other antibodies, e.g. mAB against CD25, have been successfully used for immunosuppression after liver or renal transplantation[13,14]. However, adverse reactions were associated with murine proteins limited long-term efficacy. Furthermore, the development of human anti-murine antibodies are current limitations of this approach. An approach to inhibit immune functions more selectively became feasible with the application of genetically engineered fusion proteins in animal models of organ transplantation or chronic inflammation[15–18]. For this approach cytokines or extracellular domains of integral membrane proteins were used to replace the variable regions of immunoglobulins. Fusion proteins have been shown to decrease inflammatory activity by different modes of action, including inhibition of T cell cytotoxicity, induction of apoptosis of T cells, blockade of T cell activation and blocking of co-stimulatory signals.

IMMUNOMODULATION BY CYTOKINE-IgG FUSION PROTEINS

At this point we shall turn from the general to the particular, with a discussion of one of the models of IBD, the TNBS model. One of the most useful models to study the pathogenesis of IBD is the rectal administration of 2,4,6-trinitro-benzene sulphonic acid (TNBS). This agent haptenates autologous colonic proteins with trinitrophenyl (TNP), which then induce a massive transmural infiltration of Th1 T cells producing IFN-γ (and TNF-α). These cytokines presumably cause mucosal inflammation by activating macrophages to produce inflammatory cytokines and chemotactic factors. Successful experimental trials using antibodies to IL-12 or TNF-α or antisense oligonucleotides against NF-κB indicate that the TNBS model is useful to prove new therapeutic strategies in colonic inflammation[19–21].

Elimination of CD25-positive cells as therapeutic strategy in experimental models of IBD

Compared to non-inflamed intestinal mucosa, up-regulation of the IL-2 receptor (CD25) on T cells is a typical feature of the inflamed mucosa in Crohn's disease, ulcerative colitis or pouchitis[22,23]. Lymphocyte activation by antigen or mitogen results in expression of the high-affinity trimeric IL-2 receptor complex. This receptor in turn binds IL-2, resulting in activation, proliferation, and cytokine release by T-helper cells. Therefore, a therapy that selectively eliminates acti-vated lymphocytes bearing IL-2 receptors may be of clinical efficacy in autoim-mune disease or IBD. The combination of IL-2 with a toxin as fusion protein follows this strategy. Diphtheria toxin-related ligand fusion proteins are one example of agents in which the cytotoxic portion of diphtheria toxin catalytic domain and transmembrane domain is fused to the receptor-binding portion of a known ligand. Williams *et al.* described the genetic construction and functional properties of the prototypic fusion toxin DAB_{486}-IL-2, consisting of a truncated form of diphtheria toxin fused to human IL-2[24]. This fusion protein is internalized and catalyses ADP-ribosylation of elongation factor 2, resulting in inhibition of translation, a decrease in protein synthesis, and cell death. Since activated lymphocytes produce higher levels of proinflammatory cytokines than do resting cells, selective depletion of activated lymphocytes by administration of chimaeric proteins could reduce inflammation while leaving resting and memory lymphocyte function unimpaired. Bousvaros and co-workers demonstrated that the IL-2 diphtheria toxin fusion protein specifically targets activated (CD25[+]) lamina propria lymphocytes. In these cells this fusion protein inhibited protein synthesis and IFN-γ levels by 80% in 24-h cultures[25]. In this context it is important to note that specific depletion of antigen-activated T cell clones has been demonstrated *in vivo* for IL-2–diphtheria toxin fusion protein[26]. Further, the IL-2 toxin fusion proteins have been administered with encouraging results in patients with haematological malignancies and refractory rheumatoid arthritis[27–29].

In our group we determined the anti-inflammatory effect of a recombinant immunotoxin consisting of an anti-CD25 single-chain variable fragment (scFv) fused to a deletion mutant of *Pseudomonas* exotoxin A (RFT5(scFv)ETA′) on isolated lamina propria lymphocytes of patients with IBD and in the murine model of TNBS acid-induced colitis. In our study we demonstrated a significant increase of apoptotic cells after addition of RFT5(scFv)ETA′ to mucosal lymphocytes of patients with IBD. These findings were independent of the stimulation pathway via PHA or B7.1/anti-CD3. This experiment clearly revealed the ability of the immunotoxin to selectively target and deplete activated CD25[+] lymphocytes. Depletion of activated lymphocytes *in vitro* was accompanied by a decreased release of the proinflammatory cytokine IFN-γ. IFN-γ perpetuates the process of inflammation by activating macrophages and antigen-presenting cells, which themselves activate T-helper lymphocytes. Given that LPL from intestinal mucosa of patients with IBD show increased production of IFN-γ[30], reduction of IFN-γ-producing cells by administration of RFT5(scFv)ETA′ points towards a therapeutic effect of this recombinant immunotoxin in the clinical course of IBD. Therefore, the immunotoxin seemed to be appropriate to modulate intestinal inflammation by weakening the proinflammatory response, and was thus applied in the murine model of TNBS colitis. Surprisingly, and in marked contrast to our *in-vitro* data, the administration of RFT5(scFv)ETA′ revealed no preventive, therapeutic or curative effect in mice with TNBS-induced colitis. The survival rate of RFT5(scFv)ETA′-treated mice was comparable to that of TNBS-treated mice or even worse. According to the bad clinical course of the toxin-treated mice there was no difference concerning the production of proinflammatory cytokines such as IFN-γ and TNF-α compared to the TNBS group. Moreover, we could find no differences in the production of the regulatory cytokine IL-10 between the two groups (data not shown). These data indicate that reduction of IFN-γ in CD25[+] cells, which perpetuates the inflammatory process by activating macrophages and antigen-presenting cells, is not sufficient to abrogate experimentally induced IBD in mice. In agreement with our data, Hoffmann and co-workers demonstrated that depletion of αβ CD4[+] T cells, the major constituents of mucosal infiltrates, does not influence the initiation or perpetuation of TNBS-induced colitis in rats (personal communication). Moreover, in clinical studies ablation of CD4[+] cells by administration of anti-CD4 antibody revealed only a marginal effect on chronic inflammation[31]. This supports our finding that depletion of a specific lymphocyte subpopulation is not sufficient to cure chronic IBD.

Activation of regulatory CD4$^+$ cells as a therapeutic strategy in experimental models of IBD

Thornton *et al.* demonstrated that, in certain murine models of autoimmune diseases, a subpopulation of CD4$^+$/CD25$^+$ T cells prevents inflammatory diseases[32]. In addition, Read and co-workers showed that cotransfer of CD4$^+$/CD25$^+$ T cells inhibits inflammation in transfer colitis in SCID mice[33]. These regulatory T cells were able to control inflammatory responses in the intestine[34]. Therefore, selective targeting and elimination of CD25$^+$/CD4$^+$ intestinal lymphocytes might have negative effects in IBD. Consequently, a strategy which results in the activation of mucosal regulatory cells could prevent intestinal inflammation. Recently we characterized the effects of an IL-2–IgG2b fusion protein in the TNBS model[35]. Our studies clearly show a beneficial effect of this compound with decreased mortality rate and a decrease of colonic inflammatory cell infiltration. Treatment with IL-2–IgG2b resulted in an increased systemic and colonic synthesis of the immunoregulative cytokine IL-10. The importance of this finding was demonstrated by the observation that the therapeutic efficacy of IL-2–IgG2b was abrogated after systemic neutralization of IL-10. The molecular mechanisms of IL-2–IgG2b leading to an increased IL-10 production are not well characterized. It is possible that IL-2–IgG2b directly mimics a ligand for an outside–inside signal, and actively stimulates IL-10 production. Alternatively, and we favour this hypothesis, binding of the IL-2–IgG2b to CD25 on T cells on the one hand, and on the other hand to the Fcγ receptor on macrophages, may stabilize cell–cell interactions, which results in increased synthesis of IL-10 (Fig. 1). In this context the results of Sutterwala and co-workers are of special interest. They demonstrated that ligation of macrophage Fcγ receptors can lead to a reversal of macrophage proinflammatory responses by inducing an up-regulation of IL-10 with a reciprocal inhibition of IL-12 production[36,37]. An increase of IL-10 and a decrease of IL-12 in the microenvironment of CD4$^+$ T cells, which were stimulated by the IL-2 part of the fusion protein, would result in differentiation of Tr1 cells with increased production of IL-10 and unchanged IL-4 synthesis, as we could show by flow cytometry. IL-10 is of central importance for the prevention of T-cell-mediated inflammation in the gut, as IL-10-deficient mice develop IBD[38]. In addition, IL-10 significantly inhibits the development of IBD induced by transfer of CD4/CD45RB^{high} positive T cells into SCID mice[39] or by intrarectal administration of TNBS[40]. Pender *et al.* demonstrated that IL-10 down-regulates T cell activation and mucosal damage in an experimental human fetal gut explant model[41]. However, only the addition of IL-10 in high concentrations, e.g. 10–25 ng/ml, resulted in decreased T cell and macrophage activation, cytokine production and subsequent secretion of matrix metalloproteinases by mesenchymal cells. However, mean serum levels of IL-10 after intravenous bolus injection of recombinant IL-10 were between 0.1 and 3.63 ng/ml after 6 h and 0.1 and 0.12 ng/ml after 24 h[42]. Therefore, the concentrations used in this model are far greater than the serum concentrations observed a few hours after injection. The local induction of IL-10-producing cells in the inflamed colon by fusion proteins could be a new therapeutic approach to down-regulate mucosal inflammation. This concept is further supported by the observation that administration of a

A   induction of Th1-mediated inflammation in TNBS colitis

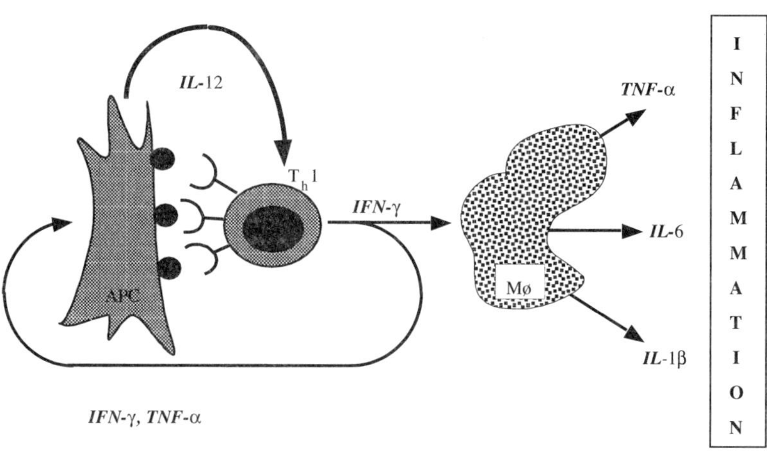

B   addition of IL-2-IgG2b in TNBS colitis

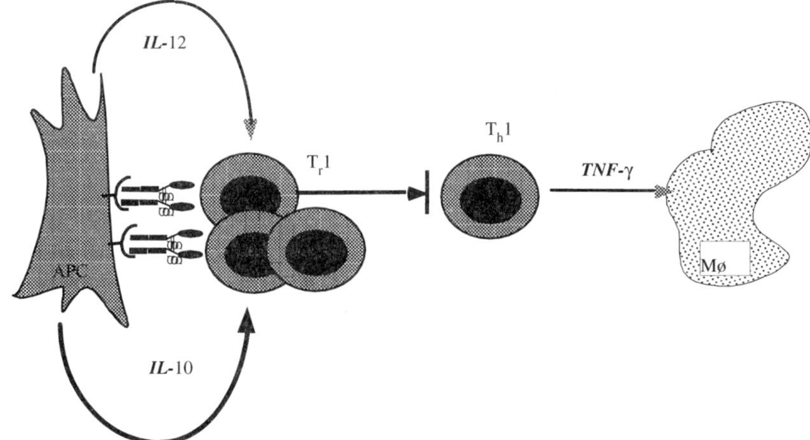

Figure 1   In TNBS colitis, antigen presentation on mucosal macrophages (APC) resulted in an increased differentiation and activation of Th1 cells. Under this condition macrophage-derived IL-12 is the key cytokine, which induces differentiation of Th0 into Th1 cells. The addition of IL-2–IgG2b fusion protein resulted in binding to Fcγ receptors on macrophages. Ligation of these receptors can lead to a reversal of macrophage proinflammatory response by inducing an up-regulation of IL-10, with reciprocal inhibition of IL-12 production. In this microenvironment, the IL-2 part of the fusion protein induces proliferation and differentiation of Tr1 cells, which act as counter-regulators of Th1-mediated inflammation

non-cytolytic murine IL-10–IgG–Fc fusion protein to mice from 5 to 25 weeks of age completely prevented the occurrence of diabetes in non-obese diabetic mice, which is another Th1-driven model. Moreover, these mice remained disease-free long after cessation of therapy[43].

CONCLUSION

As a final note, the better understanding of the immunological mechanisms that control intestinal inflammation allows us a more advantageous position with regard to the treatment of such disease states as ulcerative colitis or Crohn's disease. The specific effects of chimaeric proteins will extend the therapeutic tools for treatment of patients in the near future. However, despite the promising new perspectives of such immunomodulating strategies in gastrointestinal inflammation, excessive enthusiasm should be avoided, and possible adverse reactions of new therapies must be carefully evaluated.

Acknowledgements

Own studies are supported by grants from the German Research Council (DFG: Sta 295/3-2 and 4-1).

References

1. Fiocchi C. Inflammatory bowel disease: etiology and pathogenesis. Gastroenterology. 1998; 115:182–205.
2. Zeitz M. Pathogenesis of inflammatory bowel disease. Digestion. 1997;58(Suppl. 1):59–61.
3. Duchmann R, Neurath M, Märker-Hermann E, Meyer zum Büschenfelde KH. Immune responses towards intestinal bacteria – current concepts and future perspectives. Z Gastroenterol. 1997;35:337–46.
4. Probert CS, Chott A, Turner JR et al. Persistent clonal expansions of peripheral blood CD4+ lymphocytes in chronic inflammatory bowel disease. J Immunol. 1996;157:3183–91.
5. Gulwani AB, Akolkar PN, Minassian A et al. Selective expansion of specific T cell receptors in the inflamed colon of Crohn's disease. J Clin Invest. 1996;98:1344–54.
6. Leach MW, Bean AG, Mauze S, Coffman RL, Powrie F. Inflammatory bowel disease in C.B-17 scid mice reconstituted with the CD45RBhigh subset of CD4+ T cells. Am J Pathol. 1996;148:1503–15.
7. Claesson MH, Rudolphi A, Kofoed S, Poulsen SS, Reimann J. CD4+ T lymphocytes injected into severe combined immunodeficient (SCID) mice lead to an inflammatory and lethal bowel disease. Clin Exp Immunol. 1996;104:491–500.
8. Mosmann TR, Coffman RL. TH1 and TH2 cells: different patterns of lymphokine secretion lead to different functional properties. Annu Rev Immunol. 1989;7:145–73.
9. Weiner HL, Friedman A, Miller A et al. Oral tolerance: immunologic mechanisms and treatment of animal and human organ-specific autoimmune diseases by oral administration of autoantigens. Annu Rev Immunol. 1994;12:809–37.
10. Stallmach A, Wittig BM, Zeitz M. Modulation of gastrointestinal inflammation by chimeric proteins in experimental models. Z Gastroenterol. 2000;38:647–52.
11. Robinson M. Optimizing therapy for inflammatory bowel disease. Am J Gastroenterol. 1997;92(Suppl.):12–17S.
12. Emmrich J, Seyfarth M, Fleig WE, Emmrich F. Treatment of inflammatory bowel disease with anti-CD4-monoclonal antibody. Lancet. 1991;338:570–1.
13. Otto G, Thies J, Kraus T et al. Monoclonal anti-CD25 for acute rejection after liver transplantation. Lancet. 1991;338:195.

14. Vincenti F, Kirkman R, Light S *et al.* Interleukin-2-receptor blockade with daclizumab to prevent acute rejection in renal transplantation. N Engl J Med. 1998;338:161–5.

15. Lenschow DJ, Zeng Y, Thistlethwaite JR *et al.* Long-term survival of xenogeneic pancreatic islet grafts induced by CTLA4Ig. Science. 1992;257:789–92.

16. Bogers WM, Lang F, Parker KE *et al.* Rat interleukin-2 immunoglobulin M fusion proteins are cytotoxic *in vitro* for cells expressing the IL-2 receptor and can abolish cell-mediated immunity *in vivo*. Transplantation. 1994;58:932–9.

17. Finck BK, Linsley PS, Wofsy D. Treatment of murine lupus with CTLA4Ig. Science. 1994;265:1225–7.

18. Kunzendorf U, Pohl T, Bulfone PS *et al.* Suppression of cell-mediated and humoral immune responses by an interleukin-2–immunoglobulin fusion protein in mice. J Clin Invest. 1996;97:1204–10.

19. Neurath MF, Fuss I, Kelsall BL, Stuber E, Strober W. Antibodies to interleukin 12 abrogate established experimental colitis in mice. J Exp Med. 1995;182:1281–90.

20. Neurath MF, Pettersson S, Meyer zum Büschenfelde K-H, Strober W. Local administration of antisense phosphorothioate oligonucleotides to the p65 subunit of NF-kappa B abrogates established experimental colitis in mice. Nat Med. 1996;2:998–1004.

21. Neurath MF, Fuss I, Kelsall BL, Presky DH, Waegell W, Strober W. Experimental granulomatous colitis in mice is abrogated by induction of TGF-beta-mediated oral tolerance. J Exp Med. 1996;183:2605–16.

22. Ullrich R, Schneider T, Schieferdecker HL, Jahn HU, Riecken EO, Zeitz M. Cell activation and proliferation in the large intestine of patients with Crohn's disease or ulcerative colitis and controls. Adv Exp Med Biol. 1995;379B:1281–2.

23. Stallmach A, Schäfer F, Weber S *et al.* Increased state of activation of CD4-positive T cells and elevated interferon-γ production in pouchitis. Gut. 1998;43:499–505.

24. Williams DP, Parker K, Bacha P *et al.* Diphtheria toxin receptor binding domain substitution with interleukin-2: genetic construction and properties of a diphtheria toxin-related interleukin-2 fusion protein. Protein Eng. 1987;1:493–8.

25. Bousvaros A, Stevens AC, Strom TB, Murphy J, Lamont JT. Interleukin-2 fusion protein (DAB389IL-2) selectively targets activated human peripheral blood and lamina propria lymphocytes. Dig Dis Sci. 1997;42:1542–8.

26. Bastos MG, Pankewycz O, Rubin KV, Murphy JR, Strom TB. Concomitant administration of hapten and IL-2-toxin (DAB486-IL-2) results in specific deletion of antigen-activated T cell clones. J Immunol. 1990;145:3535–9.

27. Sewell KL, Parker KC, Woodworth TG, Reuben J, Swartz W, Trentham DE. DAB486IL-2 fusion toxin in refractory rheumatoid arthritis. Arthritis Rheum. 1993;36:1223–33.

28. Tepler I, Schwartz G, Parker K *et al.* Phase I trial of an interleukin-2 fusion toxin (DAB486IL-2) in hematologic malignancies: complete response in a patient with Hodgkin's disease refractory to chemotherapy. Cancer. 1994;73:1276–85.

29. LeMaistre CF, Saleh MN, Kuzel TM *et al.* Phase I trial of a ligand fusion-protein (DAB389IL-2) in lymphomas expressing the receptor for interleukin-2. Blood. 1998;91:399–405.

30. Fuss IJ, Neurath M, Boirivant M *et al.* Disparate CD4+ lamina propria (LP) lymphokine secretion profiles in inflammatory bowel disease. Crohn's disease LP cells manifest increased secretion of IFN-gamma, whereas ulcerative colitis LP cells manifest increased secretion of IL-5. J Immunol. 1996;157:1261–70.

31. Horneff G, Guse A, Schulze-Koops H *et al.* Human CD4 modulation *in vivo* induced by antibody treatment. Clin Immunol Immunopathol. 1993;66:80–90.

32. Thornton A, Shevach EM. CD4+ CD25+ immunoregulatory T cells suppress polyclonal T cell activation *in vitro* by inhibiting interleukin 2 production. J Exp Med. 1998;188:287–96.

33. Read S, Mauze SC, Asseman C, Bean A, Collman R, Powrie F. CD38+CD45RB(low) CD4+ T cells: a population of T cells with immune regulatory activities *in vitro*. Eur J Immunol. 1998;28:3435–47.

34. Powrie F, Leach M, Mauze S *et al.* Phenotypically distinct subsets of CD4+ T cells induce or protect from chronic intestinal inflammation in C.B-17 SCID mice. Int Immunol. 1993;51:1461–71.

35. Stallmach A, Wittig BM, Giese T *et al.* Protection of trinitrobenzene sulfonic acid-induced colitis by an interleukin-2–IgG2b fusion protein in mice. Gastroenterology. 1999;117:866–76.

36. Sutterwala FS, Noel GJ, Clynes R, Mosser DM. Selective suppression of interleukin-12 induction after macrophage receptor ligation. J Exp Med. 1997;185:1977–85.

37. Sutterwala FS, Noel GJ, Salgame P, Mosser DM. Reversal of proinflammatory responses by ligating the macrophage Fcgamma receptor type I. J Exp Med. 1998;188:217–22.
38. Kühn R, Lohler J, Rennick D, Rajewsky K, Müller W. Interleukin-10-deficient mice develop chronic enterocolitis [See comments]. Cell. 1993;75:263–74.
39. Powrie F, Leach MW, Mauze S, Menon S, Caddle LB, Coffman RL. Inhibition of Th1 responses prevents inflammatory bowel disease in scid mice reconstituted with CD45RBhi CD4+ T cells. Immunity. 1994;1:553–62.
40. Ribbons KA, Thompson JH, Liu X, Pennline K, Clark DA, Miller MJS. Anti-inflammatory properties of interleukin-10 administration in hapten-induced colitis. Eur J Pharmacol. 1997;323:245–54.
41. Pender SLF, Breese EJ, Günther U et al. Suppression of T cell-mediated injury in human gut by interleukin 10: role of matrix metalloproteinases. Gastroenterology. 1998;115:573–83.
42. Chernoff AE, Granowitz EV, Shapiro L et al. A randomized, controlled trial of IL-10 in humans. Inhibition of inflammatory cytokine production and immune responses. J Immunol. 1995;154:5492–9.
43. Zheng XX, Steele AW, Hancock WW et al. A noncytolytic IL-10/Fc fusion protein prevents diabetes, blocks autoimmunity, and promotes suppressor phenomena in NOD mice. J Immunol. 1997;158:4507–13.

Section IX
Future trends: special situations

26
Immunosuppressive therapy and pregnancy

A. U. DIGNASS

INTRODUCTION

The inflammatory bowel diseases Crohn's disease (CD) and ulcerative colitis (UC) have a high prevalence in younger patients with child-bearing potential[1,2]. Thus, uncertainties and a number of questions regarding medical treatment before and during pregnancy and the lactation period exist in inflammatory bowel disease (IBD) patients. In recent years immunosuppressants have played an increasingly important role in the medical management of patients with IBD. As a consequence the use of immunosuppressants in IBD patients with child-bearing potential has significantly increased, and represents a delicate problem in the management of younger IBD patients requiring intensive counselling.

INFLUENCE OF DISEASE ACTIVITY ON THE OUTCOME OF PREGNANCY IN IBD PATIENTS

Several studies have demonstrated that most pregnancies in women with IBD will develop normally if the patient is in remission or has only minor disease activity at the time of conception[3–6]. A meta-analysis by Miller[7], comprising more than 1300 female patients with UC and over 700 patients with CD, clearly demonstrated that normal pregnancies are observed in 83% of women with CD (71–93% in individual studies) and in 85% of women with UC (76–97% in individual studies) (Table 1). Malformations were observed in about 1% of all pregnancies and the frequency of spontaneous abortions and stillbirths was in the same range as observed in the healthy normal population (Table 1). In contrast, several studies[8–10] could demonstrate that the frequency of normal pregnancies is reduced, and the frequency of adverse outcomes of pregnancy is increased, when pregnancies take place in phases with active IBD (Tables 2 and 3). In summary, these data reflect the same outcome of pregnancies in IBD patients with inactive disease as observed in the general healthy population, and an increased risk of

Table 1 Outcome of pregnancy in inflammatory bowel diseases (meta-analysis by Miller JP)[7]

	Crohn's disease		*Ulcerative colitis*	
Number of studies	9		10	
Number of patients	748	(19–222)	1308	(46–309)
Normal births	83%	(71–93%)	85%	(76–97%)
Malformations	1%	(0–6%)	1%	(0–3%)
Spontaneous abortions	12%	(3–27%)	7%	(1–16%)
Stillbirths	2%	(0–5%)	1%	(0–3%)

Ranges in parentheses.

Table 2 Outcome of pregnancy in Crohn's disease patients with respect to disease activity (percentages)

	Normal	*Malformation*	*Prematurity*	*Stillbirths*	*Abortion*
Khosla *et al.*[8]					
Remission	82	2	n.a.	0	16
Active disease	60	0	n.a.	5	35
Nielsen *et al.*[5]					
Remission	83	n.a.	9	4	4
Active disease	49	n.a.	28	3	20

n.a. = Not available.

Table 3 Outcome of pregnancy in ulcerative colitis patients with respect to disease activity (percentages)

	Normal	*Malformation*	*Prematurity*	*Stillbirths*	*Abortion*
Willoughby and Truelove[9]					
Remission	84	2.3	n.a.	0	10.8
Active disease	71	4	n.a.	4	13
Nielsen *et al.*[6]					
Remission	92	3	6	0	8
Active disease	59	0	12	0	41

n.a. = Not available.

adverse outcome in patients with active disease, indicating that inactive IBD generally does not affect the outcome of pregnancies. Therefore it is generally recommended that women with IBD conceive at a time of minor disease activity or in remission.

GENERAL CONSIDERATIONS CONCERNING MEDICAL TREATMENT OF IBD IN PREGNANT WOMEN

The fact that adverse outcomes of pregnancy are observed more frequently in IBD patients with active disease indicates that IBD patients who plan to become pregnant, or are pregnant, should be treated adequately for active disease. Currently it is widely accepted that the standard treatment of IBD with corticosteroids and 5-aminosalicylic acid (5-ASA) derivatives is not significantly associated with malformations or adverse outcomes in pregnant IBD patients[11–14]. Therefore, corticosteroids and 5-ASA derivatives are used for the treatment of pregnant patients with active IBD and, when necessary, also to maintain remission during pregnancy. Treatment of active IBD with corticosteroids and 5-ASA derivatives during pregnancy does not significantly differ from treatment considerations in non-pregnant women, because these drugs can be used in usual dosage during pregnancy without any significantly increased adverse fetal outcomes. However, whenever possible the lowest possible dosages should be used, especially for the new 5-ASA formulations, because limited information is available concerning the adverse effects of high-dose 5-ASA treatment during pregnancy[15,16].

IMMUNOSUPPRESSIVE THERAPY IN PREGNANT IBD PATIENTS

The value of immunosuppressive therapy during pregnancy in IBD patients is less clear because of limited clinical data regarding the use of these drugs in pregnant patients with IBD, which is basically limited to case reports and small studies with limited numbers of patients[13,17–20]. Animal studies have demonstrated that very high doses of azathioprine and 6-mercaptopurine (6-MP) caused malformation of limbs, cleft palate and eye abnormalities in rats and rabbits[11]. Therapeutic doses have not been shown to cause an increase of malformation, but did cause an increase in the numbers of spontaneous abortions, and growth retardation in animals.

Significant clinical evidence regarding the use of immunosuppressants in pregnant women is provided by organ transplant patients and patients with rheumatoid arthritis with pregnancies[21–25]. The most extensive information is available regarding the use of azathioprine and 6-MP in pregnant transplant patients. These studies clearly demonstrate that normal pregnancies are observed in the majority of women treated with azathioprine and 6-MP, and that no increased incidence of stillbirths, miscarriages or fetal abnormalities is observed in patients treated with usual doses of azathioprine and 6-MP[22,25]. However, an increase of premature births and reduced weight at birth is frequently seen[21,26]. Generally, no clinically relevant immunosuppression is observed in the newborn.

Although the existing data in IBD patients are less extensive, patients with IBD do not show increased evidence of stillbirths, miscarriages or fetal abnormalities under therapy with azathioprine and 6-MP (Table 4)[11,14,17]. However, a tendency to more frequent premature births and reduced birth weight is also observed in IBD patients (Table 4). If treatment with azathioprine seems to be necessary to maintain remission of IBD, it is currently accepted that treatment with azathioprine and 6-MP be continued, following extensive discussion with the

Table 4 Effects of 6-mercaptopurine on the course of pregnancy in IBD patients (Francella et al.[30])

	6-MP terminated	Conception with 6-MP		No 6-MP
		Terminated after conception	Continued after conception	
Pregnancies	95	64	8	180
Normal	59 (62%)	39 (61%)	8	123 (68%)
Premature	5 (5%)	2 (3%)	0	4 (2%)
Spontaneous abortion	19 (20%)	13 (20%)	0	30 (17%)
Induced abortion	12 (13%)	10 (16%)	0	4 (2%)
Malformation	4 (4.2%)	3 (4.6%)	0	5 (2.8%)
Infection	3 (3%)	2 (3%)	1	2 (1%)
Neoplasia	0	1 (2%)	0	0

patient and the spouse. Informed consent should be obtained for legal reasons. In patients who do not depend on treatment with azathioprine and 6-MP this therapy should be discontinued at least 3 months before a planned pregnancy. An involuntary pregnancy under treatment with azathioprine and 6-MP is no reason to terminate a pregnancy. The effect of azathioprine and 6-MP therapy in men who wish to conceive has recently been under discussion, and the opinions are rather controversial. While experience in the transplant population does not provide evidence for increased adverse effects with respect to the outcome of the pregnancy, a recent study by Rajapakse et al.[20] reported a significantly increased incidence of pregnancy-related complications when the fathers used 6-MP within 3 months of conception. However, this study has some limitations, and the results and conclusions have caused controversy.

Little information is available regarding the use of other immunosuppressants during pregnancy. A number of case reports describe normal pregnancies following treatment with cyclosporin A and tacrolimus[11,13,14,18,19]. However, it seems to be inadequate to make general recommendations concerning use of these immunosuppressants during pregnancy, due to limited clinical evidence. Individual decisions based on the clinical situation of the individual patient are recommended. Again, the transplant literature provides more encouraging data for the use of cyclosporin and tacrolimus[24,27–29].

The use of methotrexate during pregnancy is not permitted because of well-characterized embryotoxicity and teratogenicity[11]. Because of the ill-defined long-term effects of methotrexate on male and female reproductive organs, adequate contraception for at least 6 months following methotrexate therapy is recommended. No published clinical data exist regarding the use of infliximab in humans, and only little experimental data in animals. These animal studies provide no evidence for embryotoxicity and teratogenicity. Post-marketing data from the manufacturer of infliximab report a number of normal pregnancies; however, adverse outcomes have also been observed. Because of limited data regarding the safety of infliximab adequate contraception should be recommended. Management following involuntary pregnancy under infliximab therapy should be individually discussed; elective termination of pregnancy should not be generally recommended.

References

1. Timmer A, Breuer-Katschinski B, Goebell H. Time trends in the incidence and disease location of Crohn's disease 1980–1995: a prospective analysis in an urban population in Germany. Inflamm Bowel Dis. 1999;5:79–84.
2. Timmer A, Goebell H. Incidence of ulcerative colitis, 1980–1995 – a prospective study in an urban population in Germany. Z Gastroenterol. 1999;37:1079–84.
3. Briese V, Muller H, Berkholz A. Pre-conception counseling and pregnancy in chronic inflammatory bowel diseases – Crohn disease and ulcerative colitis. Zentralbl Gynakol. 1993;115:1–6.
4. Hanan IM. Inflammatory bowel disease in the pregnant woman. Compr Ther. 1998;24:409–14.
5. Nielsen OH, Andreasson B, Bondesen S, Jacobsen O, Jarnum S. Pregnancy in Crohn's disease. Scand J Gastroenterol. 1984;19:724–32.
6. Nielsen OH, Andreasson B, Bondesen S, Jarnum S. Pregnancy in ulcerative colitis. Scand J Gastroenterol. 1983;18:735–42.
7. Miller JP. Inflammatory bowel disease in pregnancy: a review. J R Soc Med. 1986;79:221–5.
8. Khosla R, Willoughby CP, Jewell DP. Crohn's disease and pregnancy. Gut. 1984;25:52–6.
9. Willoughby CP, Truelove SC. Ulcerative colitis and pregnancy. Gut. 1980;21:469–74.
10. Woolfson K, Cohen Z, McLeod RS. Crohn's disease and pregnancy. Dis Colon Rectum. 1990;33:869–73.
11. Connell WR. Safety of drug therapy for inflammatory bowel disease in pregnant and nursing women. Inflamm Bowel Dis. 1996;2:33–47.
12. Lennard-Jones JE, Powell-Tuck J. Drug treatment of inflammatory bowel disease. Clin Gastroenterol. 1979;8:187–217.
13. Modigliani R. Drug therapy for ulcerative colitis during pregnancy. Eur J Gastroenterol Hepatol. 1997;9:854–7.
14. Subhani JM, Hamiliton MI. Review article: The management of inflammatory bowel disease during pregnancy. Aliment Pharmacol Ther. 1998;12:1039–53.
15. Diav-Citrin O, Park YH, Veerasuntharam G et al. The safety of mesalamine in human pregnancy: a prospective controlled cohort study. Gastroenterology. 1998;114:23–8.
16. Habal FM, Hui G, Greenberg GR. Oral 5-aminosalicylic acid for inflammatory bowel disease in pregnancy: safety and clinical course. Gastroenterology. 1993;105:1057–60.
17. Alstead EM, Ritchie JK, Lennard-Jones JE, Farthing MJ, Clark ML. Safety of azathioprine in pregnancy in inflammatory bowel disease. Gastroenterology. 1990;99:443–6.
18. Bertschinger P, Himmelmann A, Risti B, Follath F. Cyclosporine treatment of severe ulcerative colitis during pregnancy [letter; comment]. Am J Gastroenterol. 1995;90:330.
19. Korelitz BI. Antimetabolites in inflammatory bowel disease: long-term experience. Mt Sinai J Med. 1990;57:297–304.
20. Rajapakse RO, Korelitz BI, Zlatanic J, Baiocco PJ, Gleim GW. Outcome of pregnancies when fathers are treated with 6-mercaptopurine for inflammatory bowel disease. Am J Gastroenterol. 2000;95:684–8.
21. Marushak A, Weber T, Bock J et al. Pregnancy following kidney transplantation. Acta Obstet Gynecol Scand. 1986;65:557–9.
22. Penn I, Makowski EL, Harris P. Parenthood following renal transplantation. Kidney Int. 1980;18:221–33.
23. Plosker GL, Foster RH. Tacrolimus: a further update of its pharmacology and therapeutic use in the management of organ transplantation. Drugs. 2000;59:323–89.
24. Rayes N, Neuhaus R, David M, Steinmuller T, Bechstein WO, Neuhaus P. Pregnancies following liver transplantation – how safe are they? A report of 19 cases under cyclosporine A and tacrolimus. Clin Transplant. 1998;12:396–400.

25. Roubenoff R, Hoyt J, Petri M, Hochberg MC, Hellmann DB. Effects of antiinflammatory and immunosuppressive drugs on pregnancy and fertility. Semin Arthritis Rheum. 1988;18:88–110.
26. Pirson Y, Van Lierde M, Ghysen J *et al.* Retardation of fetal growth in patients receiving immunosuppressive therapy [letter]. N Engl J Med. 1985;313:328.
27. Armenti VT, Moritz MJ, Davison JM. Drug safety issues in pregnancy following transplantation and immunosuppression: effects and outcomes. Drug Safety. 1998;19:219–32.
28. Huynh LA, Min DI. Outcomes of pregnancy and the management of immunosuppressive agents to minimize fetal risks in organ transplant patients. Ann Pharmacother. 1994;28:1355–7.
29. Wu A, Nashan B, Messner U *et al.* Outcome of 22 successful pregnancies after liver transplantation. Clin Transplant. 1998;12:454–64.
30. Francella A, Dayan A, Rubin P, Chapman M, Present D. 6-Mercaptopurine is safe therapy for child-bearing patients with inflammatory bowel disease (IBD): A case controlled study. Gastroenterology. 2001;10:A909 (Abstr.).

27
Immunosuppressive therapy during childhood and adolescence

B. S. KIRSCHNER

INTRODUCTION

In thinking about the approach to treating children and adolescents with inflammatory bowel disease (IBD), I would like to mention four concepts, among many, that influence the choice of drug therapy. As shown in the study by Ekbom *et al.*, the frequency of pancolitis in patients with ulcerative colitis (UC) presenting at less than 15 years of age is 50% compared with 33% for those aged 15–29 years and <25% for those aged 30–39 years[1]. Furthermore, Mir-Madhjessi *et al.* have noted that proximal extension is more likely in children with rectosigmoid disease than in adults[2]. Thus, paediatric patients with UC often have more extensive disease at diagnosis. With regard to Crohn's disease (CD), Polito *et al.* compared the natural history of patients diagnosed with CD <20 years and >40 years of age[3]. Younger patients had more small bowel involvement, stricturing disease and frequency of surgery. Griffiths *et al.* have observed that final adult stature correlated with disease severity and whether remission was achieved during childhood[4]. Those with chronic severe disease had significantly lower Z-scores for height than severe disease in remission. Thus, controlling disease activity early in the course is likely to affect prognosis in this age population.

The use of immunosuppressive drugs in the treatment of IBD has greatly improved the likelihood of disease response while allowing reduction or discontinuation of corticosteroid (CS) medications in paediatric patients. As studies continue to confirm the long-term safety of these preparations, physicians who treat children and adolescents have become increasingly willing to use these drugs more frequently and for longer duration. Most of the drugs used to treat IBD have an effect on the immunoregulatory system, including the widely used 5-aminosalicylates and CS. The focus of this presentation is to review the role of other immunomodulatory agents (azathioprine, 6-mercaptopurine, methotrexate, cyclosporin, tacrolimus, thalidomide and anti-TNF-α preparations) in the management of paediatric patients with IBD.

INDICATIONS FOR CHOOSING IMMUNOMODULATORY DRUGS IN CHILDREN

While CS are effective in reducing disease activity in many children with acute UC or CD, there are clear indications for adding immunosuppressive agents. These include lack of efficacy and a wide range of potential side-effects with CS. Among paediatric patients the major indications are undesirable cosmetic appearance (such as moon facies and striae, especially in teenagers), emotional lability, reduced growth velocity, osteopenia and risk of fracture, raised intra-ocular pressure and cataract formation[5–8].

ASSESSMENT OF DRUG EFFICACY IN CHILDREN WITH IBD

One of the problems in evaluating the efficacy of drugs in paediatric populations has been the extremely low level of financial support from granting agencies and the pharmaceutical industry for clinical trials in children. More than 80% of the drugs listed in the *Physician's Desk Reference* (PDR) have never been studied in paediatric populations. With new guidelines issued by the Federal Drug Administration (FDA), there appears to be an increasing awareness of the need to study children separately from adults[9]. However, the investigations involving paediatric patients with IBD are currently often limited to small-scale pharmacokinetic studies rather than long-term studies of efficacy and safety. As a result, most of the outcome measures I will discuss have been determined retrospectively or, if prospectively, in small series of patients that would be unthinkable in adult populations.

AZATHIOPRINE (AZA) AND 6-MERCAPTOPURINE (6-MP)

AZA and 6-MP are currently among the best-studied of the steroid-sparing drugs used to manage IBD in children[10–15]. A few authors reported using these medications in paediatric patients as early as the 1970s, but many paediatric gastroenterologists were reluctant to recommend their long-term use, out of concern regarding the well-known observations of lymphoma risk in patients with systemic lupus erythematosus, until experience had accumulated regarding the safety of these drugs with long-term use in adults with IBD[16].

The success of AZA and 6-MP as CS-sparing agents in children with UC and CD has been widely recognized following the publications by Verhave and by Markowitz[10,11]. In addition to reducing CS doses, the latter group observed that the number of days of hospitalization was lower in children when they received these medications when compared with their previous course[11]. More recently, Markowitz *et al.* evaluated the efficacy of 6-MP as part of the initial therapy in children with moderate to severe Crohn's disease[15]. In this prospective, placebo-controlled multicentre trial, 55 paediatric patients (with body weights < 24 kg) were randomized to receive either 6-MP (1.5 mg/kg per day) or placebo within 8 weeks of receiving 32 mg daily of intravenous solumedrol or 40 mg daily orally of prednisone. CS doses were tapered based on the response of changes in the Harvey–Bradshaw score. The remission rate at 12 months was similar in the two groups, 89%. However, the cumulative CS dose was significantly reduced at 6, 12 and 18 months in the 6-MP group compared with the placebo group. In addition, relapse at 18 months had occurred in only 9% of the 6-MP group versus 47% of controls. Based on these findings the authors recommend that 6-MP be a part of the initial treatment of paediatric patients with newly diagnosed moderate to severe Crohn's disease. Others have documented the duration of CS-free periods, reduction in the frequency of relapses and improved gains in height and weight velocity in children with UC[17,18].

An analysis of the paediatric IBD population at our institution revealed that approximately 82% of the 95 children and adolescents who received AZA or 6-MP tolerated long-term administration[13]. Of these, 54% had no side-effects while receiving conventional doses, while 28% required dose reduction usually because of transaminase elevation (more than twice normal) or leukopenia (<4000 WBC mm^3).

It should be noted that 18% of children in our centre who received these drugs for IBD on an intent-to-treat basis were unable to continue therapy, either due to hypersensitivity (such as pancreatitis or febrile reactions) or intolerance (nausea, abdominal pain or recurrent infections). Parents and adolescent patients must be counselled to seek medical attention if there is high fever, exposure to varicella when the child has not been previously infected with this virus, herpes zoster or other protracted signs and symptoms of infectious illnesses.

The ability of these drugs to facilitate lowering or discontinuing CS therapy was confirmed in our study from the University of Chicago[13]. Eighty-seven per cent of patients who tolerate AZA or 6-MP were able to reduce their daily CS dose. Most importantly, the percentage of patients taking $\geqslant 10$ mg daily decreased from 91% to 32% correlating with a fall in the mean daily dose from 24.6 to 8.3 mg/day. In children and adolescents with remaining growth potential the goal of daily prednisone should be less than 7.5 mg daily. Doses of 5 mg daily or alternate-day CS are unlikely to interfere with linear growth or bone mineralization[8,19].

A further use of AZA and 6-MP in paediatric patients has been to control disease activity in patients whose remission had been induced by cyclosporin or tacrolimus[20–22]. Under these circumstances, as will be discussed below, AZA and 6-MP prolong remission and reduce the likelihood of colectomy in paediatric patients with UC or Crohn's colitis.

How best to select the optimal dose of AZA or 6-MP for individual patients is an area of active investigation. It has been suggested that measuring circulating 6-MP metabolite levels can predict response to therapy[12,14]. In particular, levels of 6-thioguanine (6-TG) $>235–250$ pmol per 8×10^8 RBC are reported to correlate with disease response. An analysis of 65 paediatric patients from the University of Chicago showed no significant difference between patients in remission or relapse whether 6-TG levels were above or below 235[23]. We also found no correlation between dose and 6-TG level, as had been noted by others[14,24,25]. In our subgroup of refractory patients increasing 6-TG levels were associated with a fall in the Paediatric Crohn's Disease Activity Index (PCDAI). Therefore, we find that measuring metabolite levels in non-responsive patients provides reassurance that further escalation in dose may be beneficial without precipitating significant haematological or hepatic toxicity.

METHOTREXATE (MTX)

As stated above, 18% of our patients demonstrated hypersensitivity or intolerance to AZA or 6-MP. For these patients, as well as those who are also CS-dependent or refractory, additional drug choices are necessary. Based primarily on studies by Korzarek *et al.* and Feagen *et al.*, paediatric gastroenterologists have begun to use MTX in paediatric patients with IBD[26–30]. Given the large long-term experience with MTX in children with juvenile rheumatoid arthritis (JRA), its application to IBD is being accepted by an increasing number of paediatric gastroenterologists[31].

Hepatotoxicity and the potential development of fibrosis or cirrhosis are a concern with the administration of MTX. Three studies have directly addressed this issue in children who had been receiving long-term MTX for JRA[32–34]. Graham *et al.* measured transaminase levels every 3 months in a group of 65 children with JRA who received MTX for 84–296 weeks[32]. Six patients received 2000–3000 mg cumulative doses and nine had transiently abnormal transaminase levels. Liver biopsies were performed in 12 of these children, and none had evidence of fibrosis. Kugasathan *et al.* assessed liver function and histology in a group of nine children with JRA who received MTX for more than 3 years[33]. None of these children had biochemical evidence of liver injury, and all biopsies were interpreted as normal. Most recently, Hashkes *et al.* performed 33 percutaneous liver biopsies in 25 paediatric patients with JRA[34]. Biopsies were graded on the *Roenigk Classification Scale* and correlated with biochemical abnormalities as well as duration and cumulative dose of MTX[34,35]. Of the biopsies, 82% were grade I (normal), 12% grade II (inflammation present) and 6% grade IIIA (mild fibrosis). Only the presence of abnormal transaminase levels and body mass index correlated with the Roenigk score; weekly and cumulative MTX dose as well as duration of MTX therapy did not. On the basis of these data the authors recommend performance of a liver biopsy if liver numbers were more than twice normal on at least three occasions during 1 year.

A small number of studies have been published which describe the response of children with IBD to weekly subcutaneous low-dose MTX[28–30]. Mack *et al.* administered MTX (based on $15\,mg/m^2$) subcutaneously to 14 children and adolescents with CD with either hypersensitivity reactions as described above ($n = 3$) or who were refractory ($n = 11$) to 6-MP (1.0–1.5 mg/kg per day)[28]. A fall in PCDAI from a mean of 31 to 8 was observed in nine patients (64%) within 4 weeks of therapy. CS dose decreased from a mean of 23 mg at onset to 18 mg at 1 month, 9.5 mg at 3 months, 8.0 mg at 6 months and 2.5 mg at 12 months; two patients were able to discontinue CS use. It should be noted that one patient died during an acute illness from a presumed viral infection and electrolyte abnormalities, possibly due to adrenal suppression, 3 months after starting MTX. No aetiological agent or cause could be identified before or at autopsy.

Gokhale *et al.* reported the response of 24 paediatric patients with IBD (21 CD, two indeterminate colitis (IC) and 1 UC) to MTX[30]. In this study MTX was administered based on surface area, an approach used by most rheumatologists to treat children and adolescents with JRA. In contrast to its use in JRA, MTX in our population was given subcutaneously, rather than orally, to reduce the likelihood of gastrointestinal side-effects. The dose range was $3–22\,mg/m^2$

per week with a mean of $14 \, mg/m^2$ per week. Of the 24 patients, one had a hypersensitivity reaction requiring cessation of therapy. The remaining 23 (95%) received MTX for a mean of 17.8 months. PCDAI scores decreased from 24.8 at onset to 15.1 at 6 months and 14.4 at their last clinic visit. Mean daily CS dose decreased from 19.7 to $9.8 \, mg$. As part of our approach a complete blood count and liver enzymes and function tests are performed prior to initiating MTX. We have not treated any child with acute or chronic liver disease with the exception of primary sclerosing cholangitis (PSC) with MTX. We have also not used MTX in paediatric patients with chronic lung disease, and would do so only after obtaining pulmonary function tests and consultation because of the potential risk of hypersensitivity pneumonitis. This was not seen in pulmonary function tests performed in 26 children with JRA treated with long-term MTX[31]. However, it was recently described in an 11-year-old child with JRA whose symptoms of chronic cough, fever and malaise developed 1 month after MTX had been reintroduced because of a relapse of her JRA[36]. Symptoms promptly resolved with discontinuation of MTX and initiation of CS therapy.

CYCLOSPORIN (CyA)

Following reports on the efficacy of CyA to prevent and treat graft rejection in liver transplant patients, CyA was studied in paediatric and adult patients with IBD[20,37–41]. From preliminary reports it was evident that CyA could reduce the likelihood of colectomy in paediatric patients with severely active UC who seemed destined to require colectomy[37]. However, relapse and subsequent colectomy occurred in the majority of patients[37–40]. The addition of AZA and 6-MP to the regimen of children with UC prolongs the duration of the remission in some patients[20]. Since serious adverse events may be associated with CyA use, this medication should be used only by physicians knowledgeable regarding monitoring patients for toxicity. In particular the possibility of impaired renal function, hypertension, reduction of the seizure threshold and changes in liver tests should be recognized.

CyA may be effective in treating active CD over the short term and severe perianal complications[20,21,39,41]. Mahdi *et al.* noted that seven of 10 children with severe Crohn's colitis, unresponsive to intravenous methylprednisolone and total parenteral nutrition, responded to intravenous CyA with a fall in PCDAI from 55 to 19 after 2 weeks[21]. Three children subsequently relapsed at 3–6 months and had surgery. Four patients remained well on 6-MP 3–22 months after CyA treatment. We have used CyA in CD only in highly selected patients, who were CS-dependent and refractory to AZA or 6-MP. One such patient closed multiple vulvar fistulas following CyA therapy.

Our approach has been, in most cases, to start with $4 \, mg/kg$ per day divided into two intravenous doses (i.e. every 12 h). This is the initial dose used for paediatric liver transplant patients in our centre, to prevent rejection[37]. In most instances CyA is given intravenously, but may be started orally in non-hospitalized patients with refractory UC. We adjust the dose to provide drug levels $\geq 200 \, mg/ml$, which may be higher (approximately $300 \, mg/ml$) in non-responding patients. Although some authors recommend continuous infusion, the two approaches (bolus and continuous) have never been compared with regard to the likelihood of inducing remission in UC.

A major problem with the use of CyA in children and adolescents is the marked hypertrichosis in many patients. This can be so disfiguring that children experience taunts in school and feel ostracized, some going to the point of using hair-removing agents on the face and extremities and refusing to participate in gym activities. A potential alternative to CyA is tacrolimus, which shares many of the advantages of CyA in transplant patients without the undesirable cosmetic side-effect of hirsutism[42].

TACROLIMUS (FK506)

Experience is accumulating on the potential role of tacrolimus in the treatment of refractory IBD in children[22]. In a recent study, a prospective multicentre open-label trial of tacrolimus enrolled 14 children and adolescents with severe colitis refractory to intravenous CS and total parenteral nutrition[22]. Ten patients had UC, two indeterminate colitis and two Crohn's colitis. The initial dose was 0.10 mg/kg by mouth every 12 h. Drug levels were monitored to keep tacrolimus concentrations at 10–15 ng/ml until clinical response (decreased cramping, haematochezia, cessation of transfusions and ability to tolerate oral feedings) occurred. The dose was lowered to give a blood level 5–10 ng/ml. Four weeks after discharge the prednisone taper began, and at 30–45 days 6-MP 1.5 mg/kg was added. Tacrolimus was discontinued after a total course of 60–90 days. One patient withdrew after 48 h, leaving an evaluable group of 13 patients. Nine patients (69%) responded within 14 days and went into remission, and four patients (31%) underwent colectomy. Five of the 13 patients (38%) discontinued steroids. Side-effects (while also receiving CS) were minimal and consisted of headache, tremor, hypertension and hyperglycaemia. At follow-up 1 year later five patients (38%) remained in clinical remission. Thus, as with CyA, the majority of patients who go into remission following a course of therapy for severe acute colitis still require colectomy at 1 year, although approximately 40% remain in remission on maintenance therapy with 6-MP.

In our subsequent experience with tacrolimus we have found some patients who did not respond to CyA who did go into remission with tacrolimus. Furthermore, the lack of hypertrichosis is a major benefit with regard to self-esteem and social interaction in this age group.

THALIDOMIDE

Thalidomide is thought to reduce inflammation in CD through an anti-tumour necrosis factor effect. The outcomes of thalidomide in children with IBD have not been reported, with the exception of rare anecdotal cases, usually involving severe oral ulcerations. In one child 25 mg daily was followed by improved oral ulcers within 1 week and resolution at 1 month[43]. Alternate-day thalidomide use did not prevent recurrence, and a second course was needed to heal ulcers during a subsequent relapse. Prescription use in the United States requires that all patients of child-bearing potential use contraception. Paediatricians are all too familiar with the problem of unanticipated pregnancy; therefore contraception would have to be started in patients who otherwise might not be using these agents.

ANTI-TUMOUR NECROSIS FACTOR-α ANTIBODY (ANTI-TNF-α) PREPARATIONS

In contrast to studies available for adult patients with CD, the number of prospective studies of anti-TNF-α preparations in paediatric patients is limited to very small series[44–47]. In addition, the majority of the reported patients received only one to three doses and were followed for short periods of time (mean 3 months). Thus, the dose interval or frequency, number of doses and duration of efficacy of this product is unknown in this population. To date, information is limited ragarding the optimal use of infliximab in paediatric patients. Although approved by the FDA for single administration use in refractory CD and a three-dose regimen for fistulous disease, once available it has received extensive use by practitioners, but there is limited analysis of its efficacy and safety in children and adolescents[44–47].

Hyams *et al.* reported 19 paediatric subjects who received one to three doses of 5 mg/kg per dose over 12 weeks for CS-dependent ($n = 12$) or CS-resistant ($n = 7$) CD[46]. PCDAI improved from 42.1 to 10.0 over 4 weeks, but by 8 weeks after infusion eight of the 19 (42%) had relapsed. Self-limited dyspnoea and rash occurred in three children (16%). Vasiliauskas *et al.* described the results of 23 patients from seven centres who received one to three doses of infliximab, 5 mg/kg per dose, over 6 weeks[47]. The indications were: active inflammation ($n = 22$), refractory perianal fistula ($n = 8$), CS-dependence ($n = 12$), and growth failure[13]. The Harvey–Bradshaw score decreased by <5 points by 4 weeks in 75% of children with inflammatory disease; however, 33% relapsed by 8 weeks and 50% by 12 weeks. Fistulas improved, with 57% showing complete healing. Height and weight gains were noted in eight patients followed for more than 6 months. In view of the enormous current and projected expense of this preparation, it is hoped that prospective studies will be supported to provide a basis for determining optimal efficacy of these preparations in children and adolescents with CD.

SUMMARY

As seen above, the armamentarium of available therapies for children and adolescents with IBD continues to increase. This has provided options for patients with refractory disease which often result in reduction or discontinuation of CS medications with their inherent side-effects. Clinical trials in children have traditionally lagged far behind those for adult patients, requiring those involved with the treatment of paediatric patients to extrapolate from adult populations. The recent placebo-controlled trial by Markowitz *et al.*[15] clearly demonstrates that adding 6-MP to prednisone, as initial therapy for CD, reduces CS dose and prolongs remission. As new agents become available, potential special effects in paediatric populations such as bone remodelling, growth, infectious risks, psychosocial functioning and differences in drug metabolism should be addressed.

References

1. Ekbom A, Helmick C, Zack M, Adami H-O. Ulcerative colitis and colorectal cancer – a population-based study. N Engl J Med. 1990;323:122–33.
2. Mir-Madhjessi SH, Michener WM, Farmer RG. Course and prognosis of idiopathic ulcerative proctosigmoiditis in young patients. J Pediatr Gastroenterol Nutr. 1986;5:570–6.
3. Polito JM 2nd, Childs B, Mellits ED, Tokayer AZ, Harris ML, Bayless TM. Crohn's disease: influence of age at diagnosis on site and clinical type of disease. Gastroenterology. 1996; 111:580–6.
4. Griffiths AM, Nguyen P, Smith C, MacMillan JH, Sherman PM. Growth and clinical course of children with Crohn's disease. Gut. 1993;34:939–43.
5. Tripathi RC, Kirschner BS, Kipp M *et al.* Corticosteroid treatment for inflammatory bowel disease in pediatric patients increases intraocular pressure. Gastroenterology. 1992;102:1957–61.
6. Tripathi RC, Kipp MA, Tripathi BJ *et al.* Ocular toxicity of prednisone in pediatric patients with inflammatory bowel disease. Lens Eye Tox Res. 1992;9:469–82.
7. Gokhale R, Favus M, Karrison T, Rich B, Sutton M, Kirschner BS. Bone mineral density assessment in children with inflammatory bowel disease. Gastroenterology. 1998;114:902–11.
8. Semeao EJ, Jawad AF, Stouffer NO, Zemel BB, Piccoli DA, Stallings VA. Risk factors for low bone mineral density in children and young adults with Crohn's disease. J Pediatr. 1999; 135:593–600.
9. Food and Drug Administration, Department of Health and Human Services. 21 CFR Part 201. Specific requirements on content and format of labeling for human prescription drugs; revision of 'pediatric use' subsection in the labeling; final rule. Federal Register, 13 December, 1994.
10. Verhave M, Winter HS, Grand RJ. Azathioprine in the treatment of children with inflammatory bowel disease. J Pediatr. 1990;117:809–14.
11. Markowitz J, Rosa J, Grancher K, Aiges H, Daum F. Long-term 6-mercaptopurine treatment in adolescents with Crohn's disease. Gastroenterology. 1990;99:1347–55.
12. Cuffari C, Théorêt Y, Latour S, Seidman G. 6-MP metabolite levels: a potential guide to Crohn's disease therapy. Gut. 1996;39:401–6.
13. Kirschner BS. Safety of azathioprine (AZA) and 6-mercaptopurine (6-MP) in the treatment of children and adolescents with inflammatory bowel disease. Gastroenterology. 1998;115:812–22.
14. Dubinsky M, Lamothe S, Yang HY, Targan SR, Sinnett D, Théorêt Y, Seidman EG. Pharmacokinetics and metabolite measurement for 6-mercaptopurine therapy in inflammatory bowel disease. Gastroenterology. 2000;118:705–13.
15. Markowitz J, Grancher K, Kohn N, Lesser M, Daum F and The Pediatric 6MP Collaborative Group. A multicenter trial of 6-mercaptopurine and prednisone in children with newly diagnosed Crohn's disease. Gastroenterology. 2000;119:895–902.
16. Present DH, Meltzer SJ, Krumholz MP, Wolke A, Korelitz BI. 6-Mercaptopurine in the management of inflammatory bowel disease: short and long-term toxicity. Ann Intern Med. 1989; 111:641–9.
17. Kader HA, Mascarenhas MR, Piccolo DA, Stouffer NO, Baldassano RN. Experiences with 6-mercaptopurine and azathioprine therapy in pediatric patients with severe ulcerative colitis. J Pediatr Gastroenterol Nutr. 1999;28:54–8.
18. Kappler M, Lang T, Harms H-K, Bertele-Harms R-M. Treatment with azathioprine in pediatric ulcerative colitis reduces corticosteroid usage and the need for colectomy – experience in 65 children. J Pediatr Gastroenterol Nutr. 2000;31:S77;A298.
19. Issenman RM, Atkinson SA, Radoja C, Fraher L. Longitudinal assessment of growth, mineral metabolism, and bone mass in pediatric Crohn's disease. J Pediatr Gastroenterol Nutr. 1993; 17:401–6.
20. Ramakrishna J, Langhans N, Calenda K, Grand RJ, Verhave M. Combined use of cyclosporine and azathioprine or 6-mercaptopurine in pediatric inflammatory bowel disease. J Pediatr Gastroenterol Nutr. 1996;22:296–302.
21. Mahdi G, Israel DM, Hassall E. Cyclosporine and 6-mercaptopurine for active, refractory Crohn's colitis in children. Am J Gastroenterol. 1996;91:1355–9.
22. Bousvaros A, Kirschner BS, Werlin SL *et al.* Oral tacrolimus treatment of severe colitis in children. J Pediatr. 2000;137:794–9.
23. Gupta P, Gokhale R, Kirschner BS. Clinical usefulness of 6-mercaptopurine (6-MP) metabolite levels in children with IBD. J Pediatr Gastroenterol Nutr. 2000;31:S76;A293.

24. Paerregaard A, Schmiegelow K. Measurement of thiopurine methyl transferase (TMPT) activity and azathioprine metabolites in childhood IBD treatment. J Pediatr Gastroenterol Nutr. 2000; 31:S81;A312.

25. Lowry PW, Franklin CL, Weaver AL *et al.* Cross-sectional study of IBD patients taking azathioprine (AZA) or 6-mercaptopurine (6-MP): lack of correlation between disease activity and 6-thioguanine nucleotide (6TGN) concentration. Gastroenterology. 2000;118:A4205.

26. Korzarek AR, Patterson DJ, Gelfand MD *et al.* Methotrexate induces clinical and histologic remission in patients with refractory inflammatory bowel disease. Ann Intern Med. 1989; 110:353–6.

27. Feagan BG, Rochon J, Fedorak RN *et al.* Methotrexate for the treatment of Crohn's disease. N Engl J Med. 1995;332:292–7.

28. Mack DR, Young R, Kaufman S, Ramey L, Vanderhoof JA. Methotrexate in patients with Crohn's disease after 6-mercaptopurine. J Pediatr. 1998;132:830–5.

29. Kirschner BS. Methotrexate therapy for pediatric patients with inflammatory bowel disease. Inflam Bowel Dis. 1998;4:121–3.

30. Gokhale R, Andrew H, Kirschner BS. Safety and efficacy of long-term methotrexate (MTX) in pediatric patients with inflammatory bowel disease (IBD). J Pediatr Gastroenterol Nutr. 2000;31:S-18;A64.

31. Markowitz J, Grancher K, Kohn N. Immunomodulatory therapy for IBD: changing patterns of use 1990–2000. J Pediatr Gastroenterol Nutr. 2000;31:S79;A306.

32. Graham LD, Myones BL, Rivas-Chacon RF *et al.* Morbidity associated with long-term methotrexate therapy in juvenile rheumatoid arthritis. J Pediatr. 1992;120:468–73.

33. Kugathasan S, Newman AJ, Dahms BB, Boyle JT. Liver biopsy findings in patients with juvenile rheumatoid arthritis receiving long-term, weekly methotrexate therapy. J Pediatr. 1996;128:149–51.

34. Hashkes PJ, Balistreri WF, Bove KE, Ballard ET, Passo MH. The relationship of hepatotoxic risk factors and liver histology in methotrexate therapy for juvenile rheumatoid arthritis. J Pediatr. 1999;134:47–52.

35. Roenigk HH, Auerback R, Mailbach HI, Weinstein GD. Methotrexate guidelines revised. J Am Acad Dermatol. 1982;6:145–55.

36. Cron RQ, Sherry DD, Wallace CA. Methotrexate-induced hypersensitivity pneumonitis in a child with juvenile rheumatoid arthritis. J Pediatr. 1998;132:901–2.

37. Kirschner BS, Whitington PF, Malfeo-Klein R. Experience with cyclosporin A (CyA) in severe non-specific ulcerative colitis (UC). Pediatr Res. 1989;25:117A.

38. Lichtiger S, Present DH. Preliminary report: cyclosporin in treatment of severe active ulcerative colitis. Lancet. 1990;336:16–19.

39. Brynskov J, Freund L, Rasmussen SN *et al.* A placebo-controlled, double-blind, randomized trial of cyclosporine therapy in active chronic Crohn's disease. N Engl J Med. 1989;321:845–50.

40. Treem WR, Hyams JS. Cyclosporine therapy for gastrointestinal disease. J Pediatr Gastroenterol Nutr. 1994;18:270–8.

41. Hanauer SB, Smith MB. Rapid closure of Crohn's fistulas with continuous intravenous cyclosporine A. Am J Gastroenterol. 1993;88:646–9.

42. Busque S, Demers P, Saint-Louis G *et al.* Hypertrichosis and gingival hypertrophy regression in renal transplants following substitution of cyclosporin by tacrolimus. Ann Chir. 1999;53:687–9.

43. Weinstein TA, Sciubba JJ, Levine J. Thalidomide for the treatment of oral aphthous ulcers in Crohn's disease. J Pediatr Gastroenterol Nutr. 1999;28:214–16.

44. Hadigan C, Baldassano R, Braegger CP *et al.* Pharmacokinetics of infliximab (anti-TNFα) in children with Crohn's disease: a multicenter trial. J Pediatr Gastroenterol Nutr. 1999; 29:525;A143 (abstract).

45. Baldassano R, Vasiliauskis E, Braegger C *et al.* A multicenter study of anti-TNFα chimeric monoclonal antibody (infliximab) in the treatment of pediatric patients with active Crohn's disease. Gastroenterology. 1999;116:A665 (abstract).

46. Hyams JS, Markowitz J, Wyllie R. Use of infliximab in the treatment of Crohn's disease in children and adolescents. J Pediatr. 2000;137:192–6.

47. Vasiliauskas EA, Schaffer S, Dezenberg CV *et al.* Collaborative experience of open-label infliximab in refractory pediatric patients Crohn's disease. J Pediatr Gastroenterol Nutr. 2000; 31:S227.

28
Immunosuppressive therapy and extraintestinal manifestations in inflammatory bowel disease

G. D'HAENS

INTRODUCTION

Extraintestinal manifestations (EIM) are very common in patients with inflammatory bowel disease (IBD). The majority of them occur in parallel with the inflammatory activity in the gut and respond to treatment of intestinal inflammation. A few extraintestinal problems may develop independently of gut inflammation, such as pyoderma gangrenosum, sclerosing cholangitis and axial spondylitis. In these instances the management is more complex and often frustrating, and should be designed in cooperation with dermatologists, hepatologists and rheumatologists, respectively. The majority of clinical trials in IBD use clinical scores in which EIM are only part of the total score. As a consequence the effect of the therapeutic agent on EIM alone cannot be deduced.

This chapter will review the effects on EIM of the different immunomodulatory and biological compounds commonly used to treat IBD.

PERIPHERAL ARTHRITIS

Arthritis is, after anaemia, the most common EIM associated with IBD, occurring in up to 25% of patients. It is a typical asymmetric synovitis of the larger joints which does not lead to bone destruction and deformity, and remains seronegative. Symptoms vary in intensity in parallel with gut inflammation. Treatment should be aimed at control of the intestinal inflammation, which results in disappearance of the joint symptoms. In mild IBD sulphasalazine is the agent of choice, since it is more active in arthritis than the other 5-acetylsalicylic acid (5-ASA) preparations. More severe cases require treatment with corticosteroids. As a general rule, EIM respond better/more quickly to systemic steroids than to the newer topical steroids such as budesonide. Steroid-dependent cases often respond to azathioprine/6-mercaptopurine and to methotrexate (MTX). Refractory patients can be treated with the anti-TNF antibody infliximab, which leads to a rapid resolution of joint symptoms. This is not surprising, since infliximab is also being used successfully in rheumatoid arthritis.

Arthralgia without genuine synovitis may also be drug-induced and hence not correlate with gut inflammation. Some patients report annoying joint pain during treatment with azathioprine. Infusion of infliximab can also be complicated by joint pain, either early on (within the first 3 days), which is called a 'cytokine release' syndrome, or later after 7–10 days, which represents delayed hypersensitivity. The clinician should at this point be aware of the aetiology of these problems and not intensify anti-inflammatory treatment.

AXIAL SPONDYLARTHROPATHY

Axial spondylitis and ankylosing spondylitis occur frequently in patients with IBD, predominantly with ulcerative colitis and in HLA B27-positive patients. Symptoms include morning rigidity, progressive lumbalgia and sometimes reduced thoracic expansion. This disease is chronic, and its evolution is independent of the activity or the treatment of intestinal inflammation. Although some patients experience symptom relief with sulphasalazine, the majority will remain symptomatic, even when corticosteroids and/or azathioprine or MTX are started. The first really effective therapy for spondylarthritis has been infliximab, which leads to complete resolution of back pain and improved mobility in the majority of patients.

ERYTHEMA NODOSUM (EN)

Typically, bouts of EN parallel IBD activity, without being related to the extent or duration of the disease. Approximately 70% of patients with EN also have articular problems. Treatment of EN is the same as that of an IBD attack.

PYODERMA GANGRENOSUM (PG)

PG is the most severe skin lesion that occurs in IBD. It predominantly develops in elderly patients and in patients with ulcerative colitis. An important group of patients presents with PG before their intestinal disease has been diagnosed. PG is typically seen on the extremities. It presents as a painful sterile ulceration. The relationship of the activity of IBD to the development of PG is controversial.

Local skin care is important to prevent secondary infection. Topical dapsone or intralesional corticosteroids have been successful to a limited degree. Systemic treatment with corticosteroids, azathioprine and MTX has also been rather ineffective for this disease. Better results have been reported with cyclosporin. More recently, complete and rapid healing of PG has been reported with infliximab treatment.

PSORIASIS

Psoriasis is a chronic inflammatory condition of the skin, the pathogenesis of which has many similarities with Crohn's disease. An important association between the two conditions has been reported. Psoriatic skin lesions not only improve with steroid treatment, but they also respond to cyclosporin (in general lower doses than used for ulcerative colitis) and dramatically improve and even disappear with infliximab.

OCULAR MANIFESTATIONS

The incidence of ocular complications in IBD ranges from 5% to 12%. Episcleritis and anterior uveitis represent the majority of these ocular problems. They are almost always related to important inflammation in the gut. In addition to IBD therapy, topical corticosteroids and in patients with anterior uveitis often also systemic steroids are required.

SCLEROSING CHOLANGITIS (PSC)

PSC is characterized by a chronic fibrosing inflammation of the bile ducts. It is much more frequent in patients with ulcerative colitis than in Crohn's disease, and predominantly affects male individuals. PSC is a progressive disease, even in patients whose IBD is kept 'under control'. It leads to important morbidity and significant mortality, and patients with advanced disease often require a liver transplantation.

No specific therapy has been identified that is capable of arresting or reversing PSC. Proctocolectomy does not influence the natural history of PSC. Many controlled and uncontrolled clinical trials have failed to demonstrate a therapeutic effect of colchicine, corticosteroids, azathioprine and methotrexate.

Bibliography

Curley RK, Macfarlane AW, Vickers CFH. Pyoderma gangrenosum treated with cyclosporine. Br J Dermatol. 1985;113:601–4.

Fraser SM, Sturrock RD. Evaluation of sulphasalazine in ankylosing spondylitis – an interventional study. Br J Rheumatol. 1990;29:37–9.

Javett SL. Azathioprine in primary sclerosing cholangitis. Lancet. 1971;2:663.

Knox TA, Kaplan MM. Double-blind trial of methotrexate in the treatment of primary sclerosing cholangitis. Gastroenterology. 1991:100:A4761 (abstract).

Mir-Madjlessi SH, Taylor JS, Farmer RG. Clinical course and evolution of erythema nodosum and pyoderma gangrenosum in chronic ulcerative colitis: a study of 42 patients. Am J Gastroenterol. 1985;80:615–20.

Strauss RE. Ocular manifestations of Crohn's disease: literature review. Mt Sinai J Med. 1988;55:353–6.

Van den Bosch F, Kruithof E, Baeten D, De Keyser F, Mielants H, Veys EM. Effects of a loading dose regimen of three infusions of chimeric monoclonal antibody to tumour necrosis factor α (infliximab) in spondylarthropathy: an open pilot study. Ann Rheum Dis. 2000;59:428–33.

29
Classical immunosuppressive therapy and malignancy

T. ANDUS

INTRODUCTION

Although the aetiology of Crohn's disease and ulcerative colitis is still unknown, considerable success has been achieved in the treatment of patients with inflammatory bowel disease (IBD). Whereas life expectancy was dramatically reduced in the first half of last century, for the past few years life expectancy is nearly normal in most patients[1–3].

There are several reasons for this progress. We are now able to treat active disease very effectively with drugs such as corticosteroids, antibiotics and immunosuppressants, and surgery is also much safer now. Furthermore, maintenance of remission can now be achieved in many patients by the use of immunosuppressive drugs such as azathioprine/6-mercaptopurine or methotrexate. However, the more patients are on immunosuppressive drugs for a long time, the more the question about side-effects arises. One of the most dreaded side-effects is the development of a malignancy.

The fact that immunosuppressive drugs can cause malignancies was clearly shown in patients after heart or kidney transplantation[4] several years ago. The risk for malignancies was dramatically increased in these patients, who received massive immunosuppression to prevent graft rejection (Table 1)[4].

Now the question arises: can classical immunosuppressive treatment increase the risk for neoplasms in patients with IBD? Before this question can be answered we first have to determine the risk for neoplasms in patients with IBD without immunosuppressive treatment.

MALIGNANCY IN IBD

There are many studies dealing with the risk of malignancy in IBD. These can be grouped into cohort studies of single, mostly referral centres and into regional cohort studies including all patients in a certain area. The single-centre cohort studies are often confounded by the fact that preferentially very ill patients are

Table 1 Increased incidence of non-Hodgkin's lymphoma in kidney and heart transplant recipients

Years after heart transplantation/ kidney transplantation	Patients (n)	Malignancy ratio (observed/expected)
1	7634/45 141	155/37
2	5036/35 038	90/9
3	4691/28 498	38/6
4	3325/21 540	30/6
5	2193/15 884	13/12
6	844/9851	10/4

Table 2 Malignancy in IBD

Reference, location	Patients (n)	Ratio (observed/ expected)	95% confidence interval
Ekbom et al. 1991, Uppsala[5]	CD 1655	1.2	0.0–1.6
Persson et al. 1994, Stockholm[6]	CD 1251	1.1	0.9–1.5
Palli et al. 2000, Florence[7]	CD 231	1.56	0.9–2.5
Ekbom et al. 1991, Uppsala[5]	UC 3121	1.6	1.4–1.8
Karlén et al. 1999, Stockholm[8]	UC 1547	1.4	1.1–1.6
Palli et al. 2000, Florence[7]	UC 689	0.98	0.7–1.3

treated in such specialized referral centres, whereas the regional-based cohort studies are more representative for IBD patients in general.

Overall malignancy in IBD

The overall risk for malignancy was found not to be increased in patients with Crohn's disease in three large regional cohort studies (Table 2)[5–7]. In patients with ulcerative colitis the two larger of three big regional cohort studies found a significantly increased risk for malignancy (Table 2)[5,7,8].

Colorectal cancer in IBD

The increased risk for malignancy is due to the fact that colorectal cancer is increased in patients with long-term colitis ulcerosa (especially pancolitis) (Table 3)[8–11]. This increased cancer risk seems to be related to long-term inflammation since Fonager et al. found no increased risk for colorectal carcinoma in the parents of IBD patients[12], and since treatment with 5-aminosalicylic acid preparations significantly reduces the risk for colorectal cancer[13,14]. Interestingly, in the newest regional cohort studies the colorectal cancer risk was no

Table 3 Colorectal cancer in ulcerative colitis

Reference, location	Study type	Patients (n)	Ratio (observed/ expected)	p or 95% confidence interval
Greenstein et al. 1981, Mt Sinai[9]	Hospital cohort	267	Left-sided: 8.6 Pancolitis: 26.5	$p < 0.001$ $p < 0.001$
Ekbom et al. 1992, Uppsala[10]	Regional cohort	2509	4.4	3.2–5.9
Stewenius et al. 1995, Malmö[11]	Regional cohort	471	8.6	1.8–25.1
Karlén et al. 1999, Stockholm[8]	Regional cohort	1547	4	2.7–5.8
Wandall et al. 2000, Funen, DK[15]	Regional cohort	801	1.7	0.6–3.6
Palli et al. 2000, Florence[7]	Regional cohort	689	1.8	0.9–3.3
Winther et al. 2000, Copenhagen[16]	Regional cohort	1161	0.97	n.s.

n.s. = Not significant.

Table 4 Colorectal cancer in Crohn's disease

Reference, location	Study type	Patients (n)	Incidence observed	Ratio (observed/ expected)
Ekbom et al. 1992, Uppsala[10]	Regional cohort	1469	5	1.7
Persson et al. 1994, Stockholm[6]	Regional cohort	1251	5	0.9
Mellemkjaer et al. 2000 Denmark[17]	Regional cohort	2645	15	1.1
Palli et al. 2000, Florence[7]	Regional cohort	231	2	2.5

longer significantly increased (Table 3)[7,15,16]. This is probably due to the fact that many patients are now under surveillance, and get the diseased colon out if disease activity cannot be adequately controlled by drugs, or when precancerous lesions such as dysplasia are detected by colonoscopy. This strongly suggests that prevention works in patients with IBD. Since only a minority of patients with Crohn's disease have long-term pancolitis the risk for colorectal cancer is not significantly increased in regional cohort studies of patients with Crohn's disease (Table 4)[6,7,10,17].

Small bowel cancer in Crohn's disease

Four of five large studies showed that the risk for small bowel cancer is strongly increased in patients with Crohn's disease (Table 5)[5,6,9,17,18]. Fortunately the absolute risk is very small, since clinical diagnosis is very difficult for these malignancies.

Lymphoma in IBD

Although there are some case reports concerning lymphoma in patients with IBD, speculating about causal relationship, 4 large regional cohort studies found no increased risk for lymphoma in patients with Crohn's disease (Table 6)[5–7,19]. In five large studies of patients with ulcerative colitis only the two smallest studies found a significantly increased risk for lymphoma (Table 7)[7,20] whereas the three largest studies found no significant increase (Table 7)[5,8,21].

Table 5 Small bowel cancer in Crohn's disease

Reference, location	Study type	Patients (n)	Incidence observed	Ratio (observed/ expected)
Greenstein *et al.* 1981, Mt Sinai[9]	Hospital cohort	589		85.8
Ekbom *et al.* 1992, Uppsala[10]	Regional cohort	1655	1	3.4
Munkholm *et al.* 1993, Copenhagen[18]	Regional cohort	373	2	50
Persson *et al.* 1994, Stockholm[6]	Regional cohort	1251	4	15.6

Table 6 Lymphoma in Crohn's disease

Reference, location	Study type	Patients (n)	Ratio (observed/ expected)	95% confidence interval
Ekbom *et al.* 1991, Uppsala[5]	Regional cohort	1655	0.5	0.1–1.9
Persson *et al.* 1994, Stockholm[6]	Regional cohort	1251	1.1	0.3–2.5
Palli *et al.* 2000, Florence[7]	Regional cohort	231	2.5	0.9–2.5
Lewis *et al.* 2000, UK[19]	Retrospective database	6608	1.6	0.6–3.3

Table 7 Lymphoma in ulcerative colitis

Reference, location	Study type	Patients (n)	Ratio (observed/ expected)	95% confidence interval
Ekbom *et al.* 1991, Uppsala[5]	Regional cohort	3121	1.1	0.6–1.9
Karlén *et al.* 1999, Stockholm[8]	Regional cohort	1547	1.1	0.5–2.2
Palli *et al.* 2000, Florence[7]	Regional cohort	689	2.7	1.2–5.3
Lewis *et al.* 2000, UK[19]	Retrospective database	10 398	1.2	0.6–2.2
Farrel *et al.* 2000, St James Hospital[20]	Hospital cohort	UC 515, CD 267	IBD 31	IBD 2.0–85.0

UC = Ulcerative colitis, CD = Crohn's disease.

IMMUNOSUPPRESSIVE TREATMENT IN IBD AND MALIGNANCY

Data regarding the role of classical immunosuppressive treatment and malignancy in IBD are much rarer and much less clear.

Immunosuppressive treatment and general malignancy in IBD

There are only two retrospective hospital-based studies concerning the general risk of malignancy in relation to immunosuppressive treatment. Connell et al.[22], in 755 patients with IBD after a median follow-up of 9 years, found 31 cases of malignancy. This was not significantly different from the 24 cases expected. Very recently, however, Farrell et al.[20] analysed 515 patients with ulcerative colitis and 267 patients with Crohn's disease. They found malignancies in 14 of 238 (5.9%) patients with prior immunosuppression and in 16/544 without prior immunosuppression. These data just reached statistical significance ($p = 0.04$).

Immunosuppressive treatment and colorectal cancer

Three large studies analysed the relationship between immunosuppressive treatment and the development of colorectal cancer in patients with IBD (Table 8)[20,22,23]. All three studies found no significant difference between the patients with and without prior immunosuppressive treatment.

Immunosuppressive treatment and lymphoma in IBD

Since lymphomas are frequent in patients after organ transplantation, the risk for the development of lymphoma in patients with IBD after immunosuppressive treatment has been studied. Six large studies investigated the frequency of lymphoma in patients with IBD treated with immunosuppressive drugs (Table 9)[19,20,22–25]. Overall the risk for lymphoma was very small. In three studies

Table 8 Immunosuppressive treatment and colorectal cancer in IBD

Reference, location	Study type	Patients (n)	With immuno-suppression	Without immuno-suppression	p-Value
Connell et al. 1994, St Marks[22]	Retrospective hospital database	UC 282, IC 23, CD 450	UC 8/86	UC 15/180 expected	0.54
Farrell et al. 2000 St James Hospital[20]	Hospital cohort	UC 515, CD 267	IBD 6/238 (2.5%)	IBD 9/544 (1.7%)	0.4
Fraser and Jewell 2000, Oxford[23]	Retrospective database	UC 1350, CD 855	UC 7/1299 (2.3%)	UC 28/627 (4.5%)	n.s.

UC = Ulcerative colitis; IC = indeterminate colitis; CD = Crohn's disease; n.s. = not significant.

Table 9 Immunosuppressive treatment and lymphoma in IBD

Reference	Study type	Patients (n)	With immuno-suppression	Without immuno-suppression	P*
Present *et al.* 1989, New York[24]	Retrospective hospital data	UC 120, CD 276	1/396 (Aza)		n. s.
Connell *et al.* 1994, St Marks[22]	Retrospective hospital data	UC 282, CD 450	0	0	n. s.
Korelitz *et al.* 1999, New York[25]	Retrospective hospital data	UC 170, CD 380	UC: 0, CD: 2 (6-MP)		
Farrell *et al.* 2000, St James Hospital[20]	Hospital cohort	UC 515, CD 267	4/238 (1.7%)*	0/544(0%)	0.002
Lewis *et al.* 2000, UK[21]	Retrospective database	UC 10 398, CD 6608	UC 1/628 (0.07%) (Aza), CD 0/837	0/1554(10%)	0.00–9.00
Fraser and Jewell 2000, Oxford[23]	Retrospective database	UC 1350, CD 855	IBD 3/619 (0.5%)	IBD 4/1586 (0.3%)	n. s.

Aza = Azathioprine, 6-MP = 6-mercaptopurine, n.s. = not significant.
*One CD patient took azathioprine, one UC patient took azathioprine, one UC patient took methotrexate, one UC patient took methotrexate and cyclosporin A.

the frequency of lymphoma was given in series of retrospective hospital data[22,24,25]. In the other three studies the frequency of lymphoma in patients after or during immunosuppression was compared to patients without immunosuppression[19,20,23]. Only in the smallest of the three comparative studies was a significant increase of lymphoma found in patients treated with immunosuppressive drugs compared to patients without immunosuppressive drugs[20], whereas in the two other, larger, studies no significant difference was found. This difference was due to four lymphomas, which occurred in one patient with Crohn's disease and in three patients with ulcerative colitis. Treatment consisted of azathioprine in two cases, and of methotrexate or methotrexate plus cyclosporin A in the other two cases. Since these patients were not matched for age, disease activity, course of disease or other important clinical parameters, these data neither prove nor exclude a causal relationship between lymphoma and immuno-suppressive drugs. Prospective, randomized controlled long-term trials are lacking in IBD.

IMMUNOSUPPRESSIVE TREATMENT AND MALIGNANCY IN OTHER DISEASES

Silman and co-workers treated 202 patients with rheumatoid arthritis with high doses of azathioprine (mean dose 300 mg/day)[26]. The follow-up period lasted from 1964 to 1984. They observed four lymphomas in this group. In another group of 202 patients not taking azathioprine, and matched for age, age of onset, sex, and serostatus, they observed two lymphomas. The lymphoma rates were then compared with those expected based on the incidence in the general population. This comparison suggested a five-fold increase in the rheumatoid arthritis control group and a 10-fold increase in the azathioprine-treated group.

The British and Dutch Multiple Sclerosis Azathioprine Trial Group randomized 354 patients with multiple sclerosis to receive either azathioprine 2.5 mg/kg daily or placebo in a double-masked trial[27]. They observed no lymphoma after 3 years.

Wolfe analysed 1767 patients with rheumatoid arthritis[28]. The patients were followed up for up to 25 years in an outpatient rheumatoid arthritis clinic. The incidence of lymphoma was 70/100 000 in this cohort, resulting in a standardized incidence ratio of 1.8 (95% confidence interval: 0.99–3.23). A multivariate analysis revealed the erythrocyte sedimentation rate:hazard ratio: 9.2 (2.0–42.7) and age:hazard ratio per 10 years: 2.6 (1.4–4.9), but not the methotrexate:hazard ratio 0.99 (0.3–3.0) as related to the incidence of lymphoma.

Only for cyclosporin A was a clear association found with malignancy in patients after kidney transplantation. Dantal *et al.* randomized 231 patients after kidney transplantation to receive either low-dose (75–125 ng/ml through blood concentration) or high-dose (150–250 ng/ml through blood concentration) cyclosporin A. They found a significant increase of malignancies in the high-dose group ($p = 0.034$)[29]. Most of the malignancies were skin cancers (26 versus 17) followed by breast cancers (four versus one) and lymphoma (three versus one).

CONCLUSIONS

There are no data proving that any of the classical immunosuppressive drugs can cause malignancy in IBD. However, from other diseases there are strong hints that cyclosporin A may cause malignancies. For azathioprine/6-mercaptopurine and methotrexate currently the positive effects on disease activity and quality of life outweigh the possible small risk of causing malignancy in patients with IBD[19].

References

1. Langholz E, Munkholm P, Nielsen OH, Kreiner S, Binder V. Incidence and prevalence of ulcerative colitis in Copenhagen county from 1962 to 1987. Scand J Gastroenterol. 1991;26:1247–56.
2. Munkholm P, Langholz E, Davidsen M, Binder V. Disease activity courses in a regional cohort of Crohn's disease patients. Scand J Gastroenterol. 1995;30:699–706.
3. Davoli M, Prantera C, Berto E, Scribano ML, D'Ippoliti D. Mortality among patients with ulcerative colitis: Rome 1970–1989. Eur J Epidemiol. 1997;13:189–94.
4. Oelz G, Henderson R. Incidence of non-Hodgkin lymphoma in kidney and heart transplant recipients. Lancet. 1993;342:1514–16.
5. Ekbom A, Helmick C, Zack M, Adami HO. Extracolonic malignancies in inflammatory bowel disease. Cancer. 1991;67:2015–19.
6. Persson PG, Karlen P, Bernell O *et al.* Crohn's disease and cancer: a population-based cohort study. Gastroenterology. 1994;107:1675–9.
7. Palli D, Trallori G, Bagnoli S *et al.* Hodgkin's disease risk is increased in patients with ulcerative colitis. Gastroenterology. 2000;119:647–53.
8. Karlén P, Lofberg R, Brostrom O, Leijonmarck CE, Hellers G, Persson PG. Increased risk of cancer in ulcerative colitis: a population-based cohort study. Am J Gastroenterol. 1999; 94:1047–52.
9. Greenstein AJ, Sachar DB, Smith H, Janowitz HD, Aufses AHJ. A comparison of cancer risk in Crohn's disease and ulcerative colitis. Cancer. 1981;48:2742–5.

10. Ekbom A, Helmick CG, Zack M, Holmberg L, Adami HO. Survival and causes of death in patients with inflammatory bowel disease: a population-based study. Gastroenterology. 1992; 103:954–60.

11. Stewenius J, Adnerhill I, Anderson H *et al*. Incidence of colorectal cancer and all-cause mortality in non-selected patients with ulcerative colitis and indeterminate colitis in Malmo, Sweden. Int J Colorectal Dis. 1995;10:117–22.

12. Fonager K, Sorensen HT, Mellemkjaer L, Olsen JH, Olsen J. Risk of colorectal cancer in relatives of patients with inflammatory bowel disease (Denmark). Cancer Causes Control. 1998;9:389–92.

13. Pinczowski D, Ekbom A, Baron J, Yuen J, Adami HO. Risk factors for colorectal cancer in patients with ulcerative colitis: a case–control study. Gastroenterology. 1994;107:117–20.

14. Moody GA, Jayanthi V, Probert CS, Mac KH, Mayberry JF. Long-term therapy with sulphasalazine protects against colorectal cancer in ulcerative colitis: a retrospective study of colorectal cancer risk and compliance with treatment in Leicestershire. Eur J Gastroenterol Hepatol. 1996;8:1179–83.

15. Wandall EP, Damkier P, Moller PF, Wilson B, Schaffalitzky-de-Muckadell OB. Survival and incidence of colorectal cancer in patients with ulcerative colitis in Funen county diagnosed between 1973 and 1993. Scand J Gastroenterol. 2000;35:312–17.

16. Winther KV, Jess T, Langholz E, Munkholm P, Binder V. Colorectal cancer risk in ulcerative colitis: follow-up of a population-based cohort in Copenhagen county, Denmark, 1962 to 1997. Gastroenterology. 2000;118:339.

17. Mellemkjaer L, Johansen C, Gridley G, Linet MS, Kjaer SK, Olsen JH. Crohn's disease and cancer risk (Denmark). Cancer Causes Control. 2000;11:145–50.

18. Munkholm P, Langholz E, Davidsen M, Binder V. Intestinal cancer risk and mortality in patients with Crohn's disease. Gastroenterology. 1993;105:1716–23.

19. Lewis JD, Schwartz JS, Lichtenstein GR. Azathioprine for maintenance of remission in Crohn's disease: benefits outweigh the risk of lymphoma. Gastroenterology. 2000;118:1018–24.

20. Farrell RJ, Ang Y, Kileen P *et al*. Increased incidence of non-Hodgkin's lymphoma in inflammatory bowel disease patients on immunosuppressive therapy but overall risk is low. Gut. 2000; 47:514–19.

21. Lewis JD, Bilker WB, Brensinger C, Deren JJ, Vaughn DJ, Strumia R. Are patients with inflammatory bowel disease (IBD) at increased risk for lymphoma? Gastroenterology. 2000;118:869.

22. Connell WR, Kamm MA, Dickson M, Balkwill AM, Ritchie JK, Lennard-Jones JE. Long-term neoplasia risk after azathioprine treatment in inflammatory bowel disease. Lancet. 1994; 343:1249–52.

23. Fraser AG, Jewell DP. Long-term risk of malignancy after treatment of inflammatory bowel disease with azathioprine – a 30 year study. Gastroenterology. 2000;118:A254.

24. Present DH, Meltzer SJ, Krumholz MP, Wolke A, Korelitz BI. 6-Mercaptopurine in the management of inflammatory bowel disease: short- and long-term toxicity. Ann Intern Med. 1989; 111:641–9.

25. Korelitz BI, Mirsky FJ, Fleisher MR, Warman JI, Wisch N, Gleim GW. Malignant neoplasms subsequent to treatment of inflammatory bowel disease with 6-mercaptopurine. Am J Gastroenterol. 1999;94:3248–53.

26. Silman AJ, Petrie J, Hazleman B, Evans SJ. Lymphoproliferative cancer and other malignancy in patients with rheumatoid arthritis treated with azathioprine: a 20 year follow up study. Ann Rheum Dis. 1988;47:988–92.

27. Civati G, Busnach G, Brando B *et al*. Occurrence of Kaposi's sarcoma in renal transplant recipients treated with low doses of cyclosporine. Transplant Proc. 1988;20(Suppl. 3):924–8.

28. Wolfe F. Inflammatory activity, but not methotrexate or prednisone use predicts non-Hodgkin's lymphoma in rheumatoid arthritis: a 25-year study of 1797 RA patients. Arthritis Rheum. 1998;41:188.

29. Dantal J, Hourmant M, Cantarovich D *et al*. Effect of long-term immunosuppression in kidney-graft recipients on cancer incidence: randomised comparison of two cyclosporin regimens. Lancet. 1998; 351:623–8.

30
Anti-tumour necrosis factor alpha therapy and malignancy in Crohn's disease

S. R. TARGAN and E. A. VASILIAUSKAS

INTRODUCTION

The recent development of new specifically targeted immunomodulators warrants reconsideration of malignancies in patients with Crohn's disease[1-3]. As discussed in the previous chapter, there is a great deal of controversy over whether these new therapeutics have contributed to a true increase in the number of patients with either solid tumours or lymphomas. In this brief chapter we will consider the potential contributing factors to the seemingly increased incidences of these tumours. A discussion is also provided of the mechanisms of anti-tumour necrosis factor alpha (TNF-α) mediated immunomodulation in the context of what is known about the systemic immunomodulators, such as corticosteroids and 6-mercaptopurine (6-MP). Finally, the chapter provides a review of the reported incidence of expression, or onset of malignancies, following anti-TNF-α therapy. The objective is to discuss the evidence for the association between, and incidence of, increased intestinal solid tumours and lymphomas in Crohn's disease.

It is well known that there is an increased incidence of colon cancers among patients with ulcerative colitis, and that risk of these cancers increases in association with disease duration[4-6]. For the most part the development of malignancies in ulcerative colitis has been assessed in association with symptomatic evidence of active disease[4-6]. The relationship of malignancy development to actual inflammation, as measured by inflammatory activity markers rather than clinical indicators, has not been clearly addressed.

In recent years there has been a resurgence of interest in the incidence of colonic carcinoma in Crohn's disease, mainly generated from reports of lymphomas and other cancers resulting from treatment with the newer immunomodulators[7,8]. The results of several studies on this topic suggest that the increased incidence of colonic cancer formation among patients with Crohn's disease is roughly equal to that of patients with ulcerative colitis[7,8]. One hypothesis for the increase in Crohn's disease-related cancers is that the availability of numerous immunomodulators and new therapeutics that obviate or postpone the need for surgery have extended the length of time that active, albeit subdued, inflamed regions remain *in vivo*. Another rather unlikely hypothesis is that the use of immunomodulators creates increased susceptibility to colon cancer formation.

Small bowel carcinomas are rare; however, it has been suggested that the incidence of these cancers is on the rise among patients with Crohn's disease[7]. It has been suggested that, in cases of disease with long duration, the natural history can change from being relatively quiescent to active and resistant to therapy, and that the incidence of small bowel carcinoma may increase. In a recent evaluation performed at Cedars-Sinai Medical Center, we noticed the incidence of three carcinomas from among 82 resection cases reviewed over the past 3 years. A review done at the University of Chicago has shown a similar incidence[9]. The Chicago data also suggest that a change in disease activity after a long duration, or a lack of response to therapy, may be associated with this outcome.

Despite several large studies reviewing the incidence of other lymphomas and extra-intestinal solid tumours in Crohn's disease versus a similarly matched population, conclusive evidence of increased incidence has never been presented (reviewed in ref. 10). Several studies have addressed whether there is an increased incidence of lymphoma and leukaemia in patients with Crohn's disease or ulcerative colitis. A report by Greenstein *et al.* and several recent studies by other groups, have generated conflicting data, with some suggesting an increased incidence and others showing no difference[10,11]. Problems with either a sample size or analytical approaches have prevented any study demonstrating an increased incidence[10] with a confidence interval level lower than >1.

The relationship of 'traditional' immunomodulators to the increased incidence of gastrointestinal or other malignancies has been discussed in the previous chapter. To summarize for the purposes of this chapter, it is clear that the use of azathioprine, 6-MP, or cyclosporin does not increase the incidence of lymphomas; however, there have been reported incidences of two atypical lymphomas related to the use of 6-MP. There is probably an increase in colonic as well as small bowel carcinoma in Crohn's disease; however, the use of these immunomodulators does not appear to be a causal factor.

IMMUNOMODULATORY MECHANISMS OF ANTI-TNF MODALITIES

TNF-α is a pleiotropic protein with a broad spectrum of functions within the immune system (reviewed in ref. 12). TNF-α may have differential effects depending upon whether it is locally produced in the mucosa or circulating systemically. TNF-α has a critical role in the host's protection from infectious agents. TNF-α was so named because it has been suggested that it may play a major role in the elimination of solid tumours. Thus, as with most single molecules in the immune system, there is a great deal of redundancy in the functions of TNF-α; thus its total elimination may not allow the host to be particularly susceptible to cancer formation. By contrast, total elimination of TNF-α in animal models causes these animals to be susceptible to intracellular pathogens;

however, none of these models appears to develop an increased incidence of malignancy and/or autoimmunity[13,14].

The development of anti-TNF-α modalities, particularly monoclonal antibodies, has allowed a study of the effects of TNF-α elimination on modulation of the immune system. Other broader immune modulators that inhibit T-cell and/or B-cell functions, such as the thiopurines and/or cyclosporin, the anti-TNF should have a more specific profile of inhibition. Chronic elimination of TNF-α can be achieved in experimental animals by molecular technology; at present in humans TNF-α blockade is generally accomplished by genetic manipulation and antibody technology, and this effect is transient[1]. Thus the effects of chronic absence of TNF-α in humans are unknown.

An interesting observation is that administration of anti-TNF-α monoclonal antibodies to humans has demonstrated differential effects at the site of inflammation as compared to the systemic immune compartment. In the mucosal immune compartment, studies performed in parallel with trials of anti-TNF-α in rheumatoid arthritis and Crohn's disease have reported different changes in the immune system[15–17]. Anti-TNF-α appears to inhibit T-helper-1 (Th1) responses in the mucosa while increasing the number of circulating cells with a Th1 phenotype[15]. There is not total elimination of Th1 responses; rather the Th1 response in inflamed mucosa is normalized to that which is seen in uninflamed tissues[15]. The increased number of circulating cells that potentially can produce Th1 cytokines may suggest an alteration in trafficking to the mucosa[15,16].

Other studies performed in parallel to clinical trials of anti-TNF-α have demonstrated a decrease in expression of adhesion molecules such as ICAM-1 in the mucosa without evidence of any alterations in the lymph nodes. T-cell activation in the mucosa appears to decrease, and studies have shown a possibility of decreased in NF-κB activation (reviewed in ref. 12). The fact that antibodies to TNF-α do not eliminate the potential for production of the molecule by T cells is consistent with the observation that, in general, there is not an increased incidence of severe infections in these patients[15,17]. Finally, it is apparent that, within the mucosal immune compartment, the presence of even small amounts of TNF-α has a critical role in the regulation of gamma-interferon (IFN-γ) production by Th1 T cells[17]. This rather limited down-regulation of immune responses induced by anti-TNF-α modalities suggests that the incidence of malignancies related to anti-TNF-α therapy, including solid tumours and/or lymphomas, would not be increased in Crohn's disease.

MALIGNANCY IN CROHN'S DISEASE FOLLOWING ANTI-TNF-α THERAPY

Over 30 000 US patients with Crohn's disease have been treated with at least one infusion of anti-TNF-α. The follow-up period has been relatively short (under 2 years). Anti-TNF-α was approved for acute therapy, yet many physicians are employing these agents in various ways (see Chapter 21). Given that a single infusion of anti-TNF-α may have limited down-regulatory effects (see above) this prevents a comparison with chronic elimination of TNF-α by repeated infusions. Some patients are undergoing treatment with anti-TNF-α as often as every month, and often prior to evidence of disease flares. Thus, the different regimens of treating patients with anti-TNF-α may relate to any reports of increased tumour incidence. As more patients are treated for longer periods with total elimination of anti-TNF-α, we may begin to see an increased incidence. Furthermore, the reporting system of the onset of these malignancies will be very dependent upon the individual physicians. At present there is a treatment registry being established by Centocor Inc., the producer of infliximab (Remicade™), and that will aid in assessing incidence.

No relationship has been established between anti-TNF-α monoclonal antibody therapy and the increased incidence of solid tumours, including colon carcinoma. However, we have recently observed a series of patients who have developed small bowel or colonic adenocarcinomas or squamous cell rectal tumours after several infusions of anti-TNF-α (Kam L *et al.*, unpublished). Most of these patients developed their tumours after several infusions of anti-TNF-α with time intervals of initiation of therapy to diagnosis of lesions of 5–19 months. Whether the effect of anti-TNF-α therapy on the development of tumours was to initiate the onset or accelerate their courses cannot be determined. Furthermore, whether this number of tumours is greater than the incidence of such tumours in patients with chronic Crohn's disease cannot be determined in this cohort.

There is, however, the suggestion of an increased incidence of atypical lymphomas related to the use of anti-TNF-α therapy for Crohn's disease. One patient of the 200 initially treated with anti-TNF-α developed a tumour[10]. This patient had a 30-year history of Crohn's disease treated with azathioprine and prednisone[10]. To that initial report two additional patients were reported by Bickston *et al.*[10]. One of these patients, 62 years of age, with Crohn's disease also for 30 years and treated with azathioprine and prednisone, developed lymphoma 7 months after the last infusion (Table 1). In another report a 29-year-old patient with a 4-year history of Crohn's disease treated with azathioprine, prednisone, 5-ASA derivatives and metronidazole, developed lymphoma after a single infusion, although it is unlikely that the lymphoma was related to the infusion (Table 1).

A patient followed at our centre, a 52-year-old man with a 28-year history of ileocolonic Crohn's disease complicated by complex perianal fistulas, developed Hodgkin-type lymphoma after multiple infusions of anti-TNF-α (Table 1). This patient had particularly refractory disease and underwent numerous surgical procedures for bowel obstructions and excision of fistulas. Early in his course he underwent ileal resection twice for partial small bowel obstructive symptoms. He developed peripheral neuropathy from metronidazole, leaving him with permanent residual bilateral lower extremity numbness and tingling. Since 1980 he had been maintained on prednisone and therapy with 6-MP and various 5-ASA derivatives, which provided incomplete benefit. In 1994 he participated in an anti-TNF-α receptor (rhu TNFR:Fc) trial and experienced decreased fistula drainage and closure of some fistulas. Once the trial was over his disease gradually worsened and was unresponsive to the available therapeutic options. In August of 1995 he received infliximab as part of a clinical trial, and experienced a dramatic improvement in symptoms. At 6 weeks post-infusion symptoms began to return. He subsequently received four additional 10 mg/kg doses of infliximab in November 1995 and in January, February and April 1996.

Table 1 Reported cases of lymphoma in Crohn's disease patients treated with infliximab

Reported cases	Type and location of lymphoma	Type of CD	Age (years) and gender	Disease duration (years)	Prior or concomitant immuno-suppressive therapy	Infliximab exposure		Time to diagnosis of lymphoma	
						Total number of infusions	Dose per infusion (mg/kg)	From first infusion	From last infusion
Rutgeerts et al.[3]	Intravascular duodenal B-cell non-Hodgkin's lymphoma	Unknown	61 male	30	Azathioprine, prednisone	1	10	9.5 months	9.5 months
Bickston et al.[10]	Intravascular large B-cell non-Hodgkin's lymphoma in ileal polyp and paratracheal lymph nodes	Ileocolonic perianal fistulas	62 male	30	Azathioprine, prednisone	1	10	9 months	9
Bickston et al.[10]	Nodular sclerosing Hodgkin's lymphoma in cervical, mediastinal, and thoracic lymph nodes	Ileal perianal fistulas	29 male	4	Prednisone	1	5	2 weeks	2 weeks
Current case	Nodular sclerosing Hodgkin's lymphoma in bilateral inguinal lymph nodes	Ileocolonic perianal fistulas	52 male	28	6-Mercaptopurine, anti-TNF-α receptor, prednisone, mycophenolate, thalidomide	9	5–20	4 years 7 months	12 months

The symptoms slowly returned following completion of the trial. Mycophenolate was added in place of 6-MP for approximately 7 months, without significant improvement. Due to persistent symptoms he participated in a pre-commercial release extension trial of infliximab, receiving three further 5 mg/kg infusions in August, September and October 1998. Following commercial release of infliximab he received his next and last infusion in March 1999. The degree of improvement was not as dramatic as his initial response had been. He was then treated with thalidomide for approximately 4 months, with partial but incomplete improvement in symptoms. An enlarged non-tender 2 cm left inguinal node was noted incidentally on a physical examination in March 2000. He had smoked $1\frac{1}{2}$ packs of cigarettes per day for 23 years. His medical history was otherwise unremarkable. His family history was negative for IBD and lymphoma and significant only for prostate cancer. The patient was referred for a left inguinal lymphadenectomy. A single firm lymph node ($3.0 \times 2.5 \times 1.5$ cm in greatest dimensions) was excised. The morphological and immunophenotypic findings were diagnostic of Hodgkin's lymphoma, classical type. The presence of lacunar cells and thin fibrous bands favoured a cellular phase of nodular sclerosing Hodgkin's lymphoma. Bone marrow examination revealed no evidence of lymphoma. Computerized tomography (CT) scans of the chest, abdomen and pelvis revealed no significant hilar, mediastinal, axillary, retroperitoneal or mesenteric lymphadenopathy. Liver and spleen were normal. Positron emission tomography (PET) scan with fluorodeoxyglucose revealed focal areas of increased activity in the left groin and in the right groin, consistent with neoplastic involvement. Ileocolonoscopy revealed no endoscopic inflammation. He was started on a regimen of ABVD (adriamycin, bleomycin, vincristine and dacarbazine) and has tolerated the treatment regimen well so far.

Thus, of these few reported cases, only three appear to be related to anti-TNF-α treatment, in a population of over 30 000 treated patients, and only the case reported occurred following multiple infusions. As stated above, the true incidence of lymphoma among those patients treated with multiple infusions is yet to be determined. The mechanisms of elimination of TNF-α in human studies reported above are based upon the effects after a single infusion. Any additional changes resulting from more expansive or total anti-TNF-α blockade, which may accompany multiple infusions, remains to be assessed.

Thus, the incidence of gastrointestinal tumours and lymphoma related to anti-TNF-α therapy must be closely monitored over the next several years as more and more patients undergo multiple infusions and are treated for longer periods of time. The database established by Centocor Inc. will allow us to study any increased incidence at an early time-point, and determine the parameters related to this increase. Correlation of patient profiles and their treatment regimens will help us to predict those who may be most susceptible to malignancy from administration of these very potent therapeutic modalities.

References

1. Targan SR, Hanauer SB, van Deventer SJ *et al*. Crohn's Disease cA2 Study Group. A short-term study of chimeric monoclonal antibody cA2 to tumor necrosis factor alpha for Crohn's disease. N Engl J Med. 1997;337:1029–35.

2. Present DH, Rutgeerts P, Targan S *et al*. Infliximab for the treatment of fistulas in patients with Crohn's disease. N Engl J Med. 1999;340:1398–405.
3. Rutgeerts P, D'Haens G, Targan S *et al*. Efficacy and safety of retreatment with anti-tumor necrosis factor antibody (infliximab) to maintain remission in Crohn's disease. Gastroenterology. 1999;117:761–9.
4. Goldman H. Significance and detection of dysplasia in chronic colitis. Cancer. 1996;78:2261–3.
5. Bansal P, Sonnenberg A. Risk factors of colorectal cancer in inflammatory bowel disease. Am J Gastroenterol. 1996;91:44–8.
6. Langholz E, Munkholm P, Davidsen M, Binder V. Colorectal cancer risk and mortality in patients with ulcerative colitis. Gastroenterology. 1992;103:1444–51.
7. Choi PM, Kim WH. Colon cancer surveillance. Gastroenterol Clin N Am. 1995;24:671–87.
8. Sachar DB. Cancer in Crohn's disease: dispelling the myths. Gut. 1994;35:1507–8.
9. Ruben DT, Mc Verry B, Hanauer SB. Small bowel cancer in Crohn's disease: the University of Chicago Experience. Gastroenterology. 2000;118:A757.
10. Bickston SJ, Lichtenstein GR, Arseneau KO, Cohen RB, Cominelli F. The relationship between infliximab treatment and lymphoma in Crohn's disease. Gastroenterology. 1999;117:1433–7.
11. Greenstein AJ, Gennuso R, Sachar DB *et al*. Extraintestinal cancers in inflammatory bowel disease. Cancer. 1985;56:2914–21.
12. Papadakis KA, Targan SR. Tumor necrosis factor: biology and therapeutic inhibitors. Gastroenterology. 2000;199 (In press).
13. Erickson BL, de Sauvage FK, Kikly K *et al*. Decreased sensitivity to tumour necrosis factor but normal T-cell development in TNF receptor-2-deficient mice. Nature. 1994:372:560–3.
14. Mittrucker HW, Pfeffer K, Schmits R, Mak TW. T-lymphocyte development and function in gene-targeted mutant mice. Immunol Rev. 1995;148:115–50.
15. Plevy SE, Landers CJ, Prehn J *et al*. A role for TNF-alpha and mucosal T helper-1 cytokines in the pathogenesis of Crohn's disease. J Immunol. 1997;159:6276–82.
16. Feldmann M, Elliott MJ, Woody JN, Maini RN. Anti-tumor necrosis factor-α therapy of rheumatoid arthritis. Adv Immunol. 1997;64:283–350.
17. Prehn J, Landers CJ, Targan SR. A soluble factor produced by lamina propria mononuclear cells is required for TNF-alpha enhancement of IFN-gamma production by T-cells. J Immunol. 1999;163:4277–83.

Section X
Consensus on immunosuppressive therapy

31
The use of immunosuppressors in active ulcerative colitis

M. CAMPIERI

CONSENSUS MEETING

The management of severe attacks of ulcerative colitis has for many years involved using the intensive intravenous regimen suggested by Truelove and Jewell. This approach has proved to be satisfactory in approximately 60% of patients for remission and in a further 15–20% for improvement[1]. The approach has the great advantage of establishing the time for surgery, and avoiding the side-effects of excessively long-term treatment with steroids.

The issues raised by this Consensus Conference are:

1. is there any role for immunosuppression in managing active disease? and, if so:
2. which immunosuppressor should be used?
3. in what dosage and for how long?
4. is the association necessary?
5. possible toxicity.

THE ROLE OF IMMUNOSUPPRESSION IN ACTIVE SEVERE ULCERATIVE COLITIS

The first question is: why should immunosuppressors be used in active colitis? There has been a substantial debate regarding the purposes for which they have been used. Some speakers suggested that they should be used to 'save the colon', but the majority of those attending the meeting proposed that the point is not salvage of the colon, but the overall improved condition of patients. This is actually the best answer, because the main purpose of treatment is to maintain a patient in the best condition with or without the colon!

The aim of treatment is to discover the best approach to treating those patients not responding to an intensive intravenous treatment regimen within a maximum of 10 days. In these situations use of a continuous intravenous infusion of Cyclosporin A (CyA) has been suggested. In the initial study by Lichtiger and

Present 4 mg/kg daily was suggested for a period of 10–15 days[2]. Results in the short term consist of avoiding surgery in approximately 60–80% immediately, and in the long term these figures tend to decrease to 30–40% over subsequent years[3].

Other groups have tried using lower dosages such as 2 mg/kg per day, also with positive results. Therefore it is necessary to establish the best dosage, and whether smaller dosages could be just as effective[4]. A trial is needed in this regard. It now seems that the best regimen is to amalgamate the 5-day regimen and CyA.

Other researchers have tried to use CyA as first-line treatment in patients with severe attacks of ulcerative colitis. The results are encouraging; however, a conspicuous number of side-effects have been reported[5].

Steroids can also be considered to be immunosuppressors, though their activity is mainly anti-inflammatory. We can also analyse other immunosuppressive drugs; e.g.: azathioprine (AZA) or 6-mercaptopurine (6-MP), mycofenolate, methotrexate (MTX), tacrolimus, and anti-tumour necrosis factor (anti-TNF). While we can show an unproven role for MTX and tacrolimus, the role of anti-TNF is not yet proven, and needs to be tested in clinical trials. The roles of CyA, AZA and 6-MP also remain to be proven[6].

THE ROLE OF CyA

Second choice or first choice? Traditionally the original studies pointed out the utility of using CyA if the patient does not show a clear-cut response when using only steroids, in patients having a severe attack. As regards the period of treatment, this should be approximately 2 weeks, but the main problem is whether it is better to continue with oral CyA, or to add, or substitute, another immunosuppressor such as AZA. In retrospective studies it has been documented that, when patients are receiving AZA over the long term, the percentage improvement is more than 30% and a success rate of approximately 50% can be attained over the following year[7].

There is still controversy concerning whether to add AZA at the beginning of a trial, during CyA treatment, or later. This problem needs to be answered by a prospective clinical trial.

There is consensus concerning the fact that CyA should be avoided when the level of creatinine is higher than normal, in hypertensive patients, during pregnancy, if there is a toxic megacolon, or in the case of severe infection. On this latter point many authors recommend treatment with antibiotics.

LATEST DATA CONCERNING THE ROLE OF CyA ENEMAS

Several annecdotal results have reported a trend towards a presuntive effect, but an uncontrolled trial showed no efficacy. The problem is whether some additives might have contributed to clinical inefficacy[8], since larger uncontrolled studies have shown trends towards a benefical effect[9].

CONCLUSIONS

To date the main use of immunosuppression concerns the role of CyA. The problem which needs a definite answer is whether CyA should be tested in addition to AZA. From retrospective studies it seems that when CyA is used in conjunction with AZA the results are better, but we also need to know whether the addition of AZA immediately after a course of CyA adds more benefits.

References

1. Truelove SC, Jewell DP. Intensive intravenous regimen for severe attacks of ulcerative colitis. Lancet. 1974;1:1067–70.
2. Lightiger S, Present D, Kornbluth A *et al*. Cyclosporine in severe ulcerative colitis refractory to steroid therapy. N Engl J Med. 1994;330:1841–5.
3. Hanauer SB, Baert FJ. The management of ulcerative colitis. Annu Rev Med. 1995;46:497–505.
4. Actis GC, Ottobrelli A, Pera A *et al*. Continuously infused cyclosporine at low dose is sufficient to avoid emergency colectomy in acute attacks of ulcerative colitis without the need for high-dose steroids. J Clin Gastroenterol. 1993;17:10–13.
5. D'Haens G, Suenaert P, Westhovens R, Rutgeerts P. Severe knee pain as the single symptom of CMV infection in acute ulcerative colitis treated with cyclosporin. Inflamm Bowel Dis. 1998;4:27–8.
6. Sandborn WJ. A review of immune modifier therapy for inflammatory bowel diseases: azathioprine, 6-mercaptopurine, cyclosporine, and methotrexate. Am J Gastroenterol. 1996;91:423–33.
7. Kombluth A, Present DH, Lichtiger S, Hanauer S. Cyclosporin for severe ulcerative colitis: a user's guide. Am J Gastroenterol. 1997;92:1424–8.
8. Sandborn WJ, Tremaine ZS, Schroeder KW *et al*. A placebo-controlled trial of cyclosporine enemas for mildly to moderately active left-sided ulcerative colitis. Gastroenterology. 1994;106:1429–35.
9. Winter TA, Dalton HR, Merret MN *et al*. Cyclosporin A retention enema in refractory distal ulcerative colitis and pouchitis. Scand J Gastroenterol. 1993;28:701–4.

32
Consensus on immunosuppressive therapy for ulcerative colitis: chronic active disease

D. B. SACHAR

The first question to address concerning immunosuppressive management of chronic active ulcerative colitis is what needs to be done *before* such treatment is even considered. Two preliminary steps are essential: (1) ruling out superinfection and (2) ruling out neuromotor or irritable bowel-type symptoms as the cause of the patient's complaints.

Once ulcerative colitis *per se* is clearly identified as the source of symptoms, the next step before turning to immunosuppressives is to make sure that conventional aminosalicylate therapy has been optimized. By optimization we refer to the following three considerations:

1. *Dose*. The efficacy of the aminosalicylates is almost strictly dose-related[1-3], so that no case of ulcerative colitis should be considered 'refractory' to this therapy until administration of a daily dose of at least 4.8 g (with doses up to 6 g/day currently under study).
2. *Delivery*. Medication that is prescribed is not always taken; it is therefore important to assure adherence to the prescribed regimen before it is abandoned. Moreover, the benefits of therapy with rectal 5-ASA should not be overlooked, neither for distal[4-6] nor even extensive[7] colitis.
3. *Duration*. We often fail to emphasize sufficiently to our patients the importance of oral *and* rectal 5-ASA as long-term maintenance therapies[4,5,7-9].

If aminosalicylate therapy has been optimized, but ulcerative colitis continues to relapse or to require corticosteroids for control, it is at this point that immunosuppressive treatment is clearly indicated.[10-13] What should be our management guidelines *during* immunosuppressive treatment? There are two main guiding principles. First is to start early, preferably no later than the first manifestation of steroid dependency; that is, for any relapse occurring during or soon after any course of steroid therapy, or even without waiting for relapse following any severe attack requiring hospitalization. The second guiding principle for immunosuppression is to optimize its benefits by dint of adequate dose and sufficient duration of therapy. Our specific dose recommendations are the same as for Crohn's disease. We wish also to re-emphasize the importance of not declaring azathioprine or 6-MP a failure before at least 3–4 months at maximum dose levels, as defined primarily by leukopenia or, in cases of uncertainty, by measurements of 6-TG and 6-MMP metabolite levels.

Likewise, our recommendations for duration of therapy parallel those for Crohn's disease, with stress upon the value of immunosuppressives for long-term maintenance of remission[14–16]. There appears to be no contraindication (and some theoretical albeit unproven benefit) to the continuation of 5-ASA therapy concomitant with 6-MP or azathioprine; if patients find it difficult, however, to sustain this combination, discontinuation of the 5-ASA drug should not be prohibited so long as the antimetabolite is rigorously maintained. Finally, we wish to reemphasize the importance of *not* discontinuing azathioprine or 6-MP during pregnancy, especially in women whose clinical history indicates a compelling need for these treatments to maintain remission.

Let us now suppose, however, that despite careful adherence to all the guidelines outlined above, immunosuppressive treatment with 6-MP or azathioprine has not been tolerated, or has not been effective in maintaining remission. What further steps remain *after* full-fledged trials of this therapy? We do not believe that present evidence permits recommendation of methotrexate treatment in ulcerative colitis, although thoroughly informed and determined patients might reasonably be granted such a trial. In our present state of knowledge, though, there is even less justification for encouraging the clinical use of any other advanced therapies for management of chronic active colitis, including cyclosporin, mycophenolate mofetil, anti-TNF agents, or other 'emerging' biologicals.

At this point we must recognize the rehabilitating, if not totally curative value of colectomy, whether performed with Brooke ileostomy, continent Kock ileostomy, or pelvic ileal pouch and ileoanal anastomosis. The top priority in the management of ulcerative colitis (and, for that matter, Crohn's disease as well) is *not* the avoidance of surgery, but rather the restoration and maintenance of good health. In this respect the patient's welfare surely outranks the physician's prejudices!

References

1. Hanauer S. An oral preparation of mesalamine as long-term maintenance therapy for ulcerative colitis. Ann Intern Med. 1996;124:204–11.
2. Travis SPL, Tysk C, Jârnerot G, Jewell DP. A dose-ranging study of olsalazine in ulcerative colitis. Gut. 1992;33:546–9.
3. Giaffer H, Holdsworth CD, Lennard-Jones JE *et al*. Improved maintenance of remission in ulcerative colitis by balsalazide 4 G/day compared to 2 G/d. Aliment Pharmacol Ther. 1992;6:479–85.
4. Cohen RD, Woseth DM, Thisted RA, Hanauer SB. A meta-analysis and overview of the literature on treatment options for left-sided ulcerative colitis and ulcerative proctitis. Am J Gastroenterol. 2000;95:1263–76.
5. D'Albasio G, Paoluzi P, Campieri M *et al*. Maintenance treatment of ulcerative proctitis with mesalazine suppositories. Am J Gastroenterol. 1998;93:799–803.
6. Safdi M, DeMicco M, Sninsky C *et al*. A double-blind comparison of oral versus rectal versus combination therapy in the treatment of distal ulcerative colitis. Am J Gastroenterol. 1997; 92:1867–71.
7. D'Albasio G, Pacini F, Camarri E *et al*. Combined therapy with 5-aminosalicylic acid tablets and enemas for maintaining remission in ulcerative colitis. Am J Gastroenterol. 1997;92:1143–7.

8. Marshall JK, Irvine EJ. Rectal aminosalicylate (ASA) therapy for distal ulcerative colitis. Aliment Pharmacol Ther. 1995;9:293–300.
9. Sachar DB. Maintenance therapy in ulcerative colitis and Crohn's disease. J Clin Gastroenterol. 1995;20:117–22.
10. Lobo AJ, Foster PN, Burke D *et al*. The role of azathioprine in the management of ulcerative colitis. Dis Colon Rectum. 1990;33:374–7.
11. Adler DJ, Korelitz BI. The therapeutic efficacy of 6-mercaptopurine in refractory ulcerative colitis. Am J Gastroenterol. 1990;85:717–22.
12. Kirk AP, Lennard-Jones JE. Controlled trial of azathioprine in chronic ulcerative colitis. Br Med J. 1982;284:1291–2.
13. Rosenberg JL, Wall AJ, Settles RH, Binder HJ, Levin B, Kirsner JB. A controlled trial of azathioprine in the treatment of chronic ulcerative colitis. Gastroenterology. 1973;64:973–801.
14. Fraser AG, Jewell DP. Relapse rate on and after stopping azathioprine treatment for inflammatory bowel disease. Gastroenterology. 2000;118:A786 (abstract).
15. George J, Present DH, Pou R *et al*. The long-term outcome of ulcerative colitis treated with 6-mercaptopurine. Am J Gastroenterol. 1996;91:1711–14.
16. Hawthorne AB, Logan RFA, Hawkey CJ *et al*. Randomized controlled trial of azathioprine withdrawal in ulcerative colitis. Br Med J. 1992;305:20–2.

Index

Page numbers in italics refer to figures

abortion   22, *208*, 209, *210*
absorption problems, cyclosporin   156
acetylsalicylic acid (5-ASA)   120, 222
activation function   1 (AF1)   55
activation markers, lamina propria   27
acute disease   101–4, 144–5
Adler, DJ   107
administration route   70–5, 124, 149–51, 246
adolescents   213–19
adrenocorticotrophic hormone (ACTH)   72
adverse events   120–1, 140, *140*
   see also toxicity
AF1 *see* activation function   1
Ahmad, T   68–87
allergic-type reactions   97
allopurinol   38
American College of Gastroenterology   49
5-aminosalicylates (5-ASAs)
   compliance   68–9
   Crohn's disease   74
   distal colitis   70, 73
   extensive ulcerative colitis   71–2
   optimal delivery   70–5, 246
   pregnancy   209
   response/intolerance   77–8
Andus, T   225–32
animal studies   27, 180, 200, 209
anti-interleukin-12 therapy   191–6, *193, 195*
anti-tumour necrosis factor alpha therapy
   163–76, 219, 233–8
antigen-presenting cell (APC)   18
antigens   18, 20–2, *20*, 27
antiproliferative effects   113–14
antisense to ICAM-1 *see* ISIS   2302
APC *see* antigen-presenting cell
apoptosis, T cells   191–6, *193, 195*
Arora, S   123, 124
arthritis   113, 116, *116*, 222–3, 230–1

5-ASAs *see* 5-acetylsalicylates;
      5-aminosalicylates
Ashkenazi Jewish population   3
autoimmune diseases   113, 116, *116*, 119–21,
      163, 230–1
axial spondylarthropathy   223
azathioprine (AZA)   38–42, 51
   children/adolescents   214–15
   controlled trials   108–9
   Crohn's disease   101–4
   limitations in therapy   75–6
   malignancy   *230*
   metabolism   91–2, *92*
   mycophenylate mofetil comparison   135,
      137–41
   pharmacology   91–8
   pregnancy   209, 210
   6-thioguanine nucleotides monitoring   95–7,
      96, 97
   toxicology   97–8
   ulcerative colitis   106–10
   uncontrolled trials   107–8, *108*

B cells, lamina propria   25, 31–2
bacterial flora   11–17
balsalazide   73
Baron, TH   *128*
Berin, MC   20
blood levels, cyclosporin   156–8
blood urea nitrogen (BUN)   160
Boirivant, M   191–6
Brandeis, JM   20
Brynskov, J   149–54
Budenofalk   74
BUN *see* blood urea nitrogen

C-reactive protein   172
cancer *see* malignancy

caspase-8 (FLICE)   192, *193*
CBP *see* CREB-binding protein
CD4$^+$ T cells   27, 28, 191, 197, 200, 202
CD25-positive cells   198–9
CDAI *see* Crohn's Disease Activity Index
CDP571 humanized anti-TNF alpha antibody
        165–6, 173–4, *174*
cell cycle   91
cellular anti-IL-12 mechanisms   191–6, *193*,
        195
chemokines   19, *19*
children   103, *103*, 172, 213–19
chimaeric monoclonal anti-tumour necrosis
        factor antibody *see* infliximab
Cho, JU   7–8
chromosome 6, TNF alpha gene   164
chromosome 6 (HLA region, IBD 3)   6–7
chromosome 8p22-p23   12
chromosome 12q13 (IBD 2)   5–6
chromosome 14 (IBD 4)   5, 7
chromosome 16 (IBD 1)   5
'chronic active disease' definitions   47–53
cohort studies   225–30, *227, 228*
colectomy   155–6, 160
colon cancer   233–4, 236
colorectal cancer   226–7, *227*, 229, *229*
combination therapies   70–1, 115, *115*, 166
compliance   68–9
consensus, immunosuppression   243–7
corticosteroids
    active Crohn's disease   74–5
    active distal ulcerative colitis   70–1
    children/adolescents   213, 214, 215
    compliance   69
    extensive ulcerative colitis   71–2
    host response/intolerance   78–9
    NF-κB activation *187*
corticotropin-releasing hormone (CRH)
        promoter   58, *59*
CREB-binding protein (CBP)   59
CRH *see* corticotropin-releasing hormone
        promoter
Crohn's and Colitis Foundation of America
        37, 38
Crohn's disease
    anti-TNF alpha therapy, malignancy   233–8
    AZA/6-MP   101–4
    children   213–19
    colorectal cancer *227*
    corticosteroids/salicylates   74–5
    cyclosporin   149–52
    etanercept   174–5
    glucocorticoids   119
    humanized anti-TNF antibody CDP571
        173–4, *174*
    infliximab   166, 170–5
    ISIS   2302 181–2
    lamina propria   28, *29*, 31

lymphoma   228, *228*, 229–30, *230, 237*
    methotrexate therapy   119–26
    mycophenylate mofetil   137–41
    NF-κB transcription factor   185–9, *186–7*
    pregnancy   116, 121, 207–11, *208*
    remission maintenance   75, 103–4, 121–2,
        122
    small bowel cancer   227
    steroid responses   *49, 50*
    steroid-refractory chronic   47–53, *48*
    tacrolimus/FK-506   152
    TNF alpha inhibition   163–7, 170–5
Crohn's Disease Activity Index (CDAI)   38,
        50, 51
    CDP571 humanized anti-TNF antibody
        173–4, *174*, 175
    infliximab in Crohn's disease   170, 171
    ISIS   2302 181
    mycophenylate mofetil in Crohn's disease
        137, 138, *139*
cryptopatches   25
Cryptosporidium parvum   11, 14
cyclosporin   50
    absorption problems   156
    blood levels   156–8
    children/adolescents   215, 217–18
    consensus on treatment   243–4
    Crohn's disease   149–52
    intravenous   39–40
    mechanism of action   155
    patient selection   155–6
    pregnancy   210
    ulcerative colitis   158–60
cytokine-IgG fusion proteins   198
cytokines   42
    anti-interleukin-12 therapy   191–6, *193, 195*
    anti-TNF alpha therapy, malignancy in
        Crohn's disease   233–8
    anti-TNF antibodies   163–76
    glucocorticoid downregulation   54
    ICAM-1 induction   179–84
    interleukin-2-related strategies   197–202
    intestinal epithelial cells   18, 19, *19*
    lamina propria   27, 28, *29, 30*, 31
    methotrexate effects   114, *114*
    NF-κB activation   185–9, *186–7*

DBD *see* DNA-binding site
death-induced signalling complex (DISC)
        192, *193*, 194
defensins   11–12
dexamethasone, GR regulation   61
D'Haens, G   222–4
DHFR *see* dihydrofolate reductase
Dignass, AU   207–12
dihydrofolate *113*
dihydrofolate reductase (DHFR)   80, 113, 119
diphtheria toxin   198–9

INDEX

DISC *see* death-induced signalling complex
distal disease   70–3, *73*
dizygotic twins   3
DNA   80, 91, 133, 141
  see also NF-[k]B
  transcription   58–60, *58*, *59*, 164–5
  translation   164–5
DNA-binding site (DBD)   56, 57
dosage   70–5, 246
Duchmann, R   25–35
duration of therapy   246–7

efficacy   95–7, *96*, *97*, 180–1, 214
Egan, LJ   *128*
EIM *see* extraintestinal manifestations
EN *see* erythema nodosum
enemas *see* rectal therapy
enteric β-defensin   12
enterobacteria   28
enterogenic spondyloarthropathy   28
epidemiology   3
erythema nodosum (EN)   223
erythrocyte 6-thioguanine nucleotide
  concentrations   95–7, *96*, *97*
Escherichia coli   12, 31
etanercept   166, 174–5
evidence-based standards   39, 106–10
experimental mucosal inflammation   191
extensive disease   71–2
extraintestinal manifestations (EIM)   222–4

FADD *see* Fas-associated death-domain-
  containing protein
Fas ligands   192, *193*, 194
Fas-associated death-domain-containing protein
  (FADD)   192, *193*
Feagan, BG   119–27
Fellermann, K   133–6, 144–5
fetal malformations   *208*, 209, *210*
fistulas   38–9, 51–2, 236, *237*
  cyclosporin responses   151, *151*
  infliximab   172
  tacrolimus/FK-506   152
  TNF inhibitors   165
FK506 *see* tacrolimus
FLICE *see* caspase-8
folate analogues *see* methotrexate
folic acid   *117*
formulation, salicylates   70–5
Fuss, I   191–6

Gasche, C   47–53
gastrointestinal side-effects   116–17, *116*, 140,
  140
genetics   3–10
  defensins gene expression   12, 13–14
  glucocorticoid resistance   55
  GR gene regulation   60–1

linkage leading to gene identification   7–8
NF-κB gene activation   188
thiopurine methyltransferase genetic control
  92–5, *93*, *94*, *95*
TNF alpha gene transcription/translation
  164–5
genome-wide scanning   4–5, 8
George, J   107
German Society of Gastroenterology   48
Gilat, T   128–30
glucocorticoid receptor (GRβ)   54–5, 60, 62
glucocorticoid receptor (GR)   54–63, *56*, *57*
glucocorticoid response element (GRE)   57,
  57, 58, *58*
glucocorticoids   54, 55, 119
Gonella, PA   20
gp180 expression   22
GR *see* glucocorticoid receptor
GRß *see* glucocorticoid receptor β
GRE *see* glucocorticoid response element
guanosine nucleotides   133
guidelines, American College of
  Gastroenterology   48–9
gut epithelium   18–24

HACAs *see* human anti-chimaeric antibodies
Harder, J   14
Harvey–Bradshaw scores   122, 214, 219
Hawthorne, AB   109, 125
HBD-1 gene mRNA   13, 14
HBD-2 protein   13, 14
HD-5 *see* human defensin   5
HD-6 *see* human defensin   6
hepatotoxicity   97, *97*, 120, 125, 216, 217
hereditability *see* genetics
hirsuitism   218
HLA region   6–7
HNP *see* human neutrophil peptide
Hodgkin-type lymphoma   236, *237*, 238
host responses   77–80
HPRT *see* hypoxanthine
  phosphoribosyltransferase
hsp90 expression   60
human anti-chimaeric antibodies (HACAs)
  166
human defensin 5 (HD-5)   12, 13, 14
human defensin 6 (HD-6)   12, 13, 14
human neutrophil peptide (HNP)   11
humanized anti-TNF antibody CDP571
  173–4, *174*
Hyams, JS   219
hypersensitivity, infliximab   173
hypertrichosis   218
hypoxanthine phosphoribosyltransferase
  (HPRT)   *92*

IBD 1 *see* chromosome   16
IBD 2 *see* chromosome   12q13

IBD 3 *see* chromosome 6
IBD 4 *see* chromosome 14
IECs *see* intestinal epithelial cells
IFN *see* interferon
IL-2 *see* interleukin-2
immune response 11–24, *26*
immunomodulators *see* azathioprine;
    6-mercaptopurine
IMPDH *see* inosine monophosphate
    dehydrogenase
in situ hybridization 12
individualized treatments 80
inflammatory response 179–85, 191–6, *193*,
    195
    see also cytokines
infliximab 41, 51
    axial spondylarthropathy 223
    Crohn's disease 126, 166, 170–5
    lymphomas *237*, 238
    pregnancy 210–11
inosine monophosphate dehydrogenase
    (IMPDH) 133
intercellular adhesion molecule-1 (ICAM-1)
    179–84, 235
interferon-gamma 185, 197, 198–9
interleukins 186, *186*, *187*, 188, 197–202,
    201
intestinal epithelial cells (IECs) 19–22, *19*,
    21
intestinal immune system *26*
intolerance 77–80
intravenous cyclosporin 39–40, 151–2, *151*
ISIS 2302 180–3

Janowitz, Dr Henry 37
Jewell, DP 68–87

Kaplan–Meier analysis *123*, *139*
kidney transplantation *226*
Kirschner, BS 213–21
Korelitz, D 38, 39
Kozarek, RA 121, *128*
Kruglyak, L 5

lamina propria 25–35, *26*, *30*, 188
lamina propria T-cells (LP-T cells) 27, 192,
    193, *193*, 194
Lander, ES 5
LAP *see* lingual antimicrobial peptide
LBD *see* ligand binding domain
Lichtiger, S 155–60
ligand binding domain (LBD) 56
lingual antimicrobial peptide (LAP) 12
linkage analysis 4, 5, 7–8
lipopolysaccharide (LPS) 18
logarithm of odds (LOD) 5, 6
LP-T cells *see* lamina propria T cells
LPS *see* lipopolysaccharide

lymphomas 228, *228*, 229–30, *230*
    anti-TNF alpha therapy 233–4, 236, *237*,
    238
    infliximab *237*, 238
    non-Hodgkin's *226*

Ma, Y 7
McCabe, RP 171
McGovern, DPB 68–87
macrophage protein 2 (NRAMP2) 6
maintenance therapy *see* remission maintenance
malformations, fetal *208*, 209, *210*
malignancy 225–31, *226*, 233–8
Mallow, EB 13
Marion, JF 106–10, 173
Markowitz, JF 102, 214, 219
Marth, T 191–6
Mayer, L 18–24
mechanisms of action
    anti-interleukin-12 therapy 191–6, *193*, *195*
    AZA/6-MP 91
    cyclosporin 155
    methotrexate 113–17
medication
    see also individual drugs
    compliance 68–9
    host responses/intolerance 77–80
    individualising 80
    numbers needed to harm 73, *82*
    numbers needed to treat 73, *81*
    optimization 246–7
6-mercaptopurine (6-MP)
    children/adolescents 214–15
    compliance 69
    controlled trials 108–9
    Crohn's disease 101–4
    malignancy *230*, 233–4
    metabolism 91–2, *92*
    pharmacology 91–8
    pregnancy 209, *210*
    Present, DH 37–9, 40, 41, 42
    6-thioguanine nucleotides monitoring 95–7,
    96, *97*
    ulcerative colitis 106–10, *108*
mesalamine 41, 70–1
mesalazine enemas 73
metabolism 91–2
methotrexate 40–1
    adverse events 120–1
    children/adolescents 216–17
    compliance 69
    Crohn's disease 119–26
    dihydrofolate reductase 119
    dosage/route 76–7
    host responses/intolerance 80
    pharmacology 113–17, *113–17*, 119–21
    pregnancy 210
    renal impairment 120

standards 113–30
  structure *113*
  ulcerative colitis 124–5, 128–30
6-methylmercaptopurine 76, 95–8, *96*, *97*
microsatellites 4
MMF *see* mycophenylate mofetil
molecular mechanisms 191–6, *193*, *195*
molecular structures 55–7
molecular therapy 179–204
monitoring, AZA/6-MP 95–7, *96*, *97*
monoclonal antibody (mAB) 165, 198
monozygotic twins 3
Moshkowitz, M 128–30
MTX *see* methotrexate
mucosal immunity 18–24
Mycobacterium paratuberculosis 12
mycophenolic acid (MPA) 133
mycophenylate mofetil 133–45, *140*

National Cooperative Crohn's Disease Study
  (NCCDS) 38, 42, 52, 74
National Foundation for Ileitis and Colitis 37
NCCDS *see* National Cooperative Crohn's
  Disease Study
NCoR mutations 62
neoplasms *see* malignancy
Neurath, MF 185–90, 191–6
New England Journal of Medicine 40, 41
NF-κB transcription factor 13, 14
  anti-TNF alpha therapy 235
  glucocorticoid receptor 59, 62
  mechanism of action 185–9, *187*, *189*
NNH *see* numbers needed to harm
NNTs *see* numbers needed to treat
non-allergic-type reactions 97–8
non-Hodgkin's lymphoma *226*, *237*
North American Crohn's Study Group
  (NACSG) 121, 124
novel costimulatory molecules 22
NRAMP2 *see* macrophage protein 2
nuclear localization signal 56, *56*
nuclear receptor coactivators 61–2
nuclear receptor corepressors 61–2
numbers needed to harm (NNH) 73, *82*
numbers needed to treat (NNT) 73, *81*, 102

ocular problems 224
O'Neil, DA 14
oral medication 70, 149–50, *150*
Oren, R 102, 122, 124, 128–30

p55 TNF receptor (TNFRI) 164
p65 gene transcription 185–8, *186*, *187*
p75 TNF receptor (TNFRII) 164
P-glycoprotein 79
Paediatric Crohn's Disease Activity Index
  (PCDAI) 215, 217, 219
paediatrics 103, *103*, 172, 213–19

Paneth cells 12, 13
paraesthesias, cyclosporin 160
PCDAI *see* Paediatric Crohn's Disease Activity
  Index
PCR *see* polymerase chain reaction
peri-centromeric chromosome regions 5
peripheral arthritis 222–3
peripheral blood mononuclear cells (PBMNCs)
  61, 62
Petritsch, W 137–43
Peyer's patches 25, *26*
PG *see* pyoderma gangrenosum
pharmacokinetics 92, 134
pharmacology
  see also mechanisms of action
  azathioprine 91–8
  ISIS 2302 180
  6-mercaptopurine 91–8
  methotrexate 113–17, *113–17*, 119–21
  mycophenylate mofetil 133–5
phosphodiesterase inhibitors 165
phosphorothioate oligodeoxynucleotides *see*
  ISIS 2302
placenta 22
Pneumocystis carinii 108, 149, 159
polygenic diseases 4
polymerase chain reaction (PCR) analysis 12,
  13–14
POMC *see* pro-opiomelanocortin gene
post-translational processing 164–5
PPAR-gamma ligands *189*
predictors 172–3
prednisolone 72
prednisolone and methotrexate therapy 121–2,
  122, 123–4
pregnancy 116, 121, 207–11, *208*
Present, DH 37–43
prevalence studies 3
primary sclerosing cholangitis (PSC) 217, 224
pro-opiomelanocortin (POMC) gene 58, *59*
programmed cell death *see* apoptosis
proinflammatory cytokines *see* cytokines
protein kinases *186*
PSC *see* primary sclerosing cholangitis
Pseudomonas exotoxin RFT5(scFv)ETA′ 199
psoriasis 224
purine antimetabolites *see* azathioprine;
  6-mercaptopurine
pyoderma gangrenosum (PG) 223

receptor of advanced glycation end products
  (RAGE) 186, *187*
receptor expression 19, *19*
rectal therapy 70–3, *73*, 98, 244
recurrent spontaneous abortion 22
refractory disease mechanisms 54–67
Rel homology domain 185
RclA *see* p65

relapse probability *139*
remission induction   101–3, *103*, *139*, 181–2
remission maintenance
  Crohn's disease   75, 103–4, 121–2, *122*
  distal disease   72–3, *73*
  extensive disease   73–4
  methotrexate   123
renal impairment   120
renal transplantation   134–5
reporting systems   236
resistance   55, 173
  see also hypersensitivity; intolerance
response categories, steroids   47–51, *48, 49, 50*
responses *see* host responses
restriction elements   21–2, *21*
reverse transcriptase polymerase chain reaction
  (RT-PCR)   12, 13, 14
reviews   37–43
RFT5(scFv)ETA′ *Pseudomonas* exotoxin   199
rheumatoid arthritis   113, 116, *116*, 230–1
RNase H   179
Rogler, G   54–67
Rosenberg, JL   108
RT-PCR *see* reverse transcriptase polymerase
  chain reaction
Rutgeert's, P   171

Sachar, DB   246–8
safety *see* toxicity
salicylates *see* 5-acetylsalicylates;
  5-aminosalicylates
Sandborn, WJ   91–100
Sands, BE   170–6
Satsangi, J   3–10
Schnabel, A   113–17
SCID mice   200
serum metabolites   69
sibling pair analysis   4, 5, 6, 7
side-effects *see* toxicity
significant linkage   5, 6
Silman, AJ   230
single nucleotide polymorphisms (SNPs)   8
small bowel cancer   227, *228*
SMRT mutations   62
SNPs *see* single nucleotide polymorphisms
spondyloarthropathy, enterogenic   28
spontaneous abortion, recurrent   22
Stallmach, A   197–204
standard therapy limitations   68–87
standards   91–110, 113–30
Stange, EF   50
statistical analysis   4–5
steroids
  see also corticosteroids; glucocorticoid
    receptor
  dependence/resistance   47–53, *48–50*, 121,
    122, 173–4, *174*, 182–3
  methotrexate for UC   129, *129*

stillbirths   *208, 210*
Stokkers, PC   6
Strober, W   191–6
sulphapyridine   77–8
sulphasalazine   38, 69, 73, 115, *115, 186*,
  188
surface molecules   21, *21*
susceptibility genes   3, 4
Sutherland, LR   101–5
Swedish Twin Registry   3

T cell receptor β (TCRB)   28
T cells
  see also CD4⁺ T cells
  apoptosis   191–6, *193, 195*
  clones, expansion   28
  IECs   20, *20*, 21, *21*, 22
  lamina propria   25–32, *29, 30*
T-lymphocyte-mediated immune responses
  149
TACE *see* TNF alpha converting enzyme
tacrolimus   41, 42, 152, 210, 215, 218
TAP *see* tracheal anti-microbial peptide
Targan, SR   171, 233–9
TATA-binding protein (TBP)   58
TCRB *see* T cell receptor β
tetrahydrofolic acid (THF)   113–14
thalidomide   41, 51, 165, 218–19
THF *see* tetrathydrofolic acid
6-thioguanine nucleotides   95–7, *96, 97*, 215
thiopurine methyltransferase (TPMT)   79–80,
  92–5, *92, 93, 94, 95*
thiopurines   75–6, 79–80
Thornton, A   200
TNBS *see* 2,4,6-trinitro-benzene sulphonic acid
TNF alpha converting enzyme (TACE)   164,
  165
TNF receptor fusion protein *see* etanercept
TNFRI *see* p55 TNF receptor
TNFRII *see* p75 TNF receptor
topical therapy *see* rectal therapy
toxicity
  AZA/6-MP   97–8
  cyclosporin   149, 159–60, 217–18
  extraintestinal manifestations   222–4
  6-mercaptopurine/azathioprine   38–9
  methotrexate   113–17, *116*, 120–1, 216,
    217
  mycophenylate mofetil   140, *140*
  pregnancy   207–11
TPMT *see* thiopurine methyltransferase
tracheal anti-microbial peptide (TAP)   12
transactivation   55–6, *56, 57, 58*
transcription, DNA   58–60, *58, 59*, 164–5
transforming growth factor beta   197
translation, DNA   164–5
transplants   133, 134–5, *226*
transrepression   58–60, *58, 59, 59*

INDEX

2,4,6-trinitro-benzene sulphonic acid (TNBS)
    198, 199, 200, *201*
tumour necrosis factor (TNF)   41, 163–7
twin studies   3
Tysk, C   3

ulcerative colitis
   anti-TNF antibodies   175
   AZA/6-MP   106–10
   colorectal cancer   *227, 228*
   consensus   246–7
   cyclosporin   158–60
   ISIS   2302   182
   lamina propria *30*
   lymphoma   230, *230*
   methotrexate   124–5, 128–30
   mycophenylate mofetil   144–5

NF-κB transcription factor   185–9
   steroid-refractory chronic   47–53, *48*
uncontrolled studies   107–8, *128*, 151–2, *151,*
   152

Van Deventer, SJH   163–9
Vasiliauskas, EA   233–9
Vienna classification   51
vitamin D receptor gene   6

Wehkamp, J   11–17
World Congresses of Gastroenterology   48

Yacyshyn, BR   179–84

Zeitz, M   25–35
zinc finger domains   56, *56*

Falk Symposium Series

43. Reutter W, Popper H, Arias IM, Heinrich PC, Keppler D, Landmann L, eds.: *Modulation of Liver Cell Expression*. Falk Symposium No. 43. 1987   ISBN: 0-85200-677-2*

44. Boyer JL, Bianchi L, eds.: *Liver Cirrhosis*. Falk Symposium No. 44. 1987   ISBN: 0-85200-993-3*

45. Paumgartner G, Stiehl A, Gerok W, eds.: *Bile Acids and the Liver*. Falk Symposium No. 45. 1987   ISBN: 0-85200-675-6*

46. Goebell H, Peskar BM, Malchow H, eds.: *Inflammatory Bowel Diseases – Basic Research & Clinical Implications*. Falk Symposium No. 46. 1988   ISBN: 0-7462-0067-6*

47. Bianchi L, Holt P, James OFW, Butler RN, eds.: *Aging in Liver and Gastrointestinal Tract*. Falk Symposium No. 47. 1988   ISBN: 0-7462-0066-8*

48. Heilmann C, ed.: *Calcium-Dependent Processes in the Liver*. Falk Symposium No. 48. 1988   ISBN: 0-7462-0075-7*

50. Singer MV, Goebell H, eds.: *Nerves and the Gastrointestinal Tract*. Falk Symposium No. 50. 1989   ISBN: 0-7462-0114-1

51. Bannasch P, Keppler D, Weber G, eds.: *Liver Cell Carcinoma*. Falk Symposium No. 51. 1989   ISBN: 0-7462-0111-7

52. Paumgartner G, Stiehl A, Gerok W, eds.: *Trends in Bile Acid Research*. Falk Symposium No. 52. 1989   ISBN: 0-7462-0112-5

53. Paumgartner G, Stiehl A, Barbara L, Roda E, eds.: *Strategies for the Treatment of Hepatobiliary Diseases*. Falk Symposium No. 53. 1990   ISBN: 0-7923-8903-4

54. Bianchi L, Gerok W, Maier K-P, Deinhardt F, eds.: *Infectious Diseases of the Liver*. Falk Symposium No. 54. 1990   ISBN: 0-7923-8902-6

55. Falk Symposium No. 55 not published

55B. Hadziselimovic F, Herzog B, Bürgin-Wolff A, eds.: *Inflammatory Bowel Disease and Coeliac Disease in Children*. International Falk Symposium. 1990 ISBN 0-7462-0125-7

56. Williams CN, eds.: *Trends in Inflammatory Bowel Disease Therapy*. Falk Symposium No. 56. 1990   ISBN: 0-7923-8952-2

57. Bock KW, Gerok W, Matern S, Schmid R, eds.: *Hepatic Metabolism and Disposition of Endo- and Xenobiotics*. Falk Symposium No. 57. 1991   ISBN: 0-7923-8953-0

58. Paumgartner G, Stiehl A, Gerok W, eds.: *Bile Acids as Therapeutic Agents: From Basic Science to Clinical Practice*. Falk Symposium No. 58. 1991   ISBN: 0-7923-8954-9

59. Halter F, Garner A, Tytgat GNJ, eds.: *Mechanisms of Peptic Ulcer Healing*. Falk Symposium No. 59. 1991   ISBN: 0-7923-8955-7

60. Goebell H, Ewe K, Malchow H, Koelbel Ch, eds.: *Inflammatory Bowel Diseases – Progress in Basic Research and Clinical Implications*. Falk Symposium No. 60. 1991   ISBN: 0-7923-8956-5

61. Falk Symposium No. 61 not published

62. Dowling RH, Folsch UR, Löser Ch, eds.: *Polyamines in the Gastrointestinal Tract*. Falk Symposium No. 62. 1992   ISBN: 0-7923-8976-X

63. Lentze MJ, Reichen J, eds.: *Paediatric Cholestasis: Novel Approaches to Treatment*. Falk Symposium No. 63. 1992   ISBN: 0-7923-8977-8

64. Demling L, Frühmorgen P, eds.: *Non-Neoplastic Diseases of the Anorectum*. Falk Symposium No. 64. 1992   ISBN: 0-7923-8979-4

64B. Gressner AM, Ramadori G, eds.: *Molecular and Cell Biology of Liver Fibrogenesis*. International Falk Symposium. 1992   ISBN: 0-7923-8980-8

*These titles were published under the MTP Press imprint.

65. Hadziselimovic F, Herzog B, eds.: *Inflammatory Bowel Diseases and Morbus Hirschprung.* Falk Symposium No. 65. 1992   ISBN: 0-7923-8995-6

66. Martin F, McLeod RS, Sutherland LR, Williams CN, eds.: *Trends in Inflammatory Bowel Disease Therapy.* Falk Symposium No. 66. 1993   ISBN: 0-7923-8827-5

67. Schölmerich J, Kruis W, Goebell H, Hohenberger W, Gross V, eds.: *Inflammatory Bowel Diseases – Pathophysiology as Basis of Treatment.* Falk Symposium No. 67. 1993
ISBN: 0-7923-8996-4

68. Paumgartner G, Stiehl A, Gerok W, eds.: *Bile Acids and The Hepatobiliary System: From Basic Science to Clinical Practice.* Falk Symposium No. 68. 1993
ISBN: 0-7923-8829-1

69. Schmid R, Bianchi L, Gerok W, Maier K-P, eds.: *Extrahepatic Manifestations in Liver Diseases.* Falk Symposium No. 69. 1993   ISBN: 0-7923-8821-6

70. Meyer zum Büschenfelde K-H, Hoofnagle J, Manns M, eds.: *Immunology and Liver.* Falk Symposium No. 70. 1993   ISBN: 0-7923-8830-5

71. Surrenti C, Casini A, Milani S, Pinzani M , eds.: *Fat-Storing Cells and Liver Fibrosis.* Falk Symposium No. 71. 1994   ISBN: 0-7923-8842-9

72. Rachmilewitz D, ed.: *Inflammatory Bowel Diseases – 1994.* Falk Symposium No. 72. 1994   ISBN: 0-7923-8845-3

73. Binder HJ, Cummings J, Soergel KH, eds.: *Short Chain Fatty Acids.* Falk Symposium No. 73. 1994   ISBN: 0-7923-8849-6

73B. Möllmann HW, May B, eds.: *Glucocorticoid Therapy in Chronic Inflammatory Bowel Disease: from basic principles to rational therapy.* International Falk Workshop. 1996
ISBN 0-7923-8708-2

74. Keppler D, Jungermann K, eds.: *Transport in the Liver.* Falk Symposium No. 74. 1994
ISBN: 0-7923-8858-5

74B. Stange EF, ed.: *Chronic Inflammatory Bowel Disease.* Falk Symposium. 1995
ISBN: 0-7923-8876-3

75. van Berge Henegouwen GP, van Hoek B, De Groote J, Matern S, Stockbrügger RW, eds.: *Cholestatic Liver Diseases: New Strategies for Prevention and Treatment of Hepatobiliary and Cholestatic Liver Diseases.* Falk Symposium 75. 1994.
ISBN: 0-7923-8867-4

76. Monteiro E, Tavarela Veloso F, eds.: *Inflammatory Bowel Diseases: New Insights into Mechanisms of Inflammation and Challenges in Diagnosis and Treatment.* Falk Symposium 76. 1995.   ISBN 0-7923-8884-4

77. Singer MV, Ziegler R, Rohr G, eds.: *Gastrointestinal Tract and Endocrine System.* Falk Symposium 77. 1995.   ISBN 0-7923-8877-1

78. Decker K, Gerok W, Andus T, Gross V, eds.: *Cytokines and the Liver.* Falk Symposium 78. 1995.   ISBN 0-7923-8878-X

79. Holstege A, Schölmerich J, Hahn EG, eds.: *Portal Hypertension.* Falk Symposium 79. 1995.   ISBN 0-7923-8879-8

80. Hofmann AF, Paumgartner G, Stiehl A, eds.: *Bile Acids in Gastroenterology: Basic and Clinical Aspects.* Falk Symposium 80. 1995   ISBN 0-7923-8880-1

81. Riecken EO, Stallmach A, Zeitz M, Heise W, eds.: *Malignancy and Chronic Inflammation in the Gastrointestinal Tract – New Concepts.* Falk Symposium 81. 1995
ISBN 0-7923-8889-5

82. Fleig WE, ed.: *Inflammatory Bowel Diseases: New Developments and Standards.* Falk Symposium 82. 1995   ISBN 0-7923-8890-6

Falk Symposium Series

82B. Paumgartner G, Beuers U, eds.: *Bile Acids in Liver Diseases.* International Falk Workshop. 1995 ISBN 0-7923-8891-7

83. Dobrilla G, Felder M, de Pretis G, eds.: *Advances in Hepatobiliary and Pancreatic Diseases: Special Clinical Topics.* Falk Symposium 83. 1995. ISBN 0-7923-8892-5

84. Fromm H, Leuschner U, eds.: *Bile Acids – Cholestasis – Gallstones: Advances in Basic and Clinical Bile Acid Research.* Falk Symposium 84. 1995 ISBN 0-7923-8893-3

85. Tytgat GNJ, Bartelsman JFWM, van Deventer SJH, eds.: *Inflammatory Bowel Diseases.* Falk Symposium 85. 1995 ISBN 0-7923-8894-1

86. Berg PA, Leuschner U, eds.: *Bile Acids and Immunology.* Falk Symposium 86. 1996 ISBN 0-7923-8700-7

87. Schmid R, Bianchi L, Blum HE, Gerok W, Maier KP, Stalder GA, eds.: *Acute and Chronic Liver Diseases: Molecular Biology and Clinics.* Falk Symposium 87. 1996 ISBN 0-7923-8701-5

88. Blum HE, Wu GY, Wu CH, eds.: *Molecular Diagnosis and Gene Therapy.* Falk Symposium 88. 1996 ISBN 0-7923-8702-3

88B. Poupon RE, Reichen J, eds.: *Surrogate Markers to Assess Efficacy of TReatment in Chronic Liver Diseases.* International Falk Workshop. 1996 ISBN 0-7923-8705-8

89. Reyes HB, Leuschner U, Arias IM, eds.: *Pregnancy, Sex Hormones and the Liver.* Falk Symposium 89. 1996 ISBN 0-7923-8704-X

89B. Broelsch CE, Burdelski M, Rogiers X, eds.: *Cholestatic Liver Diseases in Children and Adults.* International Falk Workshop. 1996 ISBN 0-7923-8710-4

90. Lam S-K, Paumgartner P, Wang B, eds.: *Update on Hepatobiliary Diseases 1996.* Falk Symposium 90. 1996 ISBN 0-7923-8715-5

91. Hadziselimovic F, Herzog B, eds.: *Inflammatory Bowel Diseases and Chronic Recurrent Abdominal Pain.* Falk Symposium 91. 1996 ISBN 0-7923-8722-8

91B. Alvaro D, Benedetti A, Strazzabosco M, eds.: *Vanishing Bile Duct Syndrome – Pathophysiology and Treatment.* International Falk Workshop. 1996 ISBN 0-7923-8721-X

92. Gerok W, Loginov AS, Pokrowskij VI, eds.: *New Trends in Hepatology 1996.* Falk Symposium 92. 1997 ISBN 0-7923-8723-6

93. Paumgartner G, Stiehl A, Gerok W, eds.: *Bile Acids in Hepatobiliary Diseases – Basic Research and Clinical Application.* Falk Symposium 93. 1997 ISBN 0-7923-8725-2

94. Halter F, Winton D, Wright NA, eds.: *The Gut as a Model in Cell and Molecular Biology.* Falk Symposium 94. 1997 ISBN 0-7923-8726-0

94B. Kruse-Jarres JD, Schölmerich J, eds.: *Zinc and Diseases of the Digestive Tract.* International Falk Workshop. 1997 ISBN 0-7923-8724-4

95. Ewe K, Eckardt VF, Enck P, eds.: *Constipation and Anorectal Insufficiency.* Falk Symposium 95. 1997 ISBN 0-7923-8727-9

96. Andus T, Goebell H, Layer P, Schölmerich J, eds.: *Inflammatory Bowel Disease – from Bench to Bedside.* Falk Symposium 96. 1997 ISBN 0-7923-8728-7

97. Campieri M, Bianchi-Porro G, Fiocchi C, Schölmerich J, eds. *Clinical Challenges in Inflammatory Bowel Diseases: Diagnosis, Prognosis and Treatment.* Falk Symposium 97. 1998 ISBN 0-7923-8733-3

98. Lembcke B, Kruis W, Sartor RB, eds. *Systemic Manifestations of IBD: The Pending Challenge for Subtle Diagnosis and Treatment.* Falk Symposium 98. 1998 ISBN 0-7923-8734-1

Falk Symposium Series

99.   Goebell H, Holtmann G, Talley NJ, eds. *Functional Dyspepsia and Irritable Bowel Syndrome: Concepts and Controversies.* Falk Symposium 99. 1998
ISBN 0-7923-8735-X

100.   Blum HE, Bode Ch, Bode JCh, Sartor RB, eds. *Gut and the Liver.* Falk Symposium 100. 1998
ISBN 0-7923-8736-8

101.   Rachmilewitz D, ed. *V International Symposium on Inflammatory Bowel Diseases.* Falk Symposium 101. 1998
ISBN 0-7923-8743-0

102.   Manns MP, Boyer JL, Jansen PLM, Reichen J, eds. *Cholestatic Liver Diseases.* Falk Symposium 102. 1998
ISBN 0-7923-8746-5

102B.   Manns MP, Chapman RW, Stiehl A, Wiesner R, eds. *Primary Sclerosing Cholangitis.* International Falk Workshop. 1998.
ISBN 0-7923-8745-7

103.   Häussinger D, Jungermann K, eds. *Liver and Nervous System.* Falk Symposium 102. 1998
ISBN 0-7924-8742-2

103B.   Häussinger D, Heinrich PC, eds. *Signalling in the Liver.* International Falk Workshop. 1998
ISBN 0-7923-8744-9

103C.   Fleig W, ed. *Normal and Malignant Liver Cell Growth.* International Falk Workshop. 1998
ISBN 0-7923-8748-1

104.   Stallmach A, Zeitz M, Strober W, MacDonald TT, Lochs H, eds. *Induction and Modulation of Gastrointestinal Inflammation.* Falk Symposium 104. 1998
ISBN 0-7923-8747-3

105.   Emmrich J, Liebe S, Stange EF, eds. *Innovative Concepts in Inflammatory Bowel Diseases.* Falk Symposium 105. 1999
ISBN 0-7923-8749-X

106.   Rutgeerts P, Colombel J-F, Hanauer SB, Schölmerich J, Tytgat GNJ, van Gossum A, eds. *Advances in Inflammatory Bowel Diseases.* Falk Symposium 106. 1999
ISBN 0-7923-8750-3

107.   Špičák J, Boyer J, Gilat T, Kotrlik K, Mareček Z, Paumgartner G, eds. *Diseases of the Liver and the Bile Ducts – New Aspects and Clinical Implications.* Falk Symposium 107. 1999
ISBN 0-7923-8751-1

108.   Paumgartner G, Stiehl A, Gerok W, Keppler D, Leuschner U, eds. *Bile Acids and Cholestasis.* Falk Symposium 108. 1999
ISBN 0-7923-8752-X

109.   Schmiegel W, Schölmerich J, eds. *Colorectal Cancer – Molecular Mechanisms, Premalignant State and its Prevention.* Falk Symposium 109. 1999
ISBN 0-7923-8753-8

110.   Domschke W, Stoll R, Brasitus TA, Kagnoff MF, eds. *Intestinal Mucosa and its Diseases – Pathophysiology and Clinics.* Falk Symposium 110. 1999
ISBN 0-7923-8754-6

110B.   Northfield TC, Ahmed HA, Jazwari RP, Zentler-Munro PL, eds. *Bile Acids in Hepatobiliary Disease.* Falk Workshop. 2000
ISBN 0-7923-8755-4

111.   Rogler G, Kullmann F, Rutgeerts P, Sartor RB, Schölmerich J, eds. *IBD at the End of its First Century.* Falk Symposium 111. 2000
ISBN 0-7923-8756-2

112.   Krammer HJ, Singer MV, eds. *Neurogastroenterology: From the Basics to the Clinics.* Falk Symposium 112. 2000
ISBN 0-7923-8757-0

113.   Andus T, Rogler G, Schlottmann K, Frick E, Adler G, Schmiegel W, Zeitz M, Schölmerich J, eds. *Cytokines and Cell Homeostasis in the Gastrointestinal Tract.* Falk Symposium 113. 2000
ISBN 0-7923-8758-9

114.   Manns MP, Paumgartner G, Leuschner U, eds. *Immunology and Liver.* Falk Symposium 114. 2000
ISBN 0-7923-8759-7

Falk Symposium Series

115. Boyer JL, Blum HE, Maier K-P, Sauerbruch T, Stalder GA, eds. *Liver Cirrhosis and its Development*. Falk Symposium 115. 2000   ISBN 0-7923-8760-0

116. Riemann JF, Neuhaus H, eds. *Interventional Endoscopy in Hepatology*. Falk Symposium 116. 2000   ISBN 0-7923-8761-9

116A. Dienes HP, Schirmacher P, Brechot C, Okuda K, eds. *Chronic Hepatitis: New Concepts of Pathogenesis, Diagnosis and Treatment*. Falk Workshop. 2000
ISBN 0-7923-8763-5

117. Gerbes AL, Beuers U, Jüngst D, Pape GR, Sackmann M, Sauerbruch T, eds. *Hepatology 2000 – Symposium in Honour of Gustav Paumgartner*. Falk Symposium 117. 2000
ISBN 0-7923-8765-1

117A. Acalovschi M, Paumgartner G, eds. *Hepatobiliary Diseases: Cholestasis and Gallstones*. Falk Workshop. 2000   ISBN 0-7923-8770-8

118. Frühmorgen P, Bruch H-P, eds. *Non-Neoplastic Diseases of the Anorectum*. Falk Symposium 118. 2001   ISBN 0-7923-8766-X

119. Fellermann K, Jewell DP, Sandborn WJ, Schölmerich J, Stange EF, eds. *Immuno-suppression in Inflammatory Bowel Diseases – Standards, New Developments, Future Trends*. Falk Symposium 119. 2001   ISBN 0-7923-8767-8

120. van Berge Henegouwen GP, Keppler D, Leuschner U, Paumgartner G, Stiehl A, eds. *Biology of Bile Acids in Health and Disease*. Falk Symposium 120. 2001
ISBN 0-7923-8768-6

121. Leuschner U, James OFW, Dancygier H, eds. *Steatohepatitis (NASH and ASH)*. Falk Symposium 121. 2001   ISBN 0-7923-8769-4